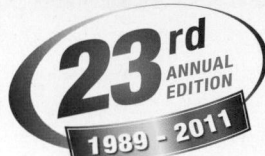

23rd ANNUAL EDITION
1989 - 2011

W9-AHQ-956

THE Calorie, Fat & Carbohydrate Counter

Contents

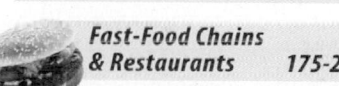
EXTRA DIET GUIDES & COUNTERS

Weight Control Tips

✅ Eat Sensibly

- Avoid fad diets. Eat 3 sensible meals daily with adequate fruit and vegetables.
- Limit portion size. Limit fats and high-fat foods, sugar, soda and alcohol. *(Sample Meal Plan ~ Page 11)*

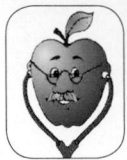

✅ Exercise Daily

- Get active and exercise every day!
- Include muscle-strengthening exercises. You'll lose more fat and keep it off. You'll also feel and look better, and you can eat a little more! *(Exercise Guide ~ Page 12)*

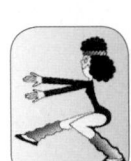

✅ Reshape Eating Behaviors

- Be aware of eating habits and behaviors that lead to overeating.
- Also focus on social and emotional situations that lead you to snack compulsively. *(Extra Notes ~ Page 14)*

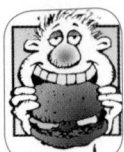

✅ Keep a Food & Exercise Journal

- A journal helps you see exactly what you eat and drink, and how much you exercise. *(Extra Notes ~ Page 15)*
- An excellent motivator and proven weight loss aid. Keeps you honest!

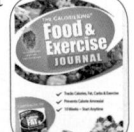

✅ Arrange Moral Support

Gain the support of family and friends. Get extra professional help if required, from your doctor, dietitian, psychologist, exercise trainer, or diet club. Beware of family saboteurs who discourage you from adopting a healthier lifestyle!

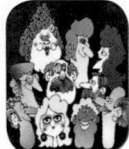

👨‍⚕️ DOCTOR CHECK-UP

Ask your doctor to check your blood pressure, blood sugar and blood cholesterol levels.

HEALTHY WEIGHTS
~ MEN & WOMEN ~
(Over 18 Years)

Based on weights with least risk of disease or death from heart disease, diabetes, stroke and cancer.

Based on Body Mass Index of 20-25

BMI calculated as: $\dfrac{\text{Weight (kg)}}{\text{Height (m)}^2}$

Height (No Shoes) Ft Ins		Healthy Weight Range (Pounds)
4'7"	~	86-108
4'8"	~	88-110
4'9"	~	92-114
4'10"	~	97-121
4'11"	~	99-123
5'0"	~	101-127
5'1"	~	105-132
5'2"	~	110-136
5'3"	~	112-140
5'4"	~	114-145
5'5"	~	119-149
5'6"	~	123-156
5'7"	~	127-158
5'8"	~	129-162
5'9"	~	134-167
5'10"	~	138-173
5'11"	~	143-178
6'0"	~	145-182
6'1"	~	149-187
6'2"	~	156-193
6'3"	~	158-198
6'4"	~	162-202
6'5"	~	170-211
6'6"	~	172-215
6'7"	~	175-220

Body Fat Distribution & Health

Moderate amounts of body fat do not compromise health. However, excess fat above the hips carries a far greater health risk than fat on or below the hips - better to be a 'pear-shape' than an 'apple-shape'.

Abdominal obesity greatly increases the risk of developing diabetes, heart disease, high blood fats, hypertension, stroke, sleep apnea, arthritis and some cancers. So-called **'cellulite'** carries no extra health risk.

Waist Circumference directly reflects the increased health risk of abdominal obesity. Waist size associated with a high health risk:
Men -- Over 40 inches **Women** ~ Over 35 inches

Body Mass Index (BMI)

BMI is a general (but not specific) indicator of body fatness. Although BMI alone is not diagnostic, the higher the BMI, the greater the health risk of developing diabetes, high blood pressure and heart disease. BMI does not apply to heavily muscled persons. BMI is used in a different way for children.

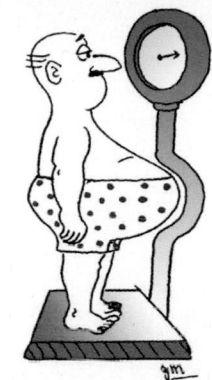

Abdominal obesity greatly increases the risk of ill-health and earlier death.

Check Your BMI: Find your height (no shoes) - look across the row to the weight nearest your own. Then track down to BMI.

Ht	WEIGHT (LBS) ~ ADULTS													
5'1"	100	106	111	116	122	127	132	137	143	148	153	158	185	211
5'2"	104	109	115	120	126	131	136	142	147	153	158	164	191	218
5'3"	107	113	118	124	130	135	141	146	152	158	163	169	197	225
5'4"	110	116	122	128	134	140	145	151	157	163	169	174	204	232
5'5"	114	120	126	132	138	144	150	156	162	168	174	180	210	240
5'6"	118	124	130	136	142	148	155	161	167	173	179	186	216	247
5'7"	121	127	134	140	146	153	159	166	172	178	185	191	223	255
5'8"	125	131	138	144	151	158	164	171	177	184	190	197	230	262
5'9"	128	135	142	149	155	162	169	176	182	189	196	206	236	270
5'10"	132	139	146	153	160	167	174	181	188	195	202	207	243	278
5'11"	136	143	150	157	165	172	179	186	193	200	208	215	250	286
6'0"	140	147	154	162	169	177	184	191	199	206	213	221	258	294
6'1"	144	151	159	166	174	182	189	197	204	212	219	227	265	302
6'2"	148	155	163	171	179	186	194	202	210	218	225	233	272	311
6'3"	152	160	168	176	184	192	200	208	216	224	232	240	279	319
6'4"	156	164	172	180	189	197	205	213	221	230	238	246	287	328

BMI 19 20 21 22 23 24 25 26 27 28 29 30 35 40

BMI Classification:

BMI Below 19
Underweight

BMI 19-24.9
Healthy Weight
(Low Health Risk)

BMI 25-29.9
Overweight
(Moderate Health Risk)

BMI 30-40
Obese (High Health Risk)

BMI Over 40
Morbid Obesity
(Very High Risk)

Interactive BMI Calculator
www.calorieking.com

Calories & Weight Loss

Calories in Food

Calories in food are derived from protein, fat and carbohydrate. Alcohol also provides calories. Vitamins, minerals and water provide no calories.

Calorie Values Per Gram

Fat/Oil	~ 9 Calories
Carbohydrate	~ 4 Calories
Protein	~ 4 Calories
Alcohol	~ 7 Calories

Note that fats have over double the calories of protein and carbohydrate. The higher the fat content of food, the higher the calories.

Sample Calculation

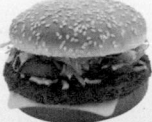

**QUARTER POUNDER®
WITH CHEESE
has 510 calories
derived from:**

26g Fat (x 9 cals/gram)	= 234
40g Carbohyd.(x 4 cals/gram)	= 160
29g Protein (x 4 cals/gram)	= 116
Total Calories	= 510

Calorie Levels for Weight Loss

Start with a calorie-controlled diet that allows a moderate weight loss of ½ - 1 pound per week. Weight loss is usually much greater in the first few weeks due to extra fluid losses.

Note: It is better to increase exercise rather than lessen food calories too drastically.

Suggested Calories for Weight Loss

Women:	Non-active	1000 - 1200
	Active	1200 - 1500
Men:	Non-active	1200 - 1500
	Active	1500 - 1800
Teenagers:		1200 - 1800

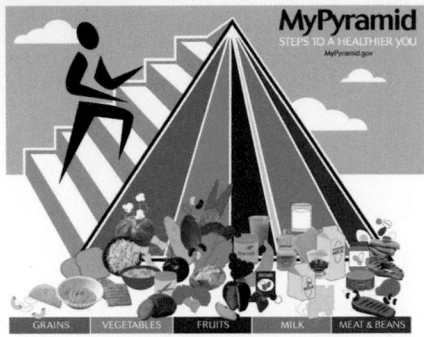

MyPyramid
STEPS TO A HEALTHIER YOU
MyPyramid.gov

GRAINS   VEGETABLES   FRUITS   MILK   MEAT & BEANS

The MyPyramid symbol represents the recommended proportion of foods from each food group and focuses on the importance of making smart food choices in every food group, every day. Daily physical activity is also important. *(More info: www.MyPyramid.gov)*

Examples of Single Serving Sizes

Grains (Eat 6 servings per day):
- 1 slice wholegrain bread (1 oz)
- ½ bun, small bagel or English muffin
- 4 small crackers or 1 tortilla
- 1 oz ready-to-eat wholegrain cereal
- ½ cup cooked cereal, rice or pasta

Vegetable (Eat 3-5 servings per day):
- 1 cup raw leafy vegetables
- 1½ cups raw chopped vegetables
- ½ cup cooked vegetables
- ½ - ¾ cup vegetable juice

Fruits (Eat 3-5 servings per day):
- 1 medium apple, orange, banana
- ½ cup canned fruit (in own juice)
- ¼ cup dried fruit
- ¾ cup fruit juice (unsweetened)
- ¼ medium avocado

Milk (2-3 servings per day):
- 1 cup (8 fl.oz) milk/soy (enriched)/yogurt
- 1½ oz cheese or ½ cup cottage cheese

Meat & Beans (Eat 2-3 servings per day):
- 2-3 oz (cooked) lean meat/poultry/fish
- 2 eggs **or** 7 oz tofu **or** ¼ cup nuts
- 1 cup (cooked) dried beans **or** chickpeas
- 4 Tbsp peanut butter **or** ½ cup nuts/seeds

Portion Size Counts!

Food portion size is critical to controlling calorie intake for weight control.

Super-sized food servings have become more common when eating out and in the home. This can mean a day's worth of calories being consumed in one meal; or a snack being equivalent to a full meal.

It is easy to underestimate portion size of foods and drinks, and unwittingly consume excess calories – even if the fat content is low or even zero!

To more accurately estimate portion size of different foods, weigh and measure your food with food scales, measuring spoons and cups. Better control of calories will result.

For a visual idea of portion sizes, visit www.CalorieKing.com. See examples (fries and cola) on this page.

Allow for Extra Calories in Packaged Food

The actual weight of packaged foods is usually 5-10% more than the label net weight (the minimum legal weight) - and in some cases up to 50% more. However, manufacturers calculate the calories based on the net weight. For actual calories, weigh the product and calculate the extra calories.

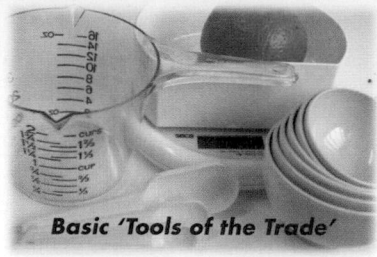

Basic 'Tools of the Trade'

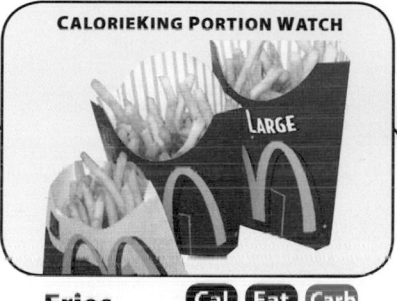

CALORIEKING PORTION WATCH

Fries	Cal	Fat	Carb
Small	250	13	30
Medium	380	20	47
Large	570	30	70

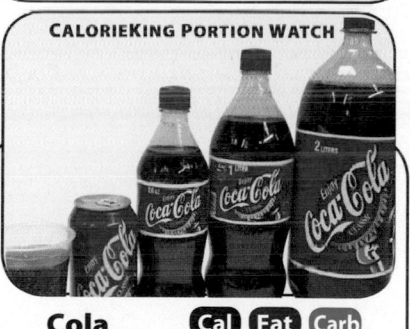

CALORIEKING PORTION WATCH

Cola	Cal	Fat	Carb
8 fl.oz Cup	100	0	25
12 fl.oz Can	150	0	37
20 fl.oz Bottle	250	0	63
1 Liter Bottle	400	0	100
2 Liter Bottle	800	0	200

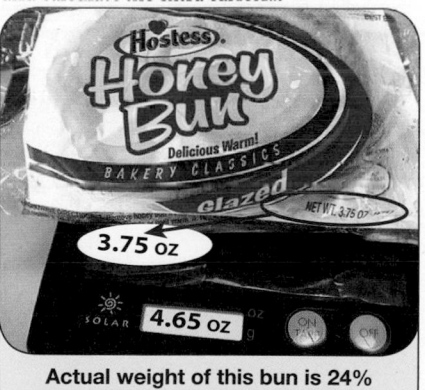

Actual weight of this bun is 24% more than the stated net weight.

Recommended Fat Intake

▶ Fat in the Diet

Fats in the diet are essential for good health. However, too much fat can contribute to obesity and a higher risk of heart disease, high blood pressure, diabetes, gallstone and certain cancers.

Dietary fat and oils have over double the calories of carbohydrates and protein.

(Example: Changing from whole-milk to non-fat milk halves the calories.)

MAXIMUM DESIRABLE FAT INTAKE (DAILY)	
Calories	**Fat**
1200 cals	30g fat
1500 cals	40g fat
1800 cals	50g fat
2000 cals	60g fat
2200 cals	70g fat
2500 cals	80g fat
3000 cals	110g fat

ZERO GRAMS TRANS FAT

*Don't be fooled by **Zero Grams Trans Fat** boldly displayed on some high-fat snacks. They are still high in fat and calories.*

Examples: Cheetos 99c pkg ~ 24g fat, 380 cals Lay's Chips (2¾ oz pkg) ~ 27g fat, 430 calories

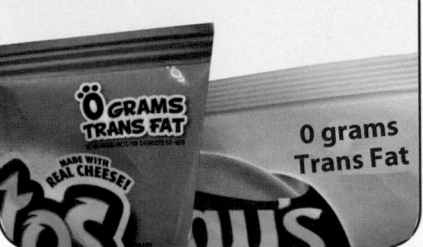

0 grams Trans Fat

▶ Beware low-fat foods

It is a mistake to think that eating low-fat or fat-free foods allows you to eat double the quantity. You can end up with even more calories than eating smaller amounts of regular-fat products.

Food products which are fat-free but high in calories include soda drinks, fruit juices, beer, alcoholic spirits, sugar and candy. Bread, rice and pasta also have negligible fat but need to be eaten in controlled amounts.

Ultimately, **it is food portion size as well as total calories that count** whether from fat, carbohydrate or protein. Remember, cows get fat on grass!

Reduced fat and fat-free foods are not necessarily low calorie. Portion size is still important.

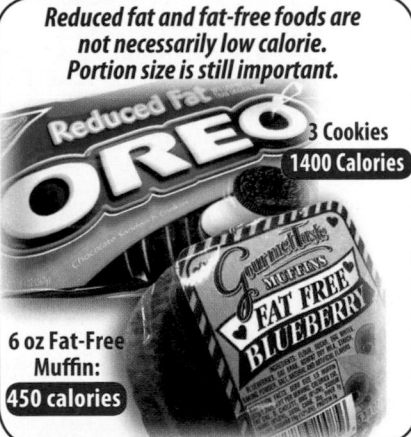

3 Cookies
1400 Calories

6 oz Fat-Free Muffin:
450 calories

FOOD LABEL MEANINGS

FDA Nutrition Claim Definitions
(All are on a Per Serving Basis)

Low Calorie: 40 Calories or less

Light or Lite: One third fewer calories or, 50% or less fat than regular product

Fat-Free: Less than half a gram of fat

Low-Fat: 3 grams or less of fat

Reduced Fat: 25% less fat than regular product

Fewer or Less Calories: At least 25% fewer calories than regular product

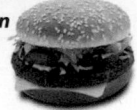

▶ Meats, Poultry, Fish

- Choose **lean cuts** of meat with little marbling. **Trim all visible fat** from meat and remove the skin from poultry. Removal of fat after cooking, is okay (to prevent dryness). Choose 'extra lean' ground beef.
- **Avoid high-fat meat products** such as salami, bacon, sausage and franks.
- **Broil or bake. Avoid frying in oil.** Allow casseroles to cool and skim off surface fat.
- **Avoid fried fish**, frozen fish in batter and canned fish in oil.

▶ Fats & Oils

- **Use minimal amounts** of all types of fat and oil. All are high in calories.
- **Choose** 'light' and 'reduced fat' spreads but still use sparingly.
- Use minimal amounts of oil when stir-frying. Use no-stick sprays like Pam.

▶ Salad Dressings & Sauces

- **Avoid regular mayonnaise and oil dressings.** Choose 'light', 'reduced fat' or 'fat-free' brands.
- **Choose** low-fat or fat-free sauces (mainly tomato-based). Avoid 'pesto', 'alfredo', 'cheese' and 'creamy' sauces.

▶ Milk, Cheese

- **Choose** low-fat or nonfat milks and yogurts. **Avoid** full-cream milk, cream, Half & Half.
- **Cheese:** Choose fat-free, and low-fat cheese. Part-skim ricotta is still high in fat. Low-fat cottage cheese is a good choice. Cheese substitutes can still be high in fat.

▶ Snacks, Cookies, Candy

- **Avoid** high-fat snacks such as potato chips, corn/tortilla chips, cheese puffs, buttered popcorn, chocolate and carob bars.

▶ Desserts/Sweets

- **Avoid high-fat desserts,** such as cake, pie, pastries, cheesecake, full-fat puddings.
- **Choose** fresh fruits, fresh fruit salad, canned fruit in water pack, low-fat ice cream. Use low-fat yogurt in place of cream.

▶ Fast-Foods & Take-Out

Check the Fast-Foods Section of this book for actual fat and calorie counts.

- **Avoid deep-fried foods** such as chicken, french fries and onion rings.
- **Pizzas:** Avoid sausage/pepperoni. Choose vegetarian topping and modest quantity of cheese. Eat a moderate serving. Eat extra salad and fresh fruit.
- **Hamburgers:** Choose medium size, lower fat burgers. Avoid bacon. Have a side salad (with fat-free dressing).
- **Delis:** Choose sandwiches/bread rolls, pitas with low-fat fillings and plain salad. Limit meat/cheese to small portions.
- **Coffees:** Avoid large sizes of latte and frappuccino. Request nonfat milk and no whipped cream. Avoid cookies and pastries.

Extra Information: www.CalorieKing.com

FRYING ADDS FAT!

The greater the surface are of potato exposed to fat or oil, the higher the fat content and calories.

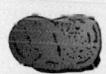 **Whole Potato (3 oz)**
0g Fat   65 Cals

 Roasted Potato (3 oz)
5g Fat   155 Cals

 Fries (Large cut, 3 oz)
12g Fat   220 Cals

 Fries (Small, 3 oz)
15g Fat   265 Cals

 Potato Chips (3 oz)
30g Fat   450 Cals

Carbohydrates ~ Friend or Foe?

Naturally-Friendly Carbs

- Carbohydrate foods in their more natural forms (not overly processed) are essential to good health. They are the main source of fuel for the body, and also provide important vitamins, minerals, antioxidants and fiber – all of which help protect against heart disease, diabetes, hypertension, constipation-related ailments and many other diseases.

- Carbohydrates even help the body produce serotonin, the 'feel good' brain chemical that helps control appetite and overeating. Too little serotonin can lead to mood swings and depression.

Carbohydrates are found in different forms in food as:

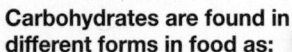

- Sugars in fruit, sugar cane, milk
- Starches in whole grains, legumes, nuts, seeds and vegetables
- Dietary fiber (See Fiber Guide ~ Page 264) Glycemic Index & Diabetes ~ Page 21

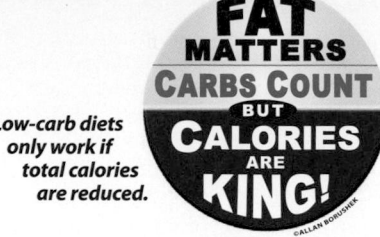

Low-carb diets only work if total calories are reduced.

FAT MATTERS CARBS COUNT BUT CALORIES ARE KING!

©ALLAN BORUSHEK

RECOMMENDED CARBOHYDRATE INTAKE

Calories (Daily)	Carbohydrate (Grams)	Percent Carbohydrate Calories
1200 cals	120g	40%
1500 cals	170g	45%
1800 cals	210g	47%
2000 cals	250g	50%
2500 cals	345g	55%
3000 cals	450g	60%

How Much Do We Need?

- As shown in the chart, well-balanced diets above 2000 calories contain 50-60% of total calories from carbohydrates.
- At lower calorie levels used for weight control (1200-1500 calories), carbohydrates account for as little as 40% of total calories. This is because protein calories have nutritional priority.
- Carbohydrates & Diabetes ~ *See Page 21*

Low-Carbohydrate Diets

- Popular low-carbohydrate diets are extreme in their recommendations to initially cut carb intake to as little as 20 grams per day – the amount in 1 thick slice of bread, or 1 medium apple, or 1 small potato.

  This greatly increases the risk of nutritional deficiencies and compromises health, particularly if fat intake is excessive through fatty meats, high-fat dairy products, and fried foods.

- While overweight Americans do need to reduce carbohydrate intake, it should be done **sensibly as part of reducing portion size and total calories.**

- Simply eating 'low-carb' food products without regard to portion size, calories or fats, will do little to promote weight loss or good health.

- **Low-carb diets (and indeed any diet) only work if total calories are reduced.**

- Refined sugars should be one of the first targets in moderating carb intake.

Extra Info ~ www.CalorieKing.com

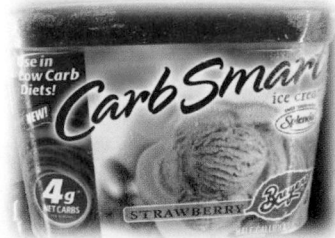

Lower carbohydrate products may still be high in calories and fat.

- Many overweight, inactive people consume over 500 calories of refined sugars per day, either self-added or as part of food products. This is equivalent to over 30 level teaspoons – a significant amount in weight control terms. Halving this amount would be reasonable and worthwhile.

Note: Naturally occurring sugars in fruits, vegetables and milk are fine when consumed in normal recommended amounts. These foods are also rich in other nutrients.

Refined sugar is referred to as having 'empty calories' because it supplies calories but negligible nutrients and no fiber.

- **Most sugar in our diet is 'hidden'** in processed foods such as soft drinks, fruit drinks, candy, cookies, cake, jam, sauces, ice cream, desserts, canned foods, and breakfast cereals.

Certainly enjoy moderate quantities of these foods, but for serious weight control, look for 'low calorie', 'diet' or 'sugar-free'.

However, be careful not to substitute sugar-rich foods with high-fat foods which might boost calories even more!

- Be aware that sugar comes in different forms such as sucrose, glucose, fructose, malt, high-fructose corn syrup, molasses, honey and maple syrup. Check the label.

- **Sugar alcohols such as sorbitol,** mannitol and maltitol are carb-based and have ½ - ¾ the calories of regular sugar. While not counted as sugar on food labels, they do add to the carb count. Excess amounts can cause bloating, gas and diarrhea.

- **Sugar-free sweeteners** such as *Equal, DiabetiSweet, NutraSweet, Splenda, Sweet'n Low* and *Stevia* make it easy to reduce sugar in drinks and recipes. Use only in moderation.

Note: Most recipes can be adapted to contain less sugar with little effect on taste or quality.

Extra Info ~ www.CalorieKing.com

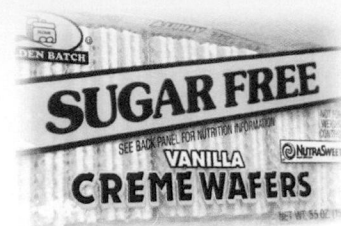

Sugar-free snacks and foods may be higher in fat and calories than the regular product.

Example ~ Creme Wafers (3):
Regular ~ 115 cals, 6g fat
Sugar-Free ~ 160 cals, 10g fat

SUGAR CONTENT OF SOME COMMON FOODS

	Teaspoons of Sugar
Coca Cola or *Pepsi,* 12 fl.oz	10
20 fl.oz size	17
Iced Tea, sweetened, 12 fl.oz	8
Chocolate Milk, 12 fl.oz	6
Honey Smacks Cereal, ¾ cup, 1 oz	4
Popcorn, caramel, 1 cup	3.5
Chocolate Bar, 1.5 oz	6
M&M's 1.7 oz pkg	7
Muffin, large, 4 oz	6
Choc Chip Cookie, 1 oz	2
Donut, Iced	6
Apple Pie, 1 piece	7
Jell-O, ½ cup	4.5
Jam, 1 Tbsp, ¾ oz	2.5
Syrup, maple, 1 Tbsp	3

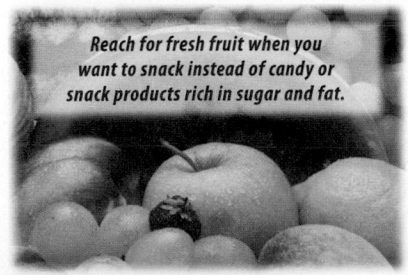

Reach for fresh fruit when you want to snack instead of candy or snack products rich in sugar and fat.

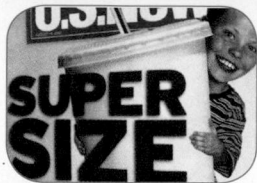

The XL Generation

Some 15% of American kids and adolescents are overweight; and childhood obesity has doubled over the last 20 years. Diabetes, high blood pressure and high cholesterol are major problem areas for overweight children and adolescents, as are depression, low self-esteem, sleep apnea and bone joint problems.

To address this problem, cooperation is required between kids, parents, schools and government. Weight control is a family and community affair.

Five Simple Tips To Get Started:

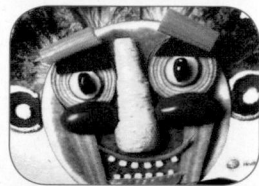

❶ Watch Soda Intake

Limit soda and sugary drinks to one serving on the weekends. Soda should not be an everyday beverage – water should be. When at restaurants or using a soda fountain, choose small servings with ice or choose diet soda instead. Schools should provide water and restrict access to soda as should parents when eating out or in the home!

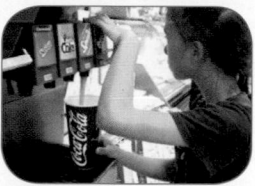

❷ Cut back on Fast-Foods and Eating Out

Many more calories are consumed when you eat out. Healthy meals prepared at home are best for the whole family.

❸ Say "No" to Super-Sizing

When meals are upsized, loads more calories are consumed. Choose sensible portion sizes when eating out and at home. Use smaller plates and choose smaller packages.

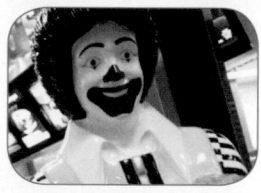

❹ Limit Between-Meal Snacking

Watch out for high-fat and high-calorie snacks – they can have more calories than a meal! Keep your eye on portion sizes and limit salty snack foods and candy to parties and special occasions. Choose fresh fruit, vegetables, nuts and low-fat milk instead.

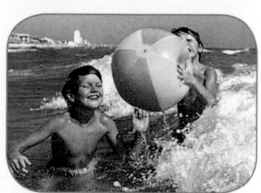

❺ Get Moving ~ Watch Less TV

Kids need at least 60 minutes of physical activity every day. It's critical for their fitness, and greatly lessens the risk of obesity.

Encourage kids to be active out of school hours. Wearing a pedometer can be highly motivational for kids to move more – as can playing dance video games such as *Dance Dance Revolution*. *Wii Fit (Nintendo)* is also useful as a fitness motivator.

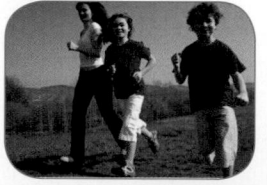

Limit TV and non-active computer games to just one hour per day. Also limit the accompanying snacks! Include exercise in family activities.

Extra information and tips ~ www.CalorieKing.com

Sample Meal Plan - 1400 Calories

For Healthy, Overweight Persons ~ Not for Persons With Any Medical Condition ~ Please Check With Your Doctor & Dietitian ~

 Breakfast (approx. 300 cal)

	1 Small Fruit or ½ oz Dried Fruit
Plus	Cereal: 1½ oz Dry (high fiber)
	or 1 cup cooked Oatmeal
Plus	½ oz Almonds/Seeds
Plus	Milk (from daily allowance) or Yogurt (low-fat)

Daily Milk Allowance (approx.160 calories)
2 cups Non-Fat Milk or 1½ cups Low-fat (1%) Milk
or equivalent Soy Drink, Yogurt, Cheese, Tofu

Fat Allowance (140 calories; 15g Fat)
4 tsp Fat or 6-8 tsp Diet Margarine or 3 tsp Oil
or 1½ Tbsp Mayonnaise or ½ medium Avocado
or 1½ Tbsp Peanut Butter or 30g Nuts/Seeds

 Breakfast ~ Choice 2

	1 Small Fruit
Plus	2 Eggs (no added fat)
	or 2 oz Cheese (low-fat)
	or 4 oz Cottage Cheese (low-fat)
	or 2 oz Lean/Canadian Bacon
Plus	1 Tomato
Plus	1 Slice Wholegrain Toast

 Lunch (approx. 440 calories)

	2 slices Wholegrain Bread (2 oz)
	or 4 Crispbreads/Crackers or 6" Pita
Plus	2 oz lean Meat, Chicken or Turkey
	or 3½oz Tuna (in water) or 2½ oz Salmon
	or 1 oz Cheese or ½ cup (4 oz) Cottage Cheese
	or ½ cup (4 oz) Ricotta Cheese (low-fat)
	or ½ cup (4 oz) Fruit Yogurt (low-fat)
	or ½ cup (4 oz) Bean Salad
Plus	Large Salad (Oil-free dressing)
Plus	1 small Fruit or ½ oz Dried Fruit

 Dinner (approx. 360 calories)

	Soup (fat-free)
Plus	3 oz lean Meat (cooked weight)
	or 4 oz Chicken Breast (no skin)
	or 3 oz Chicken Thigh/Leg (no skin)
	or 5 oz Fish (grilled, no fat)
	or ¾ cup (6 oz) Beans (Soy, Kidney, Pinto etc)/Lentils
	or Low-fat Entree (e.g. Lean Cuisine)
Plus	1 small Potato or ½ cup Rice/Pasta/Sweet Corn
	or 1 slice Wholegrain Bread
Plus	2-3 servings Vegetables/Salad
Plus	1 small Fruit + Diet Gelatin Dessert

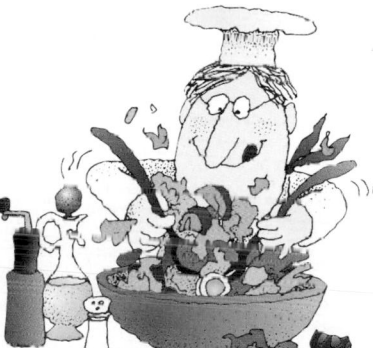

 Between Meals Water, Coffee, Tea, Diet drinks,
Fruit from main meals; Raw vegetable pieces, Milk from Daily Allowance

Exercise & Weight Control

- Persons who exercise regularly lose more weight and keep it off longer than non-exercisers.

- Exercise also improves general health and well-being. Mood, confidence and self-esteem are enhanced by a sense of control and accomplishment.

- **Exercise increases the metabolic rate** of the body even for hours after exercise - a good way to 'wake up' a sluggish metabolism and burn extra fat. Exercise compensates for any decrease in metabolic rate with increasing age and also in some heavy smokers who stop smoking.

- **Strength training** further builds muscle and aids body reshaping. You can also eat a little more food! Note: Each extra pound of muscle burns an extra 50 calories daily ~ even while you sleep! Weight from exercised muscles is okay. It is surplus fat (particularly abdominal fat) that is potentially harmful to health.

- **Avoid injury** by beginning with walking, low impact aerobics, or weight-supported exercise (e.g. swimming, cycling). Avoid competitive sports.

- **How Much?** Start with 10 - 20 minutes/day and progress to 30 - 60 minutes/day.
  Also walk up stairs instead of using elevators. Take a brisk walk at lunch. Use an exercise bike, treadmill or stair machine while watching TV. Walk the dog.

- **How Often?** While aerobic fitness requires only 3 - 4 sessions weekly, **weight control is a daily event which requires daily exercise.**

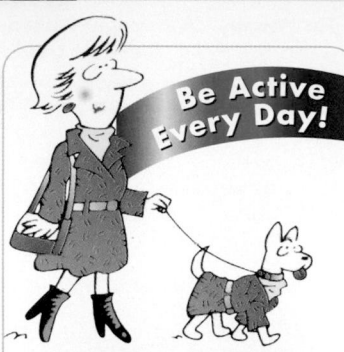

Brisk walking each day is a safe and effective way to keep trim and fit. Try it – you'll like it!
Strength-training with light weights helps to retain or rebuild muscle tissue. It enhances weight control.

FATNESS VS FITNESS

An overweight but fit person can be healthier than a thin, unfit person.

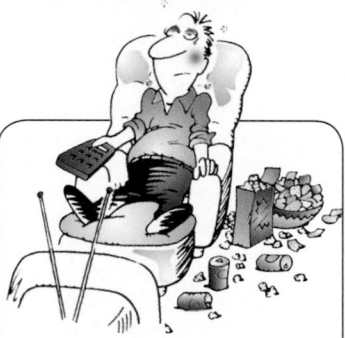

Too little exercise and too much food are the main contributors to middle-age spread.

Daily exercise and sensible eating can minimize middle-age spread. Include some strength-training to retain or build muscle.

TV CAN BE FATTENING!

- Many adults and children spend over 20 hours per week watching TV or at the computer (playing games or 'surfing') – at the same time as eating high-calorie snacks and drinks.

- Are you a TV couch potato or computer addict? Limit your TV and computer hours and plan healthy physical activities.

- At home, limit kids to just one hour daily for TV and computers. Kids need at least 60 minutes of physical activity every day.

Calories Used in Exercise

LIGHT	MODERATE	HEAVY
130 lbs ~ 3 Cals/Min	130 lbs ~ 5 Cals/Min	130 lbs ~ 8 Cals/Min
170 lbs ~ 4 Cals/Min	170 lbs ~ 6 Cals/Min	220 lbs ~ 12 Cals/Min
220 lbs ~ 5 Cals/Min	220 lbs ~ 7 Cals/Min	170 lbs ~ 10 Cals/Min

LIGHT	MODERATE	HEAVY
Walking, slow	Walking, brisk	Walking (power), Jogging
Cycling, light	Cycling, moderate	Cycling (vigorous), Spinning
Frisbee playing	Swimming, crawl	Swimming, strenuous
Gardening, light	Weight-training, light	Weight-training, heavy
Golf, social	Tennis, moderate	Wrestling/Judo, advanced
Tennis, doubles	Racquetball, beginners	Racquetball, advanced
Housework, cleaning	Aerobics, light	Tae Bo, Kick Boxing
Calisthenics, light	Football, touch	Football, training
Bowling	Basketball, Baseball	Basketball (Pro)
Ping-pong, social	Walking Downstairs	Climbing Stairs
Ice Skating, light	Snow Skiing (downhill)	Skipping Rope
Aquarobics, light	Shovelling snow	Skiing (cross country)
Skate Boarding	Dancing (ballroom)	Aquarobics, advanced
Line/Square Dancing	Rowing, moderate	Dancing (strenuous), Zumba
Tai Chi, Yoga	Volleyball, competitive	Rowing, vigorous
Volleyball		Martial Arts

Note: Only those sports or activities that are sustained over a period of time (e.g running) qualify for heavy exercise. Stop-start sports such as tennis are considered 'moderate'.

Interactive Calculations ~ www.CalorieKing.com/tools

WALKING PROGRAM

USE DISTANCE, STEPS OR TIME

Weeks	Distance	Steps Pedometer	Time
1-2	1 mile	2000	20 mins
3-5	1.5 miles	3000	18 mins
6-8	2 miles	3500	35 mins
9-10	2.5 miles	4500	45 mins
11+	3.5 miles	6000	60 mins

10,000 STEPS PER DAY

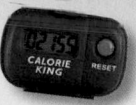

A pedometer can motivate you to be more active. It clips to your belt or waist band and registers each step.

Aim for 8,000 - 10,000 steps per day, instead of an average of only 3,000 - 4,000 steps.

For Extra Information:
www.CalorieKing.com

Reshaping Eating Behaviors

- Eating is a behavior that is largely controlled by people with whom we live or socialize, places in which we carry out our lives, and our emotions. Become aware of those situations that commonly lead to extra food being eaten.

- We may also be unaware of 'bad' eating habits that can lead to excess calorie intake; e.g. eating quickly, large mouthfuls, eating when tense or bored, finishing a large serving of food when not hungry.

Tips to help uncover and correct those 'bad' or problem eating habits:

- **Don't eat while engaged in other activities;** for example, watching TV, reading. Eat only at the table, not at the fridge or while standing.

- **Don't eat quickly.** Chewing slowly allows time to register a feeling of fullness. Don't use fingers, only utensils. Cut food into smaller pieces. Don't load your fork until the previous mouthful is finished.

- **Don't purchase problem high calorie foods.** Shop from a set list to prevent impulse buying. Avoid shopping with children.

- **Buy snack foods** in the smallest package. The larger the serving size or package, the more you are likely to eat or drink.

- **Plan meals in advance. Stick to a set menu.**

- **Plan a strategy to avoid uncontrolled eating** and drinking at social events, or when your emotions urge you to binge.

  Rehearse repeatedly in your mind exactly what you will do in such situations. Remind yourself several times each day that you are in charge of your actions and that you can be strong-willed. Seek counseling or coaching on various strategies.

- **Distract yourself** when you feel the urge to snack impulsively. Engage in some activity that will distract you from thinking about food. Examples: go for a walk, brush your teeth, phone a friend.

  If you eat out of boredom, find some new hobby or interest that gets you out of the house. Even enroll in an adult education class.

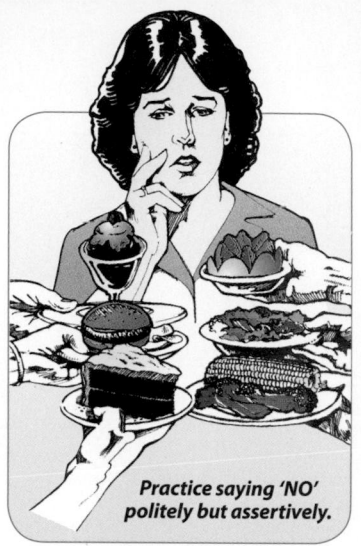

Practice saying 'NO' politely but assertively.

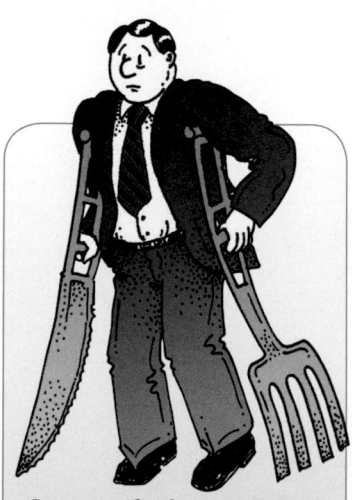

Do you use food as an emotional crutch? If so, professional counseling may be helpful.

The food journal is the most powerful proven aid for dieters. Persons who keep a food and exercise journal not only lose more weight, they also keep it off. Here are some of the reasons:

- **Recording your eating and exercise habits** jolts you into realizing just what you do eat and drink each day; and also whether you exercise sufficiently.

- **Helps you identify problem foods** and drinks with excessive calories and fat.

- **Helps identify moods**, situations and events that lead to excessive eating of unwanted calories. You can then plan to overcome or avoid them.

- **Prevents 'calorie amnesia'**, the forgetfulness that leads to rebound weight gain after successful weight loss. Recording puts you back on the right track.

- **Helps you develop greater self-discipline.** You will think twice about overindulging if you have to record it - especially if someone checks your journal regularly. It certainly keeps you honest!

- **Motivates you** to carefully plan your meals and to exercise each day.

- **Serves as a check system** for your doctor, dietitian or counselor to assess your progress and make recommendations.

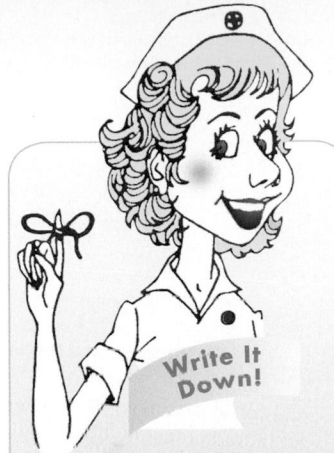

Write It Down!

"Keeping a journal gives me feedback on exactly what I eat and drink each day.

It helps prevent 'calorie amnesia' and reminds me to exercise each day.

It's a 'must' for successful weight control!"

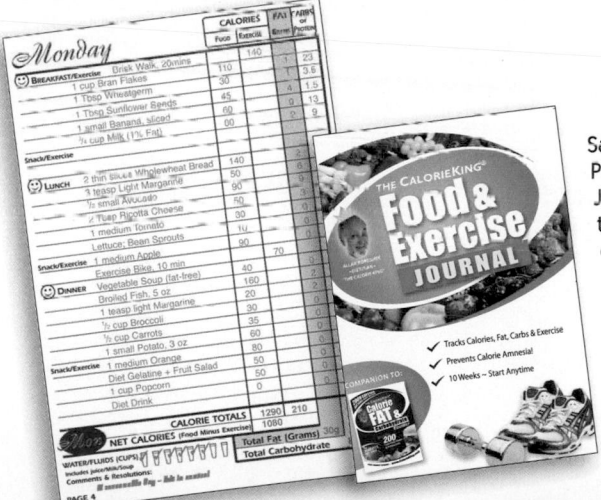

Sample Page from The Pocket Food & Exercise Journal, a 10-week journal to record food and exercise.

At day's end, exercise calories are deducted from food calories.

Includes Weekly Summary Page & Progress Checklist.

Diabetes Guide

What is Diabetes?

Diabetes is a disorder whereby the body cannot use carbohydrates (sugar and starches) properly.

- **After digestion**, sugar and starches are changed into **glucose** – the simplest form of sugar vital for body energy and growth.
- **Insulin** is the hormone which acts like a key that opens the door to body cells and allows glucose to enter.
- **Without enough insulin**, glucose builds up in the blood and passes into the urine. High blood glucose levels lead to frequent urination, extreme thirst, and tiredness.
- **Untreated diabetes increases the risk of damage to nerves and blood vessels.** This, in turn, increases the risk of heart disease, stroke, blindness, kidney damage, foot ulcers and gangrene (with amputation), impotence and other complications.

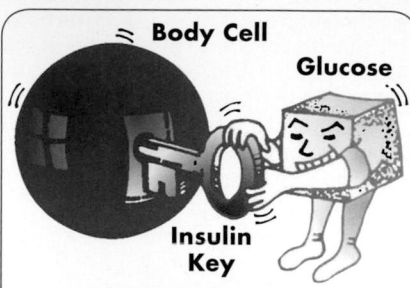

Insulin acts like a key. It opens the door to body cells and allows glucose to enter.

People with type 1 diabetes and some with type 2 have too few or no keys and require insulin injections.

Others (primarily type 2) make enough insulin but the body doesn't use it as well as it should – particularly if obese and inactive.

SYMPTOMS OF DIABETES

- Frequent urination
- Extreme thirst
- Unusual hunger
- Rapid weight loss
- Extreme fatigue
- Blurred vision
- Skin infections that are slow to heal
- Tingling/numbness in feet

DON'T IGNORE DIABETES
IT'S A SERIOUS DISEASE!

Note: Diabetes can be present even with no symptoms.

TYPE 2 DIABETES

- Occurs in 90% of diabetes cases
- Occurs mainly in adults - particularly in overweight and inactive persons
- Insulin is produced but body cells resist its action and glucose cannot enter cells
- Usually treated with meal planning and physical activity. Sometimes requires medication (pills or insulin)

TYPE 1 DIABETES

- Occurs in 10% of diabetes cases
- Usually in children and young adults
- Pancreas produces little or no insulin. Daily insulin injections (or use of an insulin pump) are necessary, as well as:
  - Matching pre-meal insulin to the amount of carbohydrate eaten
  - Weight control and regular physical activity

GESTATIONAL DIABETES

- Occurs in some women during pregnancy
- Usually disappears after the baby's birth
- Women who have had gestational diabetes still have a high risk of developing type 2 diabetes within 5 to 10 years
- Requires weight control, a healthy lifestyle and regular medical checks

Are You At Risk for Diabetes?
Pre-Diabetes ~ An Early Warning!

Pre-diabetes means that your blood glucose levels are higher than normal, but not high enough to be called diabetes.

If you have pre-diabetes, you have a higher risk for getting diabetes later on.

The good news is that you can start taking steps to prevent diabetes by making healthy lifestyle changes – such as losing weight if overweight, and being more physically active.

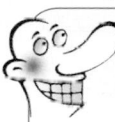

WHAT'S YOUR RISK?
Find out if you're at risk for diabetes by answering the following questions:

- ☐ I have been told I have pre-diabetes
- ☐ I have a family history of diabetes
- ☐ I am African American, Latino American, Asian American, Native American or a Pacific Islander
- ☐ I have had gestational diabetes (diabetes during pregnancy)
- ☐ I am over age 45
- ☐ I am overweight
- ☐ I get little or no physical activity
- ☐ My waist is larger than: 35 inches (for a woman) or 40 inches (for a man)
- ☐ My blood pressure is higher than 130 over 85
- ☐ My HDL (good cholesterol) is too low
- ☐ My triglycerides (blood fats) are too high

✓ CHECK YOUR RESULT

- **If you've put a check mark in two or more of the boxes,** you may be more likely to develop type 2 diabetes.
- **Talk with your healthcare provider** to see if you should have a blood test for diabetes.

BLOOD GLUCOSE CLASSIFICATION OF DIABETES

Normal:	**Below 100 mg/dl***
Pre-Diabetes:	**100-125 mg/dl***
Diabetes:	**Over 125 mg/dl***

(*Fasting Blood Glucose)

KNOW YOUR BGL
(Blood Glucose Level)
Everyone over the age of 45 should have a blood glucose test every three years

Importance of Weight Control

- **Type 2 diabetes** is more common in people who are overweight.
- **Being overweight** means that your insulin doesn't work as well to control blood glucose levels.
- **Losing just 10 to 20 pounds** can help you better manage your diabetes and lower your risk for heart disease.
- **Keys to weight control include:**
  - Following a healthy eating plan
  - Controlling food portions
  - Being physically active most days of the week
  - Keeping food records
  - Setting realistic goals
- **Work with a registered dietitian** who can help you reach a weight that's good for you.

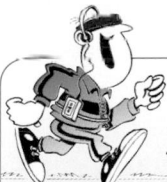

KEEP MOVING!
Every day, do at least 30 minutes of moderate intensity exercise.
(even in 5-minute sets)

It's the key to improving insulin action. Add muscle strength training 3-4 times a week to double the benefits.

Managing Diabetes

Don't battle diabetes alone. Establish a partnership with your doctor, dietitian, certified diabetes educator, and pharmacist.

Extra Support: • *Joslin Diabetes Center*
- *American Diabetes Association*
- *American Association of Diabetes Educators*
- *Juvenile Diabetes Research Foundation*
- *National Diabetes Education Program*

Hints to keep blood glucose within safe limits:

- **Control your food intake.** Know what and when you will eat. Seek referral to a dietitian for expert advice.

- **Exercise regularly.** It assists weight control and can improve sensitivity of body cells to insulin. Plan physical activity into your daily routine.

- **Monitor your blood glucose** at home and work with a blood glucose meter. It will help you become familiar with your blood glucose patterns, and the effects of food, activity and medication.

- **Take insulin or oral medication as prescribed.** If on insulin, know what action to take if hypoglycemia (low blood glucose) occurs. Also educate your family and friends.
  More Info: www.joslin.org

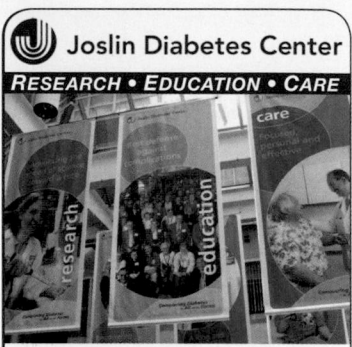

(J) Joslin Diabetes Center

RESEARCH • EDUCATION • CARE

Joslin Diabetes Center, an affiliate of Harvard Medical School, is the world's largest diabetes research center, diabetes clinic and provider of diabetes education.

MORE INFORMATION
www.joslin.org or call 800-344-4501

Be Heart Smart ~ Know Your ABC's

If you have diabetes, you are at a higher risk for heart attack and stroke than someone without diabetes. But you can fight back!

Be smart about your heart!
Take control of the ABC's of diabetes and live a long and healthy life. Talk to your healthcare provider about your ABC targets.

Ⓐ is for A1C
The A1C (A-one-C) test – short for hemoglobin A1C – measures your average blood glucose (sugar) over the last 3 months.
Suggested target: below 7%

Ⓑ is for Blood Pressure
High blood pressure makes your heart work too hard. **Suggested target: below 130/80**

Ⓒ is for Cholesterol
Bad cholesterol, or LDL, can build up and clog your arteries. **Suggested target: below 100**

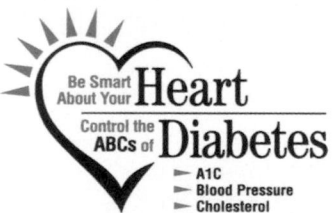

Be Smart About Your **Heart**
Control the ABCs of **Diabetes**
➤ A1C
➤ Blood Pressure
➤ Cholesterol
National Diabetes Education Program

Be smart about your heart!
Take control of the ABC's of diabetes
and live a long and healthy life.

Talk to your healthcare
provider about your ABC targets.

Take action now to lower your risk
for heart attack, stroke and
other diabetes problems.

* * *

◀ *Note: These targets are suggested by the National Institutes for Health and the American Diabetes Association*

Guidelines for choosing a healthy diet apply equally to people with or without diabetes. Eating a wide variety of foods that are mainly low in fat, low in refined sugars, and high in fiber, is recommended.

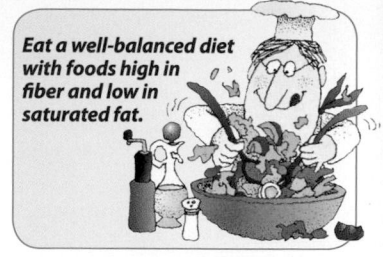

Eat a well-balanced diet with foods high in fiber and low in saturated fat.

However, actual food quantities, as well as when you eat, will also influence control of blood glucose. Your dietitian will individualize a meal plan to suit your food preferences, lifestyle and medical status.

Here are a few tips:

- **Maintain a healthy weight.** If overweight, even a modest weight loss plus daily physical activity can help manage blood glucose in type 2 diabetes.

- **Don't skip meals.** If you take insulin or an oral hypoglycemic agent, regular meals are important.

- **If on insulin,** eat meals at the same time each day. Eat a similar amount of food at each meal. Eating about the same amount of carbohydrate over the day will make best use of insulin and prevent wide variations in blood glucose levels.

- **Know how much carbohydrate you should eat** at your meals and snacks each day.

- **Choose wholegrain breads, cereals and pasta.** Eat fresh fruits, vegetables and legumes. These foods contain more fiber and slow the release of glucose into your blood after a meal.

- **Limit foods high in saturated fat, trans fat and cholesterol.** Enjoy fish, soy foods, and other foods rich in omega-3 fats. *(Extra Notes: Page 259)*

- **Limit sugars and foods high in added sugar** particularly if overweight. Small amounts of sugar as part of a meal may occasionally be okay. Check with your dietitian. *(Extra Notes: Page 9)*

- **Read the Nutrition Facts label** on foods. Check the serving size, total fat and total carbohydrate.

The Plate Method is an easy way to eat healthfully. (See next page)

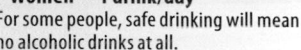

Vegetables & Salad Greens

Bread · Starch · Grain | Meat · Protein

ALCOHOL TIPS

- If you drink alcohol, have only moderate amounts:
  Men ~ 1-2 drinks/day
  Women ~ 1 drink/day
  For some people, safe drinking will mean no alcoholic drinks at all.
  (Also see Alcohol Guide ~ Page 23)

- **Drink along with your food** – especially if you use insulin or diabetes pills.

- **Do not omit any carb food** in exchange for an alcoholic drink. However, non-alcoholic beers (12 fl oz) count as one carb exchange.

- **Alcohol increases the risk of hypoglycemia** (low blood sugar) and drug interactions if you take insulin and certain types of diabetes pills.

- **Check with your doctor and dietitian.**
  Extra Info: www.joslin.org

The Plate Method – An Easy Way to Eat Healthfully

The plate method is a helpful tool to guide your food choices until you see a dietitian for your own meal plan.

For a healthy meal:

- **Fill half of your plate** with non-starchy vegetables (broccoli, green beans, carrots).
- **Fill a quarter of your plate** with carbohydrate (wholegrain bread, pasta, potato, brown rice).
- **Fill the other quarter of your plate** with 3-4 ounces of lean meat, poultry, or fish.
- **Use 1-2 teaspoons of tub margarine** or a heart-healthy vegetable oil.
- **Add** a small piece of fruit or 8 ounces of skim/low-fat milk or yogurt.

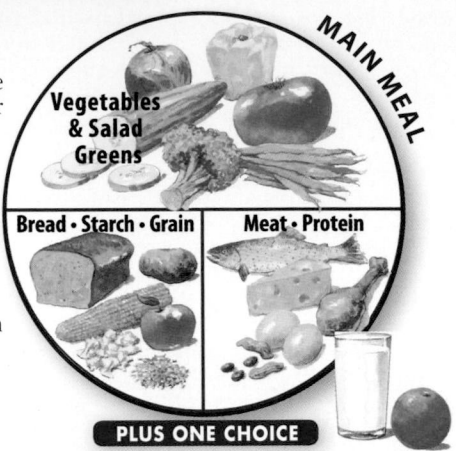

MAIN MEAL

Vegetables & Salad Greens

Bread · Starch · Grain

Meat · Protein

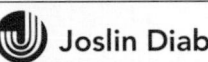

PLUS ONE CHOICE

Milk, Fruit, Dessert or other Carb Food

How Much Carbohydrate Should You Eat?

A dietitian can best determine how much carbohydrate you need at each of your meals, based on your lifestyle, food preferences, and overall diabetes control.

Until you see a dietitian, aim to keep the amount of carbohydrate you eat the same at each of your meals.

CARB CHOICES MEAL PLAN
One Carb Choice = 15 Grams of Carb

The amount in: 1 slice Bread
or ¾ cup Cereal (unsweetened)
or 1 small Potato **or** 1 small Fruit

🍅 Breakfast
- Eat 2-3 carb choices (30-45 grams)
- Include a low-fat protein source such as egg whites or skim milk.

🍅 Lunch and Dinner
- Eat 3-4 carb choices (45-60 grams carb)
- Include fruit and non-starchy vegetables. Choose small portions of low-fat protein foods.

🍅 Snacks:
If needed, eat 1-2 carb choices (15-30 grams carb).

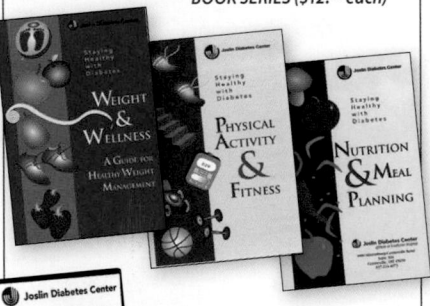
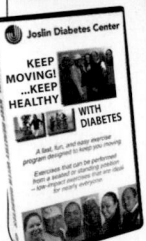

Carb Type Affects Blood Glucose

The various forms of carbohydrate affect blood glucose levels in different ways. It is difficult to predict the effect of particular foods, sugars, or meals, simply by their carbohydrate content.

Thus the same amount of carbohydrate from different foods may affect blood sugar levels very differently. Many factors affect the rate of digestion and absorption such as:

- the type of sugar, starch, and fiber
- the degree of processing and cooking (which increases digestion rate)
- the amount of protein and fat (which slow stomach emptying and digestion).

Glycemic Index (GI)

The GI is a method of ranking carbohydrate foods on a scale (0-100) according to how they affect blood glucose levels. (See next column).

The higher the GI value, the greater the food's ability to rapidly raise blood glucose levels, and the more insulin needed by the body (not desirable).

Eating low-GI foods may lead to better control of blood glucose and insulin levels (which in turn lowers the risk of damage to blood vessels and nerves). The slower digestion of low-GI foods may also help to delay hunger pangs and benefit weight control.

Note: Choosing low-GI foods is not a license to eat unlimited amounts. Calorie restriction and portion control for weight control is of prime importance.

- GI is not meant to be used by itself without regard to portion size, and other dietary recommendations for healthy eating. Foods are not good or bad on the basis of their GI.
- While GI may be a helpful tool for some people with diabetes, what is most important is to control the total amount of carbohydrate that you eat.

Extra Info: www.joslin.org
www.glycemicindex.com

LOWER-GLYCEMIC FOODS

Slower-Acting Carbohydrates
These foods are more slowly digested and absorbed. They help maintain more even blood glucose levels, as long as excessive amounts are not eaten. Use these foods regularly but still limit portion size for weight control.
Examples:

- Dried beans, peas, lentils
- Nuts and seeds
- Wholegrain breads
- Bran cereals, oats
- Sweet corn, barley, buckwheat
- Wholegrain pasta, basmati rice
- Fresh fruit: apples, avocados, bananas (firm), cherries, grapefruit, grapes, olives, oranges, peaches, pears, plums. Fresh juices.
- Vegetables: broccoli, yam, sweet potatoes, salad greens
- Milk, yogurt, soy drinks
- Dark chocolate
- Sugar alcohols (sorbitol, maltitol)

HIGHER-GLYCEMIC FOODS

Quicker-Acting Carbohydrates
These foods more rapidly raise blood glucose levels. Eat only in moderation.

- White bread, rice cakes, bagels, croissants, doughnuts
- Low-fiber cereals: Cornflakes, Rice Krispies, Froot Loops
- White potatoes, white rice
- Watermelon, ripe bananas, cantaloupe, pineapple
- Soda, sugar-sweetened sports and energy drinks
- Sugar, candy, popcorn (plain)
- Ice cream (low-fat), frozen yogurt

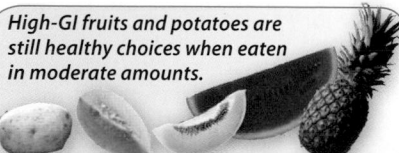

High-GI fruits and potatoes are still healthy choices when eaten in moderate amounts.

» **Calorie and fat values have been rounded off.**
Calories ~ to the nearest 5 or 10 calories.
Fat ~ to nearest half gram. **Note:** Trace amounts of fat (less than 0.3 grams) have been treated as zero.

» **Carbohydrate figures** in this book are for total carbohydrate, and not **Net Carbs** (which deducts fiber, polydextrose and sugar alcohols from total carbs).

» Because manufacturers' figures on labels are rounded off, figures in this book may differ slightly from the label. Serving sizes may also vary.

IMPORTANT DISCLAIMER

* The authors and publishers of this book are not physicians and are not licensed to give medical advice. This book is not a substitute for professional advice. Users should consult their medical professional before making any health, medical or other decisions based on the material contained herein.

* This book is a compilation of original material from other sources intended for educational purposes only. Because food manufacturers constantly change their products, only they are the authoritative source for food's most current nutritional information.

* Persons using the information herein for any medical purposes, such as matching insulin dosage to carbohydrate intake, should not rely solely on the accuracy of figures herein and should independently check food labels or contact the food manufacturer for the latest data.

* Because nutrition data for food products is subject to change, users should consult the most recent edition of this book, and the author's website www.calorieking.com for the most up-to-date information.

* **WARRANTY DISCLAIMER:**
THE AUTHOR AND PUBLISHER DISCLAIM ANY LIABILITY ARISING DIRECTLY OR INDIRECTLY FROM THE USE OF THIS BOOK. THE INFORMATION HEREIN IS PROVIDED "AS IS" AND WITHOUT ANY WARRANTY EXPRESSED OR IMPLIED. ALL DIRECT, INDIRECT, SPECIAL, INCIDENTAL, CONSEQUENTIAL OR PUNITIVE DAMAGES ARISING FROM ANY USE OF THIS INFORMATION IS DISCLAIMED AND EXCLUDED.

This information is also provided subject to Family Health Publications' Terms and Conditions found at the website, www.calorieking.com/terms and incorporated herein.

C ~ Calories
F ~ Fat (grams)
Cb ~ Carbohydrate (grams)

Abbreviations

tsp = teaspoon
Tbsp or T = Tablespoon
oz = ounce(s)
c = cup
fl.oz = fluid ounce(s)
g = gram(s)
avg = average
pkg = package

Volume Measures

(All measures are level)
3 tsp = 1 Tbsp
2 Tbsp = 1 fl.oz
½ cup = 4 fl.oz
1 cup = 8 fl.oz
2 cups = 1 Pint
2 Pints = 1 Quart
Note: 8 oz weight is not the same as 8 fl oz volume (space occupied). Dense foods weigh more per set volume. Examples:
1 cup popcorn weighs ½ oz
1 cup milk weighs 8½ oz
1 cup pudding weighs 10 oz

Metric Conversion

½ oz = 14 grams
1 oz = 28.4 grams
2 oz = 57 grams
3½ oz = 100 grams
1 fl.oz = 30 mls
1 cup (8 fl.oz) = 240 mls
33 fl.oz = 1 liter (volume)

INFORMATION SOURCES
• U.S. Dept. of Agriculture
• Food Manufacturers
• Food Industry Boards & Councils
• Author extrapolations

FEEDBACK WELCOME!
Please contact the author with your queries and suggestions.
feedback@calorieking.com

✱ **Health Hazards:** Excessive alcohol intake contributes to obesity, high blood pressure, stroke, heart and liver disease, some cancers, and even impotence. **Concentration and short-term memory** are reduced as well as athletic performance.

Other alcohol hazards include fetal alcohol syndrome, stomach upsets, menstrual problems, depression, snoring, sleep problems, work absenteeism, impaired judgement, and social/family problems.

✱ **Alcohol contributes to obesity** through its high calories and by lessening the body's ability to burn fat. Fat storage is promoted, particularly in the belly - a health danger zone. Alcohol can also stimulate the appetite.

✱ **Alcohol is potentially more harmful while dieting.** Blood sugar levels may drop with resultant fatigue and further impairment of concentration, reflexes and driving skills - and maybe even the dieter's resolve!

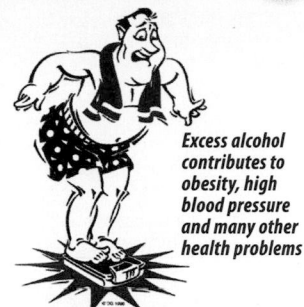

Excess alcohol contributes to obesity, high blood pressure and many other health problems

LOWER RISK ALCOHOL LIMITS

 **WOMEN:** No more than **1 drink** per day

 MEN: No more than **2 drinks** per day (Over 65 y.o. ~ 1 drink)

(At least 2 days a week should be alcohol-free)

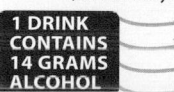 **1 DRINK CONTAINS 14 GRAMS ALCOHOL**
→ **12 fl.oz Regular Beer (5% Alc.)**
→ OR **14 fl.oz Light Beer (4.2% Alc.)**
→ OR **5 fl.oz Wine (12% Alc.)**
→ OR **1½ fl.oz Spirits (80 Proof)**

Note: You cannot save daily drinks for one occasion. Binge drinking is particularly harmful: 4 drinks for males or 3 drinks for females (within 2 hours).

For some people, **safe drinking** means no alcohol at all. Even one drink may impair driving skills, particularly if tired. For women who drink frequently, breast cancer risk is increased by 9% for each drink after the first drink.

It is advisable not to drink at all if you are:
- pregnant, trying to conceive or breastfeeding
- taking medication or have liver or heart disease (unless approved by your doctor or pharmacist)
- planning to drive, use machinery or play sports
- studying or needing to concentrate
- a child or adolescent

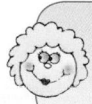 Women and adolescents are more prone to alcohol's ill-effects due to their lower body weight, smaller livers and lesser capacity to metabolize alcohol. As we age, our ability to handle alcohol decreases.

HOW TO CALCULATE ALCOHOL CONTENT

Percent alcohol on label refers to alcohol volume (ml alcohol/100ml). Note: 100ml = 3½ fl.oz

To convert to grams (weight) of alcohol, multiply the percent volume by 0.8 – since 1 ml of alcohol weighs only 0.8 grams.

EXAMPLE:
12 fl.oz Can Beer (5% alcohol)
5% alc. volume
= 5% of 12 fl.oz = 0.6 fl.oz
= 18ml alcohol (Note: 1 fl.oz = 30ml)
Weight (18ml x 0.8) = 14.4g alcohol

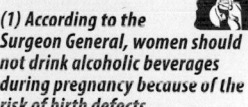

GOVERNMENT WARNINGS!

(1) According to the Surgeon General, women should not drink alcoholic beverages during pregnancy because of the risk of birth defects.

(2) Consumption of alcoholic beverages impairs your ability to drive a car or operate machinery, and may cause health problems.

EXTRA INFORMATION
Alcohol & Diabetes ~ See Page 19
Alcohol & The Heart ~ See Page 262
Tips to Avoid Harmful Drinking ~ p. 29

Quick Guide

Alc ~ Alcohol (Grams)
Cb ~ Carbohydrate

Beer

		C	Alc	Cb
Beer Contains Zero Fat				
Regular Beer (5% Alc. Vol.)				
7 fl.oz Glass		80	8.5	4
12 fl.oz Bottle/Can/Glass		140	14	10
16 fl.oz Bottle/Can		185	19	13
22 fl.oz Bottle		260	26	18
24 fl.oz Can		280	28	20
32 fl.oz Bottle		370	38	28
40 fl.oz Bottle		470	47	35
50 fl.oz Football		590	59	50
Light Beer (4.2% Alc. Vol.)				
7 fl.oz Glass		65	7	4
12 fl.oz Bottle/Can/Glass		110	12	7
16 fl.oz Bottle/Can		145	16	9
22 fl.oz Bottle		200	22	13
24 fl.oz Can		220	24	14
Non-Alcoholic Brews				
(Less than 0.5% alcohol by volume)				
Average All Brands, 12 fl.oz		70	1	14

Beer Brands

Per 12 fl.oz Serving
Percentage alcohol listed
is by volume - not by weight.

Alc ~ Alcohol (Grams)

	C	Alc	Cb
Aguila (4%)	125	11	11
Amstel Light (3.5%)	95	10	5
Anchor: Porter (5.6%)	210	15	23
Steam (4.9%)	165	14	14
Asahi: Kuronama (5.3%)	150	14	11
Select (4.7%)	140	13	11
Super Dry (4.9%)	150	14	11
Augsburger Bock (4.9%)	170	14	17
Bass (5.1%)	155	14	12
Beck's: Original (5%)	145	14	12
Premier Light (2.3%)	65	7	4
Big Sky (4.8%)	150	14	12
Black Label (5.6%)	155	16	11
Blackhook Porter (5.2%)	165	15	14
Blatz: Original (4.6%)	145	13	13
Light (3.9%)	110	11	8
Blonde (4.3%)	140	12	10
Blue Moon: Belgian (5.4%)	165	15	13
Pumpkin Ale (5.8%)	180	17	14
Spring Ale (5.4%)	160	15	12
Summer Ale (5.1%)	155	14	13
Winter Ale (5.5%)	180	15	15

Brands (Cont)

Alc ~ Alcohol (Grams)

Per 12 fl.oz Serving

	C	Alc	Cb
Budweiser: Original	145	14	11
American Ale (5.3%)	180	15	18
Chelada (5%)	185	14	20
Chelada Light (4.2%)	150	12	16
Dry (5%), (4.1%)	130	14	8
Golden Wheat (4.1%)	120	12	8
Light Golden Wheat (4.1%)	120	12	8
Ice (5.5%)	125	16	4
Ice Light (4.2%)	115	14	4
Light Lime (4.2%)	115	12	8
Select (4.3%)	100	12	3
Select 55 (2.4%)	55	6	2
Busch: Original (4.6%)	130	13	10
Ice (5.9%)	170	17	13
Light (4.1%)	95	12	3
Carlsberg (5%)	135	14	10
Castlemaine XXXX (4.7%)	140	13	9
Cerveza Aquila (3.9%)	125	11	11
Colt 45 Malt (6.1%)	175	17	11
Coors: Original (4.9%)	150	14	12
Extra Gold (5%)	150	14	13
Light (4.2%)	100	12	5
Corona: Original (4.45%)	150	14	13
Light (4.1%)	105	12	5
Dos Equis (5%)	130	14	9
Fosters: Lager (5%)	145	14	11
Premium Ale (5.5%)	145	16	12
Genesee: Regular (4.5%)	150	13	14
Genny Light (3.6%)	95	10	6
George Killian's Irish Red (5%)	160	14	15
Grolsch: Blonde (2.8%)	120	18	16
Light (3.6%)	95	11	6
Premium (5%)	145	14	10
Guinness: Draught (4%)	125	12	10
Extra Stout (6%)	175	17	14
Hamm's: Original (4.7%)	145	13	12
Special Light (3.9%)	110	12	8
Harp (5%)	150	13	13
Heineken: Original (5%)	150	14	12
Special Dark (5%)	165	14	15
Premium Light (3.5%)	100	10	7
Icehouse: Original (5%)	135	14	9
Light (5%)	125	14	7
Keystone: Ice (5.9%)	140	17	6
Light (4.2%)	105	12	5
Premium (4.4%)	110	13	6
Killian's Irish Red (5%)	160	14	15
King Cobra (6%)	135	17	5
Kirin: Ichiban (5%)	150	14	12
Light (3.3%)	95	9	8

Alcohol ~ Beers ◆ Ales (with Alcohol Counts) A

Brands (Cont)   **Beer Contains Zero Fat**

Per 12 fl.oz Serving

Alc ~ Alcohol (Grams)
Cb ~ Carbohydrate

	C	Alc	Cb
Labatt: Blue (4.7%)	125	14	9
Blue Light (4%)	110	11	8
Leinenkugel's: Original (4.6%)	150	13	14
Light (4.2%)	110	12	6
Lone Star: Original (4.7%)	135	14	12
Light (3.9%)	110	11	9
Lowenbrau Original (5.2%)	160	15	15
Magic Hat #9 (4.6% alc)	155	13	14
Magnum Malt Liquor (5.6%)	160	16	11
Michelob: Original (5%)	165	14	15
Golden Draft (4.7%)	125	14	8
Golden Draft Light (4.1%)	110	12	7
Honey Lager (4.9%)	180	14	19
Light (4.3%)	125	12	9
Pale Ale (5.6%)	185	16	9
Porter (5.9%)	195	17	18
Ultra (4.2%)	85	12	3
Ultra Amber (5%)	115	14	4
Ultra Amber Fruit (4.2%)	105	12	6
Mickey's Malt Liquor (5.6%)	160	16	11
Miller: Chill, 100 Cal, (4.2%)	100	12	4
Genuine Draft: (4.7%)	145	13	13
High Life (4.7%)	145	13	13
High Life Light (4.2%)	110	12	7
Lite (4.2%)	95	12	3
Milwaukee's Best: (4.3%)	130	12	12
Ice (5.9%)	145	17	7
Light (4.2%)	100	12	4
Minnesota's Best, Original (4.9%)	140	14	10
Molson: Canadian/Golden (5%)	135	14	11
Ice (5.6%)	160	16	12
Light (4%)	115	11	10
Molsons XXX (7.3%)	210	21	15
Moosehead Lager (5%)	140	14	11
Natural: Ice (5.9%)	160	17	9
Light (4.2%)	95	12	3
Negra Modela (5.3%)	175	15	16
Newcastle Brown Ale (4.5%)	140	13	13
Old English,"800" (5.9%)	160	17	11
Old Milwaukee: Original (4.6%)	145	13	13
Light (3.9%)	110	11	8
Ice (5.9%)	180	17	15
Old Style: Original (4.7%)	135	13	12
Light (3.8%)	110	11	8

	C	Alc	Cb
Olympia Gold Light (2.2 %)	70	6	6
Pabst: Blue Ribbon (4.7%)	145	13	12
Light (3.9%)	110	11	8
Pete's Wicked Ale (5.3%)	175	15	17
Piels (4.7%)	125	13	9
Pilsner Urquell (4.4%)	155	13	16
Red Dog (5%)	150	14	14
Red Hook: ESB (5.8%)	185	16	16
India Pale Ale (4.7%)	190	13	19
Red Stripe Jamaican Ale (4.7%)	155	14	14
Rolling Rock (4.5%)	130	13	10
Samuel Adams: Lager (4.9%)	180	14	19
Summer Ale (5.3%)	160	15	13
Sam Adams Light (4%)	120	13	10
Sapporo Premium (3.9%)	135	11	14
Schaefer: Original (4.6%)	145	13	12
Light (3.9%)	110	11	8
Schlitz: Original (4.6%)	145	13	12
Light (3.9%)	110	11	8
Schmidt's: Original (4.6%)	145	13	13
Light (3.9%)	110	11	8
Sheaf Stout (5.8%)	190	16	19
Sierra Nevada: Bigfoot (9.6%)	295	27	25
Pale Ale (5.6%)	175	16	14
Pale Bock (7%)	220	18	21
Porter (5.6%)	195	16	19
Sol Cerveza Especial (4%)	125	11	11
Southpaw Light (5%)	125	14	7
St Pauli Girl Lager (4.9%)	150	14	9
Sparks: Original (6%)	233	17	35
Light (6%)	135	17	4
Steel Reserve: High Gravity (8.1%)	220	23	16
Steel 6 (6%)	160	17	11
Stella Artois (5.2%)	155	15	12
Stroh's (4.6%)	145	13	12
Stroh's Light (3.9%)	115	11	7
Tecate: Original (4.7%)	155	13	16
Light (3.7%)	110	10	8
Tsingtao (4.7%)	155	13	16
Warsteimers: *Per 11.2 fl.oz*			
Dunkel/Verum (4.8%)	140	14	12
Weinhard's: Pale Ale (4.6%)	150	13	13
Hefeweizen (4.9%)	155	14	12
Widmer: Hefeweizen (4.7%)	165	14	13
Zeigenbock Amber (4.9%)	145	14	11

Home-Brewed Beer: Similar to regular beers, according to alcohol content.

Alc ~ Alcohol (Grams)   **Cb** ~ Carbohydrate

Non-Alcoholic Brews

Less Than 0.5% Alcohol
Average All Brands

(Busch NA, Coors NA, Haake Beck,
Kaliber, Kingsbury, O'Douls,
Old Milwaukee NA, Pabst NA,
Stroh's NA, Texas Select)

	C	Alc	Cb
12 fl.oz Can/Bottle	70	1	14
O'Doul's Amber, 12 fl.oz	90	1	18
Sharp's 12 fl.oz	60	1	12

Cider (Alcoholic)

Per 12 fl.oz

	C	Alc	Cb
Ace Cider, (5%), av. all flavors	155	14	12
Ace Joker (6.9%)	135	19	12
Hornsby's: Draft Cider (6%)	170	16	16
Hard Apple Cider (5.5%)	200	15	27
Woodchuck: Amber (5%)	200	14	21
Dark & Dry (5%)	180	14	17
Granny Smith (5%)	165	14	11
Pear (4%)	150	12	18
Raspberry (4%)	170	12	22
Wyder's: Apple (5%)	150	14	21
Pear (4%)	140	12	22
Raspberry (4%)	120	12	17

Quick Guide

Table Wines
Average All Varieties (11.5% Alc.)
(Wine Contains Zero Fat)

	C	Alc	Cb
4 fl.oz 1 small wine glass OR ½ large wine glass	100	11	3
6 fl.oz (¾ large wine glass)	145	16	4
8 fl.oz (1 large wine glass)	195	21	7
½ Carafe/Bottle, 12 fl.oz	310	34	10
1 Bottle, 750ml, 25.4 fl.oz	620	68	20

Table Wines

	C	Alc	Cb
Red: *Per 4 fl.oz*			
Burgundy/Cabernet/Merlot, av.	100	11	4
White: *Per 4 fl.oz*			
Dry (Chenin; Fume Blanc; Chardonnay)	95	11	4
Sparkling, 4 fl.oz	95	11	4
Zinfandel Sweet (Moselle/Sauterne), 4 fl.oz	85	11	2

Table Wines (Cont)

	C	Alc	Cb
Champagne: *Per 4 fl.oz Serving*			
Average 1 glass,	85	11	2
w. Orange Jce (3:1 orange)	75	8	4
w. Orange Jce (1:1 orange)	65	5	7
Cold Duck 4 fl oz	110	11	8
Korbel (12%): Brut	90	11	3
Extra Dry	90	11	4
Mulled Wine *(Gluhwein),* 4 fl.oz	180	14	20
Non-Alcoholic Wine, avg., 4 fl.oz	50	0	12
Reduced Alcohol Wine (6%):			
Average all types, 4 fl.oz	50	6	12
Sake, *Gekkeikan,* (16%), 4 fl.oz	120	15	5

Flavored Wines

Average All Brands (6% alcohol)
(Examples: Arbor Mist, Wild Vines, Boones)

	C	Alc	Cb
1 small wine glass, 4 fl.oz	80	6	10
1 large wine glass, 8 fl.oz	160	11	20
1 bottle, 750 ml (25.4 fl.oz)	510	35	64

Dessert Wines

	C	Alc	Cb
Madeira (18% alc), 2 oz	85	9	5
Marsala (18%), 2 oz	110	9	11
Port, Muscatel (18%), 2 oz	85	9	5
Sherry (15%), 2 oz			
Dry, 1 Sherry glass	90	7	7
Sweet/Cream, average	90	7	8
Vermouth, *Martini & Rossi:*			
Extra Dry (18%), 2 oz	65	9	2
Martini Rosso (16%), 2 oz	90	10	8

Cooking Wines

	C	Alc	Cb
Holland House:			
Marsala (14%), 2 Tbsp, 1 fl.oz	45	4	4
Red/White (10%), 2 Tbsp, 1 fl.oz	20	2	1
1 cup, 8 fl.oz	160	24	8
Sherry (17%), 2 Tbsp, 1 fl.oz	45	5	2

COOKING WITH WINE

For alcohol to evaporate, sufficient heat and cooking
time (at least 30 minutes) is required.
Red and white table wines would
then contain negligible residual calories.
Sweetened wines (marsala/sherry)
would contain 10 calories per 1 fl.oz.
Flambé Desserts: Only surface alcohol is burned
off, so negligible reduction in alcohol or calories.

Quick Guide

Alc ~ Alcohol (Grams)

Spirits/Liquors
Includes Bourbon, Brandy, Gin, Rum, Scotch, Tequila, Vodka, Whiskey.
Note: All spirits with same alcohol proof have similar calories and zero fat.

Average All Brands	**C**	**Alc**	**Cb**
80 Proof (40% Alcohol by Volume):			
1 fl.oz	65	9.5	0
1½ fl.oz (1 shot)	100	14	0
3 fl.oz (Double shot)	195	28	0
½ Bottle, 350 ml	770	113	0
1 Bottle, 700 ml (24 fl.oz)	1540	227	0
86 Proof (43% Alc): 1 fl.oz	70	10	0
1½ fl.oz (1 shot)	105	15	0
1 Bottle, (24 fl.oz)	1670	244	0
100 Proof (50% Alc): 1½ fl.oz	125	18	0
Shochu (Soju) ~ Izakaya Lounges			
Average all types (25% alc), 2 fl.oz	65	12	0

Flavored Spirits

	C	**Alc**	**Cb**
Captain Morgan: *Per 1.5 fl.oz*			
Original (35%)	85	12	0.5
Black Label (40%)	100	14	0
Parrot Bay (21%)	90	7.5	10
Silver Spiced (35%)	90	12	2
Malibu Rum: *Per 1.5 fl.oz*			
Original/Banana (21%)	80	7.5	30
Pineapple (21%)	75	7.5	22
Southern Comfort, (35%), 1.5 fl.oz	100	12	3

Hard Lemonade & Sodas

	C	**Alc**	**Cb**
Mike's Hard Lemonade: *Per 11.2 fl.oz*			
Original (5%), av. all flavors	235	14	32
Light (4%)	100	11	6
Mike's Hard Tea: *Per 11.2 fl.oz*			
Original (4.1%)	175	11	27
Light (3.5%)	95	9	7
Mike's Hard Punch (5.5%), 11.2 fl oz	210	15	28
Twisted Tea: *Per 12 fl.oz*			
Original (5%) av., all flavors	210	14	31
Light (4%)	115	11	9

Alcoholic Energy Drinks (with Caffeine)

	C	**Alc**	**Cb**
Sparks: *Per 12 fl.oz*			
Original (6%)	255	17	35
Light (6%)	135	17	4
Plus (6%)	260	17	35
Tilt: Green (6%), 12 fl.oz	255	17	35
Orange (6%), 12 fl.oz	285	17	42

Coolers & Premix Cocktails

Ready-To-Drink **Zero Fat Unless Indicated**	**C**	**Alc**	**Cb**
Arbor Mist: Blenders,			
all flavors (6%), 8 fl.oz	155	11	20
Bacardi Silver: *Per 12 fl.oz*			
Lemonade/Sangria, av. (6%)	270	17	41
Raz/Strawberry/Watermelon (5%)	240	14	36
Mojito: Original (5%)	230	14	34
Mango/Pomegranate (5%)	235	14	35
Ready to Pour: *Per 4 fl.oz*			
Bahama Mama (10%)	130	13	16
Hurricane (12.5%)	145	12	16
Rum Island Ice Tea (12.5%)	150	12	16
Bartles & Jaymes			
Malt Based Coolers (3.9%): *Per 12 fl.oz*			
Classic Original; Blue Hawaiian	185	11	28
Exotic Berry; Juicy Peach	210	11	34
Luscious Blackberry; Mango	230	11	40
Margarita	260	11	46
Strawberry Cosmo; Daiquiri	220	11	37
Wine Cooler (5%): *12 fl.oz*			
Classic Original	200	14	29
Blue Hawaiian; Exotic Berry, avg.	230	14	33
Other flavors, average	245	14	38
Captain Morgan Parrot Bay (5%),			
Average all flavors, 12 fl.oz	245	14	39
Daily's (6.9%):			
Bag-In-Box Cocktails (6.9%), 4.4 fl.oz	110	7	14
Single Serve Bottles, all flavors, 8 fl.oz	220	12	30
Jack Daniels Country Cocktails (5%):			
Average all flavors, 10 fl.oz	245	12	40
Jack Daniels Hard Cola (5%) 12 oz	234	14	34
Jose Cuervo Margaritas			
Original (10%), 6 fl.oz	200	14	27
Mini (10%), 6 fl.oz	210	14	24
Seagram's Escapes Coolers (3.2%)			
Bahama Mama, 12 fl.oz	150	9	39
Strawberry Daiquiri, 12 fl.oz	170	9	44
Average all other flavors, 12 fl.oz	180	9	45
Smirnoff Ice (3.2%), 11.2 fl.oz			
Light	95	9	12
Triple Black	175	9	31
Average all other flavors	200	9	36
TGI Friday's: *Per 6 fl.oz*			
On The Rocks: Margarita (7.5%)	240	14	39
Long Island Ice Tea (15%)	190	14	24
Mudslide (10%)	365	14	31
Blenders (12.5% alc): *Per 4.8 fl.oz*			
Orange Dream; Pina Colada, av.	360	14	36
Strawberry Shortcake	365	14	41

Coolers & Premix Cocktails (Cont)

Ready-To-Drink | **C** | **Alc** | **Cb**

The Club Premix Cocktails: *Per 3.4 oz Serving (½ can)*

	C	Alc	Cb
Censored on Beach; Margarita (7.5%)	105	6	17
Gin/Vodka Martini, av. (21%)	155	17	0.2
Long Island Ice Tea(15%)	145	12	16
Manhattan (17%)	115	14	5
Mudslide/Pina Colada (10%) av.	200	8	16
Screwdriver (7.5%)	95	6	14
Whiskey Sour (10%)	95	8	11

Shooters **Alc** ~ Alcohol (Grams)

Alabama Slammer	110	14	2
Amaretto Sour	120	6	19
B52	145	14	11
Beam Me Up Scotty	145	13	13
Blue Tequila	160	18	6
Jager Bomb	205	8	30
Jager Bomb (w. Sugar-Free Red Bull)	155	8	18
Jell-O Shot, 3 oz (w.1½ oz Vodka)	180	14	19
w. Diet Jell-O, 3 oz	110	14	0
Kamikaze	75	8	3
Kool-Aid	160	15	14
Orgasm	100	12	6
Peppermint Patty	195	8	11
Stinger	170	18	12
Surfer on Acid	90	7	11

Cocktail Mixers

Non Alcoholic ~ No Alcohol Added

Bacardi: *Per 8 fl.oz Prepared from 2 fl.oz concentrate*

Daiquiris, Rum runner	120	0	32
Margarita	90	0	25
Mojito	110	0	30
Pina Colada	170	0	36
Baja Bob's (Sugar Free): *Per 4 fl.oz*			
Cosmo Martini	10	0	2
Pina Colada	30	0	4
J.Cuervo: Margarita, 4 fl.oz	105	1	28
Strawberry Margarita, 4 fl.oz	115	1	20
All other flavors	0	0	0
Mr & Mrs T: *Per 4 fl.oz*			
Bloody Mary: Original	25	0	5
Bold & Spicy	35	0	7
Mai Tai	130	0	32
Margarita	100	0	26
Pina Colada	170	0	44
Strawberry Daiquiri	180	0	46
TGI Fridays: Mudslide, 2.3 fl.oz	110	0	3
Cosmo; Berrytini, 2 fl.oz	80	0	20
Strawb. Daiquiri; Margarita, 4 fl.oz	190	0	46

Cocktails **Alc** ~ Alcohol (Grams)

Made to Standard Recipes (Standard Size)
(Main Reference: The New American Bartender's Guide)

Zero Fat Unless Indicated | **C** | **Alc** | **Cb**

	C	Alc	Cb
Bacardi & Coke (w. 1½ oz Bacardi)	160	14	17
Bellini, av., 4.5 fl.oz	95	11	7
Bloody Mary (w. 1½ oz Vodka)	125	10	7
Blushin' Russian (20g fat)	405	14	23
Bourbon & Soda (w. 2 oz Bourbon)	130	19	0
Brandy Alexander (10g fat)	300	20	15
Chi Chi's: Long Island Iced Tea, 4 fl.oz	145	12	17
Mexican Mudslide, 4 fl.oz (8g fat)	240	1.5	42
Mojito, 4 fl.oz	160	11	21
Pina Colada 4 fl.oz (6g fat)	240	4	42
White Russian 4 fl.oz (7g fat)	245	1.5	43
Chupa Naranjas (w. 1½ oz Tequila)	150	16	8
Cosmopolitan	215	24	12
Daiquiri (w. 2 oz Rum) avg. all types	140	19	4
Frozen Daiquiri (w. 2 oz Rum):			
no fruit	155	19	6
with fruit (w. 1½ oz Rum)	145	14	11
Gin Martini (w. 2 oz alcohol)	140	19	0
Grasshopper	260	17	28
Harvey Wallbanger (2 oz Alc.)	200	19	17
Highball (1½ oz Whiskey)	100	14	0
Irish Coffee (contains 10g fat)	205	14	2
Kahlua Mudslide: w.milk (3g fat)	145	11	12
w. cream (12g fat)	230	11	10
Leon Drop, 4 fl.oz	130	14	10
Long Island Iced Tea (w. 3 oz Cola)	270	19	32
with Diet Cola (w. 3 oz Cola)	235	19	22
Mai Tai (with 2 oz Rum)	290	24	33
Manhattan	130	17	5
Margarita	160	18	7
Mint Julep (w.2½ oz Bourbon)	180	24	4
Moscow Mule	185	14	24
Pina Colada (contains 10g fat)	325	19	26
Red Bull & Vodka	210	14	28
with Sugar Free Red Bull	105	14	3
Screwdriver	160	14	15
Sex On The Beach	235	19	25
Spritzer (with 3 oz Wine)	65	8	2
Tequila Sunrise	200	14	25
Tom Collins (w. 2 oz Gin)	210	19	18
Vodka Soda (w. 1½ oz Vodka)	100	14	0
Vodka Tonic (w. 1½ oz Vodka)	165	14	18
Whiskey Sour (w. 2 oz Whiskey)	155	19	7
White Russian (w. 10g fat)	240	19	7
Non-Alcoholic:			
Cinderella	45	0	11
Shirley Temple (w. 6 oz Ginger Ale)	140	0	34

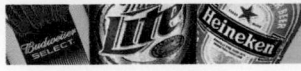
Liqueurs/Cordials

	C	Alc	Cb
Per 1 fl.oz			
Advocaat (36 Proof; 2g fat)	85	4	9
Alizé: Cognac (80 Proof)	70	9	2
Gold/Red Passion (32 Proof)	105	4	11
Amaretto (56 Proof)	100	7	14
Baileys Irish Cream (34 Proof; 5g fat)	95	4	7
Lite (30 Proof; 2g fat)	75	4	7
Benedictine (80 Proof)	90	9	5
Chambord (33 Proof)	105	4	11
Chartreuse (80 Proof)	100	9	9
Cherry Brandy (48 Proof)	80	6	9
Coffee Liqueur (53 Proof)	115	6	16
Cointreau (80 Proof)	95	9	7
Creme de Cacao (54 Proof)	100	6	15
Creme de Menthe (72 Proof)	125	9	14
Curacao (70 Proof)	95	8	6
Drambuie (80 Proof)	105	9	9
Frangelico (40 Proof)	65	5	12
Galliano (86 Proof)	100	10	8
Grand Marnier (80 Proof)	100	9	7
Kahlua (40 Proof)	90	5	15
Kirsch (68 Proof)	80	8	6
Midori (42 Proof)	80	5	11
Ouzo (80 Proof)	105	9	11
Pernod (80 Proof)	75	9	11
Sambuca (84 Proof)	100	10	11
Schnapps (100 Proof)	115	12	9
Southern Comfort (70 Proof)	65	8	3
Starbucks Liqueur:			
Coffee (40 Proof)	80	3	13
Cream (30 Proof)	85	3	9
Tia Maria (53 Proof)	120	9	15
Triple Sec (48 Proof)	60	6	10

Liqueur Coffee & Hot Drinks

Per Standard Drink			
Liqueur Coffee, avg. all types	**200**	10	10
Hot Toddy, w. 1½ oz liquor, av. all	**170**	9	19
Irish Coffee, 1½ oz whiskey & 1 oz whip	**205**	9	4
Mulled Wine (Glühwein), 4 fl.oz, av	**195**	14	25

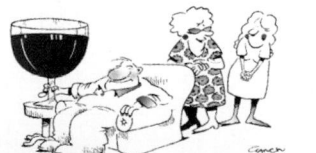

"The doctor told him to cut down to just one glass a day."

TEN HINTS TO AVOID HARMFUL DRINKING

1. **Add up the alcohol** you typically drink each day and on social occasions. How does this compare with 'low risk' amounts? (*See page 23*)

2. **Compare the alcohol content** of different drinks and select the lowest. Request half ounces of alcohol in cocktails and mixed drinks. Dilute them and keep topping off with non-alcoholic drinks.

3. **Go easy on 'Light' beers.** At 4% alcohol, on average, they are still high in alcohol compared to regular beer (5% alcohol).

4. **Try low alcohol or non-alcohol** alternatives such as fruit juices and mineral water. Take your own to parties.

5. **Before drinking alcohol,** quench your thirst with water and non-alcoholic drinks – particularly after vigorous exercise or sports.

6. **Slow the rate of drinking.** Chugging or drinking fast is the major cause of illness and death from alcohol poisoning.

7. **Avoid drinking in 'rounds'.**

8. **Have a non-alcoholic 'spacer'** between drinks (e.g. mineral water, orange juice).

9. **Don't drink on an empty stomach.** Food slows the rate of alcohol absorption.

10. **Keep track of the number of drinks** and know when to stop. Stick to a set limit.

Note: • Alcohol can be very dangerous when taken with prescription or street drugs, or when you are very tired.

Extra Info: www.CalorieKing.com

Cocktail Mixers & Extracts

	C	Alc	Cb
Angostura Bitters, ¼ tsp	2	0	0.5
Grenadine, ½ tsp	6	0	2
Lime/Lemon Juice, 2 Tbsp, 1 oz	10	0	2
Maraschino Cherry, 1 small	8	0	2
Simple Syrup, 1 Tbsp, av.	50	0	14
Sweet & Sour Mix, 2 Tbsp, 1 oz	30	0	7
Tonic Water, 8 fl.oz	80	0	22
Flavor Extracts (*McCormick*):			
Pure Lemon (83%), 1 tsp	0	3.5	0
Pure Vanilla (35%), 1tsp	0	1.5	0

Baking Ingredients

	C	F	Cb
Almond Paste:			
(Marzipan), 2 Tbsp	170	7	24
Apple Pie Filling,			
Sweetened, 9.4 oz	240	0	60
Also See Page 134			
Baking Powder: Regular, 1 tsp	5	0	2
Cream of Tartar, 1 tsp	10	0	2
Baking Mix *(Bisquick)* :			
Original, ⅓ cup, 1½ oz	160	5	26
Heart Smart, ⅓ cup, 1½ oz	140	2.5	27
Batter Mix *(Golden Dipt)*, ¼ c. mix	100	0	23
Blueberries, 1 cup, 5 oz	85	0.5	21
Butter/Margarine, ½ c., 4 oz	815	92	1
Stick, *Land O' Lakes,* ½ oz	100	11	0
Carob Flour, ½ cup	115	0.5	46
Chocolate Baking Bars: *Average all Brands*			
Sweet *(Baker's):*			
1 oz portion	120	7	16
4 oz bar	470	28	64
Semi-sweet, 1 oz	140	9	16
Bittersweet, 1 oz	140	12	14
White Baking 1 oz	160	9	16
Unsweetened, 1 oz	140	14	8
Grated, 1 cup, 4½ oz	660	69	39
Chocolate Baking Chips: *Average all Brands*			
Milk Choc./Semi Sweet 1 oz	140	8	18
½ cup, 3 oz	420	24	54
1 cup, 6 oz	840	48	108
Mini Kisses *(Hershey)*, 1 pce	5	0.5	1
Cocoa Powder, Baking: *Nestle,* 1 T.	15	1	3
⅓ cup, 1 oz	85	5	17
Hershey's, 1 Tbsp	20	0.5	3
⅓ cup, 1 oz	115	3	17
Coconut, dried:			
Unsweet., 1 oz	190	18	7
Sweetened/flaked, 1 oz	130	8	15
½ cup, 1.3 oz	195	12	22
Toasted *(Baker's)*, 1 oz	170	13	13
Coconut Cream/Milk: *See Page 89*			
Cornstarch, 1 Tbsp	30	0	7
Eggs: Large (1)	75	5	0
Jumbo (1)	90	6	0.5
Egg White: 1 Egg White	15	0	0
½ cup (4 egg whites), 4 oz	60	0	1
Flour, white:			
1 Tbsp, 0.3 oz	25	0	5.5
1 cup, 4.2 oz	400	1	88
Whole Wheat, 1 cup, 4.2 oz	400	2	84
Flavor Extracts: *Average all Brands*			
Imitation, 1 tsp	10	0	2
Pure Extract, 1 tsp	10	0	0.5
Almond, Vanilla, 1 tsp	10	0	0.5
Fruit Pectin: Swtnd, ¼ tsp	5	0	1
Unsweetened, ¼ tsp	0	0	0
Gelatin, dry, ¼ oz pkg	20	0	0
Golden Dipt, Batter Mix			
¼ cup mix, 1 oz	100	0	23
Honey, ½ cup, 6 oz	515	0	140
Lemon/Orange Peel, ¼ cup	25	0	6
Lighter Bake *(Sunsweet)*			
(Butter & Oil replacement)			
1 Tbsp, ½ oz	35	0	9
¼ Cup, 2.7 oz	140	0	36
Milk: Whole, 1 cup, 8 fl.oz	150	8	12
2%, 1 cup, 8 fl.oz	120	5	12
1%, 1 cup, 8 fl.oz	100	2.5	12
Fat-Free, 1 1 cup, 8 fl.oz	90	0.5	13
Pastry ~ *See Page 134*			
Pie Crusts ~ *See Page 134*			
Pie Fillings:			
Fruits ~ *See page 134*			
Lemon Creme, ⅓ cup	130	1.5	28
Mincemeat, 3½ oz	190	5	45
Pumpkin, 1 cup, 9.3 oz	270	1.5	60
Prune Puree, ¼ cup, 3 oz	220	0	55
Raisins, ½ cup, 2.8 oz	240	0.5	63
Rennin, 1 pkg (11g)	10	0	2
Soy Milk ~ *See Pages 49-50*			
Sprinkles, all types, 1 tsp	20	1	3
Sugar: 1 Tbsp, ½ oz	55	0	14
1 oz	110	0	28
1 cup, 7 oz	775	0	195
1 lb, 16 oz	1760	0	454
Sweeteners & Sugar Substitutes ~ *See Page 156*			
Vinegar, avg. all types, 1 oz	5	0	1
Whey, sweet, dry, 1 oz	100	0.5	21
Yeast: Active, dry, ¼ oz pkg	21	0	3
Bakers, compressed, 1 oz	30	0.5	5
Fleischmann's, 0.6 oz pkg	0	0	0

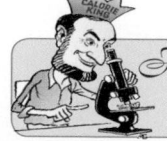

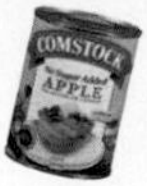

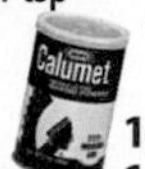

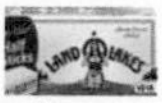

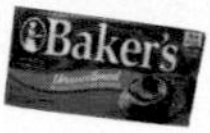

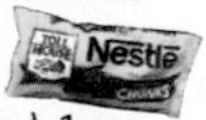

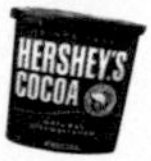

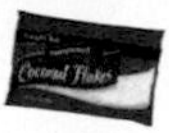

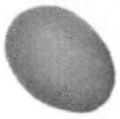

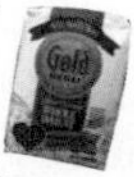

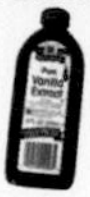

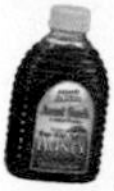

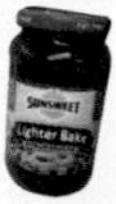

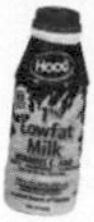

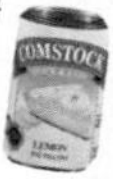

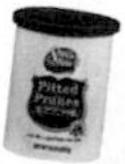

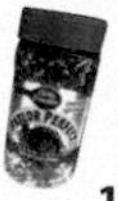

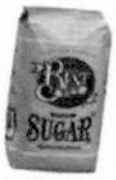

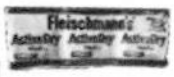

**𝒻or Full Nutritional Data
& Product Updates
~ See Author's Website
www.CalorieKing.com**

Note: Actual weight of bars is usually 5-10% more than label Net Weight. Weigh bar and allow extra calories.

Breakfast Bars   Ⓒ Ⓕ Cⓑ

Per Bar

Atkins, Day Break:			
Cinnamon Bun	160	8	18
Apple Crisp; Fruit Crumble, average	125	5	17
Choc. Chip Crisp; Cranb. Almond, av	140	6	16
Chocolate Oatmeal Fiber	130	5	24
Peanut Butter Fudge Crisp	150	7	14
Barbara's Bakery: Nature's Choice, av.	150	2	28
Fruit & Yogurt, 1.1 oz, average	150	3	28
dotFIT: *Per 2 oz Bar*			
Iced Oatmeal Blueberry	220	5	29
Iced Oatmeal Strawberry	220	5	29

Note: Carb figures include 11 grams of sorbitol and maltitol sweeteners

General Mills: Milk 'n Cereal Bars,			
Cinnamon Toast Crunch, 1.6 oz	180	4	33
Honey Nut Cheerios, 1.6 oz	160	4	28
Health Valley:			
Cobbler Cereal Bars, average, 1.3 oz	140	2.5	27
Toaster Tarts, all flavors, 1.4 oz	150	3	29
Kashi, TLC Cereal Bars, average, 1.2 oz	110	3	21
Kellogg's:			
Cinnabon Bars, all flavors,1.3 oz	150	4.5	27
Fiber Plus, Antioxidants, average	125	5	25
Pop Tarts:			
Fruit/Frosted, av., 1.8 oz	200	5	36
Low-Fat, all flav., 1.8 oz	185	3	39
Market Pantry, 1.4 oz	140	3	26
Nature's Path,			
Toaster Pastries, 1.8 oz, average	210	5	40
Nutri-Grain Bars			
Cereal Bars, average, 1.3 oz	130	3	24
Strawberry Yogurt Bar, average, 1.3 oz	140	3.5	25
Quaker: Breakfast Cookies (1), 1.7 oz	175	4.5	33
Granola Bars: *See Page 34*			
South Beach Living (Kraft)			
Protein Fit Cereal Bars, av., 1.25 oz	145	5	15
Special K Cereal Bars, average, 0.8 oz	90	1.5	18
Bliss Bar, Mocha	90	2	17
Toaster Strudel:			
Fruit flavors, average	185	8	27
Boston Cream Pie	180	7	26
Cream Cheese	185	9	25
Trader Joe's: Fig, 1.3 oz	120	2	24
Apple, Blueb./Strawberry, average	140	2.5	28

Sports & Diet Bars   Ⓒ Ⓕ Cⓑ

Per Bar

ABB, Steel Bar, average, 2.3 oz	270	8	33
AdvantEdge (EAS)			
Carb Control:			
Crisp Bar, average, 2.1 oz	240	8	27
Nutrition Bar, average, 2.1 oz	230	8	27
Anytime Health:			
Meal Replacement:			
Cookies N' Cream, 2.8 oz	310	9	42
P'nut Butter Choc Chip, 2.8 oz	310	9	42
Snack Bars: S'mores, 1.75 oz	190	6	26
Triple Choc., 1.75 oz	190	6	26
Apex Fix Crisp Bar:			
Chocolate Peanut Butter, 1.4 oz	160	4	21
Oatmeal Raisin, 1.03 oz	150	3	23
Atkins:			
Advantage: Caramel varieties, av.	170	10	21
Choc. Peanut Butter	240	12	22
Dark Choc: Alm. Coconut Crunch	180	15	16
Choc. Decadence	160	6	23
Granola flavors, av.	200	9	18
Marshmallow Mudslide	210	10	19
S'Mores	220	9	27
Sweet and Salty Almond	18	14	15
Endulge: Caramel Nut Chew	130	8	17
Choc. P'nut Butter Cups	160	13	18
Nutty Fudge Brownie	170	12	18
P'nut Caramel Cluster	140	9	12
Attune Bars:			
Chocolate Probiotic Wellness Bars: *Per 0.7 oz Bar*			
Blueberry Vanilla	100	7	9
Chocolate Crisp	90	6	12
Dark Chocolate	80	6	11
Mint Chocolate	90	6	12
Granola Probiotic, average, 1.4 oz	170	7	23
Balance: Original, average, 1.76 oz	200	7	23
Carb Well, average, 1.7 oz	195	8	23
Gold, average, 1.75 oz	210	6	23
Pure, av. all flavors	180	7	22
Barbara's Bakery:			
Crunchy Granola (2), average, 1.5 oz	190	8	27
Bariatrix Proti-Bar: (15g Protein)			
Crisp, average all flavors, 1.4 oz	160	4.5	16
Layered, average all flavors, 1.4 oz	160	5.5	15
CarbRite Diet (Doctor's), av., 2 oz	195	3.5	23
Cascadian Farms (General Mills)			
Chewy Granola: Choc. Chip, 1.25 oz	140	4	25
Harvest Berries, 1.25 oz	130	2	26

Note: Actual weight of bars is usually 5-10% more than label Net Weight. Weigh bar and allow extra calories.

Sports & Diet Bars (Cont)

Per Bar	C	F	Cb
Clif Bars:			
Original: Apricot, 2.4 oz	230	3	45
Chocolate Chip, 2.4 oz	240	5	44
Builder's, average, 2.4 oz	270	8	30
Kid Z, average, 1.26 oz	125	3.5	23
Mojo: Avg., 1.58 oz	200	10	20
Detour: Original, 3 oz	355	11	33
Biker, average, 1.76 oz	210	6	27
Lean Muscle, average, 3.17 oz	380	14	33
Lower Sugar, 3 oz	345	10	32
Oatmeal, average, 4.28 oz	455	10	60
Runner, average, 1.76 oz	205	5.5	27
Yoga,1.6 oz	370	2	28
dotFIT: *Breakfast Bars ~ Page 31*			
dotSTICK: Protein Stick (12g Prot.):			
Iced Peanut Butter Delight	190	6	26
Iced Lemon Vanilla Cream	190	6	26
EAS			
AdvantEDGE, Carb Control, av., 2.12 oz	245	8	27
Myoplex: Lite, Choc. Chip Crisp, 1.9 oz	190	4.5	28
Carb Control,			
Choc Peanut Butter, 2.46 oz	260	8	27
(Carbs include 17g sugar alcohol)			
Strength, average all flavors, 2.65 oz	280	7	25
Elevate Me!, average, 2.33 oz	235	4	35
Extend Bar, av., 1.4 oz	150	3	25
FiberPlus (Kellogg's):			
Chocolate Chip	120	4	26
Dark Chocolate Almond	130	5	24
Chocolatey Peanut Butter	130	5	24
First Endurance, EFS Bar, 2.32 oz	250	6	40
General Mills:			
Fiber One Chewy 90 Cals, av., 0.8 oz	90	2.5	17
1.4 oz, average all flavors	140	4.5	28
GeniSoy: Genisoy Bars, av., 2.2 oz	240	5.5	32
Organic Bars, 1.6 oz	160	3	25
Protein Crunch, 1.6 oz	150	5	18
Ultra Bar, 1.6 oz, 1.6 oz	160	2	27
Glenny's:			
Slim Carb, Peanut Caramel, 1.3 oz	130	2.5	19
100 Calorie, Brownies, av. all,1.06 oz	100	4	15

Per Bar	C	F	Cb
Glucerna: Meal Bars, average, 2 oz	220	7	34
Snack Bar, 1.3 oz	150	4	25
Mini Snack Bar (1)	80	2.5	12
GNC ProCrunch:			
Choc Crisp	250	4.5	36
Cookies n' Cream	250	4.5	36
Peanut Butter Crunch, 2.3 oz	260	7	34
Pro Crunch Lite, 1.2 oz	140	6	14
Gnu Foods:			
Banana Walnut, 1.6 oz	140	4	30
Cinn. Raisin; Orange Cranb., 1.6 oz	130	3	32
Choc. Brownie; P'nut Butter, av., 1.6 oz	140	4.5	30
Health Valley Chewy Granola, av.	110	1.5	22
Herbalife, Protein Deluxe!, 1.25 oz	140	4	15
HMR Benefit Bars, average, 1.4 oz	160	4	25
Jenny Craig: S'mores, 1.2 oz	130	4	22
Chocolate Caramel Peanut, 1.2 oz	150	5	19
Choc Chip Snack Bar, 1.21 oz	140	3	23
Joy Ride Bars, average, 2.8 oz	340	12	27
Kashi, GoLean Chewy, Choc. Alm	290	6	48
GoLean Crunchy!:			
Chocolate Almond	170	5	27
Chocolate Peanut	180	5	30
Average other flavors	155	3.5	27
GoLean Roll!, average, 1.95oz	190	5	28
TLC: Crunchy Granola Bars, av.,1.4 oz	170	5.5	26
Chewy Granola Bar, average, 1.2 oz	135	4	21
Fruit & Grain Bars, average, 1.13 oz	120	3	22
Keribar, Apple Peanut Butter, 1.4 oz	160	6	21
Kind Fruit & Nut Bars			
Almond & Apricot	170	11	16
In Yogurt	210	13	19
Almond & Coconut	190	14	14
Fruits & Nuts in Yogurt	210	13	20
Macadamia & Apricot	190	14	15
Sesame & Peanuts with Chocolate	230	15	19
Walnut & Date	150	7	22
Kind Plus:			
A, C & E, Cranberry & Almond	190	12	19
Omega-3, Almond & Cashew	150	9	18
Protein, Almond, Walnut, Macadamia	210	15	11

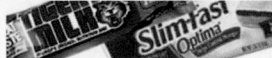
Sports & Diet Bars (Cont)

Per Bar	**C**	**F**	**Cb**
Kudos: Chocolate Chip, 1 oz	120	3.5	20
Peanut Butter, 1 oz	130	6	18
M&M's; Snickers, average, 0.84 oz	100	3	17
Larabar:			
Apple Pie, 1.6 oz	190	10	24
Banana Bread, 1.8 oz	230	11	30
Cherry Pie, 1.7 oz	200	8	30
P'nut Butter & Jelly	210	10	27
Tropical Fruit Tart	210	12	25
Lean Body: Cookie Bar, S'mores	360	13	30
Gold, Caramel Peanut, 3 oz	330	9	32
Granola Bar, average, 2.85 oz	345	12	38
Rockin' Roll, Peanut, 2.5 oz	290	16	25
Lindora: Cinnamon Crisp	160	4.5	16
Other varieties, av.	150	5	17
Luna: Bars, average, 1.7 oz	180	4.5	27
Protein, average, 1.6 oz	185	7	20
Marathon (Snickers): Energy, 2 oz	215	7	26
Protein, average, 2.8 oz	285	10	38
Market Pantry *(Target)*			
Crunchy Granola, Oat & Honey,1.5 oz	190	6	30
Sweet & Salty Bar, 1.2 oz, average	165	7	22
Medifast: Crunch, 1.13 oz	110	3	12
Maintenance Bar, 1.5 oz	160	4	22
Met-Rx: Big 100, average, 3.5 oz	380	7	51
Big 100 Colossal:			
Crispy Apple Pie	400	10	47
Peanut Butter Caramel Crunch	400	12	44
Peanut Butter Pretzel	420	12	48
Super Cookie Crunch	410	14	43
Big 100 Brownies, average	400	13	41
MLO Bio Protein: Average, 2.85 oz	315	6.5	43
Xtreme, Chocolate, 3.2 oz	320	6	44
Mojo Bars: *See Clif*			
Muscle Milk, 2.57 oz	295	11	29
Muscle Tech:			
Nitro-Tech Hardcore:			
Choc. Caramel Nut	310	8	29
S'mores; Peanut Butter	270	6	31
Strawberry Cheesecake	290	7	32
Nabisco:			
100 Calorie Granola Bars:			
Chips Ahoy, 1 oz	100	1.5	22
Nutter Butter, 1 oz	100	1.5	21
Oreo, 1 oz	100	2	21

Per Bar	**C**	**F**	**Cb**
Nature Valley			
Crunchy Granola Bars			
Apple Crisp, 1.25 oz	160	6	26
Cinnamon, 1.25 oz	180	6	29
Chewy: w/ Yogurt coating, av., 1.4 oz	140	3.5	26
Trail Mix, average, 1.25 oz	140	4	25
Nature's Path			
Granola Bars, average, 1.25 oz	150	5	26
Optimum Energy, av., 1.98 oz	220	5.5	37
Nutiva: Hempseed, 1.4 oz	210	14	11
Flax Choc., 1.4 oz	200	13	17
NutriSystem:			
Dessert Bars: Blueberry Lemon	160	5	25
Chocolate Peanut Butter	170	8	17
Nutrilite *(Amway Global)*.			
Meal Bars: Blueberry Crunch, 1.8 oz	200	7	26
Cherry Almond, 1.8 oz	200	6	26
Chocolate Crisp, 1.8 oz	190	6	26
Lemon Twist, 1.8 oz	200	7	27
Snack Bar: Caramel Creme, 0.9 oz	100	2.5	16
Cranberry Crunch, 0.9 oz	100	3	15
Fudgy Brownie w/ Almonds, 0.9 oz	100	3.5	9
Odwalla Energy Bars			
Choc. Chip Peanut, 2 oz	230	8	33
Choco-walla, 2 oz	210	5	39
Strawberry Pomegranate, 2 oz	200	2	42
Superfood, 2 oz	200	3.5	39
Average other varities, 2 oz	210	6	39
Oh Yeah! *(ISS)*, average, 3 oz	375	18	31
One Way, average 3 oz	340	12	29
Optifast, P'nut Butter			
1.6 oz bar	160	4	23
PowerBar: Enery Fruit Smoothie	220	3.5	43
Harvest Whole Grain	245	5	42
Nut Naturals, av., 1.6 oz	210	10	20
Triple Threat, average	220	6	32
Performance, Cookies & Cream, 2 oz	240	3.5	45
Pria Bars, 110 Plus, average, 1.7 oz	110	3	16
Protein Plus: Choc. Fudge Brownie	250	6	21
Cookies & Cream, 2.3 oz	260	5.5	20
PR Bar: Lemon Drop, 1.8 oz	160	7	22
Granola Crunch, 1.8 oz	210	8	20

Sports & Diet Bars (Cont)

Per Bar	C	F	Cb
Premier Nutrition:			
Premier Protein, average, 2.5 oz	280	7	24
Twisted Bar, average, 1.6 oz	190	6	21
Promax:			
Cookies 'N Cream, 2.64 oz	270	4.5	39
Choc Peanut Crunch, 2.64 oz	280	6	38
Double Fudge Brownie, 2.6 oz	280	7	38
70 Calorie Bars, 0.66 oz	70	1.5	10
Proti 15 Crisp Bar,			
Average all flavors, 1.48 oz	160	5	16
Pure Protein:			
1.75 oz Bars, av.	180	5	18
2.75 oz Bars, average	300	8	30
Pure Fit, average, 2 oz bar	225	7	25
Quaker:			
Chewy Granola Bars			
Regular, av., 0.85 oz	100	3	18
Dipps: Caramel Nut	140	6	21
Chocolate Chip, 1 oz	140	5	22
Omega-3, P'nut Butter Choc, 1.25 oz	150	5	25
25% Less Sugar, Choc. Chip, 0.85 oz	100	3.5	17
90 Calories, Dk Choc. Cherry, 1 oz	90	2	19
True Delights, average, 1.25 oz	135	4.5	23
Rebar: Original, 1.75 oz	160	0	38
Perfect 10 Energy, Lemon, 1.75 oz	210	12	24
Elev8me, Banana Nut Bread, 2.3 oz	230	4.5	34
Revival Soy Bars (Direct):			
Chocolate Temptation	270	7	32
Apple Cinnamon; Marshm. Krunch	225	3	30
Peanut Pal	240	6	28
Low Carb, average all flavors	235	8	31
Slim-Fast Bars:			
Meal Bars: Chewy Chocolate Crisp	200	6	26
Chocolate Peanut Caramel	200	7	23
Sweet & Salty Chocolate Almond	200	8	23
Snack Bars: Choc. Nougat Gone Nuts	100	5	14
Chocolatey Vanilla Blitz	100	2.5	17
Double-Dutch Chocolate	100	3.5	16
Nutty Chocolate Chew	100	3.5	15
Snickers, Marathon, av., 1.94 oz	210	7	28
South Beach Living			
Fiber Fit Granola Bars, av., 1.23 oz	120	4	25
High Protein Cereal Bars, av., 1.23 oz	145	5	15

Per Bar	C	F	Cb
South Beach Living (Cont)			
Snack Bars, average, 1 oz	100	4	14
Meal Replacement,			
average all flavors, 2.1 oz	180	6	25
SoyJoy Bars, average, 1 oz	135	6	16
Solo GI, average, 1.75 oz	200	7	26
Special K			
Bliss Bars,Raspberry, 0.8 oz	90	2	17
Protein Meal, average, 1.6 oz	180	5	25
Protein Snack Bars, average 0.9 oz	110	3	16
Steel Bar (ABB), average, 2.47 oz	270	5	35
Supreme Protein:			
Original, Caramel Nut Choc., 3.45 oz	400	15	36
Carb Conscious, Peanut Butter Crunch	390	18	26
think Bars:			
thinkThin: Protein, average, 2 oz	230	8	27
Bites, average, 0.88 oz	100	4	7
Tiger's Milk:			
Protein Rich, 1.2 oz	140	5	18
Peanut Butter, 1.2 oz	150	6	18
King Size, average, 1.9 oz	225	9	28
Trader Joe's:			
Chewy Granola Bars, 6-Packs:			
Chocolate Chip, 1.23 oz	140	4	25
Vanilla Almond, 1.23 oz	130	4	21
Fruit & Nut Bars:			
Choc. Chip, 1.6 oz	170	5	31
Trail Mix, 1.6 oz	200	6	37
Tri-O-Plex: average, 4.2 oz	420	13	45
Duo: Peanut Butter, 3.5 oz	300	10	26
Caramel Peanut Butter, 3.5 oz	340	8	45
U-Turn Protein, 2.8 oz	300	8	26
Usana:			
Nutrition Bar: Oatmeal Raisin, 2 oz	170	2.5	28
Peanut Butter Crunch, 1.5 oz	160	5	19
Vyo-Pro (AST) Choc. Brownie, 2.2 oz	200	7	24
Zoe's, Omega-3's, Chocolate Delight	190	7	27
Zone Perfect			
Classic, average, 1.76 oz	210	7	24
Dark Chocolate, average, 1.6 oz	190	6	22
Fruitified: Apple Cinn., 1.76 oz	180	2	27
Banana Nut, 1.8 oz	200	6	24
Blueberry, 1.8 oz	190	4	25
Indulgence, average, 1.6 oz	185	6	21

Cocoa & Hot Chocolate

	C	F	Cb
Cocoa (8 fl.oz cup):			
with Whole Milk	205	8.5	22
with Nonfat Milk	145	1	23
Tall (12 fl.oz): with Whole Milk	280	12	26
with Nonfat Milk	185	1	28
Hot Chocolate:			
8 fl.oz cup: With Whole Milk	180	7	26
with Nonfat Milk	140	2	17
Tall (12 fl.oz): With Whole Milk	260	10	36
with Nonfat Milk	190	2	37
Cinnabon, Mochalatta Chill, 16 oz	450	18	66
Swiss Miss Mixes, average, 1 packet	120	2.5	22

Cocoa - Chocolate Mixes

Add extra cals/fat/carbohydrate for milk
Carnation Breakfast Drinks: See Page 38

	C	F	Cb
Carnation: *Per 3 Tbsp*			
Malted Milk: Original	90	2	15
Chocolate	90	1	18
Ghirardelli			
Choc Mocha, 4 Tbsp, 1.2 oz	135	1.5	33
Double Chocolate, 4 Tbsp, 1.4 oz	140	1.5	34
White Mocha, 2 Tbsp, 0.8 oz	100	0	24
Hershey's			
Cocoa, Natural, 1 T, 0.18 oz	10	0.5	3
Horlicks, Malt Extract, 1 oz	90	2	20
Land O' Lakes: *Per 1¼ oz Package*			
Mint/Raspberry/Supreme	140	3.5	26
Nestle: *Per Single Serve Package*			
Dark Milk Chocolate	80	1	17
Carb Select: Fat-Free Hot Cocoa	25	0	5
with Marshmallows	35	0	8
Rich Milk Chocolate	80	3	15
No Sugar Added	50	0	10
Supreme Cocoa, 1 oz	120	2	22
Nesquik Powder (Nestle): *Per 2 Tbsp*			
Choc.; Strawberry, 25% less sugar	60	0	15
Chocolate; Strawb., No Added Sugar	35	1	7
Ovaltine Cocoa Mixes, average, 4 Tbsp	80	0	19
Swiss Miss: *Per Single Serve Package*			
Milk Chocolate: Made with water	120	2	23
Made with milk	210	6	31
With Marshmallows, made w/ water	120	2	23
Made with milk	210	6	33
French Vanilla	110	2	23
Marshmallow	120	2	24
Marshmallow Lovers	140	2.5	29
Rich Chocolate	110	1.5	23
Fat-Free	50	0	10
Marshmallow Lovers	70	0	13

Instant Coffee

	C	F	Cb
Powder/Granules: Regular or Decaffeinated			
1 level tsp	2	0	0.5
1 rounded tsp	4	0	1
Ground, 3 tsp	7	0	1
Brewed/Percolated, 1 cup, 8 fl.oz	4	0	1
Coffee With Milk/Cream/Creamers:			
Per Cup Coffee (8 fl.oz):			
Black	4	0	1
With Whole Milk: Dash, 1 Tbsp	15	0.5	2
2 Tbsp, 1 fl.oz	25	1	2
With 2% Milk, 2 Tbsp	20	0.5	2
With 1% Milk, 2 Tbsp	20	0.5	3.5
With Fat Free Milk, 2 Tbsp	15	0	3
With Half & Half, 2 Tbsp	50	3	2
With ¼ cup, 2 fl.oz	90	6	3
With Cream (light coffee), 2 Tbsp	65	6	2
With Coffee Mate: Liquid, reg., 1Tbsp	20	1	2
Liquid Fat Free, 1 Tbsp	25	0	5
Powder, 1 heaping tsp	15	1	2
Sugar ~ Add Extra: 1 heaping tsp	25	0	6
Single portion, 1 package	25	0	6
Sweeteners: *Equal/Splenda/Sweet N Low*			
Powder, package	0	0	0

Flavored Coffee Mixes

	C	F	Cb
Chicory: Instant Coffee, 1 tsp	5	0	1
Coffee Essence, 1 tsp	15	0	4
Caffé D'Vita: Mixes, 3 tsp	60	1.5	11
Sugar Free Mixes, 2 tsp	35	2	3
General Foods Int'l:			
Average, ½ oz	60	3	10
Sugar-free, av,. 1 tsp	30	2.5	2
Cappuccino Coolers, ½ oz	60	0	15
Hills Bros:			
Cappuccino, Fr. Vanilla			
3 Tbsp, 1 oz	120	4.5	19
Nescafé, Latte; Mocha, average, 1oz	115	3.5	21
Starbucks, VIA® Iced Coffee, 1 stick	100	0	24

Coffee Shops/Restaurants

Per 8 fl.oz Cup (Unless Indicated)

	C	F	Cb
Coffee (Regular/Percolated/Filtered)	5	0	0
Americano Drip Coffee, 1 cup	7.5	0	1
Cafe Au Lait: 1 cup, 8 fl.oz	60	3.5	5
Nonfat Milk, 1 cup, 8 fl.oz	35	0	5
Caffe Latté:			
8 fl.oz cup: With Whole Milk	110	6	9
With 2% Milk	100	3.5	9
With Nonfat Milk	70	0	10
12 fl.oz: With Whole Milk	180	9	14
With Nonfat Milk	100	0	15
16 fl.oz: With Whole Milk	220	11	18
With Nonfat Milk	130	0	19
Cafe Mocha (Mochaccino): 1 cup	150	6	20
12 fl.oz	230	9	31
16 fl.oz	290	12	41
Cappuccino:			
8 fl.oz cup: With Whole Milk	90	3.5	7
With 2% Milk	80	3	8
With Nonfat Milk	50	0	8
12 fl.oz: With Whole Milk	110	6	9
With 2% Milk	90	3.5	9
With Nonfat Milk	60	0	9
16 fl.oz: With Whole Milk	140	7	11
With 2% Milk	120	3.5	11
With Nonfat Milk	80	0	12
Mocha (with cream):			
8 fl.oz: With Whole Milk	200	11	22
With Nonfat Milk	160	6	22
12 fl.oz: Whole Milk	290	15	33
With Nonfat Milk	230	8	34
Iced Mocha (no cream):			
12 fl.oz: With Whole Milk	170	6	26
With Nonfat Milk	130	2	27
Espresso: Single (Solo)	5	0	1
Doppio (Double)	10	0	2
Espresso con Panna,			
(with dollop whipped cream), solo	30	2.5	2
Espresso Macchiato, solo	10	0	1
Frappuccino: Tall, 12 fl.oz	180	2.5	37
Grande, 16 fl.oz	240	3	48
Frappuccino Mocha			
(with Cream): Tall, 12 fl.oz	280	11	43
Grande, 16 fl.oz	380	15	57

Iced Latte: *Similar to Caffe Latte*
Starbucks: *See Fast-Foods Section ~ Page 243*

Coffee Substitute Mixes

	C	F	Cb
Roasted Cereal Beverages: (No Caffeine)			
Cafix Instant Beverage, 1 tsp	5	0	1
Kaffree Roma *(Morn. Farms)*, 1 tsp	10	0	2
Teeccino Caffe, 1 tsp	10	0	2

Irish & Liqueur Coffees

	C	F	Cb
Irish Coffee (no sugar)	175	10	0
Liqueur Coffee, average 1 fl.oz	100	5	7

Coffee Extras

	C	F	Cb
Chocolate (Cocoa) Topping, ½ tsp	5	0	1
Flavored Syrups: Regular, 2 Tbsp	80	0	20
Sugar-free, 2 Tbsp	0	0	0
Half & Half Cream, 2 Tbsp	40	3.5	1
Single serve pkg, ⅜ fl.oz	15	1.5	0.5
Light Whipped Cream, 2 Tbsp	15	1.5	1
Marshmallows, miniature (2)	5	0	1
Sugar: 1 single portion package	20	0	5
1 level tsp	15	0	4
1 heaping tsp	25	0	6
Equal/Splenda/Sweet 'N Low	0	0	0

Coffee Shop ~ Cakes, Cookies

	C	F	Cb
Cookies:			
Biscotti, 1 oz	140	6.5	18
Chocolate Chip, 3 oz	350	15	54
Oatmeal Raisin, 3 oz	350	12	56
Peanut Butter, 3 oz	410	25	39
White Chocolate Macadamia, 3⅓ oz	420	20	55
Cakes/Pastries:			
Almond Croissant, 5 oz	620	35	67
Apple Danish, 5 oz	450	18	67
Banana Walnut, 4½ oz	410	17	60
Brownie, 3 oz	390	24	42
Bundt, Chocolate, 4 oz	440	21	61
Carrot Cake, 4 oz	400	22	45
Chocolate Cake, 5 oz	530	28	65
Crumble Coffee Cake, 4½ oz	500	25	65
Cupcake, 3 oz	330	16	43
Pound Cake, av., 3 oz	330	17	40
Cinnamon Roll, 6 oz	500	15	83
Doughnuts: Sugared, 1¾ oz	220	11	27
Glazed, 2 oz	250	12	34
Pretzel, large, 4 oz	290	5	52

Starbucks Bakery Items ~ See Page 244

Bottled Coffee (Chilled)

Ready-To-Drink:

Adina: *Per 8 fl.oz Can*

Caramel Kick; Double Xxpresso	**100**	2	20
Hazelnut Hook Up; Vanilla Nutcase	**110**	2	18
Mocha Madness	**110**	2.5	20
Caribou: Espresso, 12 fl.oz	**100**	0.5	22
Regular; Vanilla, 12 fl.oz	**120**	1.5	24
Coffee Bean & Tea Leaf:			
Cafe Latte/Mocha/Vanilla, 9.5 fl.oz	**200**	3	33
Full Throttle Coffee & Energy ~ *See Page 38*			
Java Monster Energy ~ *See Page 39*			
Kahlúa, Cappuccino Shake, 10.5 fl.oz	**130**	2	24
Shock Coffee: Triple Latte, 15 fl.oz	**150**	2.5	27
Triple Mocha, 15 fl.oz can	**150**	3.5	28

Starbucks: *Per Bottle*

Frappuccino:

Caramel, 9.5 fl.oz	**200**	3	37
Coffee: 9.5 fl.oz	**200**	3	37
13.7 fl.oz bottle	**290**	4.5	53
Mocha: Regular, 13.7 fl.oz	**260**	4.5	47
Dark Choc., 13.7 fl.oz	**280**	4.5	51
Light, 9.5 fl.oz	**100**	3	12
Vanilla: 9.5 fl.oz	**200**	3	37
13.7 fl.oz bottle	**295**	4.5	55

DoubleShot:

Espresso & Cream, 6.5 fl.oz	**140**	6	18
Light Espresso & Cream, 6.5 fl.oz	**70**	4	6
Energy + Coffee, all flavors, 15 fl.oz	**210**	2.5	18

CALORIE KING TIP!

Reduce the Calories in Your Coffee Drinks:

- Request non-fat milk in place of whole or 2% milk
- Downsize to 8 fl.oz or 12 fl.oz
- Avoid cream on frappuccinos
- Replace sugar with *Equal, Splenda Stevia* or *Sweet 'N Low*
- Avoid syrup add-ons

CAFFEINE COUNTER

Moderate caffeine intake is not harmful to healthy adults. However, frequent large amounts (over 350mg/day) may cause dependency ('caffeinism') and adversely affect health. To be safe, limit caffeine to 200mg/day. Avoid if pregnant; breast feeding; a child under 8; have sleep problems or heart arrhythmia.

	Caffeine (mg)
Coffee: Instant, weak, 1 level teaspoon	30
Medium, 1 rounded teaspoon	60
Strong, 1 heaping teaspoon	100
Decaffeinated, 1 round teaspoon	2
Bags *(Folgers)*, 1 bag (6-8 fl.oz)	115
Ground, 1 Tbsp, 0.2 oz	60
Bottled (Ready-To Drink), 9.5 fl.oz	70
Coffee Shop: Brewed, 8 fl.oz	110 -150
Cappuccino: 1 cup, 8 fl.oz	75
Tall, 12 fl.oz	110
Large, 16 fl.oz	150
Decappuccino (decaffeinated)	5
Espresso: Regular/Solo	75
Double (Doppio) Espresso	150
Iced Coffee, 12 fl.oz	140
Latte, 1 cup, 8 fl.oz	75
Mocha, 1 cup, 8 fl.oz	90
Hot Chocolate, 8 fl.oz	15
Tea (Black/Green): Weak, 1 cup	20
Medium Strength, 1 cup	40
Strong, 1 cup	70
Decaffeinated Tea	0-5
Herbal Tea	0
Iced Tea, tall glass/can, 12 fl.oz	25-30
Soft Drinks: *Per 12 fl.oz Can*	
Coca-Cola, Pepsi (Regular/Diet)	35
Diet Coke; TAB; RC Cola (Regular)	45
Dr. Pepper (Reg./Diet) Sunkist Orange	40
Pepsi One; Mountain Dew; Mellow Yellow; Surge	55
Pepsi Max (Regular/Diet) Sun Drop (Reg/Diet)	70
7-Up, Fanta, Sprite, Fresca, Diet Rite Cola	0
Energy Drinks (with added caffeine): *(AMP, Adrenaline Rush, Full Throttle Monster, No Fear, Red Bull, Rockstar)*	
Average all brands: 8 fl.oz	80
16 fl.oz	160
NOS Energy, 16 fl.oz	260
Chocolate Bars: Milk Chocolate, 2 oz	20
Dark Chocolate, 2 oz	30
Cocoa/Hot Choc. Mix, 1 oz packet	5
Chocolate Milk, 1 cup, 8 fl.oz	2
Choc Chip Cookies, 2 medium, 2 oz	6
Chocolate Syrup, 2 Tbsp, 1.4 oz	5
Medicinals: *Excedrin,* Extra Strength (2)	130
NoDoz Maximum, 1 tablet	200

Extensive Caffeine Counter ~ www.CalorieKing.com

Energy/Protein Drinks

	C	F	Cb
5-hour Energy, 2 fl.oz	4	0	1
ABB:			
Anytime, Turbo Tea, 18 fl.oz	150	0	38
Energy: Adrenalyn Shot, 8.5 fl.oz	10	0	3
Ripped Force, 18 fl.oz	90	0	23
Hi-Pro:			
Pure Pro Shake, Choc Swirl, 12 fl.oz	110	1	5
Pure Pro 50, 14.5 fl.oz	240	1.5	7
Recovery: Blue Thunder, 22 fl.oz	290	0.5	40
Extreme XXL, 22 fl.oz	980	1	197
Maxx Recovery, Grape, 18 fl.oz	480	0.5	6
Accelerade, all flav., 20 fl.oz	200	0	38
AdvantEdge (EAS):			
Carb Control, 11 fl.oz	110	3	4
AllSport,			
Body Quencher, all flav., 20 fl.oz	150	0	40
AMP: Energy Drink, 16 fl.oz	220	0	58
24 fl.oz Can	330	0	87
Relaunch/Elevate, 16 fl.oz	220	0	58
Anytime Health:			
Performance Powder,			
Green Apple/Lemonade,			
2 scoops, 1 pkt, 1.73 oz	160	0	30
Whey Protein Isolate, all flavors, 1 oz	105	0	1
Arizona: AM Awake Fast Shot, 2fl.oz	10	0	3
Caution Energy, 11 fl.oz	160	0	40
Atkins: Advantage Shake, 11 oz can	160	10	4
Bally Total Fitness:			
Whey Pro, Vanilla, 1 scoop	115	1.5	3
Blast, Sugar Free, 8.3 oz	10	0	3
Bariatrix: Pudding Shakes (1)	100	2	6
Proti Anytime Drinks, avg	100	4	4
Bawls Guarana, 10 fl.oz	120	0	32
Blue Sky:			
Blue Energy, 8.3 fl.oz	120	0	29
Body Fuel (w. NutraSweet), 1 scoop	80	0	20
Bolthouse: Per 8 fl.oz			
Perfectly Protein:			
Mocha Cappuccino	180	2.5	29
Vanilla Chai Tea	160	3	25
Boost: High Protein, 8 fl.oz	240	6	33
Glucose Control, 8 fl.oz	190	7	16
Nutritional Energy, 8 fl.oz	240	4	41
Plus, 8 fl.oz	360	14	45
Kid Essentials, 8.25 fl.oz	245	9	33

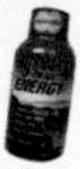

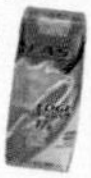

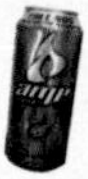

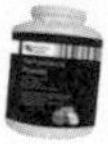

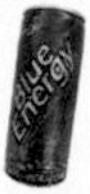

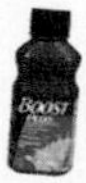

	C	F	Cb
Carnation Instant Breakfast			
Powder: All flav., 1 envelope, 1.3 oz	130	1	27
No Sugar Added, average, 0.7 oz	60	1	27
Ready-To-Drink, average, 11.5 fl.oz	260	5	41
Celebrity Juice Diet, 4 fl.oz	60	0	14
CeraSport, EX1, 8.45 fl.oz	20	0	5
Champion Lyte, Sports Drink	0	0	0
Champion Nutrition:			
Heavyweight Gainer 900, 4 scps, 5.4 oz	630	10	101
Ultramet: Original, 1 packet, 2.7 oz	280	2	24
Lite, 1 packet, 2 oz	190	1	17
Low Carb, 1 packet, 2 oz	230	6.5	6
Clif Shot Energy Gel, 1.1 oz packet	100	0	24
Cocaine Energy, 8.4 fl.oz can	70	0	18
Curves Protein Drink:			
Chocolate; Vanilla, 2 scoops, 1 oz	110	1.5	8
made with skim milk, 8 fl.oz	200	12	20
CytoSport Muscle Milk, 2 scoops	300	12	16
Designer Whey Protein, Van. Praline., 1 s.	100	2	3
Drank, Anti Energy, 8 fl.oz serve	110	0	27
EAS ~ See AdvantEdge/Myoplex			
Endura (Unipro), 2 scoops, 1.3 oz	120	0	30
Ensure: High Protein, 8 oz	230	6	31
Immune Balance, 8 fl.oz	250	6	41
Plus, 8 fl.oz bottle	350	11	50
Enterex Glucose Control, 8 fl.oz	235	9	27
FRS Energy, Orange, 11.5 fl.oz	140	0	35
Fruit₂0 (Veryfine)	0	0	0
Full Throttle: Per 16 fl.oz			
Energy, Citrus	220	0	58
Coffee & Energy:			
Caramel	230	0	58
Mocha	270	7	50
Fuze: Slenderize, 8 fl.oz	10	0	2
Refresh, 8 fl.oz	95	0	25
Vitalize, 8 fl.oz	100	0	25
Gatorade			
Thirst Quencher/Perform:			
(Lemon/Lime, AM, Fierce, Rain)			
1 cup, 8 fl.oz	50	0	14
12 fl.oz bottle	75	0	20
20 fl.oz bottle	125	0	32
24 fl.oz bottle	150	0	41
32 fl.oz bottle	200	0	52
Carbohydrate Energy, 12 fl.oz bottle	330	0	82
Endurance (Powder), made up, 8 fl.oz	50	0	14
G2 (Low Calorie), 1 cup, 8 fl.oz	25	0	7
20 fl.oz bottle	70	0	17
Nutrition Shake, all flavors, 11 oz	360	8	54
Protein Recovery Shake, 8 fl.oz	200	1	33

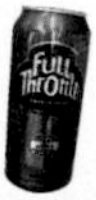

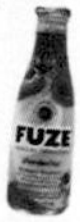

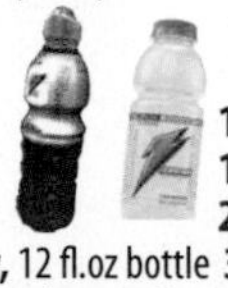

Genisoy:	C	F	Cb
Ultra XT, 3 Tbsp	150	1	20
Protein Powder, 3 Tbsp	130	1.5	5
Glaceau:			
Smartwater	0	0	0
Vitaminwater, 20 fl.oz	125	0	33
Glucerna, Shakes, 8 fl.oz	200	7	27
GNC Lean Shake: 2 scoops	180	2	30
Pro Performance			
100% Whey Protein, 1 oz	125	2.5	5
50 Gram Slam, Van., 15 fl.oz	250	1.5	9
Mass XXX, Strawb., 7 oz	750	5	126
Weight Gainer 2200 Gold, Choc., 17 oz	1840	3	402
Wheybolic Extreme 60, Van., 3 oz	280	1	7
GU Energy Gel, average, 1 packet	100	0	25
Guru Energy: Regular, 8.3 fl.oz can	100	0	25
Lite, 8.3 oz can	10	0	2
Hammer Gel, av. all flavors, 2 T., 1¼ oz	90	0	21
Hansen's: Energy Pro	120	0	32
Rumba, 8 fl.oz	130	0	32
Herbalife: Nutritional Shake, 1 pkt	90	1	13
with 8 fl.oz non-fat milk	180	1	26
Holistics (Adina), *Herbal Blends*			
Average all flavors, 14 fl.oz bottle	90	0	22
Hollywood Miracle Diet, ½ cup	100	0	25
Jarrow: Whey Protein, av., 1 scoop	95	2	2
Berry High, 1 scoop, 0.2 oz	25	0	5
Muscle Optimeal, 2 scoops, 1.65 oz	180	2	17
Java Monster, Energy· *Per 15 fl.oz Can*			
Lo-Ball	95	3	10
Loca Moca; Mean Bean	190	0	48
Original/Irish/Nut-Up/Russian	190	3	34
Jolt: Power Cola, 16 fl.oz	200	0	52
Blue Raspberry, 16 fl.oz	240	0	60
Knudsen: ReCharge, 8 fl.oz	70	0	18
Simply Nutritious, average, 8 fl.oz	120	0	30
Kombucha, Wonder Drink, 8.5 fl.oz	60	0	16
La Brada			
Drink: Lean Body, RTD, 17 fl.oz	260	9	9
Powders: Lean Body, 2.8 oz	330	8	24
Lean Body Mass 60, 6 oz	615	7	76
Carb Watchers, 2.3 oz	250	4.5	12
Lipovitan B3, 8.6 fl.oz	130	0	30
Liquid Ice: 8.3 fl.oz	130	0	29
Sugar Free, 8.3 fl oz	15	0	0
Liquid Lightning, Reg., 8.4 fl.oz	90	0	22
Max Velocity: Reg., 8.45 fl.oz can	130	0	33
16 fl.oz can	240	0	62
Sugar Free: 16 fl.oz can	15	0	1

Met-R x	C	F	Cb
Colossal RTD 15Z, 15 fl.oz can	380	14	28
Meal Replacement, 1 pkt, average	250	2	21
Protein Plus, Choc., 2 scoops	220	1.5	7
Metabol: Endurance, 2 sc.,1.83 oz	200	5	24
GlyProXTS, 1 scoop, 0.2 oz	20	0	4
Met, 2 scoops, 2.3 oz	260	3	40
Met Max, mix, 2 scoops, 2.2 oz	230	2.5	11
MLO Mus-L Blast, Choc., 4 scoops	570	3.5	112
Monster Energy: 16 fl.oz can	180	0	44
18.6 fl.oz (550ml) Can	205	0	50
Lo-Carb, 16 fl.oz	20	0	5
M-80, 16 fl.oz	180	0	46
Mixxd (with Juice), 16 fl.oz	220	0	54
MRM: Low Carb Protein, 1 scoop	120	2.5	2
Iso-holic, 1 scoop, 1 oz	115	1.5	2
Metabolic Whey, 1 scoop, 1 oz	115	2	2
Muscle Milk *(Cytosport)*:			
Powders: Regular, 2 scoops, 2.5 oz	300	12	16
Light, 2 scoops, 1.75 oz	195	6	11
Naturals, 2 scoops, 2.65 oz	350	18	12
Ready To Drink ~ See Page 48			
Muscle Tech: Meso-Tech Comp. 1 pkt	275	3	31
Mass Tech Weight Gain, 5 scoops	870	4	168
Nitro Tech Hard Core, RTD, 15 fl.oz	195	1	6
Myoplex: Original Shake, 17 fl.oz	300	7	19
Carb Control, 11 fl.oz	150	3.5	5
Deluxe Powder, 1 packet, 3.4 oz	330	3	29
Lite, 11 fl.oz	170	2	20
Powder· Original Choc. 1 pkt	300	6	22
Lite, 1 packet, 1.9 oz	180	7	24
Naturade:			
Powders: 100% Whey, Chocolate, 1 oz	110	1	11
100% Soy Natural, ⅓ cup	110	1	0
Nature's Best:			
Isopure: Original, 20 fl.oz	260	0	25
Endurance, 20 fl.oz	320	0	60
Zero Carb, 20 fl.oz	160	0	0
Carbo Power, 16 fl.oz	400	0	100
No Fear: 16 fl.oz	260	0	72
Sugar Free, 16 fl.oz	20	0	2
Noni: Tahitian/Pacific, 2 Tbsp	10	0	3
Liquid Hawaiian/Tahiti, 1 Tbsp	30	0	8
NOS: All flavors	220	0	54
Sugar Free, 16 fl.oz can	15	0	2
Nutrament *(Nestle),* 12 fl.oz	360	10	52
Nutrilite			
Protein Shakes, 11.5 fl.oz	170	6	6
Sports Drinks, Regular, 16 fl.oz	120	0	28
Whey Protein, Chocolate, 1.27 oz pkg	130	2	5
Odwalla Serious Energy, 8 fl.oz	160	0	39

Energy/Protein Drinks (Cont)

	C	F	Cb
Optifast 800:			
Ready To Drink Shakes, 8 oz	160	3	20
Powder 800 Formula, 1 pkg	160	3	20
High Protein Powder, 1 pkg	200	6	10
Optimum Nutr.: 100% Whey, 1 oz	120	1	3
100% Oats & Whey, 1 scoop, 1.85 oz	200	1.5	22
100% Soy Protein, 1.1 oz Scoop	120	1.5	1
Piranha Energy (EAS), 8.4 oz	140	0	35
PowerAde			
Regular: 12 fl.oz bottle	85	0	23
20 fl.oz bottle	125	0	35
PowerAde Zero	5	0	0
PowerBar			
Endurance, 1 scoop, 0.7 oz	70	0	17
Power Gel, average, 1.5 oz package	110	0	27
Pro-Cal 100 (R-Kane), 1 packet	100	1.5	7
Propel Enhanced Water,			
all flavors, 20 fl.oz	25	0	5
Red Bull Energy, 8.4 fl.oz	110	0	28
12 fl.oz can	160	0	40
Sugar-Free, 8.4 fl.oz	10	0	3
Shots, 2 fl.oz	25	0	6
Sugar Free, 2 fl.oz	2	0	0
Redline Energy, 8 fl.oz	0	0	0
Resource (Nestle): Breeze, 8 fl.oz	250	0	54
Diabetishield, 8 fl.oz	150	0	30
Health Shake: 4 fl.oz	200	4	35
No Added Sugar, 4 oz	200	9	22
Shake Plus, 8 fl.oz	480	16	69
Shake, Thickened, 6 fl.oz	270	6	45
Revenge: Sport (Champ. Nutr.), 0.9 oz	90	0	23
Pro-Score 100, Chocolate, 1.4 oz	150	2	3
Revival Soy Mix: Plain Soy, 1 pkg	100	1.5	2
Chocolate Day Dream, 1 package	240	2.5	36
Other varieties, average, 1 package	225	2	33
Rhino's Energy Drink, 100ml	50	0	11
Rip It Energy Fuel, Citrus X, 16 fl.oz	260	0	66
Rockstar:			
Energy Drink: 16 fl.oz	280	0	62
Sugar Free, 16 fl.oz	20	0	0
Punched, 16 fl.oz	260	0	62
Rush Energy: Regular, 8 fl.oz	140	0	31
Lite, 8 fl.oz	0	0	0
Slim-Fast			
Shake (Ready To Drink):			
Cappuccino, 11 fl.oz	190	6	25
High Protein, 11 fl.oz	190	5	24
Lower Carb Diet, average	185	9	6
Powder Shake Mix: Average, 0.9 oz	110	3	18
With 8 fl.oz fat-free milk	200	5	30

	C	F	Cb
Snapple: LYTe Water			
Av. all flavors, 8 fl.oz	0	0	0
SoBe: Per Can/Bottle			
Energize, Citrus Energy, 20 fl.oz	270	0	67
Lifewater: All flavors, 20 fl.oz	100	0	42
O-Cal, all flavours	0	0	6
Lizard Fuel, 20 fl.oz	300	0	75
Power, 20 fl.oz	250	0	63
Tsunami, 20 fl.oz	250	0	63
Vita Boom: Per 20 fl.oz			
Cranberry Grapefruit	260	0	66
Orange-Carrot	220	0	57
Spiru-Tein: Powder, average, 1.2 oz	100	0	10
Starbucks:			
Doubleshot Energy & Coffee , 15 fl.oz	205	3	34
Steaz: Energy, 12 fl.oz	130	0	34
Diet Berry Energy, 12 fl.oz	60	0	14
The Sports Club/LA:			
PTS Protein Powder,			
Choc; Mocha; Van., 2 scoops, 1.4 oz	130	4	7
Trader Joe's,			
Enhanced Water, 33.8 fl.oz	0	0	0
Twin Lab:			
Endurance Fuel, 1 sc., 1.1 oz	110	0	20
Energy Fuel, 250ml can	0	0	0
Vault: Citrus; Red, 20 fl.oz	290	0	78
Vault Zero, 8 fl.oz	0	0	0
Venom Energy: Average, 16 fl.oz	250	0	58
Low Carb, 16 fl.oz	50	0	8
Verve Energy, 8.3 fl.oz can	70	0	18
Sugar Free	5	0	1
Vitamin Water ~ See Glaceau			
Weider (Powders)			
Creatine ATP, ½ cup, 1.7 oz	210	0	37
Mega Mass 4000, 1½ cups, average	570	3.5	105
Muscle Builder, 1½ oz	170	1	22
Pure Pro Shake: Chocolate, 11.5 fl.oz	170	0.5	7
Vanilla, 11.5 fl.oz	160	0	6
Ultra Whey Pro, ⅓ cup, 1 oz	110	1.5	6
Weight Gainer, 4 scoops, 3.4 oz	380	2	71
Worldwide: Carbo Rush, 20 fl.oz	265	0	68
Pure Protein Shakes:			
35g Protein, 11 fl.oz	160	1	2
XS (Quixtar), Energy Drink, 8.4 fl.oz	10	0	1
Zico, Coconut Water, all flav., 11 fl.oz	60	0	13
Zola Acai:			
Original Juice, 12 fl.oz	185	2	44
Energy Smoothie, 12 fl.oz	185	1.5	42
Wellness Shot, 1 fl.oz	20	1	4

Quick Guide | C F Cb

Orange Juice

Average ~ Fresh or Sweetened:

	C	F	Cb
½ Cup, 4 fl.oz	55	0	13
Small Glass, 6 fl.oz	85	0	19
Regular Glass, 8 fl.oz	110	0.5	26
8¾ fl.oz Box	120	0.5	28
10 fl.oz Bottle	140	0.5	32
11½ fl.oz Can	160	0.5	37
16 fl.oz Bottle	225	1	52
20 fl.oz Bottle	280	1	64
64 fl.oz, ½ Gallon	895	4	206

Juices ~ Generic

Average All Brands: Per 8 fl.oz Unless Indicated

	C	F	Cb
Aloe Vera Juice, unsweetened, 2 oz	10	0	0
Apple Juice: 8 fl.oz	120	0	29
10 fl.oz Bottle	145	0.5	36
16 fl.oz	235	0.5	58
Carrot Juice: Fresh, 6 fl.oz	35	0	8
Sweetened, 6 fl.oz	75	0	17
Cranberry Juice, Cocktail/Blend	140	0	34
Fruit Blends, average, 8 fl.oz	110	0	27
Fruit Nectars, average, 8 fl.oz	140	0	36
Grape Juice, 8 fl.oz	155	0	38
Grapefruit Juice, 8 fl.oz	95	0	22
Lemon/Lime Juice: 1 Tbsp	3	0	1
1 cup, 8 fl.oz	50	0.5	16
Concentrate, 1 tsp	0	0	0
Noni Juice: Tahitian, 2 Tbsp, 1 fl.oz	5	0	1
Tahiti Traders, 1 fl.oz	20	0	5
Passion Fruit Juice (Fresh):			
Purple, 1 cup, 8 fl.oz	125	0	34
Yellow, 1 cup, 8 fl.oz	80	1.5	14
Papaya/Peach Nectar, av., 8 fl.oz	140	0	36
Pear Nectar, 8 fl.oz	150	0	40
Pineapple Juice, 8 fl.oz	130	0	32
Pomegranate Juice, 8 fl.oz	160	0	40
Prune Juice, 8 fl.oz	180	0	45
Strawb./Raspberry Juice, 8 fl.oz	100	0	23
Tangerine Juice, 8 fl.oz	105	0.5	25
Tomato Juice, 8 fl.oz	40	0	10
Vegetable Juice, 8 fl.oz	45	0	11
Wheat Grass Juice: 1 fl.oz 'Shot'	5	0	1
2 fl.oz 'Shot'	15	0	2

Quick Guide | C F Cb

Fruit Smoothies (Jamba Juice; Smoothie King)

Average All Brands

	C	F	Cb
Fruit Only: 8 fl.oz	115	0.5	29
12 fl.oz	175	1	43
16 fl.oz	230	1	58
24 fl.oz	350	1	78
Fruit + Non-Fat Milk/Soy:			
12 fl.oz	135	0	29
16 fl.oz	155	0	37
24 fl.oz	265	1	59
Fruit + Non-Fat Frozen Yogurt/Sherbet:			
12 fl.oz	200	0	47
16 fl.oz	265	0	63
24 fl.oz	395	0	95

Juice Brands | C F Cb

Per 8 fl.oz Unless Indicated

	C	F	Cb
Apple & Eve			
Naturally Cranberry	130	0	32
Cranberry Grape	140	0	34
Fruitables, average all flavors, 6.75 fl.oz	70	0	16
Bolthouse			
100% Juices: Carrot	70	0	14
Clementine	110	0	29
Fruit Smoothies: Per 15.2 fl.oz Bottle			
Berry Boost	210	0	57
Blue Goodness	340	0	85
C-Boost	285	0	68
Green Goodness	265	0	63
Strawberry Banana	230	0	55
Bon Dia: Per 11.5 fl.oz Bottle			
Acai: With Blueberry	200	0	47
With Manosteen	185	0	43
With Pomegranate	230	0	55
Acai Energy, average	155	0	43
Bossa Nova: Per 8 fl.oz Bottle			
Acai Juice, Original	95	0	23
Acerola/Goji/Mangostein, average	85	0	21
Bright & Early (Minute Maid)			
Orange Juice (Chilled/Frozen)	110	0	29
Campbell's			
Tomato Juice: 5.5 fl.oz can	30	0	7
8 fl.oz	50	0	10
Capri Sun			
Juice Drink, 25% Less Sugar: Per 6.75 fl.oz Pouch			
Coastal Cooler; Mountain Cooler	70	0	19
100% Juice, average, 6.75 fl.oz	100	0	24

Juice Brands (Cont)   C   F   Cb

Per 8 fl.oz Unless Indicated

Chiquita Smoothies:

	C	F	Cb
Average all flavors,			
4 oz concentrate (8 oz reconst'd)	120	0	28
12 oz Can (concentrate)	360	0	84

Clamato

	C	F	Cb
Tomato Cocktail, average	50	0	11

Crystal Geyser

Juice Squeeze: Per Bottle (12 fl.oz)

	C	F	Cb
Blackberry Pomegranate	170	0	43
Ruby Grapefruit	150	0	36
Average other flavors	140	0	32

Dannon

	C	F	Cb
Frusion Smoothie, av., 7 fl.oz	180	2.5	35
Light & Fit, 7 fl.oz bottle	70	0	14

Dole

Chilled, 100%: Per 8 fl.oz

	C	F	Cb
Orange Peach Mango	120	0	29
Pina Colada	120	0	29
Pineapple Juice	130	0	30
Pineapple-Orange Banana	120	0	30
Strawberry Kiwi	120	0	31
Average other flavors	120	0	29

Frozen Concentrates 100%:

	C	F	Cb
Average all flavors, ¼ cup	125	0	31

Five Alive *(Minute Maid):*

	C	F	Cb
Frozen Concentrate, prepared, 8 fl.oz	110	0	29

Florida's Natural

	C	F	Cb
Orange	110	0	26
Ruby Red Grapefruit	90	0	22

Frützzo: *Per 12 fl.oz Bottle*

(No Added Sugar)

	C	F	Cb
Pomegranate 100%	210	0	52
With Acai; Cherry	210	0	51
With Blueberry; Raspberry	195	0	48
Yumberry 100%			
Natural	150	0	33
Organic	120	0	25
with Blueberry; Pomegranate	165	0	39

Fuze: *Per 16 fl.oz*

	C	F	Cb
Refresh, average all flavors	180	0	48
Slenderize, av. all flavors	15	0	3
Vitalize, all flavors	200	0	50

Goya: C   F   Cb

100% Natural:

	C	F	Cb
Av. all flavors, 16 fl.oz	200	0	50

5% Juice: *Per 12 fl.oz*

	C	F	Cb
Guanabana	230	0	57
Passion & Pineapple	220	0	55
Mango Nectar, 12 fl.oz	230	0	56

Hansen's

Juice Slam: Per 6.75 fl.oz Box

	C	F	Cb
Awesome Apple	90	0	23
Other flavors	120	0	29
Organic, 1 Pouch	100	0	24
Junior Juice, 4.23 oz box	60	0	15

Natural (64 fl.oz Bottles): *Per 8 fl.oz*

	C	F	Cb
Apple, Strawberry	120	0	28
Black Grape, Pomegranate Cocktail	160	0	39
White Grape	140	0	36
Organic Blends, average	110	0	27
Fruit Smoothies, average, 12 fl.oz	175	0	44

Hawaii's Own

Frozen Concentrate: *Per 8 fl.oz, Prepared*

	C	F	Cb
10% Juice, average all varieties	110	0	28

Hi-C Juice Drinks:

	C	F	Cb
6.75 fl.oz box, average	90	0	26
Blast, 6.75 fl.oz pouch	100	0	26
Hood: Apple, 8 fl.oz	120	0	31
Fruit Punch; Orange	120	0	30

Jamba Juice: *See Fast-Foods Section*

Juicy Juice (Nestle): *Per 6.75 fl.oz Box*

	C	F	Cb
Grape	100	0	25
Average other flavors	100	0	24
4.23 fl.oz box, average	60	0	15

Kerns All Nectars

Nectars: Per 11.5 fl.oz Can

	C	F	Cb
Pear	220	0	54
Pineapple Coconut	280	8	53
Average other flavors	215	0	52

Kool Aid

	C	F	Cb
Jammers, 6.75 oz, average	90	0	24
Jammers 10	10	0	2

Kroger/Ralph's Smoothies:

	C	F	Cb
Active Lifestyle (Ralph's), average	130	0	25
Regular, average all flavors	200	2.5	38

L & A: *Per 8 fl.oz*

	C	F	Cb
All Cherry	180	0	45
All Prune Juice	180	0	41
Mixed Berry	120	0	30

Juice Brands (Cont)

	C	F	Cb
Lakewood Organic: *Per 8 fl.oz*			
Acai Amazon Berry	125	0	28
Banana Strawberry	115	0	28
Blueberry Blend	120	0	30
Cranberry Lemonade	80	0	20
Fruit Garden: Summer/Green, average	100	0	20
Blue/Purple/Red Pomegr., average	110	0	24
Goji	90	0	20
Lemonade	85	0	21
Pomegranate Blend	125	0	32
Pure: Apple	105	0	26
Blueberry	90	0	24
Carrot	90	0	20
Pink Grapefruit	90	0	22
Prune	170	0	42
Super Veggie	55	0	12
Light: Lemonade	40	0	15
Other flavors, average	60	0	21
(Note: Carbs include Erythritol natural sweetener)			
Langers: *Per 8 fl.oz*			
100% Juice (No Sugar Added):			
All Pomegranate	140	0	34
Apple Cider	120	0	28
Apple Juice	120	0	28
Mixed Berry	120	0	30
Pineapple Coconut	140	3	28
Red/White Grape Juice	160	0	40
Diet Low-Carb (25-50% Juice):			
Apple Juice Cocktail	60	0	14
Cranberry	30	0	8
Pomegranate	40	0	9
Juice Cocktails (27% Juice)			
Blueberry Cranberry	135	0	34
Cranberry Berry	135	0	34
Cranberry Grape	165	0	41
Cranberry Raspberry	150	0	36
Pomegranate	140	0	34
Pomegranate Blueberry/Cranberry	140	0	34
Strawberry Peach (20% Juice)	120	0	30
White Cranberry	120	0	28
White Cran-Raspberry	120	0	28

	C	F	Cb
Minute Maid			
Apple Juice, 15.2 fl.oz bottle	210	0	52
Cranberry, 15.2 fl oz bottle	285	0	74
Orange Juice: 100%, 8 fl.oz	110	0	27
15.2 fl.oz bottle	210	0	51
Light, 42%, 8 fl.oz	50	0	13
Fruit Punch, 6.75 fl.oz	100	0	24
Pineapple Orange, Apple, 8 fl.oz	120	0	29
Kids+Orange Juice, 6.75 fl.oz	100	0	23
Enhanced: *Per 8 fl.oz*			
Pomegranate Blueberry	120	0.5	31
Pomegranate Lemonade	110	0	31
Boxed Juices, average, 6.75 fl.oz	100	0	22
Soft Frozen: Limeade, 3 fl.oz	70	0	19
MonaVie Acai Blends			
Original; Active, 4 fl.oz	120	2	20
Mott's			
100% Apple Juice: *Per 8 fl.oz*			
Original	120	0	29
Natural	110	0	27
100% Juice Singles: *Per 14 fl.oz*			
Apple	200	0	48
Fruit Punch	230	0	16
Sunkist Orange Sensation	210	0	12
Veggie Blend	90	1	15
100% Juice Boxes: Average all flavors			
6.75 fl.oz box	100	0	24
4.23 fl.oz box	60	0	15
Mott's Plus Light,			
Apple, 8 fl.oz	130	0	15
Mott's Plus for Kids, average, 8 fl.oz	125	0	31
Mott's For Tots (47-54% Juice),			
All flavors, 6.75 fl.oz box	50	0	13
Naked Juice: *Per 8 fl.oz Unless Indicated*			
Antioxidants:			
Cherry Pomegranate Power	140	0	34
Pomegranate	150	0	37
Bare Breeze, av. all flavors	130	0	31
Probiotics, Tropical Mango, 10 fl.oz	180	0	43
Protein Zone: Mango	220	1	35
P'apple, Coconut & Banana	220	2	34
Pure Juice (100%): O-J	110	0	27
Chai Spiced Cider	120	0	30
Well Being: Berry Blast	130	0	29
Black & Blueberry	130	0	31
Mighty Mango	150	0	36
Strawberry Banana	120	0	29
Tropical	130	0	31

Juice Brands (Cont)

	C	F	Cb
Naked Juice (Cont)			
Superfood Smoothies: *Per 15.2 fl.oz*			
Acai Machine	305	5	58
Berry Veggie Machine	250	0.5	70
Blue Machine	320	0	76
Gold/Green Machine, av.	265	0	63
Power C	230	0	55
Red Machine	320	8	58
Nantucket Nectars			
Juice Cocktails: *Per 17.5 fl.oz Bottle*			
Big Cranberry	285	0	70
Carrot Orange Mango	260	0	60
Grapeade	305	0	72
Other varieties, average	260	0	65
100% Juice: *Per 17.5 fl.oz Bottle*			
Peach Orange	285	0	70
Pineapple Orange Banana	305	0	74
Pomegranate Cherry	265	0	63
Premium Orange Juice	240	0	57
Pressed Apple	260	0	65
Nectar Lemonade, 17.5 fl.oz	240	0	61
Newman's Own			
Lemonade, Regular; Pink; 8 fl.oz	110	0	27
Fruit Juice Cocktail: Gorilla Grape	140	0	34
Orange Mango Tango	130	0	33
Razzma Tazz Raspberry	120	0	28
Northland			
100% Juice: *Per 8 fl.oz*			
Cranberry; Blackberry; Raspberry	140	0	34
Cranberry Grape	140	0	36
Ocean Spray: *Per 8 fl.oz*			
Juice Cocktails:			
Cranberry Juice Cocktail	120	0	30
With Calcium	130	0	31
Ruby Tangerine	120	0	31
Ruby Red Grapefruit	110	0	28
100% Juice Blends:			
Cranberry & Concord Grape	150	0	37
Cranberry Blueberry	140	0	36
Cranberry Blends	140	0	35
Juice Drinks:			
CranApple	130	0	32
CranGrape	120	0	31
CranRaspberry/Strawberry	110	0	27
Light Juice Drinks, all flav.	40	0	10
Diet Juice Drinks:			
Cranberry Spray	5	0	2
Cranberry Grape Spray	5	0	2

	C	F	Cb
Odwalla *Per 15.2 fl.oz Bottle*			
Carrot Juice	140	0	30
Mo'Beta	300	0	74
PomaGrand Pomegranate	320	0	80
Protein Monster	300	6	35
Strawberry Lemonade	220	0	56
Super Food	250	1	57
Super Protein Original	360	1	67
Smoothies:			
Citrus C Monster	280	0	68
Mango Tango	300	2	68
Strawberry Banana	250	0	58
Orange Julius			
Originals, Orange:			
Small, 16 fl.oz	130	0.5	33
Medium, 20 fl.oz	160	0.5	41
Large, 32 fl.oz	260	1	65
Smoothies: *See Fast-Foods Section*			
Pom Wonderful			
100% Juice: *Per 8 fl.oz*			
Pomegranate: Blueberry	160	0	40
Cherry	150	0	38
Kiwi	150	0	36
Mango	140	0	35
Nectarine	130	0	31
R.W. Knudsen: *Per 8 fl.oz*			
Natural Juices: 100% Apple	120	0	30
Cranberry Raspberry	130	0	32
Grape	150	0	37
Hibiscus Cooler	100	0	25
Kiwi Strawberry	120	0	29
Mango Peach	130	0	31
Razzleberry	120	0	30
Rio Red Grapefruit	140	0	35
Other varieties, average	120	0	30
Pure Juice: Just Blackcurrant	100	0	15
Just Black Cherry	160	0	36
Just Blueberry	100	0	24
Simply Nutritious: Mega C	140	0	34
Average other varieties	125	0	30
Sparkling Essence: *Per 10.5 fl.oz*			
Average all varieties	0	0	0
Spritzers, 100% Juice: *Per 12 fl.oz Bottles*			
Black Cherry	180	0	46
Mango	170	0	42
Red Raspberry; Tangerine	200	0	47
Very Veggie, Orig, 8 fl.oz	50	0	11

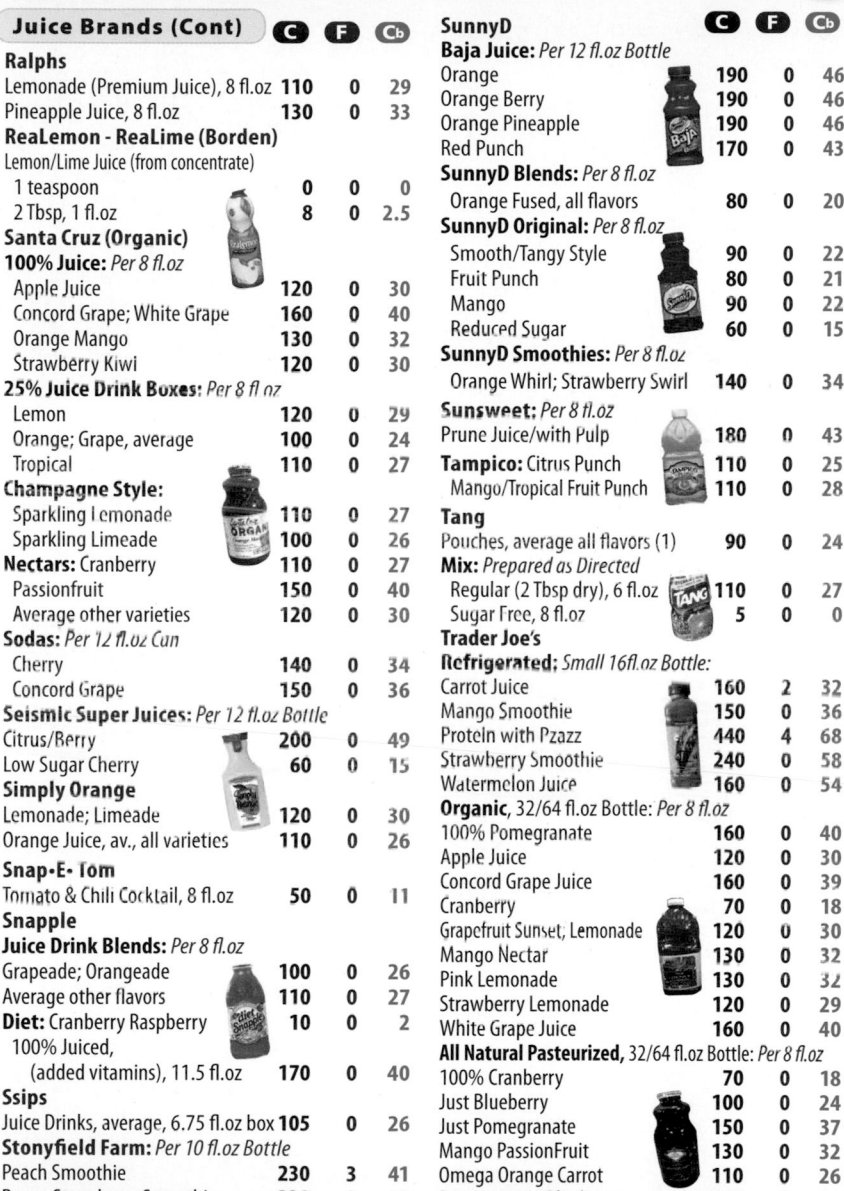

Juice Brands (Cont) — C F Cb

Ralphs

	C	F	Cb
Lemonade (Premium Juice), 8 fl.oz	110	0	29
Pineapple Juice, 8 fl.oz	130	0	33

ReaLemon - ReaLime (Borden)
Lemon/Lime Juice (from concentrate)

	C	F	Cb
1 teaspoon	0	0	0
2 Tbsp, 1 fl.oz	8	0	2.5

Santa Cruz (Organic)
100% Juice: Per 8 fl.oz

	C	F	Cb
Apple Juice	120	0	30
Concord Grape; White Grape	160	0	40
Orange Mango	130	0	32
Strawberry Kiwi	120	0	30

25% Juice Drink Boxes: Per 8 fl.oz

	C	F	Cb
Lemon	120	0	29
Orange; Grape, average	100	0	24
Tropical	110	0	27

Champagne Style:

	C	F	Cb
Sparkling Lemonade	110	0	27
Sparkling Limeade	100	0	26

Nectars: Cranberry

	C	F	Cb
Cranberry	110	0	27
Passionfruit	150	0	40
Average other varieties	120	0	30

Sodas: Per 12 fl.oz Can

	C	F	Cb
Cherry	140	0	34
Concord Grape	150	0	36

Seismic Super Juices: Per 12 fl.oz Bottle

	C	F	Cb
Citrus/Berry	200	0	49
Low Sugar Cherry	60	0	15

Simply Orange

	C	F	Cb
Lemonade; Limeade	120	0	30
Orange Juice, av., all varieties	110	0	26

Snap-E-Tom

	C	F	Cb
Tomato & Chili Cocktail, 8 fl.oz	50	0	11

Snapple
Juice Drink Blends: Per 8 fl.oz

	C	F	Cb
Grapeade; Orangeade	100	0	26
Average other flavors	110	0	27
Diet: Cranberry Raspberry	10	0	2
100% Juiced, (added vitamins), 11.5 fl.oz	170	0	40

Ssips

	C	F	Cb
Juice Drinks, average, 6.75 fl.oz box	105	0	26

Stonyfield Farm: Per 10 fl.oz Bottle

	C	F	Cb
Peach Smoothie	230	3	41
Berry; Strawberry Smoothie	230	3	39

SunnyD — C F Cb

Baja Juice: Per 12 fl.oz Bottle

	C	F	Cb
Orange	190	0	46
Orange Berry	190	0	46
Orange Pineapple	190	0	46
Red Punch	170	0	43

SunnyD Blends: Per 8 fl.oz

	C	F	Cb
Orange Fused, all flavors	80	0	20

SunnyD Original: Per 8 fl.oz

	C	F	Cb
Smooth/Tangy Style	90	0	22
Fruit Punch	80	0	21
Mango	90	0	22
Reduced Sugar	60	0	15

SunnyD Smoothies: Per 8 fl.oz

	C	F	Cb
Orange Whirl; Strawberry Swirl	140	0	34

Sunsweet: Per 8 fl.oz

	C	F	Cb
Prune Juice/with Pulp	180	0	43

Tampico: Citrus Punch

	C	F	Cb
Citrus Punch	110	0	25
Mango/Tropical Fruit Punch	110	0	28

Tang

	C	F	Cb
Pouches, average all flavors (1)	90	0	24

Mix: Prepared as Directed

	C	F	Cb
Regular (2 Tbsp dry), 6 fl.oz	110	0	27
Sugar Free, 8 fl.oz	5	0	0

Trader Joe's
Refrigerated: Small 16 fl.oz Bottle:

	C	F	Cb
Carrot Juice	160	2	32
Mango Smoothie	150	0	36
Protein with Pzazz	440	4	68
Strawberry Smoothie	240	0	58
Watermelon Juice	160	0	54

Organic, 32/64 fl.oz Bottle: Per 8 fl.oz

	C	F	Cb
100% Pomegranate	160	0	40
Apple Juice	120	0	30
Concord Grape Juice	160	0	39
Cranberry	70	0	18
Grapefruit Sunset; Lemonade	120	0	30
Mango Nectar	130	0	32
Pink Lemonade	130	0	32
Strawberry Lemonade	120	0	29
White Grape Juice	160	0	40

All Natural Pasteurized, 32/64 fl.oz Bottle: Per 8 fl.oz

	C	F	Cb
100% Cranberry	70	0	18
Just Blueberry	100	0	24
Just Pomegranate	150	0	37
Mango PassionFruit	130	0	32
Omega Orange Carrot	110	0	26
Pomegranate Blueberry	140	0	34

Juice Brands (Cont)   C   F   Cb

Per 8 fl.oz Unless Indicated

	C	F	Cb
Trader Joe's (Cont)			
Joe's Kids: *Per 6.75 oz Box*			
100% Juice: Apple	90	0	23
Apple Grape	100	0	24
White Apple	120	0	30
10% Juice, Lemonade	90	0	22
Sparkling Juices, 750ml/25.4 fl.oz Bottle: *Per 8 fl.oz*			
Blueberry	120	0	30
Cranberry	140	0	35
Pomegranate	130	0	31
Tree Top			
100% Juice From Concentrates			
Apple Berry/Grape	120	0	31
Apple Pear, 6.75 fl.oz	100	0	25
Apple/Spiced Cider	120	0	29
Kiwi Strawberry, 10 fl.oz	130	0	32
Mango Peach, 10 fl.oz	160	0	39
Ochango, 10 fl.oz	170	0	42
Orange Passionfruit	110	0	26
Tropical	120	0	29
100% Juice Fresh Pressed			
3 Apple Blend	120	0	30
Fiber Rich:			
Apple	140	0	35
Apple Apricot/Orange Banana	160	0	38
Trim			
Average all flavors, 8 fl.oz	60	0	16
Tropicana			
Coastal Groves Lemonade, av. all flav	120	0	30
Pure Premium Orange Juice	110	0	26
Pure: Indian River Grapefruit	110	0	25
Valencia without Pulp	120	0	27
Twisters: Average, 8 fl.oz	120	0	29
20 fl.oz bottle	300	0	74
V8® Juices & Drinks			
V8 100% Vegetable Juice:			
5.5 fl.oz can	35	0	7
8 fl.oz cup	50	0	10
11.5 fl.oz can	70	0	14
12 fl.oz bottle	75	0	15
V8 Spicy Hot, 12 fl.oz	70	0	14
V8 Splash, average, 8 fl.oz	70	0	19
V8 Splash Smoothies: Strawberry	90	0	20
Tropical Colada, 8 fl.oz	100	0	21
Diet V8 Splash, all flavors, 8 fl.oz	10	0	3
Fusion: All flavors, 8 fl.oz	110	0	27
12 fl.oz bottle	160	0	40

Per 8 fl.oz Unless Indicated

	C	F	Cb
Veryfine			
Apple Juice (100%)	110	0	27
Orange Juice (100%)	120	0	28
Walnut Acres: *Per 8 fl.oz*			
Organic: Apple	110	0	29
Apricot; Raspberry	130	0	32
Cherry	140	0	34
Cranberry	110	0	26
Incredible Vegetable	50	0	12
Mango Nectar	120	0	29
Welch's: *Per 8 fl.oz*			
100% Grape: Red Grape	170	0	43
100% Juice: White Grape Cherry	140	0	35
White Grape Peach	160	0	39
Cocktails (Refrigerated, 64 fl.oz Ctn):			
Guava Pineapple	140	0	36
Mango Twist	150	0	38
Strawberry Breeze	130	0	33
Light Juice (52 fl.oz Bottle),			
Grape, 8 fl.oz	50	0	13
Sparkling Juice Cocktail, 8 fl.oz	160	0	40
Concentrates (100% Juice),			
All flavors, ¼ cup, 2 fl.oz	160	0	41
Zola: *Per 12 fl.oz Bottle*			
Acai: Original	185	2	44
With Blueberry Juice	145	2	40
Smoothies: Superfood	150	0	34
Energy; Immunity, average	180	0	40

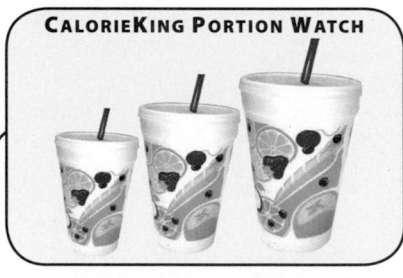

CALORIEKING PORTION WATCH

ORANGE JUICE	C	Cb
8 fl.oz	110	26
16 fl.oz	220	52
24 fl.oz	330	78
32 fl.oz	440	104

Quick Guide   **C** **F** **Cb**

Cow's Milk ~ *Average All Brands*

Whole (3.25% fat):

	C	F	Cb
2 Tbsp, 1 fl.oz	20	1	1.5
1 Cup, 8 fl.oz	150	8	12
1 Large Glass, 12 fl.oz	220	12	17
1 Pint, 16 fl.oz	295	16	22
1 Quart, 946 ml	590	32	44

Reduced-Fat (2% fat):

	C	F	Cb
2 Tbsp, 1 fl.oz	15	0.5	1.5
1 Cup, 8 fl.oz	120	5	12
1 Large Glass, 12 fl.oz	180	7.5	18
1 Pint, 16 fl.oz	245	10	23
1 Quart, 946 ml	490	20	46

Light/Low-Fat (1% fat):

	C	F	Cb
2 Tbsp, 1 fl.oz	13	0.3	1.5
1 Cup, 8 fl.oz	100	2.5	12
1 Large Glass, 12 fl.oz	150	4	18
1 Pint, 16 fl.oz	205	5	25
1 Quart, 946 ml	410	10	49

Fat Free/Skim:

	C	F	Cb
2 Tbsp, 1 fl.oz	10	0	1.5
1 Cup, 8 fl.oz	90	0.5	13
1 Pint, 16 fl.oz	180	1	26
with Oatrim Fiber (for replacement), 1 cup	85	0	12

Buttermilk: *Average All Brands*

	C	F	Cb
Reduced-Fat (2%), 1 cup	120	5	10
Low-Fat (1%): 1 cup	100	2.5	12

Lactose-Free: *Per 8 fl.oz*

	C	F	Cb
Dairy Ease: Whole	160	9	11
2% Reduced-Fat	130	5	12
Fat-Free	90	0	12
Lactaid 100: Whole	150	8	12
2% Reduced-Fat	130	5	12
1% Low-Fat	110	2.5	13
Fat-Free; Calcium Fort.	80	0	13
Real Goodness: 2% Fat	120	5	7
Fat Free 0%	80	0	7
Smart Balance, FF + Omega-3s & Vit. E	110	1	14

Lower Calorie Dairy Drinks: *Per 8 fl.oz Cup*

Calorie Countdown (Hood):

	C	F	Cb
2% Reduced-Fat	90	5	3
2% Reduced-Fat, Chocolate	90	5	5
Fat-Free	45	0	3

Goat/Sheep Milk, Kefir

Goat's Milk (Meyenberg):

	C	F	Cb
Whole, 1 cup, 8 fl.oz	140	7	11
Light/Low-Fat (1%), 8 fl.oz	100	2.5	11
Evaporated, reconst., 8 fl.oz	150	8	11

Kefir (Cultured Milk): *Per 8 fl.oz*

	C	F	Cb
Lifeway: Greek Style	200	14	12
Green	170	2	25
Lowfat, average all flavors	160	2	25
Original	160	8	15
Nancy's: Plain	110	3	14
Fruit flavors, average	180	2.5	34
Trader Joe's: Plain	110	2.5	8
Strawberry	160	2	21
Sheep's Milk, Whole, 1 cup	265	17	13

Canned & Dried Milk

	C	F	Cb
Condensed: Reg. 2 Tbsp, 1 fl.oz	130	3	23
Low-Fat (*Eagle*), 2 Tbsp	120	1.5	23
Fat-Free (*Eagle*), 2 Tbsp	110	0	24
Evaporated: Whole, 2 Tbsp	40	3	3
Whole, ½ cup	170	10	13
Low-Fat (*Carnation*), 2 Tbsp, 1 oz	25	0.5	3
½ cup, 4 fl.oz	115	2.5	14
Fat-Free, 2 Tbsp, 1 oz	25	0	4
Dried: Whole, ¼ cup, 1 oz	160	9	12
Skim/Non-Fat, ⅓ cup	80	0	12
Made up, 1 cup, 8 fl.oz	80	0	12
Buttermilk (sweet cream), 1 oz	110	2	14
Non-Fat, 1 Tbsp	25	0	3
Malted (*Carnation*), dry, 1 Tbsp	30	0.5	6

Soy/Non-Dairy Drinks ~ *See Page 49*

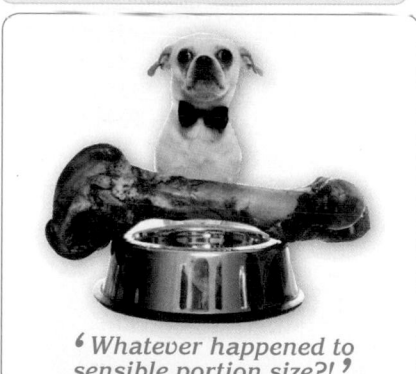

' Whatever happened to sensible portion size?! '

Quick Guide

C F Cb

Chocolate Milk
Average All Brands: Per Cup (8 fl.oz)

	C	F	Cb
Whole Milk (3.3%): 1 cup	210	8	26
1 Pint, 16 fl.oz	415	17	52
Reduced-Fat (2%), 1 cup	190	5	30
1 Pint, 16 fl.oz	380	10	60
Low-Fat (1%), 1 cup	160	2.5	26
1 Pint, 16 fl.oz	315	5	52

Brands ~ Flavored Milk

Ready-To-Drink: Per 8 fl.oz Cup Unless Indicated

	C	F	Cb
Albertson's, Choc Milk	200	2.5	34
Alta Dena: Chocolate, 8 fl.oz	260	9	37
Pint/16 fl.oz	520	18	74
Low-Fat Chocolate, 8 fl.oz	200	3	32
Pint/16 fl.oz	400	6	64
Chug: *Per 12 fl.oz Bottle*			
Chocolate; Cookies 'n' Cream, 12 fl.oz	420	12	68
Vanilla, 12 fl.oz	440	11	75
Hood: Chocolate, 8 fl.oz	230	9	31
Low-Fat (1%), Chocolate	170	3	28
Horizon Organic: Low-Fat Chocolate	170	3	27
Reduced-Fat Vanilla	190	4.5	30
Kroger, Choc Milk, Low-Fat, 1%	180	2.5	33
Land O Lakes			
Grip 'n Go: Choc. (2% red-fat), 12 fl.oz	290	8	43
Strawberry, (1% low fat), 12 fl.oz	260	4	42
Muscle Milk (*Cytosport ~ Hi Protein*):			
17 fl.oz Box: Chocolate	330	16	13
Average other flavors	310	12	16
11 fl.oz Box: Choc./Choc Malt, av	230	11	11
Average other flavors	210	10	9
14 fl.oz Bottle: Chocolate	240	9	14
Average other flavors	220	9	11
Lite: Chocolate	170	4.5	12
Cafe Late; Vanilla, average	160	4.5	11
Nesquik: *Per 16 fl.oz Bottle*			
Chocolate	400	10	65
Fat-Free	320	0	64
Strawberry	400	10	66
Prairie Farms, Choc., 16 fl.oz bottle	440	16	58
Quaker, Milk Chillers, 14 fl.oz bottle	245	9	32
Ralphs, Chocolate, Low-Fat, 8 fl.oz	210	2.5	36
Skinny Cow, Chocolate, Fat-Free	150	0	26

Brands ~ Flavored Milk (Cont)

Ready-To-Drink: Per 8 fl.oz Cup Unless Indicated

	C	F	Cb
Starbucks:			
Vanilla Frappuccino, 13.7 fl.oz	290	4.5	53
Yoo-Hoo:			
Chocolate: 6½ fl.oz box	100	0	23
9 fl.oz bottle	145	1	32
15½ fl.oz bottle	250	2	55
Lite Chocolate, 9 fl.oz bottle	70	1	15
Double Fudge: 9 fl.oz bottle	160	1	34
15½ fl.oz bottle	270	2	64
Strawberry, 15½ fl.oz bottle	250	1	55

Bottle Coffee Drinks ~ See Page 37

Shakes

	C	F	Cb
Arby's:			
Chocolate; Jamocha, 17 fl.oz	620	17	108
Vanilla, 17 fl.oz	540	17	85
Burger King:			
Chocolate:			
Value, 12 fl.oz	340	9	60
Small, 16 fl.oz	440	11	78
Medium, 22 fl.oz	650	16	119
Large, 32 fl.oz	960	23	176
Other flavors ~ *See Page 186*			
Denny's:			
Chocolate; Strawberry, 12 fl.oz	560	26	76
Vanilla, 12 fl.oz	560	26	76
Hardees:			
All flavors, average, 16 fl.oz	700	33	86
McDonalds:			
Average all flavors:			
12 fl.oz cup	430	10	75
16 fl.oz cup	570	13	101
21 fl.oz cup	760	18	132
32 fl.oz cup	1140	26	200

Other Restaurants ~ See Fast-Foods Section

Smoothies

Smoothies:
Made Up Ready-To-Drink
(8 fl. oz Milk/Soy + Fruit): *Per 12 fl.oz*

Average all types:

	C	F	Cb
With Whole Milk	300	8	50
+ Ice Cream, 1 scoop	400	13	62
With Non-Fat Milk	240	0	50

Fruit Smoothies ~ See Page 41
Freshens; Jamba Juice; TCBY: See Fast-Foods

Rice & Cereal Drinks

Per 8 fl.oz Cup	C	F	Cb
Almond Breeze (*Blue Diamond*)			
Regular	60	2.5	8
Chocolate	120	3	22
Vanilla	90	2.5	16
Unsweetened: Original; Vanilla	40	3	2
Chocolate	45	3.5	3
Almond Dream			
Enriched: Original	50	2.5	6
Unsweetened	30	2.5	1
Amazake, Oh So Original	150	0	34
Better Than Milk			
Rice Vegan Mix:			
Original, 2 Tbsp powder, 0.67 oz	100	2.5	16
Vanilla, 2 Tbsp powder, 0.67 oz	80	2	8
Cacique,			
Horchata Rice Drink	160	3.5	31
Don Jose:			
Horchata Rice Drink	140	4	25
Cereal Match	100	3	17
EdenBlend, Rice & Soy	120	3	18
Kern's, Horchata	140	3	26
Pacific			
Rice Drinks:			
Low-Fat Plain/Vanilla	130	2	27
Organic Oat: Original	130	2.5	24
Vanilla	130	2.5	25
Nut Drinks: Hazelnut, Original	110	3.5	18
Almond: Original, Low-Fat	60	2.5	8
Vanilla, Low-Fat	70	2.5	11
Organic: Original	60	2.5	8
Chocolate, Single Serve	100	3	19
Vanilla, Single Serve	70	2.5	11
Rice Dream			
Original/Enriched	120	2.5	23
Carob	150	2.5	30
Heartwise: Original	130	2	27
Vanilla	140	2	30
Horchata	160	2.5	32
Vanilla; Vanilla, Enriched	130	2.5	27
Supreme: Chocolate Chai	160	3	35
Vanilla Hazelnut	140	2.5	29
Trader Joe's:			
Rice Drinks:			
Original, Organic	120	2.5	23
Vanilla	130	2.5	26
WestSoy: Plain Rice	110	2.5	20
Vanilla Rice	110	2.5	20

Note: Rice/Oat/Nut drinks are very low in protein. Unless enriched with protein (and calcium), they are not suitable for infants as a substitute for milk or calcium-enriched soy drinks.

Soy Milk ~ Ready-To-Drink

Per 8 fl.oz Cup	C	F	Cb
365 Organic (*Whole Foods*):			
Original, unsweetened	70	4	4
Chocolate	140	3.5	22
Vanilla	90	3.5	10
Light: Original	70	1.5	9
Vanilla	70	1.5	10
Bolthouse Farms:			
Perfectly Protein:			
Mocha Cappuccino	180	2.5	29
Purely Chocolate	160	2.5	27
EdenBlend, Organic	120	3	18
Edensoy: Original	140	5	14
Carob; Chocolate, average	175	4	29
Vanilla	150	3	24
Light: Original	100	2	15
Vanilla	110	1	22
Extra: Original	130	4	13
Vanilla	150	3	23
8th Continent:			
Original	80	2.5	7
Chocolate	140	3	22
Vanilla	100	3	11
Fat-Free: Original	60	0	8
Vanilla	70	0	11
Light: Original	50	2	2
Chocolate	90	1.5	12
Kidz Dream			
Smoothies: Berry Blast	100	2	17
Orange Cream	120	2	21
Lifeway			
Kefir, Low-Fat, Peach/Strawberry	160	2	25
O Organics (*Safeway*):			
Plain	90	3.5	8
Chocolate	150	4	23
Vanilla Soy	100	3	9
Odwalla:			
Super Protein: Originalq	190	1	35
Chocolate	170	3.5	24
Vanilla Al'Mondo	190	6	25
Protein Monster, Vanilla	200	3.5	24
Pacific			
Enriched: Plain, Low-Fat	80	3	9
Vanilla, Low-Fat	110	2.5	15
Organic, Original, Unsweetened	90	4.5	4
Ultra (*Extra Protein/Calcium*): Plain	120	4	11
Vanilla	130	4	14

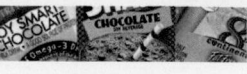

Soy Milk ~ Ready-To-Drink

Per 8 fl.oz Cup	C	F	Cb
Silk			
Original	100	4	8
Chocolate	150	3	25
Heart Health	80	1.5	10
Plus DHA Omega-3	110	5	8
Unsweetened	80	4	4
Vanilla	100	3.5	10
Very Vanilla	130	4	19
Light: Original	70	2	8
Chocolate	90	1.5	15
Vanilla	80	2	10
Slim-Fast (Soy-Based) ~ See Page 40			
So Nice:			
Fortified: Original	80	3	7
Chocolate	150	3	24
Natural	80	4	3
Strawberry	110	3	15
Omega 3, Vanilla	120	4	15
Prebiotic, Original	120	3	18
Soy Dream			
Shelf Stable Enriched: Original	100	4	8
Chocolate	150	4	21
Classic Vanilla	140	4	18
Vanilla	120	4	14
Soy Slender: Plain	60	3	3
Average other flavors	70	3	4
Trader Joe's:			
Soy Milk: Original	110	2	13
Vanilla	100	2	16
Organic: Original	130	3	17
Chocolate	120	3	17
Vanilla	130	3	19
Organic Unsweetened	70	3.5	3
Chocolate Soy Milk, 8 fl.oz box	130	2.5	23
WestSoy			
Lite: Plain	60	2	6
Vanilla	70	2	8
Low-Fat: Plain	90	1.5	14
Vanilla	120	1.5	21
Non-Fat: Plain	70	0	10
Vanilla	80	0	12

Soy Milk ~ Ready-To-Drink (Cont)

Per 8 fl.oz Cup	C	F	Cb
WestSoy (Cont)			
Longevity, Plain	90	3.5	10
Plus: (25% Less Sugar):			
Plain	90	3.5	7
Vanilla	100	3.5	10
Unsweetened:			
Almond; Organic Plain	90	4.5	5
Chocolate; Vanilla	100	4.5	6
Soy Shakes, Chocolate; Vanilla, av.	170	3.5	29

Soy Powder Mix

1 oz (¼ cup) mix makes 8 fl.oz Cup	C	F	Cb
Soy Protein Isolate, 1 oz dry	95	1	0
Better Than Milk:			
Original, 2 Tbsp	70	1	16
Vanilla, 2¾ Tbsp	75	2	15
Light, 2 Tbsp	75	2.5	7
Genisoy (Powder Shakes):			
Per 3 Rounded Tbsp			
Plain; Natural: 1 oz	110	1.5	0
Ultra-XT, 1.3 oz	130	1.5	5
Chocolate: 1.2 oz	130	0.5	16
Ultra-XT, 1.4 oz	150	1	20
Vanilla: 1.2 oz	130	1	17
Ultra-XT, 1.4 oz	150	1	20
Now, Soy, ¼ cup, 0.78 oz	95	4.5	7
Revival Soy Shakes: *Per Packet*			
Plain, Unsweetened	100	1.5	2
Vanilla Pleasure	220	2	31
Average other flavors	230	2	33
Whole Foods			
Choc.with Spirulina, 1 oz	100	1	10
Vanilla with Spirulina, 1 oz	100	0	11

Coconut Milk Drink

	C	F	Cb
So Delicious: *Per 8 fl.oz cup*			
Original	80	5	7
Vanilla	90	5	9
Unsweetened	50	5	1

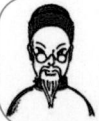

Confucious say:
'Man who eat with one chopstick never have problem with obesity'

Quick Guide

Cola Drinks
Average All Brands
Includes *Coca-Cola* and *Pepsi*

	C	**F**	**Cb**
8 fl.oz Cup/Can	100	0	26
12 fl.oz Can	150	0	39
16 fl.oz Bottle	200	0	52
20 fl.oz Bottle	250	0	65
24 fl.oz (Pepsi)	300	0	84
1-Liter Bottle (34 fl.oz)	400	0	100
2-Liter Bottle (68 fl.oz)	800	0	200

Other Soda Drinks *(Average All Brands)*

	C	F	Cb
Club Soda, 12 fl.oz	0	0	0
Cream Soda, 12 fl.oz	190	0	48
Diet/Low Cal Drinks, 12 fl.oz	5	0	1
Ginger Ale, 12 fl.oz	125	0	31
Lemon Lime, 12 fl.oz	150	0	37
Orange, 12 fl.oz	180	0	45
Pink Lemonade, 12 fl.oz	180	0	45
Root Beer, 12 fl.oz	150	0	39
Tonic Water, 12 fl.oz	125	0	2
Mineral Water: Plain, 12 fl.oz	0	0	0
Sweetened/flavored, 12 fl.oz	150	0	37
With Fruit Juice, 12 fl.oz	120	0	30
Soda Water/Seltzer: Plain/Diet	0	0	0
Sweetened/flavored, 12 fl.oz	155	0	39
With Fruit Juice, 12 fl.oz	160	0	40
Soft Frozen Lemonade, 12 fl.oz	300	0	75

Fountain, Movie Theater & Take-Out

Average All Flavors

	C	F	Cb
Small Cup, 12 fl.oz: No Ice	160	0	40
With ⅓ Ice	120	0	30
Regular, 16 fl.oz: No Ice	215	0	53
With ⅓ Ice	160	0	40
Medium, 22 fl.oz: No Ice	295	0	73
With ⅓ Ice	220	0	55
Large, 32 fl.oz: No Ice	430	0	105
With ⅓ Ice	320	0	80

(Note: ⅓ Cup of Ice = ¼ Cup Liquid)

Soft Drinks Brands

Per 12 fl.oz Unless Indicated

	C	F	Cb
A&W:			
Root Beer	180	0	46
Diet Cream Soda/Root Beer	0	0	0
Albertson's:			
Super Chill: Cola	165	0	44
Root Beer	180	0	48

Soft Drink Brands (Cont)

Per 12 fl.oz Unless Indicated	**C**	**F**	**Cb**
Barq's, Root Beer	160	0	45
Big Red, 20 fl.oz	260	0	63
Blue Sky: Cola; Or. Creme	160	0	43
Black Cherry Soda	140	0	37
Grape; Lemon Lime, av.	130	0	36
Raspberry; Root Beer, average	165	0	44
Bubble Up, 8 fl.oz	110	0	28
Cactus Cooler, 12 fl.oz	150	0	40
Canada Dry: *Per 8 fl.oz*			
Ginger Ale	90	0	25
Tonic Water	90	0	24
Capri Sun:			
Juice Drinks, all flavors, 6 fl.oz	60	0	16
Coca-Cola: *Per 12 fl.oz*			
Classic/Caffeine Free	140	0	39
Diet Coke, all flavors	0	0	0
Cherry Coke/Vanilla Coke	155	0	42
Coca-Cola Zero	0	0	0
Country Time, Lemonade, 12 fl.oz	135	0	36
Crush:			
Orange/Grape: 12 fl.oz	195	0	53
20 fl.oz bottle	320	0	86
Strawberry, 20 fl.oz	290	0	77
Diet Orange, 20 fl.oz	35	0	10
Dad's: Orange Cream Soda	180	0	46
Root Beer, 12 fl.oz	165	0	41
Diet Rite, Pure Zero	0	0	0
Dr Pepper: Regular	150	0	40
Cherry	165	0	59
Diet, all flavors	0	0	0
Fanta, all flavors	175	0	48
Fresca: Original Citrus	0	0	0
Blackcherry Citrus	0	0	0
Peach Citrus	0	0	0
GuS, average all flavors	95	0	23
Hansen's: Diet Soda	0	0	0
Natural Cane Sugar:			
Cola; Root Beer	160	0	40
Pomegranate	130	0	35
Hawaiian Punch, Fruit Juicy Red	180	0	45
Henry Weinhard's: Root Beer	170	0	43
Cream flavor, average	175	0	42
Hires, Root Beer	170	0	45
IBC: Root Beer	160	0	43
Cream Soda; Black Cherry	180	0	48
Icee: Coca-Cola; Barq's	100	0	27
Minute Maid: Fruit Punch	175	0	48
Lemonade	100	0	25

Per 12 fl.oz Unless Indicated

	C	F	Cb
Jarritos, all flavors, 12.5 fl.oz	170	0	43
Jelly Belly, all flavors	180	0	42
Jolt: Cola, 16 fl.oz	200	0	54
Blue Raspberry, 16 fl.oz	240	0	30
Grape, Orange, 16 fl.oz	210	0	52
Jones Soda: Cola	160	0	40
Whoopass, 16 fl.oz	200	0	52
Other flavors, average	185	0	46
Mello Yello, Regular	175	0	48
Minute Maid: Fruit Punch	160	0	44
Lemonade Regular/Pink			
12 fl.oz can/bottle	150	0	42
20 fl.oz Bottle	275	0	70
Orangeade	160	0	43
Mountain Dew:			
Live Wire; Code Red	170	0	46
Diet flavors	0	0	0
Mug Root Beer	160	0	43
Natural Brew: Draft Root Beer	180	0	44
Ginseng Cola; Outrageous Ginger Ale	170	0	42
Vanilla, Cream	170	0	42
Nehi, Royal Crown Peach	190	0	51
Orangina: 10 fl.oz bottle	120	0	32
Pepsi: Regular/Caffeine Free	150	0	41
Diet Pepsi; Jazz	0	0	0
One	0	0	0
Wild Cherry; Vanilla	150	0	42
Perrier, Carbonated Water	0	0	0
Pibb, Xtra	150	0	39
RC Cola, Regular	160	0	43
Reed's, Ginger Brew,			
average all varieties	145	0	38
7·UP: Regular; Cherry	150	0	39
Diet varieties	0	0	0
7·UP Plus	15	0	3
Safeway/Vons: Go 2 Cola	160	0	40
Cherry Cola	160	0	40
Ditto Lemon Lime	160	0	40
Parker's Cream Soda	170	0	42
Parker's Root Beer	180	0	47
Santa Cruz, Sparkling, average	135	0	33
Schweppes: Seltzer	0	0	0
Tonic Water; Ginger Ale, average	130	0	35
Shasta: Cream Soda	190	0	47
Cherry Cola	180	0	45
Dr. Shasta	150	0	38
Club Soda; Diet, all flavors	0	0	0
Tiki Punch; Pineapple; Or.	200	0	50
Ginger Ale	130	0	33
Other flavors, average	170	0	41

Per 12 fl.oz Unless Indicated

	C	F	Cb
Sierra Mist, Lemon Lime	150	0	39
Sprite: Regular	145	0	40
Zero	5	0	0
Squirt, Ruby Red	170	0	45
Stewarts: Root Beer	160	0	40
Grape; Orange 'n Cream	190	0	48
Sun Drop: Regular, 20 fl.oz bottle	325	0	81
Cherry Lemon, 20 fl.oz bottle	300	0	78
Sunkist: Orange	190	0	52
Diet Sunkist	0	0	0
TAB	0	0	0
Thomas Kemper: Root Beer	160	0	40
Other flavors, average	160	0	40
Trader Joe's:			
Sparkling:			
French Berry Lemonade,			
1 cup, 8 fl.oz	130	0	31
1 Bottle, 33.8 fl.oz	520	0	124
Lime Ade, 1 cup, 8 fl.oz	110	0	28
1 Bottle, 33.8 fl.oz	440	0	108
Pink Lemonade, 8 fl.oz	130	0	31
1 Bottle, 33.8 fl.oz	520	0	124
Vernor's, Ginger Soda	150	0	39
Virgil's Root Beer	160	0	42
Walgreens:			
Orchard Grape Soda, 20 fl.oz	300	0	84
Cola; Zesty Lem. Lime, av., 20 fl.oz	225	0	65
Root Beer, 20 fl.oz	225	0	75
Welch's,			
Sparkling Juice Cocktail	240	0	60
365 Organic (Whole Foods):			
Spritzers, all flavors	110	0	28

Powdered Soft Drink Mix

Per 8 fl.oz Prepared, Unless Otherwise Stated

	C	F	Cb
Capri Sun, Sport, 6.75 fl.oz	60	0	16
Cool Splashers, 8 fl.oz	60	0	16
Country Time: Lemonade	60	0	16
Other flavors, average	80	0	19
Lite	35	0	8
Crystal Light, 8 fl.oz	5	0	0
Flavor Aid, ⅛ package	0	0	0
Kool-Aid: All flavors	60	0	16
Unsweetened, 6 fl.oz	0	0	0
Propel, ½ package	10	0	3
Tang, Regular, 2 Tbsp, 0.9oz	105	0	28

Quick Guide

Teas

	C	F	Cb
Regular: Bag, Loose or Instant			
Brewed, 1 cup, 8 fl.oz	2	0	0.5
(Add extra for sugar/milk)			
Herbal: Average all varieties, 1 cup	2	0	0
Bigelow, all flavors	0	0	0
Celestial Seasonings:			
All flavors	0	0	0
Bubble Tea, average, 12 fl.oz	175	0	41
Chai Tea: *Cafe D' Vita,* 2 Tbsp	120	3.5	21
Starbucks: See Fast-Foods Section			

Iced Tea
Average All Brands

	C	F	Cb
Sweetened: 8 fl.oz	100	0	25
12 fl.oz	150	0	38
16 fl.oz	200	0	50
Unsweetened: 8 fl.oz	2	0	0

Iced Tea Mixes

Per 8 fl.oz Made-Up

	C	F	Cb
4C Iced Teas:			
Sweetened, av. all flavors	70	0	18
Totally Light, all flavors	0	0	0
Crystal Light Sugar Free	5	0	0
Lipton: Instant, unsweetened	0	0	0
Instant Raspberry	80	0	19
Lemon	70	0	18
Peach; Raspberry, Sugar Free	5	0	1
Iced Tea To Go	0	0	0
Nestea			
Lemonade Tea, 1⅓ Tbsp	60	0	15
Lemon flavored Iced Tea, 1⅓ Tbsp	60	0	15
Sugar Free Lemon Iced Tea, 2 tsp	5	0	2
Unsweetened Tea, 2 tsp	0	0	0

Bottled & Canned Teas

Arizona: *Per 8 fl.oz*	C	F	Cb
Black with Ginseng	60	0	15
Green Tea(s)/Asian Plum	70	0	18
Diet Green Tea (with Sorbitol)	5	0	2
Peach/Raspberry	70	0	18
Sweet Tea	90	0	23
Fuze, all flavors, 16 fl.oz	120	0	30
Gold Peak, Lem. ,16.9 fl.oz bottle	170	0	44
Hansen's: Green Tea: Reg., 16 fl.oz	120	0	30
Peach; Pomegranae, 16 fl.oz	180	0	44

Bottled & Canned Teas (Cont)

Honest Tea: *Per 16.9 fl.oz*	C	F	Cb
Black Forest Berry/Peach/Lori's Lemon	65	0	17
Lipton Brisk			
Av. all flavors, 12 fl.oz can	130	0	33
20 fl.oz bottle	215	0	55
Lipton Iced Tea			
Lemon; White w/Raspb., 16.9 fl.oz	120	0	32
Green Tea with Citrus:			
16.9 fl.oz bottle	170	0	44
20 fl.oz bottle	200	0	53
Diet, all flavors	0	0	0
Sparkling, av. all flavors, 16 fl.oz	120	0	32
Minute Maid, Pomeg. Tea, 8 fl.oz	40	0	9
Nantucket, Lemon Tea 16 fl.oz	160	0	44
Nestea Iced Tea			
With Lemon: 8 fl.oz	90	0	23
16.9 oz Bottle	180	0	45
20 fl.oz Bottle	210	0	52
Diet Green/Lemon	0	0	0
Pom Pomegranate:			
Pomegranate Tea, 16 fl.oz	140	0	34
Pomegranate Lychee, 16 fl.oz	140	0	36
Pomegranate Peach Passion, 16 fl.oz	160	0	38
Light flavors, average, 16 fl.oz	70	0	34

Note: Carbs figure for Light flavors includes Erythritol natural sweetener which has negligible calories.

Sbarro, 16 fl.oz Bottle	180	0	48
Snapple: Diet/Unsweetened Teas	0	0	0
Iced Tea Blends, all flav., 16 fl.oz	200	0	50
Black Teas, average, 8 fl.oz	40	0	10
Green; White, 8 fl.oz	60	0	15
Red Tea, 8 fl.oz	40	0	10
SoBe, Green, 20 fl.oz	250	0	63
Ssips, Lemon Iced, 6¾ fl.oz	80	0	21
Steaz: Peach/Mint, 16 fl.oz	80	0	20
Sparkling Organic, 16 fl.oz	135	0	35
Tazo, Organic Blac, 13.8 fl oz	60	0	15
TeaZazz: Orig./Peach, 20 fl.oz	50	0	12
Green Tea Lemon, 20 fl.oz	60	0	15
Trader Joe's: *Per 8 fl.oz*			
Organic Tea & Lemonade	100	0	25
Pomegranate Green Tea	60	0	15
Unsweetened *(Kettle/Green)*	0	0	0
Turkey Hill: Iced Tea, 16 fl.oz	180	0	42
Fruit flavors, average, 16 fl.oz	205	0	50
365 Organic *(Whole Foods):*			
Berry Black Tea, 16 fl.oz	60	0	14
Lemon Green Tea, 16 fl.oz	40	0	10
White Jasmine Tea, 16 fl.oz	30	0	8

Note: Most breads have similar calories on a weight basis. However, volume may vary.

For example, 1 oz of bread may equal 1 slice regular bread or 2 slices of a lighter bread.

It is best to weigh bread used and calculate using: 1 oz bread = 70 calories, 14g carb.

Quick Guide

Bread

	C	F	Cb
White or Wheat ~ Average Per Slice			
Thin or Light, ¾ oz	50	0.5	10
Sandwich slice, 1 oz	70	1	14
Thick or Large slice, 1½ oz	105	1.5	21
Thick/Home-made, 2 oz	140	2	28
Extra Thick/Home-made, 3 oz	210	3	42
Whole Loaf: 16 oz	1120	16	224
24 oz Loaf	1680	24	336
With Seeds or Nuts:			
Sandwich slice, 1½ oz	130	5	18
Thick slice/Home-made, 2½ oz	215	8	30
Toast ~ Has same calories as bread used			
1 Slice (1 oz fresh)			
with 2 tsp regular spread	140	9	12
with 2 tsp "light" spread	105	5	12
with 1 Tbsp regular spread	170	12	12
with 1 Tbsp "light" spread	120	7	12

Breads

Per Slice Unless Indicated

	C	F	Cb
12-Grain, 1½ oz	110	1.5	22
Batard (8 oz), thick slice, 2 oz	150	0.5	28
Bran style/Dark, 1 oz	70	1	14
Bread with Soy Isoflavones, 1.2 oz	80	2.5	13
Buttermilk, average, 1½ oz	110	1	22
Caraway Rye, 2 oz	150	2	28
Challah, ¾ oz	85	1.5	17
Chapati, 1 oz	110	3	18
Ciabatta, 2 oz	130	1	26
Cornbread, average, 3 oz	220	6	37
Cracked Wheat Sourdough, 1½ oz	130	0.5	27
Croissants: *See Page 134*			
Crustless Bread, regular slice, ¾ oz	40	0.5	8.5
Crusts Only, regular slice, ¼ oz	30	0	7
English Toasting, 2 oz	140	1.5	27
'Enriched' Breads, average, 1 oz	60	1	12
Flax & Grain, 1½ oz	120	3	19
Flax & Sunflower Round, 1.2 oz	90	2	18

Breads (Cont)

Per Slice Unless Indicated

	C	F	Cb
Foccacia: Plain, 2 oz portion	150	2.5	28
Cheese & Garlic; Pesto, 2 oz	160	6	21
Tomato & Olive, 2 oz	150	5	21
French Stick/Baguette, 1 oz	70	1	15
French Toast, 1.6 oz	140	2	26
Sticks *(Aunt Jemima)*,1 oz	90	2	17
Garlic Bread/Toast:			
Small slice + 1 tsp spread, ¾ oz	80	5	7
Med. slice + 2 tsp spread, 1½ oz	160	10	14
Thick slice + 3 tsp spread, 1.8 oz	220	14	20
Pepperidge Farm, 1 slice, 1.4 oz	160	10	15
Hemp Bread, 1.2 oz	95	2	12
Italian Bread, 2 oz	140	1	28
Light Bread, averaage, 0.8 oz	40	0.5	8
Lower Carb (higher Protein/fiber),			
average all brands, 1 oz	60	1.5	9
MultiGrain, 1.5 oz	100	2	19
Naan Flatbread, ½, 2 oz	160	3.5	29
Nut/Health Nut, 1.35 oz	90	1.5	18
Oatmeal/Oatbran Bread, 1½ oz	90	0.5	19
Pita: Average all types,			
Small (4" diam) 1.1 oz	90	0	18
Large (6½" diam) 2 oz	140	1.5	27
Extra Large (9" diam) 4 oz	300	1.5	60
Popovers (1), no butter	130	2	18
Poppyseed (Vienna), 0.8 oz	55	1	10
Pumpernickel: Large slice, 1.35 oz	80	0	15
Cocktail/Party size	30	0.5	6
Raisin Bread, 1 oz	80	1	15
Raisin Walnut, 1 oz	70	0.5	15
Roman Meal, 1.1 oz	80	1	15
Rye: Average, 1 thin slice, 1 oz	80	1	14
1 thick slice, 2 oz	150	2	25
Cocktail size, 0.4 oz	25	0.5	4
Sandwich Bread, 1 oz	70	1	12
Sandwich Pockets, 2 oz	140	1.5	27
Sourdough, 1½ oz	120	1	25
Sourdough French, 1 oz	75	0	14
Spelt, 1.6 oz	130	1	26
Sprouted 7-Grain, 1.5 oz	110	0.5	18
Squaw, 1.1 oz	85	0.5	13
Sweet Hawaiian Bread, 1.3 oz	110	2	19
Tacos/Tortillas: *See Page 172*			
Turkish/Middle Eastern, 1 oz	80	1.5	16
Wheat-Free Breads: Spelt, 1.6 oz	130	1	26
Brown Rice with Fruit Juice, 1.5 oz	110	2	21
Healthseed Rye, 1.6 oz	90	1	20
Millet, 1.5 oz	100	1	20
Whole Wheat: Thin, 1 oz	70	1	14
Thick, 1.7 oz	130	2	23

Bread Brands

Per Slice Unless Indicated

	C	F	Cb
Ener-G: Gluten-Free Breads			
Brown Rice Bread, 1.3 oz	130	6	18
Light Brown Rice, ¾ oz	50	2	7
Corn Loaf, ¾ oz	40	1.5	7
Light Tapioca, ¾ oz	45	1.5	7
Ezekiel:			
Sprouted Grain: Low Sod., 1.2 oz	80	0.5	15
Sesame, 1.2 oz	80	0.5	14
Francisco International			
Sourdough, Round Loaf, 1.6 oz	110	0.5	22
Nature's Path:			
Manna: Carrot Raisin; Millet Rice	130	0	28
Cinnamon Date	150	0	29
Fig Fennel Flax	120	1.5	26
Fruit & Nut	140	1	27
Sunseed	160	2	29
Whole Rye	150	0	32
Oroweat:			
100% Whole Wheat, 1.35 oz	90	1	17
9 Grain DHA, 1.35 oz	90	1	17
Country Buttermilk, 1.35 oz	100	1.5	19
Honey Wheat Berry, 1.2 oz	80	1	17
Pepperidge Farm:			
100% Whole Wheat, Very Thin	110	2	20
15 Grain, Small Slice	70	1.5	13
Farmhouse Soft Hearty White	120	1.5	22
Light Style, average	130	1	26
Frozen Breads,			
Garlic Bread: Parmesan, 2.5"	160	6	23
Premium Roasted	160	7	19
Texas Toast	150	7	18
Sara Lee:			
45 Calories & Delightful Wheat	45	0.5	9
Honey Wheat, 1 oz	80	1	14
Hearty & Delicious:			
100% Multigrain, 1.5 oz	120	1.5	21
Soft & Smooth, 100% Whole Wheat, 1 oz	80	1	13
Schwan's, Frozen: *Per Serving*			
Cheese Stuffed Breadsticks, 2 oz	160	7	18
Five Cheese Garlic French Bread, 3.4 oz	330	20	26
French Baguette Bread, ¼ loaf, 1.7 oz	130	0	25
Trader Joe's:			
Fat-Free Multi-Grain, 1.1 oz	70	0	15
Gourmet White, 1.5 oz	120	3.5	19
Soft 10 Grain, 1.5 oz	90	1.5	16
Sprouted Rye, 1.2 oz	90	1	15
Wonder: Classic White Sandwich, 1 oz	70	1	14
Light White, ¾ oz	40	0	9
Smartwhite, 1 slice, 0.92 oz	50	0.5	11

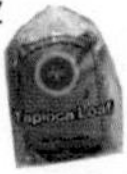

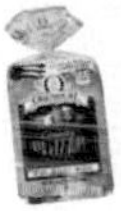

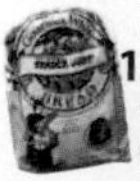

Biscuits, Bread Rolls & Buns

	C	F	Cb
6" Roll, Plain, average 2½ oz	200	1	38
Biscuits/Rolls: Average, 2½" diameter			
Commercially Baked	130	6	17
Prepared from Recipe	210	10	27
Refrigerated Dough, Baked	95	4	13
Brown 'n Serve, average, 1 oz	70	1	13
Ciabatta Roll, 3½ oz	230	4	41
Dinner Rolls:			
1 small, 1 oz	90	1.5	17
1 medium (3" diam), 1½ oz	110	1	23
Frankfurter/Hot Dog: 1¼ oz	110	1.5	21
1½ oz size	130	2	25
French: 1 med, 1.3 oz	110	1.5	22
1 large, 3 oz	230	2.5	42
Hamburger: Regular, 1½ oz	110	1.5	22
Large, 3 oz	210	3	40
Hoagie/Submarine, Plain, 2⅓ oz	200	1	38
Kaiser Rolls:			
Small, 2 oz	200	2.5	35
Large, 3½ oz	350	4	61
Refrigerated Dough, Baked: *Pillsbury*			
Buttermilk Biscuit (3), 2.25 oz	150	2	29
Crescent Roll, Original, 1 oz	110	6	11
Grands! Flaky Layers Bisc., Original	180	8	25
Traditional Dinner Roll, 1.4 oz	100	1.5	20
Sourdough Roll, 1¼ oz	110	1	21
Wheat Rolls: Small, 1.2 oz	100	1	17
Medium, 1¾ oz	130	1.5	23
Large, 3½ oz	260	3	46

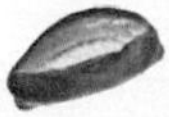

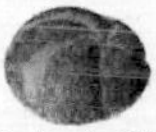

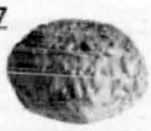

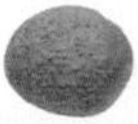

Breadsticks, Croutons

	C	F	Cb
Breadsticks: Salt Sticks, plain, 1 oz	110	1	20
Fresh baked (1), 2 oz	180	2.5	34
Stella D'oro: Sesame (1)	50	2	7
Original, 1 piece	45	1	7
Croutons: Seasoned, 2 Tbsp, ¼ oz	35	1.5	4
Zesty Italian (*Pepp. Farm*), 6 croutons	30	1	5

Bread Products

	C	F	Cb
Bread Crumbs, dry:			
Plain or seasoned, 1 oz	110	1.5	20
1 cup, 3½ oz	385	5	70
Corn Flake Crumbs, 1.1 oz	120	0	29
Graham Cracker Crumbs, 1 oz	110	2.5	20
Keebler, 3 Tbsp, 0.65 oz	70	1.5	13
Bread Dough: Frozen, 1 slice, 2 oz	140	2	26
Refrigerated, French, 1" slice	60	1	13
Wheat; White, 1" slice	80	2	14
Coating Mixes: Average, 2 Tbsp., 1 oz	100	0.5	20
Stuffing: Average, dry mix, 1 oz	110	1	10
Prepared, ½ cup, 4 oz	180	9	11

Quick Guide

Bagels
	C	F	Cb
Average All Brands			
Plain/Onion:			
1 mini/bagelette, 1 oz	75	0.5	15
1 small bagel, 2 oz	145	1	29
1 medium bagel, 3 oz	230	1.5	45
1 large bagel, 4 oz	285	2	56
Bagel Chips *(New York Style)*,			
4 slices, ¾ oz	100	4.5	12
Pizza Bagel Bites, 4 pieces, 3.1 oz	200	6	29
Bagel Crisps *(New York Style)*, 7 pieces	140	6	17
Bagel Thins *(Thomas')*, 1, 1.6 oz	110	1	24

Bagel Brands ~ *Per Bagel*
	C	F	Cb
Controlled Carb Gourmet			
High Fiber Bagel, average, 2 oz	160	5	22
Individual Wrapped, 2 oz	80	6	18
Zero Net Carbs, 2 oz	120	2	14
Costco Bakery: Plain	330	1.5	70
Cinnamon Raisin	340	1.5	73
Wholegrain	300	5	56
Enjoy Life, all types, 3.2 oz	275	6	50
Lenders: Original, plain, frozen, 2 oz	140	0.5	29
New York, plain, frozen, 3.3 oz	230	1	48
Premium, plain, refrigerated, 2.9 oz	210	1.5	43
Sara Lee: Mini, average, 1.3 oz	100	0.5	20
Plain, 3.35 oz	260	1	50
Blueberry, 3.7 oz	280	1	54
Cinnamon Raisin, 3.7 oz	270	1	54
Everything, 3.7 oz	280	3.5	50
Onion, 3 oz	270	1	52
Western, The Alternatives, av., 2 oz	110	0	25

Bagel Spreads
	C	F	Cb
Cream Cheese:			
Plain: 2 Tbsp, 1 oz	80	8	2
2 oz mini-tub	160	16	4
Reduced Fat: 2 Tbsp, 1 oz	60	5	2
2 oz mini-tub	120	10	4
Flavors: Lox, 1 oz	75	6	1
Raisin Walnut, 1 oz	90	6	8
Strawberry, 1 oz	60	3	7
Sundried Tomato, 1 oz	80	7	2
Vegetable, 1 oz	60	6	1

English Muffins
	C	F	Cb
Average All Brands			
Plain/Whole Wheat:			
Regular, 2 oz	133	1.5	26
Heavier, 2.5 oz	155	2	31
Super Size, 3.2 oz	190	2	38
Raisin-Cinnamon, 2.2 oz	140	1	29

Note: Actual weight of packaged muffins can be 10-15% heavier than stated net weight.

Rice Cakes
	C	F	Cb
Reg. size, av.1 cake, 0.32 oz	35	0	7.5
Hain, Mini, plain, 10 pieces	70	2	12
Lundberg, all types, 0.65 oz	70	0.5	14
Quaker, Apple Cinnamon, 0.45 oz	50	0	11

Taco Shells & Tortillas
	C	F	Cb
Tacos: Mini Size (1)	25	1.5	2
Regular size, all types (1)	50	2	7
Large (1)	90	4	13
Salad Shell, flour *(Del Oro)*, 1.4 oz	230	17	10
Tortilla (Soft Taco), each	85	2	15
Corn Tortilla: 6", 1 oz	55	0.5	11
Flour Tortilla: 8", 1.75 oz	145	3	26
Low-Fat	110	1.5	22
Burritos, 1 tortilla, 2.3 oz	190	5	32
Low-Fat	110	1.5	22
Tostada Bowl (Rio Rancho), 6" 1.25 oz	180	9	22
Tostada Shells, (1)	55	3	6
La Tortilla Factory			
Fat Free Flour Tortillas:			
Burrito size, 2.5 oz	120	0.5	34
Soft Taco, 1.8 oz	90	0	24
Low-Fat Low Carb Tortillas:			
Large, 2.2 oz	80	3	19
Original; Flavors, 1.26 oz	50	2	11
Smart & Delicious:			
Traditional; Whole Wheat 2 oz	100	1.5	24
Mission Foods			
Tortillas: *Per 1, 6" Tortilla*			
Carb Balance, Flour; Whole Wheat	80	2	12
Small Flour, 0.65 oz	110	2.5	18
96% Fat Free, 1 oz	90	1	17
Extra Thin Yellow Corn, 0.65 oz	40	0.5	8
Life Balance, Flour; Whole Wheat	125	3.5	19
Multigrain Flour, 1.4 oz	130	3	19
White Corn, 0.74 oz	45	1	18

Breakfast Cereals

Quick Guide

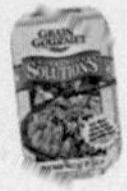

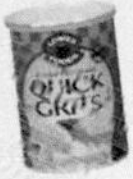

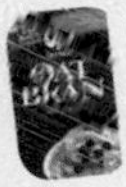

Cooked Cereals

	C	F	Cb
Buckwheat Groats, roasted:			
Dry, ⅓ cup, 3 oz	205	2	61
Cooked, 1 cup, 6 oz	155	1	34
Bulgur: Dry, ½ cup, 2½ oz	240	1	53
Cooked, 1 cup, 6½ oz	150	0.5	34
Corn/Hominy Grits:			
Dry: ¼ cup, 1.4 oz	145	0.5	31
3 Tbsp, 1 oz	110	0.5	23
Cooked, ¾ cup, 6½ oz	110	0.5	23
Instant, 1 packet, dry, 0.8 oz	75	0	18
With Imitation Bacon Bits, 1 oz	100	0.5	22
Cream of Rice, cooked, ¾ cup, 6½ oz	95	0	21
Cream of Wheat:			
Regular, cooked, ¾ cup, 6½ oz	100	0.5	21
Quick, cooked, ¾ cup, 6½ oz	95	0.5	20
Instant, cooked, ¾ cup, 6½ oz	110	0.5	24
Farina: Cooked, ¾ cup, 6 oz	85	0	18
Millet, dry, ¼ cup, 1¾ oz	190	2	36
Oat Bran: Raw, ⅓ cup, 1 oz	70	2	19
Cooked, ½ cup, 3¾ oz	45	1	13
Oatmeal: Dry, ⅓ cup, 1 oz	105	1.5	18
Regular, cooked, ¾ cup, 6 oz	110	2	19
1 cup, 8 oz	145	2.5	25
Instant: Regular, dry, average, 1 oz	105	1.5	18
Flavored, dry, average, 1½ oz	150	2	32
Wheat Hearts, 1 oz dry, ¾ cup cooked	110	0.5	24

Brans, Wheat Germ, Add-Ons

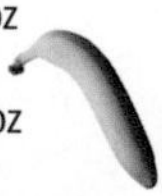

	C	F	Cb
Bran: Wheat, unprocessed,			
1 Tbsp, 0.10 oz	5	0	2
Rice Bran: Raw, 1 Tbsp, 0.18 oz	15	1	2.5
¼ cup, 1 oz	95	6	15
Oat Bran: Raw, 1 Tbsp, 0.18 oz	10	0.5	4
⅓ cup, 1 oz	70	2	19
Wheat Germ: Raw, 1 Tbsp, ¼ oz	25	0.5	4
¼ cup, 1 oz	105	3	15
Fruit: Dried, average, 1 oz	70	0	18
Banana, ½ medium	55	0	14
Prunes in Syrup (5), 3 oz	90	0	23
Honey, 1 Tbsp, ¾ oz	65	0	17
Lecithin Granules, 1 Tbsp, 0.35 oz	55	4	0.5
Nuts, Almonds (6), ¼ oz	40	4	1.5
Bee Pollen Granules, 1 Tbsp, 0.28 oz	25	1	2
Psyllium Husks, 1 Tbsp, 0.18 oz	15	0	4

Hot/Cooked Cereals ~ Brands

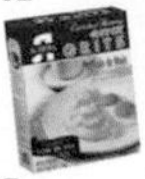

Per Serving, Dry Mix only

	C	F	Cb
Albers Grits, ¼ cup, 1.4 oz	140	0.5	31
Bobs Red Mill,			
10 Grain, ¼ cup, 1.4 oz	150	4.5	27
Country Choice,			
Quick Oats, ½ cup, 1.4 oz	150	3.5	27
Dr McDougall's			
Big Cup Organic Oatmeal: *Per Cup*			
Grains: W/ Cranb, Muesli, 3.1 oz	320	4	62
With Peach Raspberry 3 oz	300	4	62
4 Grain with Real Maple, 2.55 oz	260	3	52
Organic Instant Oatmeal: *Per Packet*			
Original, 1 oz	120	2	21
Light Apple Cinnamon, 1.95 oz	120	1.5	24
Light Maple Brown Sugar, 1.34 oz	150	2	28
Erewhon: Barley Plus, ¼ cup, 1.7 oz	170	1	37
Brown Rice Cream, ¼ cup, 1.6 oz	170	1	36
Instant Oatmeal, 1.25 oz pkg, av.	130	2.5	25
McCann's Instant Irish Oatmeal			
Apple & Cinnamon, 1.23 oz	130	1.5	27
Maple & Brown Sugar, 1.5 oz	160	2	32
Original, 1 oz package	100	2	19
Steel Cut Oats, ¼ cup, 1.4 oz	150	2.5	27
Nabisco: Cream of Wheat, Farina, 1 oz	120	0	23
Malt-O-Meal: Orig., 3Tbsp, 1.2 oz	130	0.5	27
Maple Brown Sugar, ¼ cup	170	0	37
Natures Path:			
Oatmeal: Apple Cinnamon, 1.7 oz	210	2.5	40
HempPlus, 1 packet, 1.4 oz	160	2.5	30
Maple Nut, 1.7 oz	210	4	38
NutriSystem: *Per Packet*			
Oatmeal, Apple Cinnamon	130	1.5	26
Ocean Spray,			
Oatmeal, all flavors, 1.51 oz	160	2	33
Quaker:			
Instant Oatmeal: *Per Packet Unless Indicated*			
Regular, Organic 1 oz	100	2	19
Cinnamon & Spice, 1.62 oz	170	2	35
Maple Brown Sugar, 1.45 oz	160	2	31
Peaches & Cream, 1.23 oz	130	2	27
Raisin, Date & Walnut, 1.3 oz	140	2.5	27
Old Fashioned Oats, ½ cup, 1.4 oz	150	3	27
Quick Oats, ½ cup, 1.4 oz	150	3	27
Grits: Instant, all types, 1 oz	100	0	21
Quick, ¼ cup, 1.3 oz	130	0.5	27
Silver Palate, Oatmeal, 1.4 oz	160	3	

Updated Nutrition Data ~ www.CalorieKing.com
Persons with Diabetes ~ See Disclaimer (Page 22)

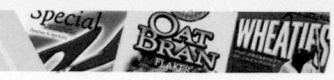

Quick Guide

Cold Cereals
Average All Brands

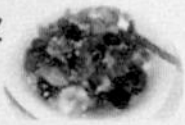

	C	F	Cb
Bran Flakes, ¾ cup, 1 oz	95	0.5	24
Corn Flakes, 1 cup, 1 oz	100	0	24
Granola, ¼ cup, 1 oz	150	7.5	16
Oat Bran Cereal, ½ cup, 1½ oz	145	3	25
Puffed Rice, 1 cup, ½ oz	55	0	13
Puffed Wheat, 1 cup, ½ oz	45	0	10
Raisin Bran, ½ cup, 1 oz	90	0.5	22
Rice Crisps, 1 cup, 1 oz	105	0.5	24
Shredded Wheat, 1 biscuit, 1 oz	85	0.5	20
Sugar-frosted Flakes, ¾ cup, 1 oz	115	0	28
Wheat Flakes, ¾ cup, 1 oz	105	1	24

Breakfast/Cereal Bars/Pop Tarts: *See Page 31*

Ready-To-Eat Cereal

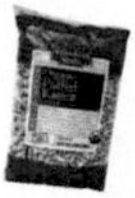

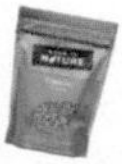

	C	F	Cb
Arrowhead Mills : *Per Cup*			
Flakes: Amaranth, 1.2 oz	140	2	26
Kamut, 1.1 oz	120	1	25
Maple Buckwheat, 1.5 oz	170	1	35
Oat Bran, 1.2 oz	140	2.5	24
Rice, sweetened, 1.7 oz	180	1	40
Spelt, 1.1 oz	120	1	24
Granola, Crunchy Oat Bran, 1.7 oz	210	8	33
Puffed: Corn, ½ oz	60	1	12
Kamut, ½ oz	50	0	11
Millet, ½ oz	60	0.5	11
Rice, ½ oz	60	0	14
Wheat, ½ oz	60	0	12
Shredded Wheat: Original, 1.7 oz	190	1	38
Sweetened, 1.8 oz	200	10	42
Back to Nature: *Per ½ Cup, Unless Indicated*			
Granola: Apple Blueberry, 1.7 oz	200	2.5	39
Choc. Delight, 1.8 oz	220	6	37
Classic Granola, 1.7 oz	200	3	39
Cranberry Pecan, 1.7 oz	200	5	35
Honey Almond with Flax, 1.5 oz	190	7	29
Organic Cherry Vanilla, 1.7 oz	200	4	38
Sunflower & Pumpkin Seed, 1.65 oz	200	7	31
Wild Blueberry Walnut, 1.5 oz	190	6	30

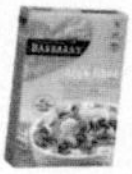

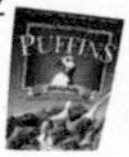

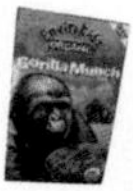

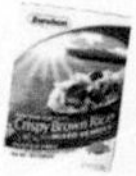

Barbara's Bakery

	C	F	Cb
Cherry Vanilla, 1.7 oz	200	4	38
Classics, Organic & Sweetened:			
Breakfast O's, average, 1 cup, 1 oz	120	2	22
Brown Rice Crisps, 1.1 oz	120	1	25
Corn Flakes, 1 cup, 1.1 oz	110	1	25
High Fiber::			
Original, 55g	180	1.5	42
Flax & Granola, 1 cup, 2 oz	200	3	43
Pomegranate, 1 cup, 2 oz	190	1.5	42
Puffins: Original, ¾ cup	90	1	23
Cinnamon, ⅔ cup, 1 oz	100	1	26
Peanut Butter, ¾ cup, 1 oz	110	2	23
Wild Puff, average, ¾ cup	120	1	26
Shredded Oats:			
Cinnamon Crunch, 1 cup, 2 oz	230	3	43
Bite Size: Vanilla Almond, 1 cup, 2 oz	220	3	42
Breadshop Granola:			
Honey Gone Nuts, 1.85 oz	240	10	33
Average other flavors, 1.8 oz	210	8	34
Cascadian Farm			
Hearty Morning, ¾ cup, 1.9 oz	200	3	43
Honey Nut O's, 1 cup, 1 oz	110	1	25
Multi Grain Squares, ¾ cup, 1 oz	110	1	25
Oats & Honey Granola, ⅔ cup, 2 oz	230	6	42
Purely O's, 1 cup, 1.1 oz	110	1	24
Raisin Bran, 1 cup, 1.9 oz	180	1	43
Ener-G, Rice Bran, ½ cup, 2.4 oz	220	14	34
EnviroKidz: *Per 1 oz*			
Amazon Frosted Flakes	120	0	27
Gorilla Munch	120	0	27
Koala Crisp	110	1	25
Leapin Lemur	120	1.5	25
Panda Puffs	130	2.5	24
Erewhon			
Aztec Crunchy Corn & Amaranth, 1 oz	110	0	26
Corn Flakes, 1 cup, 2 oz	130	0	30
Crispy Brown Rice: 1 cup	110	0	25
With Mixed Berries, 1 cup	120	0.5	27
Gluten Free, 1 cup, 1 oz	110	0.5	25
Kamut Flakes, ⅔ cup, 1.2 oz	110	0	25
Raisin Bran, 1 cup, 1.8 oz	170	1	40
Rice Twice, ¾ cup, 1 oz	120	0	26

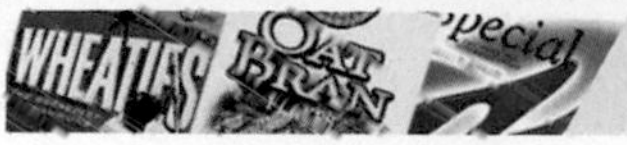

Ready-To-Eat (Cont)

	C	F	Cb
Ezekiel 4.9 Flourless Cereals			
Almond ½ cup, 2 oz	200	3	38
Golden Flax, ½ cup, 2 oz	180	2.5	37
Original, ½ cup, 2 oz	190	1	40
General Mills			
Basic 4, 1 cup, 1.9 oz	200	2	43
Cheerios: Per ¾ Cup			
Apple Cinnamon, 1 oz	120	1.5	24
Berry Burst, Triple Berry, 1 oz	100	1	22
Chocolate, 1 oz	100	1	23
Frosted, 1 oz	110	1	23
Fruity, 1 oz	100	1	23
Honey Nut, 1 oz	110	1.5	22
Multi Grain, 1 oz	110	1	23
Oat Cluster Crunch, 1.1 oz	100	1	22
Original, 1 oz	100	2	20
Yogurt Burst, all flavors, 1 oz	120	1.5	24
Chex: Corn, 1 cup, 1 oz	120	0.5	26
Chocolate, ¾ cup, 1.1 oz	130	2.5	26
Honey Nut, ¾ cup, 1.1 oz	120	0.5	28
Multi-Bran, ¾ cup, 1.6 oz	160	1.5	39
Rice, 1 cup, 1 oz	100	0	23
Wheat, ¾ cup, 1.6 oz	160	1	38
Cinnamon Toast Crunch, ¾ cup, 1 oz	130	3	25
Cocoa Puffs, ¾ cup, 1 oz	100	1.5	23
Count Chocula, ¾ cup, 1 oz	110	1	23
Fiber One: Original, ½ cup, 1 oz	60	1	25
Honey Clusters, 1 cup	160	1.5	42
Golden Grahams, ¾ cup, 1 oz	120	1	26
Honey Nut Clusters, 1 cup, 2 oz	210	1	49
Kix: 1¼ cups, 1 oz	110	1	25
Berry Berry, ¾ cup, 0.9 oz	100	1	22
Lucky Charms, average, ¾ cup, 1 oz	110	1	22
Oatmeal Crisp, Almond, 1 cup, 2 oz	240	4.5	47
Raisin Nut Bran, ¾ cup, 1.75 oz	180	3	38
Reese's Puffs, ¾ cup, 1 oz	120	3	22
Total: Cinn. Crunch, 1 cup	190	2.5	40
Plus Omega-3s, 1.8 oz	200	3.5	39
Raisin Bran, 1 cup, 1.9 oz	160	1	40
Wheaties, ¾ cup, 1 oz	100	0.5	22

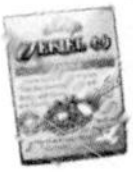

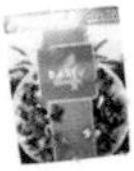

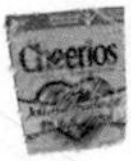

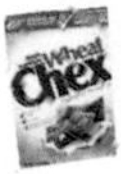

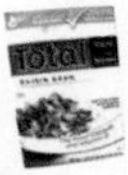

	C	F	Cb
Glucerna			
Crunchy Flakes:			
'n Strawb., ¾ cup, 1.1 oz	100	0.5	25
'n Almonds, ¾ cup, 1.1 oz	100	1	24
'n Raisins, ¾ cup, 1.2 oz	110	0.5	28
Health Valley			
Organic Flakes:			
Amaranth Flakes, 1 cup, 1 oz	100	1	23
Blue Corn Flakes, ¾ cup, 1.1 oz	100	0	24
Cranberry Crunch, ¾ cup, 1.8 oz	190	4	38
Fiber 7, Multigrain Flakes, 1 c., 1.7 oz	160	1	37
Golden Flax, 1 cup, 1.75 oz	190	3.5	37
Oat Bran Flakes, 1 cup, 1.75 oz	190	1.5	39
With Raisins, 1 cup, 1.9 oz	200	1.5	43
Crunch-Ems!, Rice; Corn, 1 cup, 1 oz	110	0	27
Heart Wise, 1 cup, 2 oz	200	3	37
Heartland			
Granola: Original, ½ cup, 2.25 oz	240	6	40
Balanced Blend, ⅔ cup, 1.8 oz	210	3	41
Low-Fat Raisin, ½ cup, 2 oz	200	3	40
Kashi			
7 Whole Grain: Flakes, 1 cup, 1.8 oz	180	1	41
Honey Puffs, 1 cup, 1.1 oz	120	1	25
Nuggets, ½ cup, 2 oz	210	1.5	47
Puffs, 1 cup, 0.67 oz	70	0.5	15
Whole Wheat Biscuit:			
Autumn Wheat, 1 cup, 1.9 oz	180	1	43
Cinnamon Harvest, 1 cup, 1.9 oz	180	1	43
Island Vanilla, 1.9 oz	190	1	44
Kashi U, Blackcurrant & Walnuts, 1 c.	200	3.5	42
GoLEAN, Original, 1 cup, 1.8 oz	140	1	30
Crunch!: Plain, 1 cup, 1.9 oz	190	3	37
Honey Almond Flax, 1 cup, 1.9 oz	200	4.5	36
Good Friends: Orig., 1 cup, 1.9 oz	160	1.5	42
Cinna-Raisin Crunch, 1 cup, 1.8 oz	170	1.5	41
Granola: Apple Orchard, ½ cup, 1.9 oz	220	7	38
Cocoa Beach, ½ cup, 1.9 oz	230	9	36
Mountain Medley, ½ cup, 1.9 oz	220	7	38
Summer Berry, ½ cup, 1.9 oz	220	6	39
Heart to Heart:			
Honey Toasted Oat, ¾ cup, 1.2 oz	120	1.5	
Oat Flakes & Blueberry Clusters, 1 c.	200	2	
Warm Cinnamon Oat, ¾ cup, 1.2 oz	120	1	
Mighty Bites, Honey Crunch, 1 cup	120		
Vive, Toasted Graham & Van., 1¼ cups	17		

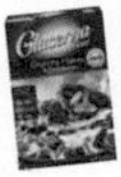

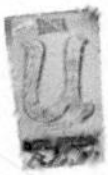

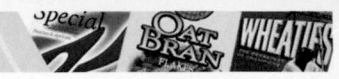

Ready-To-Eat (Cont) | C | F | Cb

Kellogg's

	C	F	Cb
All-Bran: Original, ½ cup, 1.1 oz	80	1	23
Bran Buds, ⅓ cup, 1.1 oz	70	1	24
Complete Wheat Flakes, ¾ cup, 1.1 oz	90	0.5	23
Strawberry Medley, 1 cup, 1.9 oz	170	1.5	44
Apple Jacks, 1 cup, 1 oz	100	0.5	25
Cocoa Krispies, ¾ cup, 1.1 oz	120	1	27
Corn Flakes: Original, 1 cup, 1 oz	100	0	24
Simply Cinnamon, 1 cup, 1.1oz	120	0	27
Corn Pops, 1 cup, 1.1 oz	120	0	29
Cracklin' Oat Bran, ¾ cup, 1.8 oz	200	7	35
Crispix, Original, 1 cup, 1 oz	110	0	25
Crunch, Raisin Bran, 1 cup, 1.9 oz	190	1	45
FiberPlus:			
Berry Yogurt Crunch, 1.9 oz	170	1	43
Cinnamon Oat Crunch, 1.1 oz	110	1.5	26
Froot Loops:			
Original, 1 cup, 1 oz	110	1	25
Marshmallow, 1 cup, 1.1 oz	110	1	25
Frosted Flakes, ¾ cup, 1.1 oz	110	0	27
Red. Sugar, 1 cup, 1.1 oz	120	0	28
Granola, Low-Fat:			
with Raisins, ⅔ cup, 2.1 oz	230	3	48
without Raisins, ½ cup, 1.7 oz	190	2.5	40
Honey Smacks, ¾ cup, 1 oz	100	0.5	24
Mini-Wheats: Frosted Big Bite (5)	180	1	41
Frosted: Bite Size (24), 2.1 oz	200	1	48
Blueberry Muffins (24)	180	1	43
Unfrosted (30), 2.1 oz	200	1.5	46
Mueslix, ⅔ cup, 2 oz	200	3	40
Nutri-Grain Bars: See Page 31			
Product 19, 1 cup, 1.1 oz	100	0	25
Raisin Bran: Regular, 1 cup, 2.1 oz	190	1	46
Extra, 1 cup, 1.9 oz	190	3	44
ice Krispies: Orig. 1¼ cups	130	0	29
rosted, ¾ cup, 1.1 oz	110	0	27
oa, ¾ cup, 1.1 oz	120	1	27
¾ cup, 1.1 oz	120	1.5	26
rt,			
s, 1 cup, 1.8 oz	190	0.5	43

Kellogg's (Cont) | C | F | Cb

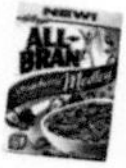

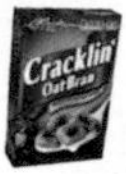

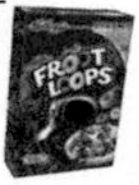

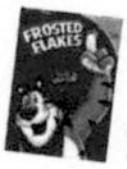

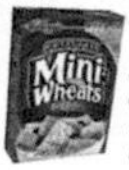

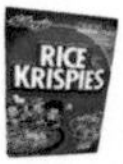

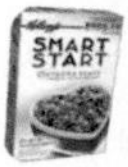

	C	F	Cb
Smorz, 1 cup, 1.1 oz	120	2	25
Special K: Original 1 cup, 1.1 oz	120	0.5	23
Blueberry, ¾ cup, 1.1 oz	110	0	26
Fruit & Yogurt, ¾ cup, 1.1 oz	120	1	27
Red Berries, 1 c., 1.1 oz	110	0	27
Vanilla Almond, ¾ cup	110	1.5	25
Low Fat Granola, ½ cup, 1.8 oz	190	3	39

Kozy Shack
Ready Grains: *Per 7 oz Pkg*

	C	F	Cb
Apple & Cinnamon	210	2	38
Maple Brown Sugar	190	2	32
Original	180	2.5	29
Strawberry	210	2	37

Malt-O-Meal

	C	F	Cb
Apple Zings, 1 cup, 1.1 oz	130	1	30
Blueb. Muffin Tops, ¾ cup	130	3.5	24
Cocoa Dyno-Bites, ¾ cup	120	1	26
Coco Roos, ¾ cup, 1 oz	120	1.5	26
Colossal Crunch, ¾ cup, 1.1 oz	120	1.5	26
Frosted Flakes, ¾ cup, 1 oz	120	0	28
Frosted Mini Spooners, 1 cup	190	1	45
Golden Puffs, ¾ cup, 1 oz	110	0	24
Honey Nut Scooters, 1 cup, 1 oz	110	1.5	24
Raisin Bran, 1 cup, 1.7 oz	220	1.5	49

Nature's Path

	C	F	Cb
Heritage, average, ¾ cup, 1 oz	120	1	24
Honey'd Cornflakes, ¾ cup, 1 oz	120	0	26
Multigr. Oatbran Flakes, ¾ cup, 1 oz	110	1	24
Flax Plus, Multibran ¾ cup, 1 oz	110	1.5	23
Maple Pecan Cr., ¾ cup	220	7	38
Pumpkin Raisin Cr., ¾ cup	210	4.5	40
Raisin Bran, ¾ cup, 2 oz	190	2.5	41
Kamut Puffs, 1 cup, ½ cup	50	0	11
Optimum, Blueberry Cinn. 1 cup 2 oz	200	3	38

New England Natural Bakers

	C	F	Cb
Muesli, ½ cup, 2.1 oz	220	5	40
Granola Pouches:			
Crispy Fruity, ⅔ cup, 1.9 oz	250	9	39
All Natural: Banana Wallnut, ½ cup	260	12	34
Honey Nut Cinnamon, ½ cup	270	12	35

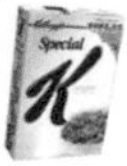

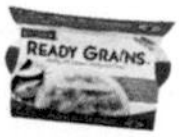

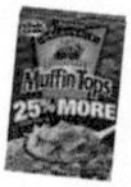

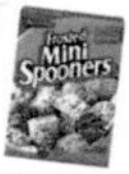

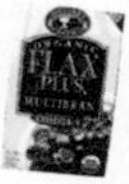

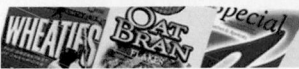

Ready-To-Eat (Cont)

	C	F	Cb
New Morning			
Cocoa Crispy Rice, ¾ cup, 1 oz	120	0.5	26
Fruit-e-O's, Organic, 1 cup, 1 oz	120	1.5	25
Oatios: Original, 1 cup, 1 oz	110	2	22
Apple Cinnamon, 1 oz	120	1	18
NutriSystem: *Per Packet*			
Granola, Low-Fat	160	2.5	31
NutriCinnamon Squares	120	0.5	23
NutriFlakes (40% Bran Flakes)	110	1	23
NutriFrosted Crunch	120	0.5	24
Peace			
Crisps, av. all varieties,1.95 oz	225	2.5	46
Hearty Raisin Bran, 1.95 oz	190	2	43
Granola, average all varieties ⅔ cup	240	6	41
Post			
Alpha Bits, 1 cup, 1 oz	110	1	23
Bran Flakes, ¾ cup, 1 oz	100	0.5	24
Grape-Nuts: Original, 2 oz	200	1	48
Flakes, ¾ cup, 1 oz	110	1	24
Great Grains, 3/4 cup, 2 oz, average	205	4	38
Honey Bunches of Oats:			
With Almonds, ¾ cup	130	2.5	25
With Vanilla Bunches, 1 cup	220	3	46
Average other varieties, ¾ cup	120	1.5	25
Honeycomb, Original, 1½ cups	130	1	28
Just Bunches: Cinn./Honey, av., ⅔ cup	250	7	43
Pebbles: Cocoa; Fruity ¾ cup, 1 oz	120	1	26
Raisin Bran, 1 cup, 2.1 oz	190	1	46
Selects: Banana Nut Crunch 2.1 oz	240	6	44
Cranberry Almond Crunch, 1.8 oz	200	3	40
Waffle Crisp, 1 cup, 1 oz	120	2.5	25
Quaker			
100% Natural Granola:			
With Honey, ½ cup, 1.8 oz	210	6	35
With Honey & Raisins, 1.8 oz	210	6	38
Low-Fat, ⅔ cup	210	3	45
Oat Bran, 1¼ cup, 2 oz	210	3	43
Oatmeal Squares, Brown Sugar, 1 c.	210	2.5	44
Cap'n Crunch: Regular, ¾ cup, 1 oz	110	1.5	23
Crunch Berries, ¾ cup, 1 oz	100	1.5	22
Peanut Butter, ¾ cup, 1 oz	110	2.5	21

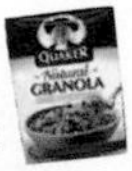

Quaker (Cont)	C	F	Cb
Crunchy Corn Bran, ¾ cup, 1 oz	90	1	23
Honey Graham Oh's, ¾ cup	110	2	23
King Vitaman, 1½ cup, 1.1 oz	120	1	26
Life, all types, ¾ cup, 1.1 oz	120	1.5	26
Sweet Home Farm			
Honey Nut Granola, ½ cup, 1.9 oz	250	10	37
Low-Fat Granola, ½ cup, 1.9 oz	210	3	44
Trader Joe's			
Clusters: Raisin Bran, 1 cup, 2 oz	190	3	41
Super Nutty Toffee, ¾ cup, 2 oz	250	9	38
Average all other flavors			
⅔ cup, 1.3 oz	145	3.5	26
1 cup, 2 oz	220	5	39
Cornflakes, 1 cup, 1.1 oz	110	0	26
Golden Flax Cereal, ¾ cup, 1.7 oz	200	3.5	37
Granola: Mango Passion, 2 oz	240	8	37
Pecan Praline, ½ cup, 1.65 oz	210	7	31
Trek Mix, ⅔ cup, 2 oz	240	8	37
High Fiber, ⅔ cup, 1 oz	80	0.5	23
Honey Nut O's, ¾ cup, 1 oz	120	1.5	24
Joe's O's, 1 cup, 1 oz	110	1.5	22
Morning Lite, 1 cup, 1.85 oz	170	2.5	40
Shredded Wheats, Bite Size, 1 c., 1.7 oz	180	1	38
Triple Berry O's, ¾ cup, 1 oz	110	1	25
Toasted Oatmeal Flakes, ¾ cup, 1.1 oz	110	1	23
Wheats, average, 1 cup, 2 oz	200	1	42
Twigs, Flakes & Clusters, 1 cup, 1.9 oz	170	1.5	41
Udi's, Granola, Au Naturel, ½ cup, 2 oz	240	8	38
Uncle Sam			
Cereal with Real Mixed Berries, 1 cup	190	4.5	39
Original, ¾ cup, 1.95 oz	190	5	38
Weetabix:			
2 biscuits, 1.3 oz	125	1	26
Crispy Flakes: Original, ¾ c., 1.1 oz	110	0.5	24
and Fiber, 1¼ cup, 2 oz	170	1.5	44
Whole Foods (365)			
Corn Flakes, 1 cup, 1 oz	110	0	26
Honey Puffed Wheat, 1 oz	110	0	24
Frosted Flakes, ¾ cup, 1 oz	110	0	27
Oat Bran Flakes, 1 cup, 2 oz	220	2.5	44
Raisin Bran, 1 cup, 2 oz	200	0.5	44
Shredded Wheat, 1 cup, 1.7 oz	180	1	
Frosted, 1 cup, 2 oz	210	1	

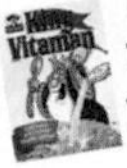

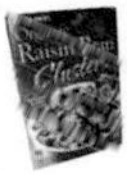

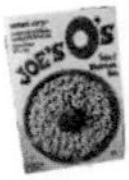

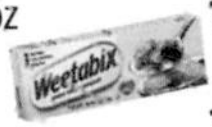

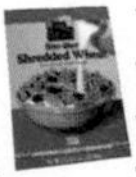

Ready-to-Eat

	C	F	Cb
Angel Food: Plain, w/o oil, 2 oz	145	0	33
Plain with oil, 2 oz	145	1	27
with Cream Frosting	255	7	45
Almond Croissant, 5 oz	620	35	67
Apple Danish, 5 oz	450	18	67
Apple Pie: *See Pies/Tarts Page 134*			
Baklava, 1½" square, 1.75 oz	200	10	27
Banana with Butter Cream, 2 oz	230	9	37
Banana Walnut, 3 oz	270	11	40
Bear Claw, 4½ oz	540	24	71
Black Forest, 3 oz (1/12)	345	11	59
Brownie: Small, 2" Square, 1 oz	130	8	14
Large, 3 oz	390	24	42
Bundt, average all types			
1 slice 3 oz (1/10)	300	13	42
Mini-Bundt, 5 oz	500	22	70
Cannoli	375	17	44
Carrot Cake: Plain, 3 oz	300	16	37
with Cream Cheese Frosting	400	22	48
Cheesecake: Small serving, 3 oz	235	13	26
Large serving, 5 oz	395	21	44
with Low-Fat Cheese/Fruit, 3 oz	170	4	28
Cheesecake Factory: 1 slice	630	45	53
Denny's Cheesecake, 1 slice	580	38	51
Chocolate Cake:			
Plain, w/o frosting, 1/12 of 9", 3½ oz	340	14	51
with chocolate frosting, 4 oz	415	18	62
Chocolate Croissant, 4¼ oz	470	26	54
Chocolate Eclair with Custard, 3½ oz	260	16	24
Chocolate Fudge Cake, 3 oz	270	12	40
Chocolate Meringue, 1/6 pie	320	13	48
Churros, 1 stick, 1½ oz	125	5	18
Cinnamon Crumb Cake, 2½ oz	260	9	40
Cinnamon Roll: Small, 2 oz	220	8	34
Regular, 4 oz	440	16	68
Large, 6 oz	660	24	102
Brands ~ *See Page 67*			
Coffee Cake, 2 oz	180	6	30
Concha: Small, 2 oz	240	9	33
Large (5" diameter), 5½ oz	615	23	85
Cream Puff (custard fill), 4.6 oz	335	20	30
Creme Horns, each, 3 oz	210	5	36
Crumble Coffee Cake, 4½ oz	500	25	65
Danish Pastry:			
Small, 2½ oz	250	14	25
Large, 5 oz	500	28	50
onuts: *See Page 66*			
lair, Choc., Custard fill, 3½ oz	260	16	24
Bars, average, each	160	3	31

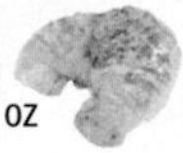
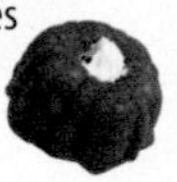
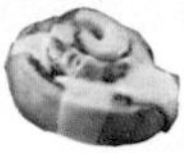
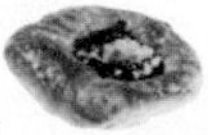

Ready-to-Eat (Cont)

	C	F	Cb
Fruit Cake, Dark/Light, 2 oz	185	5	34
Fudge Nut Brownie, each, 3½ oz	380	18	54
Gingerbread: From mix, 3" square	210	4	41
Honey Bun, each, 2.7 oz	310	15	39
Jelly Roll, 1/12 roll, 1.8 oz	150	2	32
Key Lime Pie, 4.3 oz	400	25	41
Kolacky, Apricot/Raspberry, ½ oz (1)	60	3.5	8
Lady Fingers, 3 oz	310	4.5	59
Lemon Cake, 4 oz	440	24	49
Lemon Poppy Seed Creme, 1.6 oz	180	9	23
Marble Cake, 1 slice, 4 oz	430	23	50
Mississippi Mud Pie, 4 oz	480	22	67
Mud Cake, 1 piece, 4½ oz	380	20	44
Muffins: *See Page 67*			
Palmier Cookie, large, 4½ oz	490	25	62
Pineapple Upside Down, 2½ oz	230	9	36
Peach Melba, 3½ oz	300	8	52
Pecan Sticky Roll, 6½ oz	690	22	91
Pecan Twirls, 1 piece, 1.3 oz	170	7	26
Pies & Tarts: *See Page 134*			
Pound Cakes: Iced Lemon, 3½ oz	360	17	50
Marble, 3¾ oz	350	13	53
Raspberry Rugulah,			
1 piece, 1.2 oz	110	9	7
Scone, fruit, 2 oz	200	9	30
Sponge: Plain, 2½ oz	220	10	33
with Cream & Strawberry Jam	390	12	69
with Chocolate Frosting	290	12	45
Starbucks Cakes ~ Page 244			
Strawberry Creme, 4.7 oz	400	27	33
Strudel Bites, ¾ oz	60	2.5	9
Strudel, fruit, average, 4.4 oz	300	17	32
Sweet Roll, average, 1½ oz	150	6	23
Swiss Rolls, (2)	270	12	38
Tiramisu, 4.4 oz	440	22	34
Turnovers, fruit, average, 3 oz	290	15	35

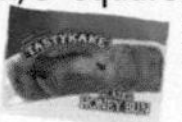

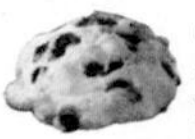
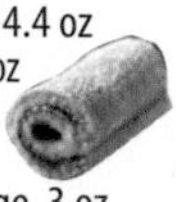

Cupcakes

	C	F	Cb
Average all Varieties			
Regular:			
Cake only, 1½ oz	140	5.5	20
Cake + Icing, 2½ oz	260	13	34
Large *(Muffin Size):*			
Cake only, 2½ oz	235	9	34
Cake + Icing, 5 oz	520	27	67
Mini (2-Bite):			
Cake only, 0.4 oz	40	1.5	5.5
Cake + Icing, 1 oz	110	5.5	13
Icing Only: Per 1 oz	115	7	13
Thick/Tall amount, 2½ oz	290	17	32
Very Berry	350	10	58

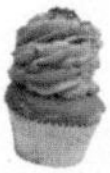
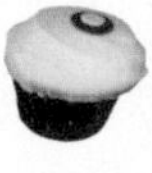
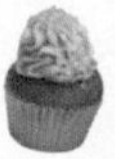

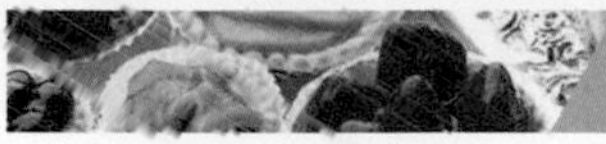

Cakes ~ Brands

	C	F	Cb

Albertson's Bakery
Ring Cakes: *Per ⅛ Cake*

	C	F	Cb
Angle Food, 2 oz	160	0	36
Butter, 3 oz	310	16	39
Chocolate, 3 oz	300	14	38

Cake Slices:

Banana Nut Loaf	310	16	37
Butter Creme	110	6	20
Creme Cake (2), 3.17 oz	300	12	43
Cinnamon Streusel (2), 3.17 oz	350	18	43

Bimbo

Concha, Vanilla, 2.1 oz	260	11	35
Mini Pound Cake, 1.76 oz	170	4.5	29
Pecan Pound Cake, 2.25 oz	260	11	36
Raisin Pound Cake, 2.25 oz	240	9	38

Bon Appetit

Banana Bread	440	25	49
Cheese Coffee Cake, 4 oz	480	26	56
Walnut Brownie, 3.5 oz	380	18	54
Sliced: Cheesecake, 4 oz	430	24	49
Lemon Cake, 4 oz	430	24	49
Marble Cake, 4 oz	430	24	50
Danish: Apple (1), 5 oz	420	22	50
Bear Claw (1), 5 oz	480	26	54
Cheese & Berries (1), 5 oz	500	28	52
Vienna Cream (1), 5 oz	480	28	54
Claim Jumper: Carrot Cake, 4.6 oz	450	24	54
Choc. Motherload Cake, 5.3 oz	520	27	73

Cheesecake Factory: *See Fast-Foods Section*

Entenmann's

Cheese-Filled Crumb Coffee, 1.9 oz	200	10	25
Chocolate Fudge, ⅛, 2.5 oz	270	11	40
Crumb Coffee, ⅒, 2 oz	260	13	34
Louisiana Crunch, ⅑	330	14	49
Pecan Danish Ring, ⅛	240	15	24
Raspb. Danish Twist, ⅛	220	11	29

Enten-Minis:

Butterscotch (2), 2 oz	250	10	37
Carrot (2), 2.8 oz	330	15	46
Choc. Creme Cupcake (2), 2.8 oz	310	11	50
Sponge Creme Cupcake (2), 2.3 oz	260	12	36

Muffins/Sweet Rolls: *See Page 67*

Glenny's
100 Calorie Brownie: *Per Brownie*

Regular, 1.4 oz	100	4	12
Blondie, 1.4 oz	100	4	15
Peanut Butter, 1.4 oz	100	4	15

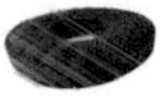

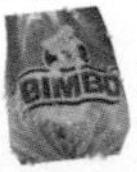

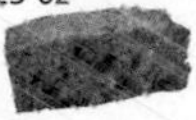

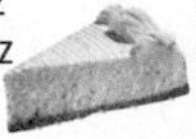

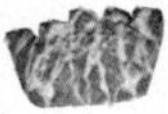

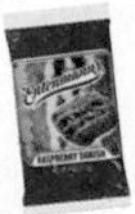

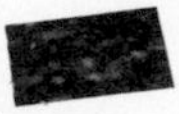

Great American Cookies
Cookie Cakes: *Per Slice*

	C	F	Cb
By the Slice, 4.6 oz	580	27	83
Heart Shaped, 3.5 oz	440	21	64
M&M, 1 slice, 4 oz	500	24	73

Hershey's:

Brownies: Hershey's	380	18	56
Reese's	380	18	54

Hostess:

100 Calorie Packs, Coffee Cakes, Cinnamon Streusel (3)	100	3	21
Cinnamon Streusel Cake (1)	170	5	29
Chocodiles	240	11	33
Cup Cake: Choc. (1), 1.76 oz	180	6	30
Orange (1), 3.74 oz	410	14	68
Ding Dongs (2), 2.82 oz	360	19	47
Ho Ho's (3), 3 oz	370	17	54
Snoballs (2)	360	11	61
Suzy Q, 2 cakes, 4 oz	460	19	70
Twinkies, 1 cake, 1.5 oz	150	4.5	27
Fried Twinkie	360	28	26

Zingers:

Chocolate (1)	150	5	25
Devils Food (3)	440	15	74
Raspberry (3)	480	20	71
Vanilla (3)	470	16	81

Kroger

Cinnamon Rolls: with Icing	160	6	22
Reduced Fat	140	3.5	24

Little Debbie

100 Calories: Choc. Cake (1), 1 oz	100	3	17
Yellow Cake w. Icing (1), 1 oz	100	3	18
Brownies, Fudge (1), 2.15 oz	280	12	40
Chocolate Cup Cake	210	8	33
Coffee Cakes (1)	200	6	35
Devil Cremes (1) 1.65 oz	200	9	29
Devil Squares, 2 cakes, 2.2 oz	260	11	38
Fancy Cakes (2)	300	13	44
Frosted Fudge , 1.5 oz cake	190	9	27
Star Crunch (1)	150	6	22
Smores (1)	190	7	30
Strawberry Shortcake Rolls, 2.1 oz	240	9	40
Swiss Cake Rolls (2), 2.15 oz	270	12	39
Zebra Cakes, 2 cakes, 2.6 oz	320	14	

Nemo's

Banana Cake, 3 oz	300	12	
Chocolate Cake, 3 oz	300		
Carrot Cake, 3.6 oz	390		

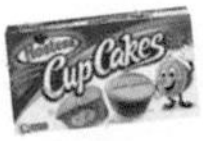

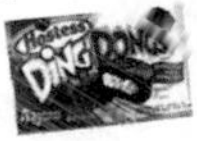

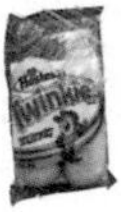

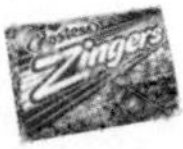

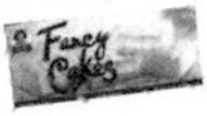

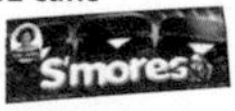

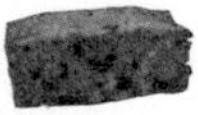

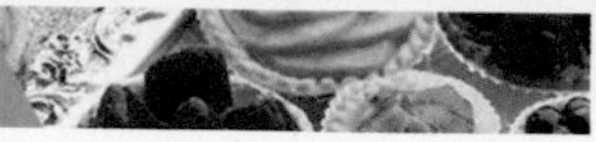

C Cakes, Pastries ~ Packaged

Cakes ~ Brands (Cont)

Item	C	F	Cb
Oreo			
Cakesters,			
2-cake package, 2 oz	250	12	36
Pillsbury			
Sweet Moments Brownies (Frozen):			
Bite Sized, Choc. Caramel/ Fudge, 3 pcs	180	9	25
Molten Lava: Chocolate Caramel, 1 pc.	360	18	48
Chocolate Fudge, 1 piece	370	19	47
Pepperidge Farm			
3-Layer Cakes:			
Chocolate Fudge, ⅛ cake	230	10	33
Coconut, ⅛	240	10	35
Fudge/Golden, ⅛ cake, av.	230	9	34
Dumplings: Apple (1)	230	11	29
Peach (1)	250	11	34
Turnovers (Frozen): Apple, 3.15 oz	270	15	31
Raspberry, 3.15 oz	280	15	34
Safeway Select			
Molten Chocolate Lava Cake, 4½ oz	440	26	50
Sara Lee			
Cheesecake: *Per Slice*			
French Strawberry, ⅙	320	18	37
New York Style Classic, ⅙ cake	480	30	47
Original Cream Cherry, ¼ cake	320	11	50
Original Cream, ¼ cake	320	17	36
Original Cream Strawberry, ¼ cake	310	11	49
Coffee Cakes:			
Banana, ⅕ cake	280	10	46
Carrot, ⅙ cake	340	18	41
Deluxe Cinnamon Rolls with Icing (1)	260	12	33
Pecan Cake, ⅙ cake	190	10	22
Layer Cakes: *Per ⅛ Whole*			
Chocolate Gold, ⅛ cake	320	14	46
Layer Coconut, ⅛ cake, 2.7 oz	290	12	44
Layer Double Chocolate, ⅛ cake	290	9	49
Layer Vanilla, ⅛ cake	260	14	32
Pound Cakes: *Per ¼ of Cake*			
All Butter	300	16	35
Free & Light	220	4	41
Strawberry Swirl	225	7.5	38
ites: *Per* Serving			
riginal: (1)	20	1	3
(25)	440	27	44
wberry (1)	20	1	2
	430	25	45
oc. Fudge Brownie (1)	90	4	12

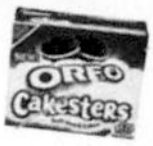

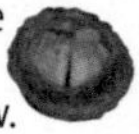
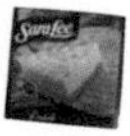
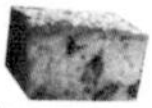
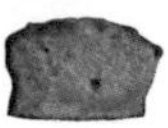

Item	C	F	Cb
Smart Ones (Weight Watchers)			
Brownie à la Mode	200	4	36
Chocolate Eclair	140	4	24
Choc. Chip Cookie Dough Sundae	170	3	32
Double Fudge Cake	170	4	31
Key Lime Pie, 3.3 oz	190	4.5	33
Mint Choc Chip Sundae, 2½ oz	150	3	28
Mocha Fudge Sundae, 2½ oz	160	4	27
Peanut Butter Sundae, 2½ oz	170	5	28
Strawberry Shortcake, 3½ oz	170	6	25
Starbucks: *See Page 244*			
Tastykake			
Creme Filled Cupcakes:			
Chocolate: (3), 3.5 oz	390	15	59
with Vanilla Icing (3), 3.5 oz	390	15	60
Crumb Topped Koffee (3), 3.5 oz	370	17	52
Kandy Kake (3), 2 oz	270	16	30
Krimpets, Butterscotch (3), 3 oz	350	10	60
Trader Joe's			
Bakery:			
Almond Ring Cake, ⅛, 1.8 oz	250	13	30
Apple Streudel, ⅙, 3.5 oz	240	12	32
Apricot Almond Tart, ⅙, 4 oz	450	24	56
Bundt, Tripple Chocolate, ½	340	21	41
Cheesecake Brownie Bites (1)	110	7	9
Flourless Choc. Cake, 1 pce, 2 oz	260	17	23
Lemon Cake, ⅛, 3.25 oz	350	19	43
Mini Carrot Cake, 5 oz	450	19	68
Whoopie Pie (1), 2.5 oz	350	14	54
Bread Cake:			
Banana Bonanza, ⅙, 2.65 oz	250	9	39
Carrot Zuccini, 1/11, 2 oz	170	3.5	39
Walnut Streusel Coffee, 1/12, 2 oz	180	8	25
Loaf Cakes:			
Cranberry Pumpkin, ⅛, 2 oz	140	2	30
Pumpkin Nut, ⅐, 2.65 oz	270	10	43
Frozen Dessert:			
Apple Raspb. Turnovers, 3.17 oz	280	14	34
Cheesecake: Plain, 3.5 oz	320	19	30
Choc Chip, 3.5 oz	350	20	36
Triple Choc, 3.5 oz	340	19	34
Tuxedo, 3.5 oz	320	17	34
Chocolate Ganache, ⅛, 3.5 oz	420	26	50
Choc Lava Cake (1), 3.8 oz	360	23	40
Karat Cake, ⅛, 2.9 oz	320	19	37
N.Y. Style Cheesecake, ⅐, 4.5 oz	400	28	32
Tiramisu Torte, ⅐, 3.2 oz	230	12	24
Tarts: Apple, ⅙, 3.5 oz	210	8	33
Raspberry, ¼, 4.83 oz	290	10	51

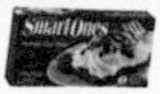
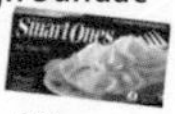
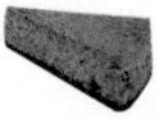

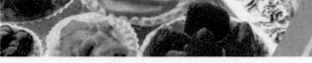

Cakes ~ Mixes

Prepared As Directed

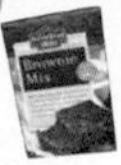

Arrowhead Mills	C	F	Cb
Dessert Mix, Brownie, 1/20 pkg	150	8	21
Organic Cooking Mix, Choc. Chip, 0.7 oz	90	4	16
Gluten Free: Brownie, 1/20 pkg	160	9	21
Choc Chip (1), 0.7 oz	110	3.5	16
Betty Crocker			
Cakes (Super Moist): *Per 1/12 Cake*			
Butter Recipe Yellow	250	12	35
Carrot	260	14	35
Cherry Chip	230	7	35
Chocolate varieties	270	13	34
Devil's Food	260	13	35
White	220	6	35
Other flavors, average	270	13	35

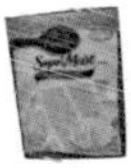

If using No Cholesterol Recipe, deduct 40 cals and 4g fat.

	C	F	Cb
Other Cakes: Pound Cake, 1/8	290	13	48
Gingerbread Cake, 1/8	220	6	39
Pineapple Upside Down, 1/6	390	12	65
Sunkist Lemon Bar (1)	140	4	24
Brownie Mix: *Per 1/20 Pkg*			
Dark Chocolate Fudge	160	10	24
Fudge	170	6.5	23
Low-Fat Fudge, 1/18 pkg	140	3	28
Supreme: Original	160	7	26
Chocolate Chunk	180	8	25
Peanut Butter; Walnut, average	180	10	23
Triple Chunk	180	8	25
Pouch Mix: *Per 2 Cookies*			
Chocolate Chip	170	8	21
Double Chocolate Chunk	150	6	21
Oatmeal	160	7	22
Oatmeal Chocolate Chip	160	8	21
Peanut Butter	150	8	20
Rainbow Chocolate Candy	160	7	22
Sugar Cookie	160	8	21
Walnut Chocolate Chip	170	9	21
Warm Delights: *Per Bowl*			
Cinnamon Swirl, 3.3 oz	390	10	72
Lemon Swirl, 3.6 oz	380	9	72
Molten Caramel, 3.4 oz	360	10	64
Molten Chocolate 3.4 oz	370	12	61

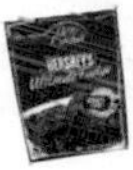

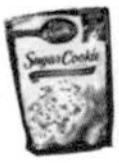

Duncan Hines	C	F	Cb
Brownie Mix: *Per 1 oz Brownie, Prepared*			
Decadent, Caramel Turtle	150	7	23
Premium: Chewy Fudge	170	8	24
Milk Chocolate	170	9	22
Cake Mix: *Prepared, 1/12 Pkg.*			
Moist Deluxe Cake:			
Banana Supreme	270	12	36
Classic Yellow	270	12	36
Coconut Supreme	250	11	34
Dark Choc. Fudge/Devil's Food	290	15	35
French Vanilla	270	12	34
Jell-O No Bake Cheesecakes: *Prep'd As Directed*			
Cherry, 1/8 pkg	300	13	48
Homestyle Chsecake, 1/6	360	15	45
Real Cheesecake, 1/6 pkg	360	18	40
Strawberry, 1/8 pkg	300	13	48
Krusteaz: Cinn. Crumb Cake, 1"	220	7	38
Lemon/Key Lime Bar, 2" bar	150	3.5	29
Pillsbury			
Moist Supreme: *Per 1/12 Pkg, Dry Mix Only*			
Classic White/Yellow	170	3.5	35
Devils Food	160	2.5	35
Brownie Mix: *Dry Mix Only*			
Caramel Swirl, 1/12 pkt, 1.2 oz	130	2.5	27
Cheesecake Swirl, 1/18 pkt, 0.85 oz	100	2.5	20
Chocolate Extreme, 1/16 pkt, 1 oz	120	3	22
Mint Chocolate, 1/15 pkt, 1 oz	110	2.5	22

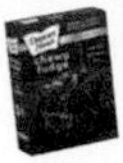

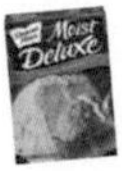

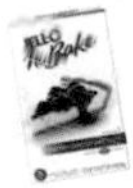

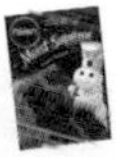

Cake Frostings

Betty Crocker	C	F	Cb
Rich & Creamy, av., 2 T.	140	5	23
Whipped, all flavors, 2 T.	100	4.5	15
Duncan Hines:			
Creamy Homestyle, av. all flav., 2T.	140	6	23
Whipped, avg., 3 Tbsp	150	7	22
Pillsbury: *Per 2 Tbsp (approx. 1/12 Tub)*			
Creamy Supreme: Choc Fudge	140	6	21
Classic White	140	6	23
Milk Choc	140	6	21
Vanilla; Vanilla Funfetti	150	6	25
Red. Sugar: Choc. Fudge, 2 Tbsp	100	6	17
Vanilla, 2 Tbsp	120	7	18
Whipped Supreme, avg all flavors	100	5	14

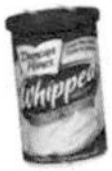

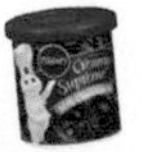

Quick Guide   C   F   Cb

Donuts
Average All Brands

	C	F	Cb
Plain, 1¾ oz	210	12	25
Sugared, 1¾ oz	220	11	27
Glazed, 2 oz	250	12	34
Chocolate Iced, 2 oz	260	14	29

Donuts ~ Brands   C   F   Cb

Albertson's

	C	F	Cb
Donut Holes: Glazed Old Fash. (4)	260	16	26
Powdered Sugar (4) 1.7 oz	210	12	24
Gem Donuts: Plain Cake (3) 1.6 oz	190	12	20
Cinnamon Sugar (3), 1.83 oz	240	15	23
Glazed (1), 1.6 oz	140	6	21

Bon Appetit

	C	F	Cb
Cherry Donuts (1) 2 oz	280	18	28
Mini Donuts: Chocolate (4)	270	16	29
Powdered; Crumb, average (4)	245	12	33

Dolly Madison

	C	F	Cb
Regular, 1¾ oz	270	12	40
Donut Gems,			
Powdered Mini's (4), 2 oz	230	11	31

Dunkin' Donuts

	C	F	Cb
Apple N' Spice	240	11	32
Blueberry Cake	330	18	38
Boston Kreme	280	12	38
Chocolate Frosted Cake	340	19	38
Chocolate Glazed Cake	280	15	33
Cinnamon Cake	290	18	30
Glazed Cake	320	18	37
Jelly Filled	260	11	36
Old Fashioned Cake	280	18	27
Powdered Cake	300	18	30
Sugar Raised	190	9	22
Vanilla Kreme Filled	320	17	37

Entenmann's

	C	F	Cb
Crumb, 2 oz	350	12	36
Frosted Devil's, 2.36 oz	310	18	36
Glazed Buttermilk, 2¼ oz	270	13	37

Donuts ~ Brands (Cont)   C   F   Cb

Entenmann's (Cont)

	C	F	Cb
Plain, 1½ oz	190	11	21
Rich Frosted, 2 oz	300	20	30

Pop'ems (bite size): *Per 4 pieces*

	C	F	Cb
Frosted, 2.1 oz	320	23	28
Glazed, 1.83 oz	220	10	30
Popettes: Cinnamon (4), 2 oz	250	13	31
Glazed Krullers (2), 1.62 oz	210	12	25

Hostess

	C	F	Cb
Dunkin Stix (3)	490	25	63
Donut Bites, 1 pouch, 2.3 oz	300	15	39
Regular: Plain, 1.4 oz	160	9	18
Choc. Frosted, 2 oz	240	14	27
Powdered, 1.7 oz	190	9	25
Old Fashioned Glazed, 2.1 oz	260	13	33
Donettes: Frosted (4) 2.15 oz	270	17	29
Crumb (3), 2 oz	220	9	32
Crunch (6), 4 oz	360	16	32
Krullers (3), 2.25 oz	270	14	34
Powdered (4), 2.15 oz	230	11	31

Krispy Kreme

	C	F	Cb
Chocolate Glazed Cruller	290	15	37
Chocolate Iced Glazed	250	12	33
Chocolate Iced Kreme Filled	350	20	39
Chocolate Iced w. Sprinkles	270	12	38
Cinnamon Twist	240	15	23
Glazed Cruller	240	14	26
Glazed Kreme Filled	340	20	39
Maple Iced Glazed	240	12	32
New York Cheesecake	340	20	34
Original Glazed	200	12	22
Powdered Cake	290	14	37
Traditional Cake Doughnut	230	13	25
Glazed Doughnut Holes, Orig., (5)	200	11	25

Little Debbie

	C	F	Cb
Donut Sticks (2), 1.65 oz	230	14	25

Tastykake

	C	F	Cb
Cinnamon, 1.8 oz	210	11	26
Mini: Coated, 3 oz	380	22	42
Powdered Sugar (6) 2½ oz	280	13	37

Quick Guide | C | F | Cb

Muffins: Ready-To-Eat
Average All Types:

	C	F	Cb
Small, 1 oz	80	3	12
Medium, 2 oz	160	6	24
Large, 3 oz	240	9	36
Extra Large, 4 oz	320	12	48
Giant, 6 oz	480	18	72
Super Size, 8 oz	640	24	96

Brands ~ Ready-To-Eat

	C	F	Cb
Albertsons: *Mini Muffins, Per 1.76 oz*			
Banana Nut (2)	200	12	20
Blueberry (2)	180	10	21
Honey Raisin Bran (2)	170	7	24
Awrey's: Blueberry, 2.5 oz	240	12	31
Raisin Bran, 1.5 oz muffin	160	8	23
Controlled Carb Gourmet			
Almond Blueberry Muffins, 3 oz	210	15	27
Entenmann's:			
Little Bites, Blueberry, 1 pkt,	180	8	25
Chocolate Chip, 1 packet	190	9	26
Hostess: Mini, 1 pouch, average	260	15	30
Fruit Pie/Tart, average, 4.5 oz	480	20	69
Muffin Loaf: Blueberry, 3.8 oz	440	19	62
Banana Nut, 3.8 oz	460	24	56
100 Calorie Packs:			
Cinnamon Streusel	100	3	21
Twinkie Bites (3)	100	2.5	18
Little Debbie: Banana Nut (1), 1.9 oz	210	9	30
Blueberry (1), 1.9 oz	190	8	27
Chocolate Chip (1), 1.9 oz	210	9	28
My Favorite Muffin:			
Chocolate Chip, 6 oz	635	33	81
Fat-Free, Blueberry; Cherry Pie, 6 oz	325	0	78
Otis Spunkmeyer: *Per Whole 4 oz Muffin*			
Banana Nut	440	22	58
Chocolate Chip	440	22	56
Wild Blueberry	400	16	56
Starbucks: *See Fast-Foods Section*			
Trader Joe's:			
Apple Craberry, ½ 68g	110	2.5	19
Banana Chocolate Chip, 4 oz	400	18	57
Blueberry Bran, ½, 68g	110	2.5	19
Carrot, 4 oz	320	11	52
Cranberry Mango Blueberry, ½, 68g	110	2.5	19
Triple Berry (1), 4 oz	310	11	49
Mini: Blueberry, 0.8 oz	110	6	12
Bran w. Raisin, 0.8 oz	80	3	13
Weight Watchers: Blueb., 2.5 oz	190	2.5	42
Double Chocolate, 2.5 oz	180	3	41

Muffin Mixes | C | F | Cb

Prepared: Per Muffin

	C	F	Cb
Betty Crocker: Apple Streusel	230	8	37
Banana Nut	210	10	27
Cinnamon Streusel	210	9	28
Wild Blueberry	180	8	26
Pouch Mix: Choc Chip	130	3.5	22
Blueb.; Lemon Poppyseed, avg.	120	2.5	23
Cornbread	160	9	24
Krusteaz: Banana Nut	220	3.5	32
Choc Chip	180	4	34
Lem. Poppyseed	170	4	30
Oatbran (1)	180	4.5	31
Sunmaid: English, Honey Raisin	170	0.5	36
Trader Joe's: Triple Berry, ½2	150	2	28

Sweet Rolls & Buns | C | F | Cb

Note: It is best to weigh for accuracy as actual
weight can be 10-50% higher than label weight·

	C	F	Cb
Bimbo, Bimbolete (1), 2.2 oz	240	9	36
Bon Appetit, Cinn. Roll, 5 oz	690	40	78
Cinnabon: Classic	815	32	117
Caramel Pecanbon	1100	47	156
Minibon, 1 roll	340	13	49
CinnaPretzel	750	6	156
Cinnabon Stix (5) w/out frosting	410	23	46
with Frosting	590	34	66
Cloverhill Bakery			
Jumbo Honey Bun, 4.75 oz	600	35	64
Entenmann's: Cinn. Bun (1), 3 oz	330	13	49
Hostess:			
Cinnamon Sweet Roll (1)	200	6	34
Honey Bun, Glazed:			
Net weight, 3.75 oz	410	22	50
Actual weight, 4.65 oz	510	27	62
Iced/Frosted, 3.5 oz	410	24	42
Little Debbie:			
Honey Buns, 1.76 oz	230	13	26
Pecan Spinwheels, 1 oz	100	4	16
McDonald's: Cinnamon Melts, 4 oz	460	19	66
Pillsbury: Cinnamon Roll, w. Icing	140	5	23
Reduced Fat (1) 1.5 oz	130	3.5	24
Ralph's, Cinnamon Roll, 2.5 oz	290	11	44
7-Eleven, Iced Honey Bun, 4.75 oz	520	24	71
Zen Bakery: Cinn. Raisin Roll (1), 3.2 oz	230	2	48

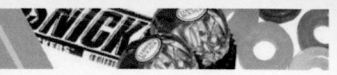

Quick Guide

Chocolate **C** **F** **Cb**
Average All Brands
Milk Chocolate, regular:

	C	F	Cb
Plain/Nuts/Fruit, average, 1 oz	**155**	**10**	**16**
1½ oz Bar	**225**	**15**	**24**
2 oz Bar	**310**	**20**	**32**
4 oz Block	**620**	**40**	**64**
8 oz Block	**1240**	**80**	**128**
1 Pound, 16 oz	**2480**	**160**	**256**
Dark/White Chocolate, 1 oz	**155**	**9**	**17**
Sugar Free *(Hershey's)* 1 piece, 0.3 oz	**40**	**2**	**5**

Chocolate-coated:

	C	F	Cb
Almonds, 5-6, 1 oz	**155**	**9**	**16**
Clusters, Nut, 3 pieces, 1.2 oz	**210**	**14**	**20**
Coffee Beans, 1.4 oz	**220**	**13**	**22**
Creme/Cordial Centers, 1.26 oz	**170**	**6**	**28**
Fudge, 1.5 oz	**220**	**13**	**27**
Macadamias, 10 pieces, 1.4 oz	**220**	**16**	**21**
Mints, 1 medium, ½ oz	**55**	**1**	**11**
Nougat & Caramel, 1 oz	**150**	**9**	**15**
Peanuts, 12 medium, 1 oz	**150**	**10**	**15**
Raisins, 28 medium, 1 oz	**110**	**4**	**19**

Cooking Chocolate:

	C	F	Cb
Sweet/Semi-sweet, 1 oz	**140**	**9**	**16**
4 oz Bar *(Baker's)*	**480**	**28**	**64**
Chips: 1 Tbsp, ½ oz	**70**	**4**	**9**
½ cup, 3 oz	**420**	**24**	**54**
Unsweetened, 1 oz	**140**	**14**	**8**
Carob: Plain, 1 oz	**150**	**9**	**16**

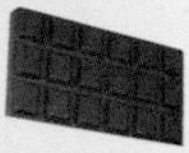

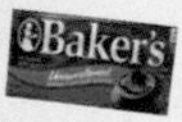

Brands & Generic **C** **F** **Cb**

Per Piece/Serving

	C	F	Cb
3 Musketeers: 1 bar, 2.13 oz	**260**	**8**	**46**
Minis, 7 pieces, 1.4 oz	**170**	**5**	**32**
100 Calorie Bars *(Hershey's)*, 0.6 oz	**100**	**6**	**11**
100 Grand: 1.5 oz bar	**190**	**8**	**30**
Super Size, 2.8 oz	**360**	**14**	**58**
Snack Size (1), ¾ oz	**100**	**4**	**15**
Abba Zabba, 2 oz bar	**250**	**5**	**48**
After Dinner Mints, 1 small	**25**	**1.5**	**3**
After Eight Mint *(Nestlé)*, each	**35**	**1.5**	**4**
Air Head, 1 bar, ½ oz	**60**	**1**	**15**
Almond Joy: 2 bars, 1.6 oz	**220**	**13**	**26**
King Size, 2 bars, 1.62 oz	**230**	**13**	**27**
Snack, 0.6 oz bar	**80**	**4.5**	**10**
Egg (1), 1.1 oz	**150**	**8**	**18**
Pieces (46), 1.4 oz	**200**	**10**	**27**

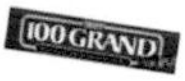

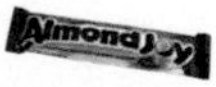

Brands & Generic (Cont)

Per Piece/Serving **C** **F** **Cb**

	C	F	Cb
Almond Roca, 3 pieces, 1.27 oz	**200**	**15**	**17**
Almonds, sugar-coated (15), 1.4 oz	**190**	**7**	**27**
Almond Clusters *(Trader Joe's)*,			
2 pieces, 1.2 oz	**210**	**14**	**15**
Altoids *(C & B)*, 3 pieces	**10**	**0**	**2**
Andes, Thins, av., all flav. (8), 1.4 oz	**200**	**13**	**22**
Anthon Berg: Cognac, each	**180**	**8**	**25**
Creamy Mint (4), 1.4 oz	**180**	**6**	**31**
Marzipan with Madeira, 1.4 oz	**175**	**7.5**	**26**
Marzipan Brod	**120**	**7**	**13**
Atomic Fireball, 1 piece, 0.3 oz	**35**	**0**	**9**
Baby Ruth: King Size, 3.7 oz bar	**500**	**24**	**66**
2.1 oz bar	**280**	**14**	**39**
Fun size, 2 bars	**170**	**8**	**24**
Minis, 4 bars	**210**	**9**	**30**
Baci *(Perugino):* 1 piece, ½ oz	**75**	**6**	**7**
3 pieces, 1½ oz	**230**	**17**	**22**
Baskin-Robbins:			
Sugar Free, 4 pieces, 0.6 oz av	**40**	**1**	**15**
Big Hunk, 2 oz	**230**	**3**	**47**
Bit-O-Honey, 1.7 oz	**180**	**3.5**	**39**
Chews, 6 pieces, 1.4 oz	**150**	**3**	**32**
Bliss *(Hershey's):* Milk/Dark Choc. 6 pcs	**210**	**14**	**25**
Dark Chocolate Bar (1), 1.25 oz	**160**	**12**	**21**
Milk Choc: Meltaway Center, 6 pieces	**220**	**15**	**24**
Bar (1), 1.25 oz	**180**	**12**	**20**
Blow Pops, ea., 0.6 oz	**60**	**0**	**17**
Bon Bons, 3 pieces	**65**	**0**	**15**
Boston Baked Beans, 11 pieces, ½ oz	**70**	**2**	**11**
Brach's: Almond Supremes (11)	**210**	**13**	**21**
Bridge Mix, 16 pieces, 1.4 oz	**180**	**9**	**26**
Chocolate Peanut Cluster, 3 pieces	**210**	**14**	**19**
Double Dippers (15), 1.4 oz	**210**	**14**	**19**
Maple Nut Goodies (8)	**190**	**9**	**27**
Milk Maid Caramel (4), 1.37 oz	**160**	**4.5**	**27**
Orange Slices (30), 1.6 oz	**150**	**0**	**37**
Special Treasure Butter Toffee (3)	**50**	**1**	**11**
Breath Savers, all types, each	**5**	**0**	**2**
Bubble Gum: *See 'Gum' Page 75*			
Bulls Eyes, 3 pieces, 1.2 oz	**130**	**3**	**23**
Buncha Crunch: ⅓ cup, 1.4 oz	**180**	**8**	**26**
Movie Box, 3.2 oz	**450**	**20**	**65**
Burnt Peanuts, 31 pieces, 1.4 oz	**170**	**6**	**29**

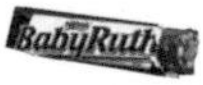

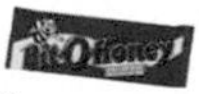

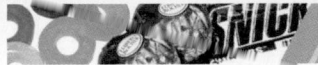

Brands & Generic (Cont)

Per Piece/Serving	C	F	Cb
Butterfinger: 2.1 oz bar	270	11	43
King Size (3), 3.7 oz	480	18	75
Fun Size, (1), 0.75	100	4	15
Giant, (Pieces in Chocolate),			
¼ Bar, 1.1 oz	150	8	21
Miniatures: 1 piece, 0.35 oz	45	2	7.5
4 pieces, 1.4 oz	180	8	29
Snack Pack, 4 bars, 1.4 oz	180	7	29
Crisp Bar: Original, 2.1 oz	270	11	43
King Size, 2 oz	310	17	38
Minis, 2 bars	210	11	25
Snackerz: Single, 1 pouch, 1.25 oz	170	8	23
Fun Size, 2 pouches, 1.2 oz	150	7	21
King Size, 10 pieces, 1.4 oz	190	8	25
Butter Mints, 7 pieces, 0.46 oz	50	0	12
Butterscotch: 3 pieces	60	0	15
Chips (Hershey's), 1 f.	80	4	10
Discs (Walgreens), 3 pieces, 0.63 oz	70	0	17
Cadbury: Caramello Bar, 1.6 oz	220	10	29
Dairy Milk Bar, 7 pieces, 1.4 oz	200	11	23
Mini Eggs, 12 pieces, 1.4 oz	190	8	28
Candy Apple, medium, 6.5 oz	280	0	60
Candy Cane, medium, 5", ½ oz	40	0	10
Candy Corn, 20 pieces	150	0	38
Candy Jar Mix (Jewel) (3), 0.6 oz	60	0	14
Candy Necklaces,each, 0.7 oz	80	0	20
Caramello Bar (Cadbury), 1.6 oz	220	10	29
Caramels: each, 0.35 oz	40	1	8
Chocolate, each, 0.23 oz	25	0.3	6
Creams: 3 pieces, 1¼ oz	130	3	23
Caramel Popcorn, ⅔ cup	150	6	23
Cella's Cherries, 3 pieces, 1.52 oz	160	6	27
Certs, Breath Mints, 1 piece	5	0	2
Charleston Chew: 1 bar, 1.4 oz	160	4.5	30
Mini, 1.5 oz	190	6	34
Charms: Blow Pop	60	0	17
Flat Pop, ½ oz	50	0	14
Chew-ets Peanut Chews:			
Original, 4 pieces,1.65 oz	230	12	29
Chewz, 1 roll, 1 oz	120	1	28
Chick O Stick, 2 oz	240	9	42
Chocolate Parfait Nips, 2 pieces	60	2	11

Per Piece/Serving	C	F	Cb
Chunky Bar (Nestlé),			
King Size, 2½ oz	370	21	41
Chupa Chups, 1 Pop	50	0	12
Cinn. Buttons (Walgreens), 3 pieces	60	0	18
Cinnamon Disks (Walmart), 3 pieces	70	0	18
Circus Peanuts, Marshmallow (Spangler),			
5 pieces, 1.35 oz	150	0	38
CocoaVia, Original, 0.8 oz	100	6	12
Coconut Stacks, 8 pieces	290	13	37
Coffee Go, Candie, 4 pieces	60	1	12
Coffee Rio-Gold, Sugar Free, (4)	45	1.5	10
Conversation Hearts (Necco), 1 large	10	0	3
Cookie Dough Bites, 1.4 oz	200	10	27
Cote d'Or: Dark 86% Coca, 3.5 oz	605	55	19
Dark 70%, Orange, 3.5 oz	575	46	34
Dark Raspberry, 3.5 oz	580	46	34
Milk Intense, 3.5 oz	575	40	45
Cotton Candy, 1 oz	110	0	28
Cough Drops: See Page 75			
Cracker Jack, ½ cup, 1 oz	120	2	23
Creme Savers: See Lifesavers			
Crisped Rice, Choc Chip, 1 bar, 1 oz	115	4	20
Crows, 11 pieces, 1.4 oz	130	0	33
Crunch: Original, 1.55 oz bar	220	12	29
Fun Size, 1.34 oz	210	10	29
Miniatures: 6 pieces	180	9	25
Buncha Crunch, ⅓ cup, 1.3 oz	180	8	26
Crunch Crisp, 1.72 oz	240	13	32
Dots, 11 dots, 1.4 oz	130	0	33
Double Dip Stick, 1 stick	16	0.5	3
Dove			
Milk Choc: Singles Bar	200	12	22
Large Tablet Bar, 3.53 oz	540	33	60
Choc. Covered Almonds, 5 pieces	230	15	19
Promises: Plain, 1 piece, 0.3 oz	45	2.5	5
With Caramel, 1 piece, 0.3 oz	40	2	5
With Peanut Butter, 1 piece, 0.3 oz	40	2	5
Dark Choc: Singles Bar, 1.3 oz	190	12	22
Large Tablet Bar, 3.53 oz	510	33	60
Choc. Covered Almonds, 13 pieces	210	15	19
Promises: W/ Raspberry Cream, 1 pce	40	3	5
With Tiramisu, 1 piece, 0.3 oz	40	2	5
Sugar Free, all flavors, 5 pieces	190	15	22
Dum Dum Pops (Spangler), 1 pop	20	0	5

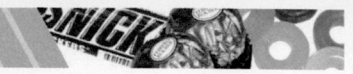

Brands & Generic (Cont)

Per Piece/Serving	C	F	Cb
English Toffee, 1 piece, 0.42 oz	70	4	6
Eda's Sugar Free, all flav., 5, ½ oz	40	0	15
5th Avenue: 2 oz bar	260	12	38
King Size bar	440	20	64
Fannie May: Single Wrapped Pieces			
Mint Meltaway, 1.51 oz	230	15	24
Mint Milk, 1.55 oz	190	6	32
Pixie (1), 1.51 oz	210	12	24
Trinidad, 1 piece, 1.5 1oz	200	12	23
Fast Break *(Reese's):* 2 oz bar	260	12	35
3.5 oz bar	460	22	62
Ferrero Rocher: each	75	5	5
3 pieces, 1.3 oz	220	16	16
Rondnoir (4), 1.4 oz	220	14	21
Fifty 50 Snack Bars:			
Almond, 7 pieces, 1.4 oz	210	17	18
Crunch Bar, 7 pieces, 1.1 oz	140	12	16
Dark Choc, 7 pieces, 1.4 oz	170	14	21
Milk Choc., 7 pieces, 1.4 oz	190	16	19
Peanut Butter, 1.2 oz	200	14	21
Fluffy Stuff *(Charms)*,1.4 oz	150	0	40
Fondant: Choc-coated, 1.2 oz	125	3	27
Mint, 1 oz	105	0	25
Fran's: Gold Bar Almond, 1.6 oz	250	14	27
GoldBite Almond, 0.8 oz	120	7	13
Frooties, 12 pieces, 1.4 oz	160	3.5	32
Fruit Drops, each, ¼ oz	20	0	4
Fruit Gems *(Sunkist)*, (4), 1.4 oz	130	0	33
Fruit Leathers, average, 0.5 oz	50	0.5	12
Fruit Pastilles *(Rowntree)*, 1 roll	185	0	45
Fruit Rolls, 1 roll	80	1	17
Fruit Roll-Ups, ½ oz	50	1	12
Fruit Runts *(Walgreens)*, 12 pieces	60	0	14
Fudge: Chocolate/Vanilla (1), 1 oz	120	4	20
With Nuts (1), 1 oz	145	9	15
Choco. Marshmallow, 1 oz	130	5	20
With Nuts, 1 oz	135	6	19
Peanut Butter, 1 oz	115	3	19
Ghirardelli:			
Squares: Dark Choc. (4), 1.6 oz	220	17	23
Milk & Caramel (3), 1.6 oz	220	12	27
3 oz Bars: Dark Choc., 4 squares	220	17	23
Filled, Peanut Butter, 4 squares	250	17	22
Intense Dark: Twilight Delight, 3 pcs	200	17	17
Evening Dream, 3 pieces	190	15	20

Per Piece/Serving	C	F	Cb
Godiva:			
Bars: Milk/Dark, av., 1½ oz	230	14	26
Extra Dark: 75%, 1½ oz	230	17	18
85%, 1.4 oz	260	21	14
Chocoiste:			
Dark Choc, Cherries (12)	190	7	30
Milk Choc, Cashews (14)	230	15	19
Hearts: Dark Ganache (4)	200	12	23
Milk Praline (4)	220	13	23
Go Lightly: Choc Lovers Asst. (2)	220	16	28
Bags: Assorted Taffy, 5 pieces	130	3	36
Vanilla Caramels, 5 pieces	150	6	32
Sugar Free Mint Creme Crunch (4)	150	5	33
Hard Candy (4), ½ oz	45	0	15
Goobers Peanuts, 1 package, 1.4 oz	200	13	21
Good & Plenty *(Hershey's)* 1.4 oz	140	0	35
GooGoo Clusters, 1 bar, 1.8 oz	230	12	30
Gum Drops: *1 small*, 0.1 oz	15	0	3
5 pieces, 0.63 oz	75	0	15
Gummi: Bears (22) 1.4 oz	150	0	34
Chewy Sweet Tarts (4), 1.5 oz	160	0	36
Novelties (Walgreens), 7	140	0	34
Worms (1), 13 pieces, 1.4 oz	130	0	31
Guylian:			
Bars: Dark Chocolate, 0.3 oz	55	4	3
Milk Choc. w/ Hazelnuts, 0.3 oz	55	4	3
White Choc. w/ Hazelnuts, 0.3 oz	60	4	6
No Sugar Added Bars:			
Milk Chocolate, 3 squares	150	11	16
54% Cocoa, Dark Choc., 3 squares	140	11	16
Seashell: Bar, 1.4 oz	210	13	21
Boxed, Originals (1), 0.35 oz	60	4	6
Truffles (1), 0.4 oz	70	5.5	5
Heath: Original (1), 1.38 oz	210	13	24
King Size, 2.8 oz	410	22	49
Snack Size, 3 pieces, 1.5 oz	230	14	27
Hershey's:			
Milk Chocolate: 1.55 oz	210	13	26
Giant 7 oz, (3 pces), 1.3 oz	180	11	22
King Size:, 2.6 oz	370	22	44
Cacao Reserve:			
Milk Choc. (35% cacao),			
4 blocks, 1.4 oz	220	15	21
Dark Choc. (65% cacao), 1.3 oz	160	13	19
Extra Dark (60% cacoa):			
Cranberry, Blackb. & Alm. (4)	180	14	21
Pomegranate, 4 pieces, 1.4 oz	170	12	23
Raspberry, 4 pcs, 1.4 oz	180	14	21
Candy-Coated Eggs:			
Milk Choc (8), 1.2 oz	170	8	27
With Almonds, (8) 1.2 oz	200	12	18

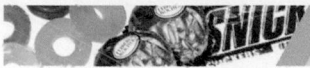

Brands & Generic (Cont)

Per Piece/Serving

	C	F	Cb
Hershey's (Cont):			
Pot of Gold Chocolate Asst.			
Carmel (4), 1.4 oz	190	10	25
Chocolate (4), 1.4 oz	200	12	23
Nuts (4), 1.4 oz	210	13	23
Pecan Caramel Clusters (4), 1.4 oz	200	12	23
Special Dark Choc.: 1.45 oz bar	180	12	25
With Almonds, 1.45 oz bar	190	14	22
King Size, 2.6 oz	330	22	45
Pieces (50), 1.4 oz	180	8	29
Snacksters, 1 package, 0.7 oz	100	3.5	15
Sugar Free: Milk Choc. 5 pcs, 1.4 oz	160	13	24
Peanut Butter Cups Minis (5)	180	13	27
Special Dark Chocolate (5), 1.4 oz	190	15	23
York Peppermint Patties, 3 pieces	120	8	24
Honeycomb: Plain, 1 oz	115	0	27
Choc-coated, 2 pieces	180	7	31
Hot Tamales,			
20 pieces, 1.4 oz	150	0	36
Hugs ~ *See Kisses*			
Jawbreakers *(Sathers)*, (15), 0.6 oz	60	0	16
Jellies, 2 medium, 1 oz	130	0	33
Jells, Raspberry *(Joyva)*, 3 pcs, 1.55 oz	160	0	38
Jelly Beans: Small, 37 beans, 1.4 oz	120	0	35
Regular, 13 beans, 1.4 oz	150	0	37
1 bean	10	0	3
Sugar Free, 35 beans	80	0	37
Jumbo, 1 bean	20	0	5
Jewel, 13 beans, 1.4 oz	140	0	36
Sathers/Walgreens, 13 beans	150	0	37
Wonderbeans, 33 beans	100	0	24
Jelly Bellys: Each	4	0	1
35 beans, 1.4 oz	140	0	37
Sugar Free Beans/Sours (35), 1.4 oz	80	0	37
Jelly Rings *(Jewel)*, 5 pieces, 1.4 oz	110	0	26
Jolly Rancher:			
Gummies, 10 pcs	120	0	28
Hard Candy, 3 pcs	70	0	17
Jelly Beans, 30 pieces, 1.4 oz	140	0	36
Lollipops (1), 0.55 oz	60	0	16
Screaming Sours, 3 pieces, 2 oz	200	0	49
Soft & Chewy, 1 packet, 2 oz	200	0	49
Sour Blasts, 4 pieces, ½ oz	50	0	13
Jujubees, all types (52), 1.4 oz	110	0	28
Juju Bears, 5 pieces	130	0	34
Juju Mix *(Sathers)*, 11 pieces, 1½ oz	150	0	36
Jujyfruits, 16 pieces, 1.4 oz	120	0	32

Per Piece/Serving

	C	F	Cb
Junior Caramels: 13 pieces, 1.48 oz	190	6	33
Mini, 2 boxes, 1 oz	130	4	23
Junior Mints: 1.83 oz	220	4	45
16 pieces, 1.4 oz	170	3	35
Kissables, 39 pcs, 1.4 oz	180	9	28
Kisses:			
Milk Choc, 1 piece, 0.16 oz	25	1.5	2.5
9 pieces, 1.4 oz	200	12	25
With Almonds (9), 1.4 oz	210	14	21
Caramel Filled 9 pieces, 1.5 oz	190	9	27
Cherry Cordial, 9 pieces, 1.5 oz	180	7	30
Special Dark, 9 pieces, 1.4 oz	180	12	25
Kit Kat: 4-piece bar, 1.5 oz	210	11	28
King Size, 8 pieces, 3 oz bar	420	22	56
Snack Size, 3 pcs, 1.48 oz	210	11	27
Extra Krispy Bar (1)	220	12	29
White Choc, 4 piece, 1½ oz	220	12	26
Kraft, Caramels (5), 1.4 oz	160	3.5	31
Kudos: *See Page 33*			
Lance, Peanut Bar, 2.3 oz package	340	19	29
Lemon Drops (4), 0.6 oz	60	0	16
Sugar Free *(Walgreens)* (3), 0.6 oz	50	0	17
Lemonhead (26), 1.4 oz	140	0	36
Licorice: Average all types, 1 oz	100	0	25
Bites *(Switzer)*, each	10	0	3
Chews *(Panda)*, each	10	0	3
Tid Bits, each	10	0	1.5
Twists: Black/Red, avg. 1 pce	35	0	8
Sugar Free, 1 piece	13	0	2.5
American Licorice Co.: Extinguisher (1)	160	1.5	37
Red Vines, 7 pieces, 1.4 oz	140	0	33
Sip-n-Chew, 1 package 1 oz	100	1	23
Snaps, 31 pieces, 1.4 oz	140	0.5	33
Sour Punch, 6 pieces, 1.4 oz	150	0.5	34
Super Ropes, 1 piece, 2 oz	200	0	46
Super String, 1⅓ pieces	140	0	34
Sugar Free Red Twists, 7 pieces	90	0	25
Young & Smiley: Strawberry (11)	150	1.5	33
Traditional Black, 11 pieces	140	1.5	32
Lifesavers: Large size, 1 candy	15	0	3
Regular, all flavors, 1 candy	10	0	2.5
1 Roll (14 candies), 1.14 oz	140	0	35
Creme Savers: 3 pieces, 0.5 oz	60	1	11
Sugar Free, 4 pieces	45	1.5	13
Gummies (4), 0.5 oz	45	0	11
Pep-o-mint (4), ½ oz	60	0	
Fruit Splosion (10), 1.4 oz	130	0	
Sugar-Free Delites: *Per Candy*			
Orchard Fruits; Summer Blend	7	0	
Butter Toffee; European Collect.	10		

Brands & Generic (Cont)

Per Piece/Serving	C	F	Cb
Lik-m-aid (Nestlé), Wonka Fun Dip, 1 pkg	50	0	13
Lindt: Lindor Truffles, average, (1)	75	6	5
Milk Chocolate Bars: Raspb. (5)	200	10	25
Truffles, 7 pieces	240	18	18
Classic Recipe, Hazelnut (10)	230	16	20
70% Cocoa, 4 pieces	220	17	13
Lollipops: Mini, ¼ oz	25	0	6
Small, ½ oz	50	0	12
Medium, 1 oz	100	0	25
Giant (4" diam), 7 oz	790	0	198
Look Bar, 1.5 oz	190	6	49
M & M's:			
Milk Chocolate: 1 pce	5	0.1	0.5
20 pieces, 0.6 oz	70	3	10
1.7 oz package	240	10	34
13 pieces, 1.5 oz	210	9	30
Almond Choc., 1.3 oz	200	11	21
Minis, 1 tube, 1.08 oz	150	7	21
Peanut: 1.63 oz pkg	250	13	30
Fun Size, 18g pkg	90	4.5	11
Peanut Butter, 1.6 oz package	240	14	26
Dark Chocolate: 1.69 oz pkg	240	11	33
Peanuts, 1.5 oz	220	12	25
Premiums: Chocolate Trio, 1.5 oz	230	14	25
Mint Thrills, 1.5 oz	240	14	25
Pretzels, 1.14 oz	150	5	24
Mamba, 9 pieces, 1½ oz	170	2.5	36
Marshmallow Egg, 1 egg, 1 oz	120	3	22
Mary Jane, (Necco), 5 pces, 1.4 oz	160	3.5	32
Marshmallows: Firm/Soft, 1 oz	90	0	23
Regular size, 4 pieces, 1 oz	100	0	24
Mini-Marshmallow, ⅔ cup, 1 oz	95	0	24
Choc-coat. Twists (Joyva), each	95	2	10
Fluff, 2 Tbsp, 0.63 oz	60	0	15
Kraft: Mini, 1 oz	90	0	23
Creme, ½ oz	45	0	11
Jet-Puffed, 5 pcs, 1 oz	100	0	24
Funmallows, ⅔ cup, 1 oz	100	0	24
Marzipan, 2 Tbsp, 1.4 oz	160	4	29
Mauna Loa, Milk Choc., 1.35 oz	200	15	21
Mexican Hats (7), 1.34 oz	120	0	30
Mentos: Regular (1)	10	0	3
Sugar Free (1)	5	0	2.5
Mike & Ike:			
Orig.: 1 pkg, 2.1 oz	220	0	55
23 pieces, 1.4 oz	140	0	36
...uds, 13 pieces, 1.4 oz	170	6	28
...'s (Storck), 6 pieces, 1.4 oz	170	3	35

Per Piece/Serving	C	F	Cb
Milky Way:			
Bars: Single, 2 oz	260	10	41
Fun Size (2), 1.2 oz	150	6	24
To Go, 1.8 oz	230	9	36
Miniatures (5), 1.52 oz	190	7	30
Midnight Bar: (1), 1.76 oz	220	8	36
Minis (5), 1.4 oz	180	7	29
Simply Caramel, 1.9 oz	250	11	37
Mints: Uncoated, 3 pieces	70	0	17
1 mint	7	0	1
1 large mint	15	0	3
Mon Cheri (Ferrero), 4 pcs, 1.59 oz	260	18	20
Mounds: 1.7 oz bar	230	13	29
Snack (2), 1.2 oz	160	9	20
King Size, 3½ oz	460	26	58
Minis, 3 pieces, 1.45 oz	190	11	24
Mr Goodbar, 1.73 oz bar	250	17	25
King Size, 2.6 oz bar	380	26	38
Mrs Fields Choc, 2 pieces, 1.16 oz	160	6	26
Munch Bar, 1.42 oz	220	15	18
Necco Candy Wafers (40) 2 oz	220	0	56
Newman's Own:			
Milk Chocolate, Caramel Cups (3)	160	8	21
Dark Chocolate: Caramel Cups (3)	160	9	21
Peanut Butter Cups (3)	180	12	17
Nips, all flavors, 2 pieces, ½ oz	60	2	11
Nougat: 3 pcs, 1.48 oz	170	1	39
Choc. Covered, 1 oz	125	4	22
Nuggets: Milk Chocolate, 4 pieces	200	12	25
w/ Toffee & Almonds, 4 pieces, 1.3 oz	200	13	21
Special Dark w/ Almonds, 4 pieces	180	13	20
Nutrageous Bar (Reese's), 1.8 oz	260	16	28
Oh Henry!, 2.2 oz bar	300	17	26
Orange Slices:			
Jewel, 3, 1½ oz	140	0	35
Walgreens, 4 pieces, 1.6 oz	160	0	39
Pastel Mints (Walgreens), 20 pieces	60	0	14
PayDay Bar: 1.8 oz bar	250	13	29
King Size, 3.4 oz bar	440	24	50
Snack Size, 0.7 oz	90	5	10
Avalanche, 1.8 oz bar	250	13	29
Peanut Bar, 1.6 oz bar	235	15	21
Peanut Butter Cups: See Reese's; Newman's Own			
Peanut Brittle: 1 piece, 1½ oz	190	5	32
Sugar Free (Russell Stover)			
4 pcs, 1.3 oz	140	10	24
Peanuts, choc-covered, 14 pieces	230	14	23
Pearson's Mint Patties (5), 1.34 oz	150	2.5	31
Peppermints, 7 small, 0.5 oz	60	0	15
Brach's, 3 pieces	60	0	16

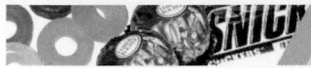

Brands & Generic (Cont)

Per Piece/Serving	C	F	Cb
Pez, 1 roll	35	0	9
Planters: Choc. Peanuts , 1.4 oz	210	15	18
Double Peanut Bar, 1.6 oz	220	13	21
Pops ~ *See Lollipops*			
Pop Rocks, 0.34 oz package	35	0	9
Pot of Gold:			
Assortment: Caramel, 4 pieces	190	10	25
Nut, 4 pieces	210	13	23
Pretzels: Choc-covered, Mini (6)	200	9	25
White Choc Bites (23), 1.4 oz	200	9	25
Pretzel Flipz *(Nestlé)*, 8 pcs, 1.4 oz	130	5	20
Raisinets: Milk Choc. 1 pkg, 1.6 oz	190	8	30
King Size, 2.8 oz	330	13	56
Movie Pack, 3.5 oz	380	16	64
Dark Choc., ¼ cup, 1.6 oz	180	8	32
Reese's			
Clusters, 3 pieces, 1½ oz	220	12	24
Crispy Crunchy Bar: 1.7 oz	260	18	22
2 pieces, 1.2 oz	170	10	19
King Size, 3.1 oz	480	32	40
Fast Break, 2 oz bar	260	12	35
Peanut Butter Chips, 1 Tbsp, ½ oz	80	4	8
Peanut Butter Cups: 2 cups, 1.5 oz	200	12	22
King Size (1), 2.8 oz	400	24	44
Mini, 5 pieces, 1.55 oz	220	13	25
8-Pack, 1 piece, ½ oz	80	4.5	9
Snack Size, 1 piece, 0.74 oz	110	6.5	12
Sugar Free: 5 pieces, av., 1.38 oz	180	13	27
Caramel Filled (2),1.4 oz	150	11	27
Big Cup: Regular, 1.4 oz	200	12	22
King Size (2), 2.8 oz	400	22	24
White Chocolate (2), 1.5 oz	220	13	22
Pieces: Regular, 51 pieces, 1.4 oz	190	9	25
Special Dark (50), 1.4 oz	180	8	29
Sticks: 1.5 oz	220	13	23
King Size (1), 3 oz	440	26	46
Snack Size (1), 0.6 oz	90	5	9
Snacksters, 1 package, ¾ oz	100	4	14
Whipps, (40% less fat), 1½ oz	230	9	37
Rice Krispies Treats *(Kellogg's):*			
1 bar, av. all varieties, 0.8 oz	90	2.5	17
Riesen, Choc. Chew, 4 pieces, 1.26 oz	170	6	28
Rocky Road: Milk/Dark 1.8 oz bar	240	11	34
Roca Thins, all flavors, 4 pieces	210	15	23
Rolo: All types, per roll, 1.7 oz	220	10	33
Bites, 7 pieces, 1.4 oz	190	9	29
Root Beer Barrels (3) 0.63 oz	60	0	17

Per Piece/Serving	C	F	Cb
Russell Stover Candy:			
Boxed Chocolates: Chocolate Coated			
Assorted (2), 1.13 oz	150	7	23
Cherry Cordials (3), 1.34 oz	150	5	25
Dairy Cream Caramels (2), 1.16 oz	150	7	22
Elegant Collection (3), 1.59 oz	210	10	29
French Choc. Mints (4), 1.34 oz	220	13	22
Nut, Chewy & Crisp Centers, (2)	160	8	21
Pecan Delights (2), 1.83 oz	270	16	32
Sugar Free: Assort. Candies (3), 1.55 oz	180	12	26
Pecan Delights (2), 1.7 oz	220	17	26
Bags: Caramel (3), 1.3 oz	180	8	25
Coconut (3), 1.5 oz	200	10	26
Mint Patty (3), 1.5 oz	180	7	30
Pecan Delight (2), 1.2 oz	180	11	20
Salt Water Taffy *(Brach's)*, (5)	170	2.5	36
Seashells *(Guylian)*, 4 shells, 1.6 oz	260	17	24
See's Candies:			
Almond Royal, 5 pieces, 1.3 oz	190	13	18
Butterscotch Chews (5), 1.5 oz	210	12	27
Krispy's: Caffe Latte, 5 pieces 1.3 oz	180	8	27
Mint, 5 pieces, 1.3 oz	170	8	27
Little Pops:			
Butterscotch (4), 0.5 oz	60	2	12
Cafe Latte (4), 0.5 oz	50	1.5	9
Chocolate (4), 0.5 oz	60	3	10
Vanilla (4), 0.5 oz	50	2	9
Lollypops, average, 0.7 oz	90	3	17
Milk Molasses Chips, 6 pieces, 1.4 oz	180	8	27
Milk Peppermints, 2 pieces, 1.23 oz	150	4	28
Peanut Brittle Bar, 1 oz	150	10	15
Peanut Butter Patties, 1.2 oz	170	10	16
Peppermint Twists (3), 0.53 oz	60	0	15
Raisins, Dark/Light (28), 1.4 oz	170	7	29
Toffee-ettes, 3 pieces, 1.6 oz	270	21	18
Sugar Free: Dark Bar, 1.5 oz	180	16	24
Dark Walnut Clusters, 1.5 oz	230	21	17
Peanut Brittle, 1.5 oz	170	14	17
Skittles:			
Original, 2.17 oz	250	2.5	56
Sour, 1.8 oz	200	2	44
Tropical; Wild Berry, 2.17 oz	250	2.5	56
Fun Size, 1 bag, 0.5 oz	60	1	14
Tear & Share, 4 oz bag	420	4.5	93
Skor Toffee Bar (1), 1.4 oz	200	12	25
Smarties:			
Candy Rolls (1), ¼ oz	25	0	6
Giant, 2 pieces, ¼ oz	25	0	6

Brands & Generic (Cont)

Per Piece/Serving	C	F	Cb
Snack Barz (Hershey's) (1), 2.1 oz	280	13	36
Snickers: 2.07 oz bar	280	14	35
King Size, 3.29 oz	440	22	56
Amond Bar, 1.76 oz	240	11	32
Creme Egg (1), 1 oz	150	8	17
Fudge Bar, 1.78 oz	250	13	31
To Go Bar, 1.65 oz	220	11	28
Dark Chocolate Bar (1), 1.65 oz	250	12	31
Miniatures, 4 pieces, 1.27 oz	170	9	22
Sno Caps, ¼ cup, 1.4 oz	180	8	30
Soft 'N Chewy Butter Toffee, each	30	0.5	5
Sorbee: Choc., ½ bar, 1.4 oz	180	12	25
Crystal Light Hard Candy, 4 pieces	25	0	13
(Note: Carb figures include Isomalt which has fewer calories than sugar.)			
Sour Patch: All types, 1.5 oz	150	0	37
1 straw	20	0	5
Spearmint Leaves: Jewel (5), 1.4 oz	140	0	35
Walgreens, 4 pieces, 1.62 oz	160	0	39
Spree Candies: Original, 15 pieces	50	0	13
Chewy Spree, 8 pieces	60	0	13
Starburst: Candy Canes, 0.5 oz	70	0	18
Fruit Chews, each	20	0.4	4
8 pces, 1.4 oz	160	3.5	34
Jellybeans, 1.5 oz	150	0	37
Jellybean Egg, 2 oz	200	0	51
Tropical Fruit (8), 1.4 oz pack	160	3.5	34
Starlight Mints, 3 pieces, 0.56 oz	60	0	15
Suckers (Walgreens) (1), 0.39 oz	45	0	11
Sugar Babies, Original, 1.4 oz	160	1.5	37
Sugar Coated Peanuts, 1 oz	120	8	10
Sunbursts Sunflowers (Kimmie):			
Coffee Break Tube, 1.41 oz	200	11	22
Candy Bar Bag, 1.7 oz	190	9	27
Sunburst Milk, 1.4 oz	210	11	23
Swedish Fish (7), 1.48 oz	150	0	38
Sweet 'N Low: Chews (1)	20	0.5	5
Coffee Cremes (1)	40	3	6
Wafer Bars, average, 3 pieces	140	7	23
Mint Cremes, 3½ pieces	120	9	22
Symphony:			
Milk Choc. 1.5 oz bar	220	14	23
Large Block, 3 pieces, 1.27 oz	190	11	21
With Almonds & Toffee (1), 1½ oz	220	14	23

Per Piece/Serving	C	F	Cb
Taffy, 1 piece, 1 oz	60	0	17
Take 5 (Hershey's): Original, 1.55 oz	200	11	25
King Size, 2.25 oz	300	16	37
Snack Size, 2 pcs	210	11	26
3 Musketeers: Original, 2.13 oz	260	8	46
Fun Size, 3 pcs, 1.6 oz	190	6	34
Minis, 7 pcs, 1.4 oz	170	5	32
Mint Bar, 2 pcs, 1.2 oz	150	5	26
Truffle Crisp, single pack, 2 bars	170	9	20
Tang-a-Roos, 1 roll	25	0	6
Terry's Choc Orange (5), 1.5 oz	230	12	27
Dark Choc Orange (5), 1.5 oz	240	13	28
Tic Tac, all varieties, each	2	0	0
Toblerone: 1.23 oz bar	180	9	23
1.8 oz bar	260	13	32
3.5 oz bar	510	30	63
Toffees, Regular, 1 oz	160	9	18
Toll House Milk Choc. Morsels, 1Tbsp	70	4	9
Tootsie Pops (1), 0.6 oz	60	0	15
Tootsie Roll: 2.25 oz roll	245	2	55
Mini Chews, 1.4 oz	140	3	28
Truffles: Regular, 1 piece, 0.42 oz	60	4	6
Large (Godiva), ¾ oz	110	6.5	12
Extra Large (J.Schmidt), 1½ oz	220	13	24
Turtles (Nestlé): Average, each	80	4.5	10
Sugar Free, 3 pieces, 1.34 oz	150	11	20
Twists (Sugar Free): Licorice; Strawberry,			
7 pieces, 1.4 oz	90	0	25
Twix: 2 cookies, 2 oz	280	14	37
4 To Go	480	24	64
Fun Size, 0.5 oz	80	4	10
Java, 2 cookies	280	15	36
Minis, 3 pcs, 1 oz	150	8	20
Caramel, 0.85 oz	130	6	16
Peanut Butter 4 To Go	480	28	48
Peanut Butter, 1.8 oz	280	17	28
Twizzlers: Cherry Bites (17), 1.4 oz	140	0.5	32
Cherry Nibs, 2.2 oz package	220	1.5	50
Pull 'n' Peel Cherry (2), 1.66 oz	160	1	37
Twists Strawberry, 1.6 oz	160	0.5	36
U-No Bar 1.5 oz	250	17	22
Weight Watchers (Whitman's):			
Butter Cream Caramel (3)	150	8	23
Caramel Medallions (3)	160	9	24
Coconut (3)	150	9	23
English Toffee Squares (3)	150	9	21
Mint Patties (3)	150	9	23
Peanut Butter Cups (4)	180	8	31
Pecan Crowns (3)	160	10	24

Brands & Generic (Cont)

Per Piece/Serving	C	F	Cb
Werther's: Original (3), 0.56 oz	70	1.5	14
Chewy Caramel (6), 1.31 oz	170	6	28
Caramelts (7), 1.4 oz	190	7	28
Sugar-Free (5)	40	1	15
Whatchamacallit Bar, 1.6 oz	230	12	28
King Size, 2.6 oz	370	20	45
Whitman's: Sampler (4), 1.75 oz	240	11	34
12 oz Box, 4 pieces, 1.59 oz	220	12	27
Sugar Free, 10 oz Box, 3 pcs, 1.42 oz	180	12	25
Reserve, 7 oz Box, 2 pieces, 1.16 oz	160	9	21
Whoppers, av. all flav., 18 pieces	190	8	31
Wonka: Wonka Bar (1), 7.6 oz	360	19	49
Exceptional Bars, av. all, 4 pcs	200	13	23
Gobstopper, 0.5 oz	60	0	14
Laffy Taffy: Orig., 5 bars, 1.5 oz	160	2	36
Stretchy & Tangy, 1½ oz	165	4	33
Nerds, 1.8 oz	170	0	44
SweetTarts (8) ½ oz	50	0	13
Yogurt Candy,			
Coated Raisins, 27 pieces, 1.4 oz	180	8	28
York Peppermint Pattie:			
Regular, 1.4 oz	140	2.5	31
Fun Size, 0.6 oz	60	1	14
King Size, 1.45 oz	150	3	33
York Mints (3)	10	0	3
Zachary Choc. Peanuts, 1.48 oz	240	15	21
Zagnut, 1.52 oz bar	200	8	31
Zero Bar: 1.8 oz bar	230	8	37
King Size, 3.4 oz	400	14	68
Zingos, 3 pieces, 0.07 oz	5	0	2

Gum ~ Per Piece

	C	F	Cb
Bazooka, each	15	0	4
Beechies	6	0	2
Big League Chews	10	0	2
Double Bubble Ball	20	0	5
Bubble Yum	25	0	6
Sugarless	10	0	3
Candilicious	30	0	2
Carefree (Sugarless/Regular)	5	0	2
Chiclets, 1 piece	5	0	1
Clorets, 1 stick	10	0	2
Dentyne	5	0	0.5
Estee, bubble/regular	5	0	2
Extra (Wrigley's), Sugar-Free	5	0	2
Freshen-Up	10	0	3
Hubba Bubba: Regular	20	0	5
Sugar-free, average	14	0	0.5
Ice Breakers	10	0	2
Jolt Gum, 2 pieces	15	0	3
Super Bubble	15	0	4
Trident, Original; White	5	0	1
Wrigley's, all flavors	10	0	2

Carob Candy C F Cb

Per Piece/Serving	C	F	Cb
Carob: Plain/Natural, 1 oz	155	9	15
Carob Coated: Raisins, 1 oz	130	8	15
Almonds/Peanuts, 1 oz	150	10	14
Malt Balls, 1 oz	135	8	15
Caramels, 1 oz	110	4	18
Dates, 1 oz	125	5	20
Soybeans	145	9	16
Trail/Party Mix, 1 oz	150	9	15
Carob Chips, unsweetened, 1 oz	155	9	15

Cough Drops C F Cb

	C	F	Cb
Beech Nut, 1 drop	10	0	2
CVS, Sour Lemon Throat Drops			
Diabetic Tussin, 1 drop	0	0	0
Halls: Defense Vit. C, 1 drop	15	0	4
Sugar Free, 1 drop	5	0	3
Fruit Breezers, 1 drop	15	0	4
Menthol Drops, 1 drop	15	0	4
Sugar Free, 1 drop	5	0	4
Plus, 1 drop	20	0	5
Listerine Lozenge (Amer. Chicle)	10	0	2
Luden's Throat Drops, all flavors, 1	10	0	2
Sugar Free, 1 drop	0	0	0
Pine Bros, 1 cough drop	10	0	2
Ricola: Cough Drops (1)	10	0	3
Sugar-Free Lemon Mint (2)	0	0	1
Rite Aid, Menthol Cough (1)	10	0	3
Robitussin: Regular, 1 drop	15	0	3
Honey Cough, 1 drop	40	0	10
Sugar Free Throat, 1 drop	10	0	3
Sunny Orange Vit. C, 1 drop	10	0	3
Rolaids Sodium Free, 1	5	0	1
Sathers Peppermint Lozenges, 1	15	0	3
Squibb Cough/Throat Loz.'s, 1	15	0	4
Sucrets (Beecham) Lozenges, 1	10	0	2
Wintergreen Loz. (Walgreens), 1	15	0	3

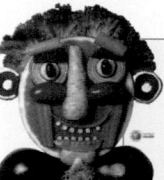

Eat at least 5 servings of fruit and vegetables every day . . . and Enjoy Better Health!

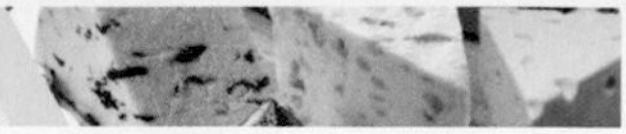

Quick Guide   **C** **F** **Cb**

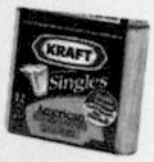

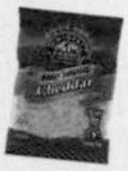

Firm/Hard Cheeses
(American, Cheddar, Colby, Swiss)

Regular Cheese:

	C	F	Cb
Thin Deli slice, ¾ oz	90	7	0
1 oz slice/piece	115	9	0.5
8 oz package	915	75	3
16 oz (1lb) package	1830	150	6
Cubes: 1" cube, ¾ oz	85	7	0.5
1¼" cube, 1 oz slice	115	9	0.5
Diced: 1 cup, 4½ oz	530	40	2
Grated: 1 Tbsp, ¼ oz	30	2.5	0
Shredded: Cheddar, ¼ cup, 1 oz	115	9	0.5
1 cup, 4 oz	455	37	1.5
Cheddar, Reduced-Fat, ¼ cup, 1 oz	80	6	1
Mozzarella: ¼ cup, 1 oz	85	6.5	0.5
Part-Skim, ¼ cup, 1 oz	70	5	1
Sliced: 1 thin (3½" square), ¾ oz	85	7	0.5
Rectangular (7"x 4"x ⅛ "), 1½ oz	170	14	0.5
Round (3¼" diameter x ⅛ "), ¾ oz	85	7	0.5
Semi-circular, 1¼ oz			
(5½" long, 3½" radius, ⅛" thick)	140	12	0.5
Fat-Free: Average all brands, 1 oz	40	0	2
Low-Fat: Average all brands, 1 oz	50	2	0.5
Reduced Fat: Average all brands, 1 oz	80	5	0.5

Cheese   **C** **F** **Cb**

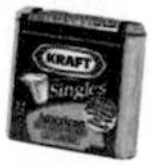

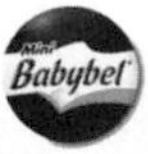

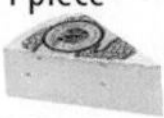

Per 2 Tbsp, 1 oz Unless Indicated

American:

	C	F	Cb
Regular: 1 slice, 1 oz	105	9	0.5
Alpine Lace,			
Deli, 25% Red. Fat, 0.8 oz	70	5	1
Kraft, 0.67 oz slice	60	4.5	1
Land O'Lakes, 0.8 oz slice	80	7	1
Light: *Kraft* (2% Milk), 0.67 oz	45	2.5	2
Fat-Free: *Kraft,* 0.7 oz slice	30	0	2
Borden, 1 slice, 0.7 oz	30	0	3
Babybel, Mini *(Laughing Cow):*			
Original/Bonbel (1), ¾ oz	70	6	0
Light Original (1), ¾ oz	50	3	0
Gouda (1), ¾ oz	80	6	0
Blue/Bleu, Light, 0.75 oz	35	1.5	2
Bonbel *(Laughing Cow),* 1 piece	70	6	0
Camembert	85	7	0
Caraway	105	8	1
Castello *(Wegman's),* av., 1 oz	120	12	0

Cheese (Cont)   **C** **F** **Cb**

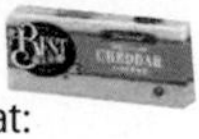

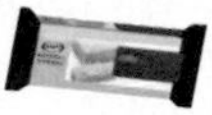

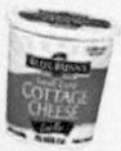

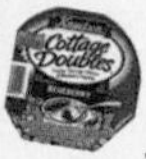

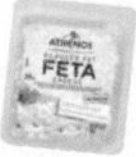

Per 2 Tbsp, 1 oz Unless Indicated

Cheddar: (Also see 'Quick Guide')

	C	F	Cb
Regular	115	9	0.5
Alpine Lace	90	7	0
Reduced-Fat/Low-Fat:			
Borden, Shredded, ¼ cup, 1 oz	80	6	1
Cabot Vermont, 50% Light, 1 oz	70	4.5	0.5
Fat-Free, Kraft, 0.7 oz slice	30	0	2
Cheese Balls *(Kaukauna),* average	100	7	4
Cheese Curds: Fresh, ¼ cup, 1 oz	110	9	0
Breaded & Fried ~ *See Page 78*			
Cheese Logs *(Kaukauna),* average	100	7	4
Cheshire	110	9	1.5
Colby: Regular	110	9	0.5
Reduced-Fat *(Kraft)*	80	6	0
Colby-Jack, regular	110	9	1
Cottage Cheese: *Average All Brands*			
Creamed (4% milk fat): 2 Tbsp, 1 oz	30	1	1.5
½ cup, 4 oz	120	5	6
With fruit, ½ cup, 4 oz	130	4	15
Reduced-Fat (2%): 2 Tbsp, 1 oz	25	0.5	1
½ cup, 4 oz	100	2	4
Low-Fat (1%): 2 Tbsp, 1 oz	20	.5	1
½ cup, 4 oz	80	1	3
Fat-Free/Non-Fat: 2 Tbsp, 1 oz	20	0	1
(Jewel), ½ cup, 4 oz	80	0	5
Fiber One, 1% Fat, ½ cup, 4 oz	80	2	8
Friendship: 1% Low-Fat Pineapple, 4 oz	120	1	16
Nonfat with P'apple, ½ cup, 4 oz	110	0	17
Pot Style 2%, ½ cup, 4 oz	90	2.5	3
Hood w. Chive/Onion, 4 oz	90	1	5
Knudsen:			
Free: Non-Fat, ½ cup, 4.oz	80	0	7
2% Milk Fat, ½ cup., 4 oz	100	2.5	6
Cottage Doubles, av., 5.5 oz carton	150	2.5	18
On the Go! Free, 4 oz carton	70	0	7
Low-Fat, 4 oz carton	90	2.5	6
Lactaid: Low-Fat, ½ cup, 4 oz	80	1	7
Light N' Lively: Fat-Free, 4.4 oz	80	0	8
Low-Fat, ½ cup, 4.4 oz	80	1.5	6
Cream Cheese: *See Page 79*			
Edam, Regular	100	8	0.5
Farmer *(Friendship)*	50	2.5	0
Feta: Regular	75	6	1
Crumbled, ½ cup, 2½ oz	190	15	3
Red.-Fat *(Athenos)*	60	4	1
Fontina	110	9	0.5
Gjetost (Goat's Milk, fresh)	130	8	12

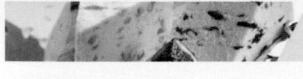

Cheese (Cont)   C F Cb

Per 2 Tbsp, 1 oz Unless Indicated

Item	C	F	Cb
Goat's Milk Cheese:			
Chevre, Soft	80	6	1
Chavril: Regular	60	4.5	0.5
Semi-Soft	100	8.5	1
Hard	130	10	0.5
Gorgonzola	100	8	0.5
Galbani Dolcelatte	95	8	1
Gouda	100	8	0.5
Gruyere	115	9	1
Havarti *(Land O'Lakes),* 0.75 oz	80	7	0
Italian Pasta Blend *(Sargento)*	90	6	2
Jarlsberg *(Wegman's)*	100	8	0
Jarlsberg Reduced Fat, shredded	70	3.5	0
Labneh (Lebanese Cream Chse), 1.8 oz	70	4	4
Lactose Free Cheese *(Lifetime)*			
Jalapeno Jack	105	8	2
Fat Free Cheddar	40	0	1
Limburger	95	8	0
Mascarpone *(Wegman's)*	130	13	1
Mexican:			
Cacique: Cotija	110	9	0
Queso Fresco	80	6	0
Queso Quesadilla	70	5	2
Ranchero	80	6	0
Chi-Chi's, Salsa Con Queso, Mild	45	3	4
Kraft, 4 Cheese; Taco, shredded	100	8	1
Sargento, Shredded	110	9	1
Supremo Chihuahua: Queso Bianco	100	8	0
Queso Oaxaca; Queso Del Caribe	85	6.5	1
Monterey Jack: Regular	110	9	0
Kraft 2% Milk Reduced Fat	80	6	1
Alpine Lace, Co-Jack	70	5	0
Weight Watchers	90	6	1
Mozzarella:			
Regular	85	6.5	0.5
Land O'Lakes/Polly-O, average	90	6	1
Shredded	90	7	1
Light: *Polly-O Lite,* Shredded	60	2.5	1
Kraft 2% Milk Fat, Reduced Fat	70	4	1
Part Skim: *Alpine Lace* 25% Red.	60	4	1
Borden/Kraft, Shredded	80	5	1
Polly-O, String (2% milk)	70	5	1
Fat-Free: *Polly-O*	35	0	1
Kraft, shredded	45	0	2
Muenster: Regular	105	9	0.5
Low-Fat	85	5	1
Myzithra, grated, 4 T. 1 oz	80	4	2

Cheese (Cont)   C F Cb

Per 2 Tbsp, 1 oz Unless Indicated

Item	C	F	Cb
Parmesan: Fresh/Block	110	7.5	1
Grated (Packaged): 1 Tbsp	20	1.5	0
1 oz quantity	120	8	1
½ cup, 1¾ oz	215	14	2
with Romano *(Frigo),* grated	110	7	0
Kraft Reduced-Fat Topping, 1 Tbsp	20	1	2
Pizza Cheese, shredded:			
Regular *(Kraft)* ¼ cup, 1 oz	90	7	1
Port de Salut	100	8	0
Port Wine (Kaukauna)	90	6	4
Provolone: Regular	100	7.5	0.5
Reduced-Fat: *Alpine Lace,* 0.8	60	4.5	0
Sargento, 1 slice, 0.67 oz	50	3	1
Puh *(Kondele),* average	95	7	1
Quark: 40% fat	47	3	1
20% fat	32	1.5	1
Skim/Non-Fat	22	0	1.5
Queso: Anejo/Asadero/Blanco	105	9	1
Chichuahua/De Papa	110	9	2
Ricotta Cheese:			
Whole Milk	50	3.5	1
½ cup, 4½ oz	215	16	4
Part Skim,	40	2	1.5
½ cup, 4½ oz	170	10	6
Light/Low-Fat	25	1	1.5
½ cup, 4½ oz	125	5	6
Fat-Free, ½ cup, 4½ oz	100	0	10
Baked Ricotta, 2 oz portion	130	9	3
Romano: Block/Loaf	110	8	1
Grated (Package):	120	9	1
1 Tbsp, 0.2 oz	20	1.5	0
Roquefort	105	9	0.5
Sheep's Milk	45	3	1
Smoked: *Wegman's*	100	8	0
Tillamook, Smoked Cheddar	110	9	0
Stilton *(Wegman's)*	110	10	0
String *(Frigo/Kraft/Sargento)*	80	6	0.5
Light String-Ums *(Kraft)*	80	4.5	1
String Lite *(Frigo)*	60	2.5	0.5
Light *(Sargento),* 0.75 oz	50	2.5	1
Swiss: Regular	110	8	1.5
Reduced-Fat: *Alpine Lace,* 0.8 oz	70	4.5	1
Kraft, 2% Milk, 0.7 oz slice	50	2.5	2
Tilsit	100	7.5	0.5
Tybo	100	7	0.5
Vermont *(Cabot)*	110	9	0
Wensleydale	100	8	0.5
Whey Cheese	125	8	9

Cheese Products | C | F | Cb |

Item	C	F	Cb
Cheese Food:			
Average all flavors: ¾ oz slice	70	5	2
1 oz slice	95	7	2.5
Alouette:			
Soft Spreadable: Per 2 Tbsp., 0.8 oz			
Garlic & Herbs	80	8	1
Light	50	4	2
Light Garlic & Herbs	50	4	2
Peppercorn Parmesan	80	8	1
Cabot, 50% Red-Fat Ched., av., 1 oz	70	4.5	0
Cracker Barrel, Extra Sharp Ched., 1 oz	120	10	0
Handi-Snacks: *(Kraft)*			
Breadsticks 'n Cheez, 1.1 oz	110	4.5	14
Ritz Crackers 'n Cheez, 1 oz package	100	6	11
Kraft:			
American: Singles 1 sl., ¾ oz	45	2.5	2
Fat-Free, 1 slice, 0.7 oz	25	0	2
Easy Cheese,			
American, 2 Tbsp, 1.2 oz	90	6	2
Snack Pack Cubes:			
Colby & Monteray Jack, 2%, 1.5 oz	160	13	1
Kraft Natural:			
Cheese Sticks: Cheddar (1), 1 oz	120	10	0
Mozzarella, 1 stick, 1 oz	80	5	0
Colby Jack, Red. Fat (1), 1 oz	90	6	0.5
2% Reduced Fat, 1 oz	90	6	1
Laughing Cow:			
Wedges: Original Creamy Swiss (1)	50	4	1
Light Varieties, 1 wedge	35	2	2
Mini Babybel ~ See Page 76			
Lifetime:			
Cholest. Reducing,1 Slice, 0.7 oz	30	1	2
Block, 1" cube, 1 oz	45	1.5	1
Precious, Cheddar Chse Sticksters, 1 oz	110	9	1
Rondele:			
Spreadable: All Flavors, 2 Tbsp., 1 oz	70	7	1
Light, Garlic & Herb, 2 Tbsp., 1 oz	50	4	2
Sargento:			
Chef Style: Cheddar, shred., ¼ cup, 1 oz	110	9	1
Mozzarella, shredded, ¼ cup	80	6	1
Snack Bars, Mild Cheddar (1)	90	7	1
Sticks, Pepper Jack (1), 0.74 oz	80	6	0
Smart Beat, Fat-Free,			
All varieties, 0.6 oz slice	25	0	3
Velveeta: Original, ¾ oz	60	4	2
Extra Thick, 1.2 oz	100	7	3
Shredded, ¼ cup, 1.3 oz	130	9	3
WisPride:			
Port Wine: Ball/Cup, 1.1 oz	90	7	4
Cup, Lite, 2 Tbsp, 1.1 oz	70	3.5	5

Cheez Whiz | C | F | Cb |

Item	C	F	Cb
Original, 2 Tbsp, 1.1 oz	90	7	4
Light, 2 Tbsp, 1.1 oz	80	3.5	6
Salsa Con Queso, 2 Tbsp, 1.1 oz	90	7	4

Cheese Curds

Item	C	F	Cb
Fresh: ¼ cup, 1 oz	110	9	0
1 cup, 4 oz	440	36	0
Breaded & Fried:			
A&W, 5 oz	570	40	27
Culver's, 6.7 oz	670	38	54

Cheese Substitutes

Item	C	F	Cb
Galaxy:			
Grated Parmesan Flavor, 2 tsp, 0.18 oz	15	0	0
Oat/Rice Slices, 1 slice, 0.7 oz	40	2	1
Veggy: American, 1 slice, ½ oz	40	2.5	0.5
Mozzarella Flavor, 1 slice, ½ oz	40	2.5	0.5
Lifetime, Swiss Rice Chunk, 1" cube	95	7	2
Lisanatti: Almond Cheese, average	50	1	3
Rice Cheese, average, 1 oz	60	3	2
Mori Nu:			
Tofu: Silken Soft, 1" slice, 3 oz	45	2.5	2
Firm, 1" slice, 3 oz	50	2.5	2
Soya Kaas: Cheddar, 1 oz	70	4	1
Fat-Free, all varieties, 1 oz	40	0	2
Soy-Sation, Shredded Cheese, av., 1 oz	70	4	2
Tofutti, Better Than Cream Cheese, 1 oz	85	5	9
Trader Joe's: *Per Slice*			
Soy Cheese:			
Cheddar Flavor, 0.7 oz	45	2	3
Mozzarella Flavor, 1 oz	70	4	3
Yogurt Cheese, 1 slice, 1 oz	100	8	0

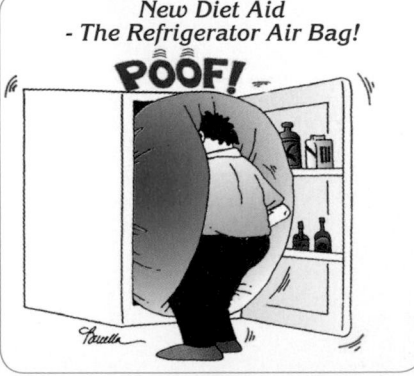

New Diet Aid - The Refrigerator Air Bag!

POOF!

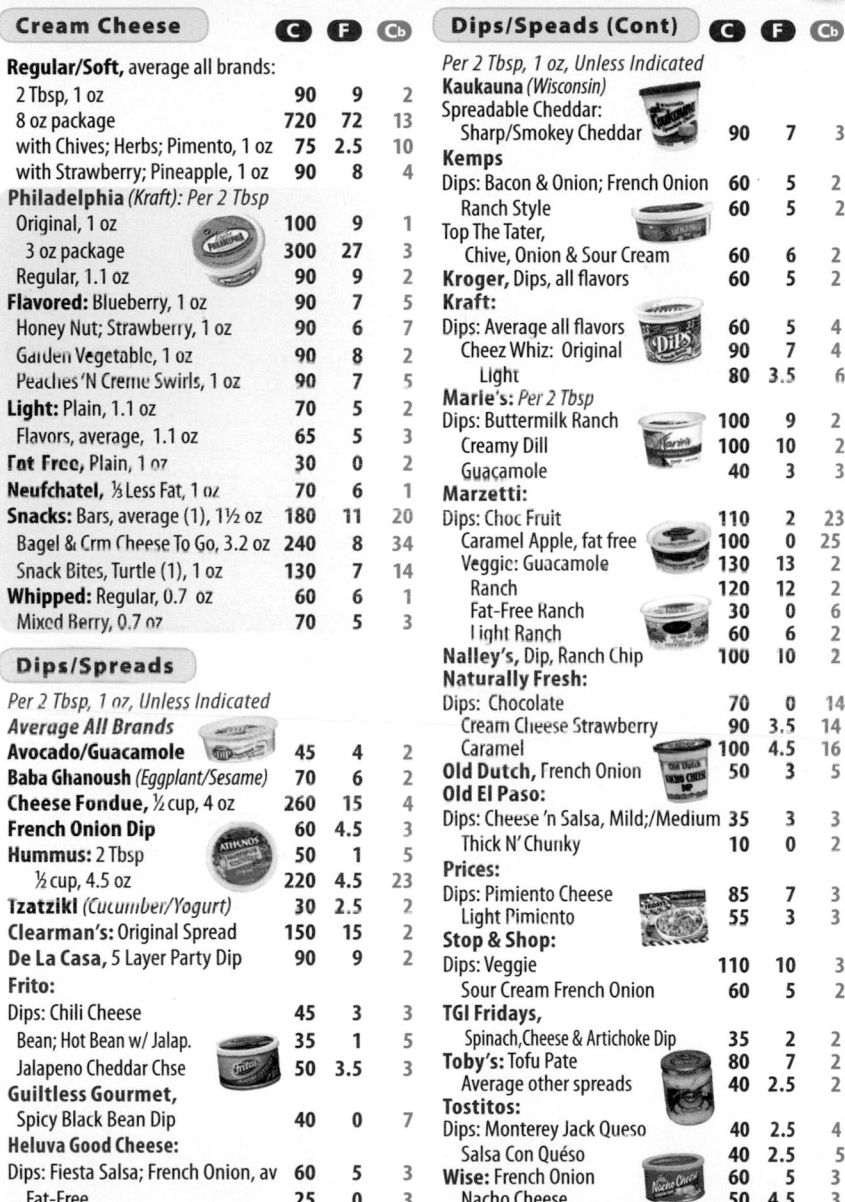

Cheese ~ Cream Cheese ◇ Dips (C)

Cream Cheese   C   F   Cb

Regular/Soft, average all brands:

	C	F	Cb
2 Tbsp, 1 oz	90	9	2
8 oz package	720	72	13
with Chives; Herbs; Pimento, 1 oz	75	2.5	10
with Strawberry; Pineapple, 1 oz	90	8	4
Philadelphia (Kraft): Per 2 Tbsp			
Original, 1 oz	100	9	1
3 oz package	300	27	3
Regular, 1.1 oz	90	9	2
Flavored: Blueberry, 1 oz	90	7	5
Honey Nut; Strawberry, 1 oz	90	6	7
Garden Vegetable, 1 oz	90	8	2
Peaches 'N Creme Swirls, 1 oz	90	7	5
Light: Plain, 1.1 oz	70	5	2
Flavors, average, 1.1 oz	65	5	3
Fat Free, Plain, 1 oz	30	0	2
Neufchatel, ⅓ Less Fat, 1 oz	70	6	1
Snacks: Bars, average (1), 1½ oz	180	11	20
Bagel & Crm Cheese To Go, 3.2 oz	240	8	34
Snack Bites, Turtle (1), 1 oz	130	7	14
Whipped: Regular, 0.7 oz	60	6	1
Mixed Berry, 0.7 oz	70	5	3

Dips/Spreads

Per 2 Tbsp, 1 oz, Unless Indicated
Average All Brands

	C	F	Cb
Avocado/Guacamole	45	4	2
Baba Ghanoush (Eggplant/Sesame)	70	6	2
Cheese Fondue, ½ cup, 4 oz	260	15	4
French Onion Dip	60	4.5	3
Hummus: 2 Tbsp	50	1	5
½ cup, 4.5 oz	220	4.5	23
Tzatziki (Cucumber/Yogurt)	30	2.5	2
Clearman's: Original Spread	150	15	2
De La Casa, 5 Layer Party Dip	90	9	2
Frito:			
Dips: Chili Cheese	45	3	3
Bean; Hot Bean w/ Jalap.	35	1	5
Jalapeno Cheddar Chse	50	3.5	3
Guiltless Gourmet,			
Spicy Black Bean Dip	40	0	7
Heluva Good Cheese:			
Dips: Fiesta Salsa; French Onion, av	60	5	3
Fat-Free	25	0	3

Dips/Speads (Cont)   C   F   Cb

Per 2 Tbsp, 1 oz, Unless Indicated

	C	F	Cb
Kaukauna (Wisconsin)			
Spreadable Cheddar:			
Sharp/Smokey Cheddar	90	7	3
Kemps			
Dips: Bacon & Onion; French Onion	60	5	2
Ranch Style	60	5	2
Top The Tater,			
Chive, Onion & Sour Cream	60	6	2
Kroger, Dips, all flavors	60	5	2
Kraft:			
Dips: Average all flavors	60	5	4
Cheez Whiz: Original	90	7	4
Light	80	3.5	6
Marie's: Per 2 Tbsp			
Dips: Buttermilk Ranch	100	9	2
Creamy Dill	100	10	2
Guacamole	40	3	3
Marzetti:			
Dips: Choc Fruit	110	2	23
Caramel Apple, fat free	100	0	25
Veggie: Guacamole	130	13	2
Ranch	120	12	2
Fat-Free Ranch	30	0	6
Light Ranch	60	6	2
Nalley's, Dip, Ranch Chip	100	10	2
Naturally Fresh:			
Dips: Chocolate	70	0	14
Cream Cheese Strawberry	90	3.5	14
Caramel	100	4.5	16
Old Dutch, French Onion	50	3	5
Old El Paso:			
Dips: Cheese 'n Salsa, Mild;/Medium	35	3	3
Thick N' Chunky	10	0	2
Prices:			
Dips: Pimiento Cheese	85	7	3
Light Pimiento	55	3	3
Stop & Shop:			
Dips: Veggie	110	10	3
Sour Cream French Onion	60	5	2
TGI Fridays,			
Spinach,Cheese & Artichoke Dip	35	2	2
Toby's: Tofu Pate	80	7	2
Average other spreads	40	2.5	2
Tostitos:			
Dips: Monterey Jack Queso	40	2.5	4
Salsa Con Quéso	40	2.5	5
Wise: French Onion	60	5	3
Nacho Cheese	50	4.5	3

79

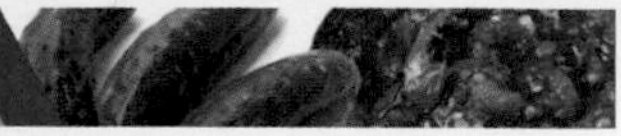

Condiments, Sauces | C | F | Cb

Average of Brands & Homemade

	C	F	Cb
Apple Sauce: *Also see Page 102*			
Sweetened, ¼ cup, 2½ oz	55	0	13
Unsweetened, ¼ cup, 2 oz	25	0	7
Barbecue Sauce: Avg., 2 Tbsp, 1 oz	40	0	10
Bull's Eye, Original, 1 oz	60	0	14
Bearnaise Sauce, ¼ cup, 2½ oz	190	19	5
Buffalo Wing Sce: Honey Mustard, 1 T.	40	3	3
Average other varieties, 1 Tbsp	25	2	2
Catsup (Ketchup), regular, 1 Tbsp	15	0	4
Cheese, h/made, ¼ cup, 2½ oz	150	10	12
Chef-Mate, Hot Dog, ¼ cup	70	2.5	9
Chili Sauce: *Heinz,* 1 T., ½ oz	20	0	5
Del Monte, 1 Tbsp, ½ oz	20	0	5
Cocktail Sauce, ¼ cup	110	0	15
Fat-Free *(Walden Farms)* 1 Tbsp	0	0	0
Cranberry, all types, ¼ cup, 2½ oz	110	0	27
Demi Glaze Gold, 2 tsp	30	0.5	3
Honey Mustard *(French's)* 1 tsp	5	0	1
Horseradish: 1 tsp	2	0	0
Kraft, 1 tsp	15	1.5	1
Ketchup: Regular, 1 T., ½ oz	15	0	4
Heinz One-Carb, 1 Tbsp	5	0	1
Mole: *Doña Maria,* 2 Tbsp, 1 oz	200	13	10
Rogelio Bueno 2 Tbsp, 1 oz	160	11	12
Mushroom Sauce, ½ cup, 2 oz	50	2	5
Mustard, average, 1 tsp	5	0	0.5
Pesto Sauce, ¼ cup, 2 oz	90	5	8
Pizza Sauce, cnd., ¼ cup, 2 oz	30	0	6
Seafood Cocktail Sce, ¼ cup	60	0	15
Soy Sauce: Avg., 1 Tbsp	10	0	1
Kikkoman Lite Soy, 1 Tbsp	10	0	1
Sour Cream Sce, ½ cup	250	15	22
Spaghetti Sce, ½ cup, 4½ oz	135	6	19
Steak Sauce: A1, 1 Tbsp, ½ oz	15	0	3
Lea & Perrins, 1 Tbsp, ½ oz	20	0	5
Carb Well *(A1)* 1 Tbsp, ½ oz	5	0	1
Strawb. Puree Sce, Unsweet., 2 T.	10	0	2
Sweet & Sour Sauce:			
Contadina, 1 Tbsp	40	1	8
Kraft, 1 Tbsp	60	0	13
La Choy, 2 Tbsp, 1.2 oz	60	0	14
Tabasco Sauce, 1 tsp	2	0	0
Taco Sauce, average, 2 Tbsp, 1 oz	10	0	1
Tartar Sauce: Heinz, 2 Tbsp, 1 oz	120	11	4
America's Choice, 2 Tbsp, 1 oz	160	17	1
Hellmann's, Regular, 2 Tbsp, 1 oz	80	7	4
McCormick, Fat-Free, 2 Tbsp, 1 oz	30	0	7
Teriyaki Sauce *(Kikkoman)*1 T., ½ oz	15	0	2
Vinegar, White or Wine, 2 Tbsp	4	0	1
White Sauce, ½ cup, 5 oz	130	7	10
Worcestershire Sauce, 1 tsp	5	0	1

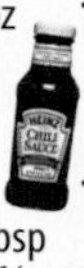

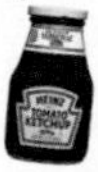

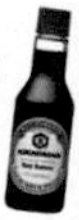

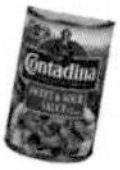

Pickles & Relish | C | F | Cb

Average All Brands

	C	F	Cb
Bread & Butter Pickles, 4 sl., 1 oz	25	0	6
Chutney, 2 Tbsp, 1¼ oz	50	0	11
Dill Pickle:			
Slices, 4 slices, 1 oz	4	0	1
1 large,			
(3¾"x 1¼" diam.), 2¼ oz	12	0	3
Extra lrg (4"x 1¾" diam.), 5 oz	30	0	6
Halves: Small, 1 oz	3	0	0.5
Large, 2½ oz	8	0	2
Sweet, small, ½ oz	22	0	6
Gherkins, sweet, 1 medium, 1 oz	30	0	7
Green Chiles, chopped, 2 Tbsp	5	0	1
Horseradish, 1 Tbsp	10	0	2
Jalapenos, pickled (2), 2 oz	10	0.5	2
Jalapeno Relish, 1 Tbsp, ½ oz	5	0	1
Mustard, avg. all brands, 1 tsp	5	0	0.5
Peppers, Hot/Mild (1), 1.6 oz	20	0	4
Pickled: Beets, ½ cup, 4 oz	75	0	19
Onions, 1 medium, ¾ oz	10	0	2
Cocktail Onion, 1 onion	2	0	0
Red Cabbage, ½ cup, 3 oz	65	0	15
Pickles: Sweet, 2 Tbsp, 1 oz	35	0	5
Large (3"x ¾ diam.), 1¼ oz	40	0	10
Pickle in a Pouch, 1 large	12	0	3
Relishes: Sandwich Spread, 1 tsp	20	1	5
Cranberry-Orange, 1 Tbsp	30	0	7
Hot Dog *(Heinz),* 1 Tbsp, ½ oz	17	0	3
Sweet Pickle, 1 Tbsp, ½ oz	20	0	5
Sweet Cauliflower, 1 oz	35	0	8
Sauerkraut, Drained, 1 cup, 5 oz	25	0	6

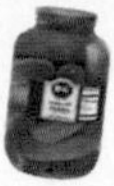

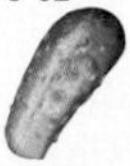

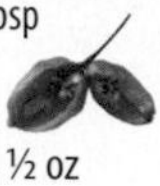

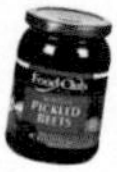

Salsa

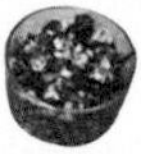

Average all Types:

	C	F	Cb
Regular, without oil, 2 Tbsp, 1 oz	15	0	3.5
Made with oil, 2 Tbsp, 1 oz	40	3	8
La Victoria, 2 Tbsp, 1 oz	10	0	2
Old El Paso, 1 Tbsp, 1 oz	10	0	3
TGI Friday's, 1.2 oz	15	0	4

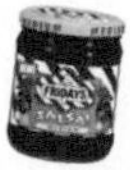

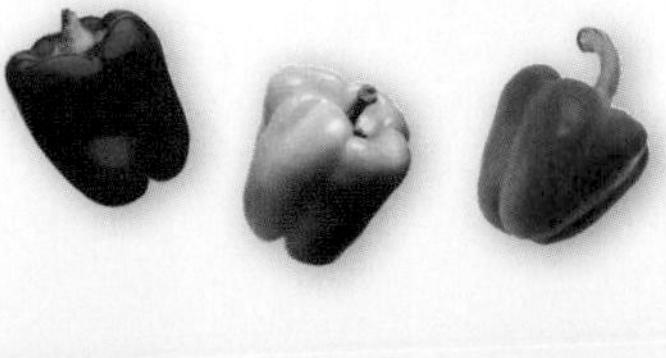

Quick Guide　C　F　Cb

Cookies

Average All Brands: Per Cookie

	C	F	Cb
Biscotti: Small, 0.5 oz	70	3	10
Regular, 1 oz	140	6.5	18
Chocolate Chip Cookies:			
Small/Thin 0.5 oz	70	3.5	9
Regular, 1 oz	140	7	18
Large, 2.5 oz *(Mrs Fields)*	330	16	46
Extra Large, 4 oz	555	28	73
Oatmeal/Oatmeal Raisin:			
Small/Thin 0.5 oz	65	2.5	10
Regular, 1 oz	130	5	20
Large, 2.5 oz *(Mrs Fields)*	330	14	44
Extra Large, 4 oz	510	20	78
Peanut Butter:			
Small/Thin 0.5 oz	70	3.5	9
Regular, 1 oz	135	7	17
Large, 2.5 oz *(Mrs Fields)*	330	17	41
Extra Large, 4 oz	540	27	67
Low-Fat Cookies			
Choc Chip (Low-Fat), (1), ½ oz	65	2	10
Oatmeal Raisin (Fat-Free), (1), 1 oz	95	0.5	22
Peanut Butter (Low-Fat), (1),1 oz	105	5	15

Quick Guide　C　F　Cb

Crackers

Average All Brands: Per Cracker

	C	F	Cb
Cheese Crackers: Plain, 1"square	5	0	0.5
Small, octagonal	10	0	1
Round (2" diam.)	15	0	1.5
Sandwich (Peanut Butter)	35	1.5	4
Graham, 2½" square	30	0.5	5
Melba Toast, plain, 1 piece	20	0	4
Oyster & Soup Crackers, ½ oz	60	2	10
(40 small oysters/20 lge hexagons)			
Rice Crackers: 1 small	9	0	1.5
Rice Snacks, Oriental-Style, 1 oz	130	2.5	23
Saltines, 5 crackers	65	2	11
Snack-type, 1 round cracker	15	0	2
Soda Crackers *(Saltine),* 2	25	1	4.5
Water Cracker *(Carr's):* Regular	30	0	7
Small, 1 cracker	15	0	3
Wheat, thin	9	0.5	1.5
Zweiback Toast, 1 piece	35	1	6

Brands　C　F　Cb

Per Cookie/Cracker (Unless indicated)

Albertsons

	C	F	Cb
Animal Crackers (6), 1 oz	130	3.5	22
Chocolate Chip:			
Original (3), 1 oz	150	7	20
Chewy (2), 1 oz	130	6	18
Chunky, 0.6 oz	80	3.5	10
Chocolate Sandwich Cremes (3) 1.1oz	150	6	25
Double Filled (2) 1 oz	140	6	21
Fudge Graham (3), 1 oz	140	7	19
Fudge Wafer (3), 1 oz	140	8	18
Graham Crackers: Cinnamon (2)	130	3	25
Honey (2), 1 oz	140	3	24
Low-Fat Honey (2), 1 oz	110	1	22
Marshmallow Ring (1), 1 oz	130	6	20
Milk Chocolate Chip, 2.5 oz	310	14	30
Striped Shortbread (3), 1.1 oz	160	7	21
Sugar, 2.5 oz	270	9	22
Triple Chocolate, 2.8 oz	310	12	33
White Chocolate Chip, 2.5 oz	280	11	37
Vanilla Wafers (9), 1.1 oz	140	4.5	24

Annie's

Cheddar Bunnies

	C	F	Cb
Regular: 1 oz Snack Pack	140	6	19
7½ oz Box	1125	50	140
Sour Cream & Onion, 1 oz	140	6	18
White Cheddar, 1 oz	140	6	18
Whole Wheat, 1 oz	130	6	17
Bunny Classics: Buttery Rich, 1 oz	140	5	20
Cheddar, 1 oz	140	7	18
Saltine, 1 oz	140	3	22
Bunny Grahams: Friends, 1 oz	130	4.5	21
Chocolate, 1 oz	130	4.5	22

Austin

Crackers: *Per Package*

	C	F	Cb
Cheese with Cheddar Cheese	190	10	23
Cheese with Peanut Butter	190	10	23
Sandwich:			
Chocolatey Peanut Butter Flavored	190	8	26
Grilled Cheese Flavored, 1.38 oz	190	9	24
PB & J Flavored, 1.38 oz	190	8	26
Toasty Crackers w/ P'nut Butter, 1.3 oz	190	9	23
Zoo Animal Crackers, 1 oz	120	1.5	23
Sandwich Cremes: *Per Package*			
Lemon OHs!; Vanilla Cremes, 1.2 oz	170	7	24

Per Cookie/Cracker, Unless Indicated

	C	F	Cb
Barbara's Bakery:			
Cookies: Fig Bars (2), av., 1.35 oz	120	0	28
Snackimals (10), average	120	4	19
Crackers:			
Rite Lite Rounds (5)	60	2	11
Wheatines (4)	60	1	11
Blue Diamond:			
Nut Thins ~ Crackers			
Average all flavors: 17 crackers, 1.1 oz	130	3	23
½ Package, 2.2 oz	260	6	46
1 Package, 4.25 oz	520	12	92
Brent & Sam's:			
Chocolate Chip Pecan, 1 oz	140	8	15
Key Lime White Chocolate, 1 oz	130	7	16
Oatmeal Raisin with Pecans, 1 oz	130	7	16
Triple Chocolate Bliss (2), 1 oz	110	5	14
White Chocolate Macadamia (2), 1 oz	130	7	14
Carr's:			
Crackers:			
Poppy & Sesame (4)	80	5	9
Table Water (5)	70	1.5	13
Whole Wheat (2)	80	4	10
Cookies, Ginger Lemon Cremes (2)	130	5	20
Cheez·It ~ *See Sunshine, Page 87*			
Chips Ahoy! ~ *See Nabisco, Page 85*			
Country Choice			
Ginger Snaps (5)	140	5	22
Sandwich Cremes (2), average	130	5	19
Soft Baked, average all flavors	100	4	16
Vanilla Wafers (7)	140	5	22
Dr. Kracker:			
Crackers, Flatbread, average all flavors	100	4	11
Snacker: Klassic 3-Seed (8)	120	5	13
Seeded Spelt (8)	120	6	12
Spelt Sunflower Cheese (8)	100	6	12
Average other flavors (8)	120	5	15
Erin Baker's:			
Original Breakfast Cookies: *Per 3 oz*			
Mocha Cappuccino	300	6	53
Peanut Butter	320	11	47
Peanut Butter & Jelly	320	9	52
Vegan Peanut Butter Choc. Chunk	330	10	52
Minis: *Per 1 oz Cookie*			
Peanut Butter	110	3	16
Other flavors, average	100	2	18
Organic Brownie Bites, average	95	2	18

Per Cookie/Cracker, Unless Indicated

	C	F	Cb
Famous Amos:			
(Bite Size Cookies)			
Chocolate Chip: 4 cookies, 1 oz	150	7	20
1.4 oz Snack bag	210	10	28
3 oz (99cents) bag	450	21	60
12 oz bag	1800	84	240
15 oz box	2250	105	300
Chocolate Chip & Pecans (4)	150	8	18
Sandwich Creme:			
Chocolate (3), 1 oz	170	7	25
Vanilla (3), 1 oz	170	7	25
Chocolate: 3 cookies, 1.2 oz	170	7	25
2.2 oz bag	310	9	33
14 oz package	1980	82	290
Fig Newtons ~ *See Nabisco, Page 85*			
Girl Scouts:			
Cookies: Caramel DeLites (2)	140	7	19
Do-si-dos (2)	110	5	16
Peanut Butter Sandwich (3)	160	6	26
Samoas (2)	150	8	19
Shortbreads (4)	120	4.5	19
Thanks-A-Lot (9)	150	6	22
Thin Mints (4)	160	8	22
Goldfish ~ *See Pepperidge Farm, Page 86*			
Grandma's: *Per Package*			
Peanut Butter Sandwich Creme (5)	210	10	28
Rich 'N Chewy, Choc Chip (6)	240	12	32
Vanilla Sandwich Creme (5)	190	8	28
Van./Choc. Mini Sandwich Creme (9)	150	7	22
Homestyle Big Cookies: *Per Cookie*			
Chocolate Chip (1)	190	9	25
Fudge Choc. Chip (1)	150	6	25
Oatmeal Raisin (1)	150	5	25
Peanut Butter (1)	170	9	20
Great American Cookies:			
Cookies: Chewy Pecan Supreme	240	13	30
Chewy Chocolate Supreme; Sugar	200	9	29
Double Fudge;/Reese's, average	225	10	33
Oatmeal Walnut Raisin	230	10	33
Original M&M/Reese's	240	12	32
Peanut Butter M&M	250	14	29
Snickerdoodles	240	11	33
White Chunk Macadamia	250	14	30
Double Doozies: Original	690	34	94
M&M Big Bite	340	17	46
Cookie Cakes: 16" Cookie	460	22	67
16" M&M Cookie	500	24	73
Heart Shaped	440	21	64
Sliced Cookie Cake, 1 slice	580	27	83

Per Cookie/Cracker, Unless Indicated

Health Valley: **C** **F** **Cb**

Cookies:

	C	F	Cb
Cookie Cremes Sandwich (2), average	125	5	19
Oatmeal Raisin Cookie	90	3.5	14
Mini: Chocolate Chip (4)	120	6	16
Chocolate Chocolate Chip (4)	130	7	16

Crackers:

	C	F	Cb
Original Grahams: Amaranth Bran (6)	120	3	22
Oat Bran (6)	120	3	22
Rice Bran (6)	110	3	19
Organic: Bruschetta Vegetable (4)	70	3	10
Cracked Pepper; Sesame (4)	70	3	10
Stoned Wheat; Whole Wheat av., (4)	70	3	9

Joseph's Lite Cookies:

Crispy Bite Size: *Sugar Free, Per 4 Cookies*

	C	F	Cb
Almond; Chocolate Peanut Butter	95	5	13
Chocolate Mint	95	5	14
Choc. Walnut; Pecan Chocolate Chip	95	5	13
Chocolate Chip	95	5	13
Lemon; Peanut Butter, average	95	4	15
Oatmeal Choc Chip w. Pecans	95	5	14
Oatmeal; Pecan Shortbread, average	95	5	15

Kashi:

TLC Cookies: *Per Cookie*

	C	F	Cb
Happy Trail Mix, Chewy	140	5	21
Oatmeal: Dark Choc.	130	5	20
Raisin Flax	130	4.5	20

Crackers:

	C	F	Cb
Heart To Heart Whole Grain:			
Original (7)	120	3.5	22
Roasted Garlic (7)	120	3.5	22
Party:			
Mediterranean Bruschetta (4)	120	4	18
Roasted Garlic & Thyme (4)	130	4.5	18
Stoneground 7 Grain (4)	130	5	17
TLC:			
Country Cheddar (18)	130	4.5	20
Fire Roasted Vegetables (15)	120	3.5	21
Honey Sesame (15)	120	3	22
Original 7 Grain (15)	120	3.5	21
Toasted Asiago (15)	130	4	21
Snack Packs: Original 7 Grain (15)	120	3.5	21
Variety Pack, 1 package, av.	130	3.5	21

Per Cookie/Cracker (Unless indicated)

Keebler: **C** **F** **Cb**

Crackers:

	C	F	Cb
Club: Original (4)	70	3	9
Reduced Fat (5)	70	2	12

Grahams:

	C	F	Cb
Original (8)	120	3.5	22
Cinnamon (8)			
Honey (8)	135	4	23

Town House:

	C	F	Cb
Original (5)	80	4.5	10
Reduced Fat (6)	60	1.5	11

Wheatables:

Crackers.

	C	F	Cb
Original Gldn. Wheat (17)	140	6	20
Toasted Honey Wheat (17)	140	6	20
Nut Crisps, all flavors, (16)	140	6	20

Cookies:

	C	F	Cb
Cheesecake Middles, Orig./Choc, (3)	130	7	17

Chips Deluxe:

	C	F	Cb
Chocolate Lovers; Coconut	80	4.5	10
Original (2)	160	8	19
Rainbow	80	4	10
Rainbow Mini's 1.4 oz package	200	10	27
Soft & Chewy (2)	150	7	22
Country Style Oatmeal (2)	130	6	19
Danish Wedding (4)	130	6	18
E.L. Fudge: Original	90	3.5	13
Double Stuffed (2)	180	9	24

Fudge Shoppe:

	C	F	Cb
Deluxe Grahams (3)	140	7	18
Fudge Sticks (3)	150	8	20
Fudge Stripes (3)	150	7	21
Mini's, 1 package	200	9	27
100 Calorie Package	100	3.5	16
Grasshopper (4)	150	7	20
Gripz, average, 1 pouch	125	5	17
Iced Animal (6)	140	4.5	22

Sandies Cookies:

	C	F	Cb
Choc Chip Pecan (2)	170	10	18
Pecan Shortbread (2)	160	10	18
100 Calorie Package	100	3.5	16
Vienna Fingers: Regular (2)	150	6	22
Reduced Fat (2)	140	4.5	24
Wafers: Vanilla (8)	140	5	22
Mini Vanilla (18)	140	6	21

Per Cookie/Cracker, Unless Indicated

Kroger

	C	F	Cb
Cookies: Chip Mates			
Original (3), 1.5 oz	160	8	22
Chewy (2), 1 oz	130	6	20
Chunky (2), 1 oz	130	6	18
Olde Sthrn Pecan Shortbread (2),1 oz	150	9	15
Sugar Wafers (4), 1.1 oz	160	7	24
Vanilla Wafers (7), 1.1 oz	130	3.5	23
Crackers:			
Grahams, Original; Honey (4)	120	3	20
Saltines, Original, (5), 0.5 oz	60	1.5	10
Kid-O's			
Mint (2) 1 oz	140	6	22
Chocolate Lovers (2), 1 oz	140	6	21
Double Filled Sandwich (2) 1 oz	140	6	21
Chocolate Sandwich (3) 1.15 oz	150	6	25

Lance: *Per Package of 6*

	C	F	Cb
Cookies:			
Nekot, Peanut Butter	240	11	32
Strawberry Cookies	230	10	33
Crackers, Malt	190	10	19
Sandwich Crackers:			
Nip Chee, Cheddar Cheese	190	9	23
Toastchee: Peanut Butter	220	12	23
Reduced-Fat	190	8	23
Toasty, Peanut Butter	180	9	19

Little Debbie

	C	F	Cb
Fig Bar	160	3	31
Marshmallow Pie, average	180	7	28
Marshmallow Treat	160	4	31
Oatmeal Creme Pie , 1.34 oz	170	7	26
Nutty Bar (2), 2 oz	310	18	33
Crackers: Cheese w/ Peanut Butter (4)	130	6	15
Peanut Butter Toasty (4)	130	6	16

Lu

	C	F	Cb
Le Petit Beurre (4)	140	4	24
Le Petit Ecolier, average (2)	130	6	17
Pim's, Orange (2)	100	3	16

Macaroni & Cheese, *(Nabisco)*

	C	F	Cb
Average all flavors	150	7	18

Manischewitz

	C	F	Cb
Chocolate Macaroon	45	2	8
Matzo Cracker, Miniatures (10)	110	0	25
Tam Tam Crackers: Everything (10)	130	5	19
Onion (10)	140	5	21

Per Cookie/Cracker, Unless Indicated

Miss Meringue

	C	F	Cb
Chocolettes (10), average	130	3.5	24
Macaroons			
Traditional Recipe, 1.3 oz	180	10	20
Madeleines			
Chocolate (2), 1.2 oz	160	9	18
Traditional Recipe (2), 1.2 oz	160	9	19
Meringue Classiques			
Cappuccino (4), 1.1 oz	110	0	26
Mint Chocolate Chip (4), 1.1 oz	120	1.5	25
Triple Chocolate (4), 1.1 oz	120	1.5	25
Vanilla Rainbow/Van. (4), 1.1 oz	110	0	27
Meringue Minis			
Chocolate (13), 1.1 oz	110	0	26
Chocolate Chip (12), 1.1 oz	130	1.5	27
Mint Chocolate Chip (12), 1.1 oz	120	1.5	26
Orange Creamsicle (13), 1.1 oz	110	0	27
Vanilla; Rainbow Van. (13), 1.1 oz	110	0	27
Sugar-Free Chocolate (13), 0.5 oz	40	0	8
Sugar-Free Vanilla (13), 0.5 oz	35	0	9

Mother's

	C	F	Cb
Chocolate Chip (4), 1 oz	150	7	20
Circus Animal (6), 1 oz	150	7	20
Coconut Cocadas (5), 1.2 oz	160	8	21
Double Fudge (2), 1.3 oz	170	7	27
English Tea (2), 1.3 oz	180	7	27
Macaroons (2), 1 oz	170	11	17
Oatmeal (2), 1 oz	130	5	19
Taffy (2), 1.3 oz	180	8	27
Vanilla Creme (2), 1.3 oz	180	7	26
Iced: Lemonade (4), 1 oz	150	7	19
Oatmeal (1), 14 oz bag	150	6	23

Mrs Fields Cookies: *Fast-Foods Section ~Page 219*

Murray Sugar Free Cookies

	C	F	Cb
Fudge-Dipped: Grahams (4)	140	8	19
Mint Cookies (4)	130	7	17
Vanilla Wafers (4)	150	10	19
Creme Sandwiches:			
Lemon; Chocolate; average	130	6	20
Oatmeal (3)	140	7	21
Peanut Butter (3)	150	9	16
Shortbread (8)	130	5	21
Shortbread Pecan (3)	160	11	18
Vanilla Wafers (9)	130	5	24
Vanilla Creme Wafers (4)	130	8	19

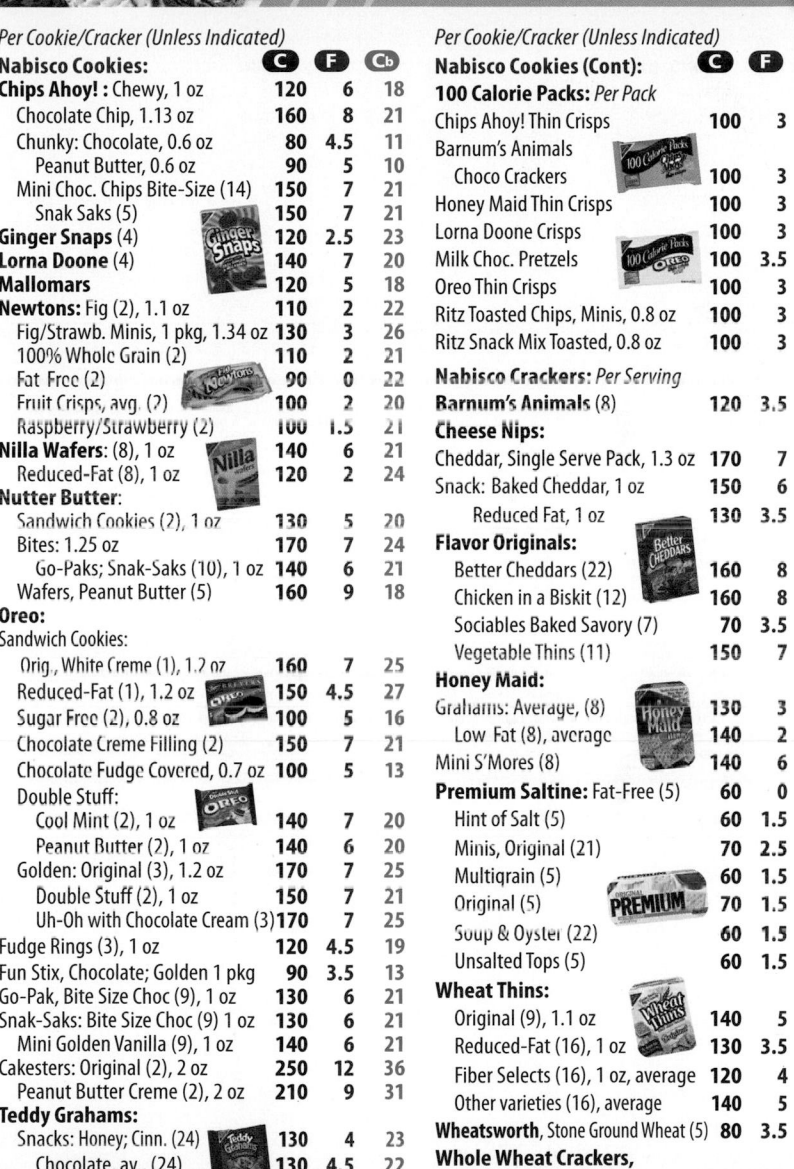

Per Cookie/Cracker (Unless Indicated)

Nabisco Cookies:	C	F	Cb
Chips Ahoy! : Chewy, 1 oz	120	6	18
Chocolate Chip, 1.13 oz	160	8	21
Chunky: Chocolate, 0.6 oz	80	4.5	11
Peanut Butter, 0.6 oz	90	5	10
Mini Choc. Chips Bite-Size (14)	150	7	21
Snak Saks (5)	150	7	21
Ginger Snaps (4)	120	2.5	23
Lorna Doone (4)	140	7	20
Mallomars	120	5	18
Newtons: Fig (2), 1.1 oz	110	2	22
Fig/Strawb. Minis, 1 pkg, 1.34 oz	130	3	26
100% Whole Grain (2)	110	2	21
Fat Free (2)	90	0	22
Fruit Crisps, avg. (2)	100	2	20
Raspberry/Strawberry (2)	100	1.5	21
Nilla Wafers: (8), 1 oz	140	6	21
Reduced-Fat (8), 1 oz	120	2	24
Nutter Butter:			
Sandwich Cookies (2), 1 oz	130	5	20
Bites: 1.25 oz	170	7	24
Go-Paks; Snak-Saks (10), 1 oz	140	6	21
Wafers, Peanut Butter (5)	160	9	18
Oreo:			
Sandwich Cookies:			
Orig., White Creme (1), 1.2 oz	160	7	25
Reduced-Fat (1), 1.2 oz	150	4.5	27
Sugar Free (2), 0.8 oz	100	5	16
Chocolate Creme Filling (2)	150	7	21
Chocolate Fudge Covered, 0.7 oz	100	5	13
Double Stuff:			
Cool Mint (2), 1 oz	140	7	20
Peanut Butter (2), 1 oz	140	6	20
Golden: Original (3), 1.2 oz	170	7	25
Double Stuff (2), 1 oz	150	7	21
Uh-Oh with Chocolate Cream (3)	170	7	25
Fudge Rings (3), 1 oz	120	4.5	19
Fun Stix, Chocolate; Golden 1 pkg	90	3.5	13
Go-Pak, Bite Size Choc (9), 1 oz	130	6	21
Snak-Saks: Bite Size Choc (9) 1 oz	130	6	21
Mini Golden Vanilla (9), 1 oz	140	6	21
Cakesters: Original (2), 2 oz	250	12	36
Peanut Butter Creme (2), 2 oz	210	9	31
Teddy Grahams:			
Snacks: Honey; Cinn. (24)	130	4	23
Chocolate, av., (24)	130	4.5	22
Snak Saks,			
Mini Choc Chip/Honey (47), av.,	130	4	22

Per Cookie/Cracker (Unless Indicated)

Nabisco Cookies (Cont):	C	F	Cb
100 Calorie Packs: *Per Pack*			
Chips Ahoy! Thin Crisps	100	3	18
Barnum's Animals			
Choco Crackers	100	3	17
Honey Maid Thin Crisps	100	3	16
Lorna Doone Crisps	100	3	16
Milk Choc. Pretzels	100	3.5	16
Oreo Thin Crisps	100	3	16
Ritz Toasted Chips, Minis, 0.8 oz	100	3	17
Ritz Snack Mix Toasted, 0.8 oz	100	3	16
Nabisco Crackers: *Per Serving*			
Barnum's Animals (8)	120	3.5	22
Cheese Nips:			
Cheddar, Single Serve Pack, 1.3 oz	170	7	22
Snack: Baked Cheddar, 1 oz	150	6	19
Reduced Fat, 1 oz	130	3.5	21
Flavor Originals:			
Better Cheddars (22)	160	8	18
Chicken in a Biskit (12)	160	8	19
Sociables Baked Savory (7)	70	3.5	9
Vegetable Thins (11)	150	7	20
Honey Maid:			
Grahams: Average, (8)	130	3	24
Low Fat (8), average	140	2	28
Mini S'Mores (8)	140	6	21
Premium Saltine: Fat-Free (5)	60	0	13
Hint of Salt (5)	60	1.5	12
Minis, Original (21)	70	2.5	10
Multigrain (5)	60	1.5	10
Original (5)	70	1.5	11
Soup & Oyster (22)	60	1.5	11
Unsalted Tops (5)	60	1.5	11
Wheat Thins:			
Original (9), 1.1 oz	140	5	22
Reduced-Fat (16), 1 oz	130	3.5	22
Fiber Selects (16), 1 oz, average	120	4	22
Other varieties (16), average	140	5	22
Wheatsworth, Stone Ground Wheat (5)	80	3.5	10
Whole Wheat Crackers,			
Reduced Fat (7), 1.1 oz	120	2.5	23
Zwieback, 1 piece, 0.3 oz	35	1	6

Per Cookie/Cracker (Unless Indicated) **C** **F** **Cb**

Newman's Own Organics

	C	F	Cb
Alphabet Cookies (10) average	120	3	22
Champion Chip: Chocolate Chip (4)	160	7	21
Expresso Chocolate Chip (4)	150	7	21
Wheat-Free & Dairy-Free (4)	160	8	21
Other varieties, average	160	8	21
Fig Newman's: Fat-Free, 2 bars	120	0	28
Low-Fat, 2 bars	140	2	28
Wheat/Dairy-Free, 2 bars	120	1.5	26
Newman-O's: Original (2)	130	4.5	20
Choc. Creme (2); Mint Creme (2)	130	4.5	20
Ginger-O's (2)	120	4.5	19
Wheat-Free & Dairy-Free (2)	130	4.5	21
Oreo Cookies ~ *See Nabisco, Page 85*			

Peek Freans

	C	F	Cb
Assorted Creme (2)	140	6	19
Nice Biscuits (2)	160	6	25
Shortcake (2)	140	7	18

Pepperidge Farm

Cookies

	C	F	Cb
American Classics, Chocolate Chunk,			
Chesapeake, Dark Chocolate Pecan	130	6	17
Montauk, Milk Chocolate	130	6	18
Nantucket: Dark Chocolate	130	6	18
Double	140	7	19
Sausalito, Milk Chocolate	130	6	17
Tahoe, White Choc. Macadamia	130	6	17
Brussels (3)	150	7	20
Brussels Mint (3)	190	10	22
Chessmen (3)	120	5	18
Distinctive Collection:			
Ginger Family (4)	160	5	26
Golden Orchard (3)	140	6	21
Geneva (3)	160	9	19
Homestyle: Ginger Man (4)	130	3.5	21
Oatmeal	140	6	21
Shortbread (2)	130	6	17
Sugar (3)	150	7	21
Milano: Original (3)	180	10	21
Milk Chocolate (3)	170	9	21
Soft Baked Cookies:			
Montauk Milk Chocolate	140	6	22
Oatmeal Raisin	130	4.5	23
Sanibel Snickerdoodle; Mystic Sugar	140	5	22
100 Calorie Pouches: *Per Packet*			
Chessmen	100	3.5	15
Dark Chocolate Chunk	100	3.5	15
Goldfish	100	3.5	14
Oatmeal Raisin	100	3	16

Pepperidge Farm (Cont)

Crackers

	C	F	Cb
Cheese Crisps (20)	140	6	19
Entertaining Quartet (4)	70	2.5	10
Golden Butter (4)	70	2.5	11
Harvest Wheat (3)	80	3.5	11
Wheat Crisps (17), 1 oz	140	5	21
Goldfish: Grahams (50)	130	4	22
Average all flavors: 1 oz (55)	140	5	20
1.5 oz pouch	210	9	27
2 oz carton	280	10	40
Pretzel Thins:			
Everything (11)	120	0.5	25
Simply (11)	110	0	21
Snack Sticks:			
Artisan Cheese (11)	130	4	20
Toasted Sesame (12)	140	5	20

Ritz

	C	F	Cb
Crackers: Orig., ½ oz	80	4.5	10
Reduced-Fat, ½ oz	70	2	11
Honey Butter (5), 06 oz	80	4	10
Peanut Butter, 1.4 oz package	190	9	24
Real Cheese, 1.4 oz package	200	11	22
Roasted Vegetable, 0.6 oz	80	3.5	10
Whole Wheat, ½ oz	70	2.5	11
100 Calorie Snack Mix, 1 pkg, 0.8 oz	100	3	16
Crackerfuls: Garlic Herb, 1 oz	140	7	17
Other Varieties, 1 oz	130	7	17
Ritz Bits Sandwiches: Cheese, 1 oz	150	9	17
Carry Me Pak , 2 oz	290	17	33
Cheddar Cheese, 1 oz packs	130	7	17
Cheese Go-Pak (13), 1 oz	150	9	17
Peanut Butter, 1.25 oz	170	10	20
Peanut Butter Go-Pak, 1 oz	160	8	18
Peanut Butter 2 Go, 1.38 oz	190	9	24
Single Serve, 1.5 oz	220	13	24
Ritz Chips: Toasted Original, 1 oz	130	4.5	21
Cheddar; Sour Crm & Onion, 1 oz	130	6	19

Safeway Select

	C	F	Cb
Homestyle: Choc. Chunk Brownie	120	5	19
Oatmeal Raisin, 1 oz	130	6	18
Indulgent: Double Choc Chunk, 1 oz	130	7	18
Milk Choc. Macadamia Nut, 1 oz	140	8	17
Pecan Choc Chunk, 1 oz	140	9	16
White Choc. Macadamia Nut, 1 oz	140	8	17
Tuxedos: Chocolate (3), 1.3 oz	180	7	26
Cinnamon Bun; Vanilla (3) 1.3 oz	180	8	26
Mint Chip Creme (2), 1 oz	140	7	20
Vanilla Creme Wafers (4)	150	8	20

Snackwell's

	C	F	Cb
Creme S'wich (2) 1 oz	110	3	20
Creme Sandwich, 12 Packs 1 pkg	210	5	38
Devil's Food Cake, Fat-Free, ½ oz	50	0	12
Lemon Creme Sandwich Sugar Free (3)	130	6	23
Shortbread Sugar Free (3) 1 oz	130	6	21

South Beach Living
Cookies: *Per Package*

	C	F	Cb
Peanut Butter	100	5	15
Oatmeal Choc. Chip	100	5	16

Stella D'Oro

	C	F	Cb
Almond Toast (2)	100	2	20
Anginetti, 1 oz	130	3.5	22
Anisette Sponge Low-Fat (2)	95	1	19
Anisette Toast Low-Fat (3)	125	1	27
Biscotti, average, ¾ oz	95	4	13
Breakfast Treats: Chocolate Cookie	90	3	15
Original	90	3	15
Original Mini, 1 oz	120	3.5	21
Viennese Cinnamon	90	2.5	16
Coffee Treats: Almond Toast (2)	100	2	20
Angel Wings, 1 oz	170	12	14
Anisette Sponge (2)	90	1	18
Anisette Toast, 1.1 oz	130	1	27
Banana Walnut Toast, 1 oz	100	2	19
Blueberry; Cinnamon Toast, 1 oz	100	1	20
Roman Egg Biscuits, 1.1 oz	130	4	21
Continental Cookie Collection, 1 oz	130	4.5	20
Egg Jumbo, 1.1 oz	120	1.5	26
Lady Stella Assortment, 1 oz	130	4.5	20
Margherite (2)	130	5	20
Margherite Mini, 1.1 oz	150	5	24
Swiss Fudge (2) 1.1 oz	170	9	22

Streit's

	C	F	Cb
Wafers: Chocolate (3)	160	9	19
Vanilla (3)	170	11	18
Rolls, Chocolate (3)	105	6	12

Sunshine

	C	F	Cb
Krispy: Original; Whole Wheat (5)	60	1.5	11
Oyster & Soup, 16 crackers	60	1.5	11
Wheat (5)	60	1.5	11
Cheez-It: Original (27), 1 oz	150	8	17
Reduced-Fat (29), 1 oz	130	4.5	20

Also See Snacks ~ Page 150

Per Cookie/Cracker (Unless Indicated) **C F Cb**

Trader Joe's

	C	F	Cb
100 Calorie Packs, average	100	2.5	18
Cherry Granola (2), 1 oz	110	4	18
Chocolate Almond Lacey's (2)	170	12	16
Chocolate Chip: Small (4), 1.1 oz	140	7	18
Large, Singles , 1.7 oz	280	14	35
Caramel Cashew (3), 1 oz	140	7	16
Dark Choc Chunks with Almonds (3)	140	7	17
Dunkers: Choc Chip (2), 1.2 oz	160	7	21
Choc Coated Choc. Chip (2), 1.3 oz	190	9	25
Ginger Snaps (5), 1 oz	140	6	21
Joe Joe's S'wich Cremes, Choc./Vanilla (2), 1 oz	130	5	20
Lemon Crisps (5)	120	4	19
Meringues: Low-Fat, Chocolate (4)	120	1.5	25
Fat-Free Vanilla (4)	110	0	27
Very Mini Meringues, Van. (100)	100	0	24
Oatmeal Raisin, 1.8 oz	270	12	35
Pecan Southern Style (4), 1 oz	150	9	15
Righteous Rounds Choc Chip (5), 1 oz	130	4	20
Thins: Meyer Lemon (9), 1 oz	160	5	25
Triple Ginger (9), 1 oz	140	4.5	24
Triple Choc Chunk, 1 oz	140	7	20
Ultimate Vanilla Wafers (5), 1 oz	120	6	15
Water Crackers (4)	60	1	12

Triscuit *~ See Page 85 (Nabisco)*

Whole Wheat Crackers: *Per Serving*

	C	F	Cb
Original (15), 1 oz	120	4.5	19
Thin Crisps, Orig. (15), 1 oz	130	5	21
Roasted Garlic (8), 1oz	120	4.5	20

Voortman

	C	F	Cb
Chunky Chip Cookies (1), ¾ oz	100	4.5	14
Sugar Free Cookies:			
Chocolate Chip (2), 1.4 oz	160	10	26
Fudge P'nut Butter Wafers (3), 1 oz	140	8	20
Lemon Wafers (3), 1 oz	130	8	17
Vanilla Wafers (3), 1 oz	130	8	17
Vanilla Wafers: Regular (3), 1.1 oz	140	6	20

Zesta:

	C	F	Cb
Crackers: Whole Grain Wheat (5)	60	1.5	11
Fat Free (5)	60	0	13
Original (5)	60	1.5	11

365 *(Whole Foods):*

	C	F	Cb
Choc Chip (5), 1 oz	130	6	19
Classic Fig Bars (2), 1.3 oz	140	2.5	27
Lady Fingers (5), 1.1 oz	120	1.5	25
Lemon Wafers (5), 0.9 oz	120	5	17
Oatmeal (6), 1 oz	130	4.5	20
Sandwich Cremes (2), average	130	5	20
Sugar (5), 1.1 oz	130	4	22

Thaw, Bake & Serve | C | F | Cb

Pillsbury Cookies: *Per Cookie Unless Indicated*
Refrigerated Cookie Dough
Big Deluxe Classics:

	C	F	Cb
Oatmeal Raisin	150	6	24
Peanut Butter Cup	170	8	22
White Chunk Macadamia Nut	170	9	22
Other varieties	170	8	23
Ready To Bake: Sugar Cookie (2)	170	8	22
Chocolate Chip with Walnuts (2)	170	9	22
Chocolate Chunk Chip (2)	180	9	23
Peanut Butter with Reese's Pieces (2)	170	8	22
S'mores (1); Chocolate Candy (2)	160	7	23
Create n Bake: Peanut Butter	120	6	16
Chocolate Chip	130	6	18
Peanut Butter	120	6	16
Sugar	120	5	18
Refrigerated Dough:			
Cinnamon Roll (1)	140	5	23
Flaky Cinnamon Twists with Icing (1)	180	9	22
Flaky Supreme with Icing (1)	370	19	48
Grands Flaky Supreme, Cinnamon Rolls with Icing (1)	310	9	54
Simply Bake Bars:			
P.B. Choc.; Turtle Supreme, 1/12 pkg	150	8	19

Toll House (Nestlé): *Per Cookie Unless Indicated*
Refrigerated Dough:

	C	F	Cb
Chocolate Chunk (2)	180	9	23
Jumbo Chocolate Chip (1)	180	9	23
Mini Brownie Bites (3)	160	8	20
Mini Chocolate Chip (3)	160	8	21
Walnut Chocolate Chip (2)	180	9	22
Ultimates Refrigerated Dough			
Chocolate Chip Lovers	180	9	23
Choc. Chips & Chunks with Pecans	190	10	22
Peanut Butter Chips & Choc Chunks	180	9	23
Triple Chocolate Decadence	170	8	23
Turtle	180	9	23
White Chocolate Macadamia Nut	190	10	22

Crispbreads | C | F | Cb

Per Crispbread Unless Indicated

	C	F	Cb
Finn Crisp: Original, Rye	40	0	10
Other types	19	0	3
Kavli Norwegian:			
Crispy Thin (3)	50	0	11
Hearty Thick (2)	60	0	12
Malsovit Meal Wafers	75	4	7
New York Flatbread Crisps	35	0	7
Ry-Krisp: Natural (2)	50	0	11
Seasoned (2)	60	1	11
Sesame (2)	60	2	10
Ryvita: Dark/Light (2)	70	0	16
WASA: Crisp'n Light 7 Grain (3)	60	0	13
Fiber	30	1	7
Hearty, 0.5 oz	45	0	11
Light Rye (2), 0.5 oz	60	0	14
Multi Grain, 0.5 oz	45	0	10
Whole Wheat, 0.5 oz	50	1	10

Matzos

Manischewitz

	C	F	Cb
Egg 'n Onion Matzo, 1 oz	100	1	23
Mandelin (9)	35	2	4
Matzo Meal, 1/4 cup	130	0	28
Matzo Farfel, 1 cup, 2.7 oz	180	0.5	60
Passover Egg Matzos, 1.1 oz	120	0	28
Tam Tam Crackers, Onion (10)	140	5	21
Thin Salted; Thin Tea Matzos, 0.9 oz	100	0	22
Unsalted, 1 oz	90	0	20
Whole Wheat, 1 oz	110	0.5	23
Crackers: Miniatures (10)	110	0	25
Passover Egg Matzo (11)	110	0	20
Streit's			
Mediterranean Matzos, 1 Matzo, 1 oz	90	0.5	18
Unsalted Matzos, 1 Matzo, 1 oz	100	0	23

    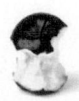

Quick Guide

Cream
Average All Brands
Half & Half Cream:

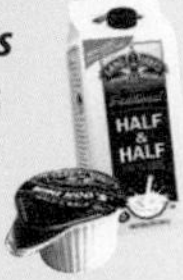

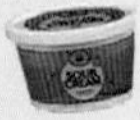

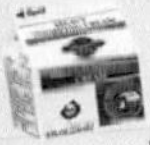

	C	F	Cb
1 Tbsp, 0.5 oz	20	1.5	0.5
2 Tbsp, 1 oz	40	3	1
¼ cup, 2 oz	80	6	2
Single Serve Cup, ⅜ fl.oz	15	1.5	0.5
Light: Coffee/table (20% fat): 1 Tbsp	30	3	0.5
2 Tbsp, 1 oz	60	6	1

Sour Cream:

	C	F	Cb
Regular: 1 Tbsp, 0.5 oz	25	2.5	1
1 cup, 8 oz	490	48	10
Low-Fat/Light: 1 Tbsp, 0.5 oz	20	1.5	1
2 Tbsp, 1 oz	40	3	2
Fat-Free: Average, 2 Tbsp, 1 oz	25	0	4
Hood, 2 Tbsp, 1 oz	25	0	4
Kroger, 2 Tbsp, 1 oz	20	0	3
Naturally Yours; Oak Farm, 2 Tbsp	20	0	3
Knudsen, 2 Tbsp, 1 oz	30	0	5

Sour Cream Substitute:

	C	F	Cb
Albertson's, 2 Tbsp, 1 oz	60	5	2
Tofutti Sour Supreme, 2 Tbsp, 1 oz	85	7	9

Whipping Cream:
Heavy (37% fat):

	C	F	Cb
1 l.fluid/2 T. whipped	50	5.5	0.5
¼ cup whipped	100	11	1
½ cup fluid/1 cup whipped	400	44	3.5
Light (30% fat):			
1 Tbsp fluid/2 Tbsp whipped	45	4.5	0.5
½ cup fluid/1 cup whipped	350	37	4

Coconut Cream/Milk

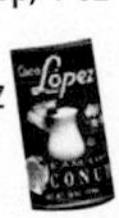

Coconut Cream (Canned),

	C	F	Cb
Plain/unsweetened: 2 Tbsp, 1 oz	75	6.5	3
½ cup, 4 oz	285	26	12
Sweetened: *Coco Lopez,* 1 oz	130	5	21
½ cup, 4 oz	520	20	84

Coconut Milk (Canned):

	C	F	Cb
Natural Value: Reg., ¼ cup, 2 fl.oz	120	11	5
Lite, ¼ cup, 2 fl.oz	55	5	1
Thai Kitchen: Lite, ¼ cup, 2 fl.oz	45	4	1
Premium, 2 fl.oz	120	10	4
Coconut Water (Center), 1 cup	45	0.5	9

Whipped Toppings
Average All Brands

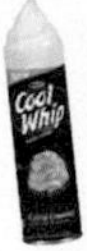

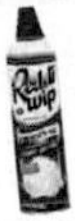

	C	F	Cb
Cream (Pressurized): 2 Tbsp	20	1	1
¼ cup	45	4	2
½ cup	90	8	4
Cream Topping: Lite, 2 Tbsp	20	1	3
Cool Whip: Extra Creamy, 2 Tbsp	25	2	2
Lite, 2 Tbsp, ¼ oz	15	1	2
Free, 2 Tbsp, 0.32 oz	15	0	3
Kraft: Dream Whip, 2 Tbsp	10	0	2
Reddi-Wip: Original, 2 Tbsp, 0.28 oz	15	1	0.5
Chocolate, 2 Tbsp, 0.28 oz	15	1	1
Extra Creamy, 2 Tbsp, 0.28 oz	20	1.5	0.5
Fat-Free, 2 Tbsp, 0.28 oz	5	0	1

Creamers (Non-Dairy)

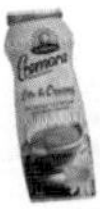

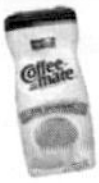

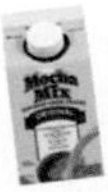

Powder:
Coffee-Mate/Cremora/N-Rich

	C	F	Cb
Original: 1 tsp	10	0.5	1
1 heaping tsp	25	2	2
Lite, 1 tsp	10	1.5	2
Flavors: 4 tsp	60	3	8
Fat-Free, Average, 4 tsp	50	0	11

Liquid/Refrigerated: *Per Tablespoon*
Coffee-Mate

	C	F	Cb
Unflavored: Original, 1 Tbsp	20	1	2
Fat-Free, 1 Tbsp	10	0	2
Low-Fat, 1 Tbsp	10	0.5	1
Flavors: Average all flavors, 1 Tbsp	35	1.5	5
Fat-Free, all flavors, 1 Tbsp	25	0	5
Hood, Country Creamer, 1 Tbsp	20	1.5	2

International Delight:

	C	F	Cb
Average all flavors, 1 Tbsp	40	1.5	7
Fat-Free French Vanilla, 1 Tbsp	30	0	7

Kroger
Coffee, Fat-Free & Lactose Free:

	C	F	Cb
French Vanilla, 1 Tbsp	30	0	6
Hazelnut, 1 Tbsp	35	1.5	6
Mocha Mix: Original, 1 Tbsp	20	1.5	2
Fat-Free, 1 Tbsp	10	0	1
Lite, 1 Tbsp	10	0.5	1
Silk: Original, 1Tbsp	15	1	1
French Vanilla; Hazelnut, 1 Tbsp	20	1	3

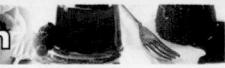

## Ready-To-Serve	C	F	Cb
Instant Pudding, Regular, ½ cup	170	4	30
Reduced Calorie: *Estee*	70	0	12
Jell-O Snacks, sugar-free, ½ cup	60	1	13
Royal Flan,Vanilla sugar-free, ½ cup	80	0	21
Hunt's Snack Pack: *Per 3.5oz Cup*			
Puddings, average all flavors	120	3.5	21
Jell-O Puddings:			
Pudding & Pie Filling: *Per ¼ Package*			
Cook & Serve, average, prepared	150	3	26
Instant, regular, average, dry	100	0	23
Fat & Sugar Free, average, dry	30	0	8
Pudding Snacks: Fat-Free, 4 oz	100	0	23
Cheesecake Snack, Strawb. 3½ oz	130	2	26
Mousse Temptations, average, 2.3 oz	60	3	10
Smoothie Snacks, 4 oz	100	2.5	18
Kozy Shack Puddings:			
Regular :			
Chocolate, ½ cup, 4 oz	140	3.5	24
Key Lime, ½ cup, 4 oz	110	0	25
Low-Fat (1% Milk), 6-Pack,			
Average, 1 pudding cup	110	1	20
No Sugar Added, 4-Pack: *Per 1 Pudding Cup*			
Chocolate; Tapioca	65	1	11
Vanilla	90	3	10
Gelatin, Simplywell, 4 oz, av all	100	1	17
Rice: *Per ½ Pudding Cup, 4 oz*			
Original	130	3	22
Cinnamon Raisin	140	3	24
European Style	130	3.5	22
No Sugar Added, 1 pudding cup	70	0.5	14
Soy, average, 1 cup	115	2	22
Flans: Creme Caramel, 1 cup	150	3.5	27
Restaurant Style, 1 cup	190	6	28
Frozen Desserts: Cream Puffs (6)	260	20	15
Chocolate Truffle Rolls (8)	240	13	27
Mini Eclairs (5)	250	16	23
Mini Napoleons (5)	280	14	35
Tiramisu, 1 cup	220	10	29
Kraft Handi Snacks: *Per Cup (3.5 oz)*			
"Doubles", average all flavors	100	1	22
Rice Pudding	140	6	19
Vanilla Pudding	90	1	20
Choc. Pudding, Fat-Free	90	0	21

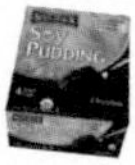

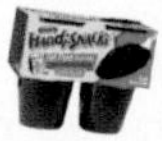

## Ready-To-Serve (Cont)	C	F	Cb
Kroger: *Per Container*			
Butterscotch, 3½ oz	110	2	22
Chocolate, 3½ oz	110	2.5	21
President's Choice			
Key Lime Pie (36 oz), ⅛ pie, 4.5 oz	440	20	59
Mississippi Mud Pie (36 oz), ⅛, 4.5 oz	405	22	49
Swiss Miss Pudding Snacks: *Per 4 oz Cup*			
Chocolate, Low-Fat	130	2	26
Chocolate Vanilla Swirl	140	3.5	27
Creamy Vanilla	140	3.5	24
Milk/Dark Chocolate	150	3.5	27
Old Fashioned Tapioca	140	3.5	24

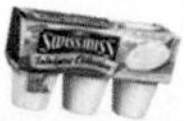

## Homemade Puddings			
Apple Tapioca, ½ cup	150	0	32
Bread Pudding, ½ cup	250	8	40
Blancmange, ½ cup	140	5	19
Chocolate, ½ cup	190	6	30
Crème Brûlée, ½ cup	400	35	16
Plum Pudding, 2 oz	170	3	32
Rice with Raisins, ½ cup	200	4	38
Sponge Pudding, 3½ oz	340	16	45
Tapioca Cream, ½ cup	110	4	15
Trifle, ½ cup	180	7	26

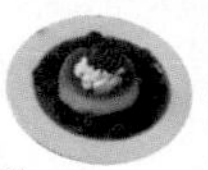

## Custards			
Custard Mix: Dry, ⅙ package	85	1	17
Prepared with 2% milk, ½ cup	140	3.5	21
Jello Flan, with 2% milk, ½ cup	140	2.5	20
Royal-Flan: Prep. with 2% milk, ½ cup	130	2.5	18
Homemade Custard			
Baked: Plain, ½ cup, 4½ oz	150	7	16
with skim milk, artif. sweetened	70	3	4
Boiled, ½ cup	165	7	18

## Meringues			
Meringue Swirl, ½ oz	50	0	8
Meringue Shell, 1 oz shell	100	0	16

## Gelatin • Parfait • Jell-O			
Gelatin Mix: *Jell-O, Royal ~ Made Up*			
Regular, all flavors, ½ cup	80	0	18
Sugar Free/Low Calorie, ½ cup	10	0	0
Creme Gelatin/Parfait: *Per ½ Cup*			
Ida Mae, ½ cup	60	2	10
Reser's, Dessert Parfait, 3.88 oz	100	2	19
Gel Snacks *(Jell-O):* Regular, 3.5 oz	90	0	22
X-Treme Snacks:			
Cherry/Raspb., 3½ oz	70	0	17
Watermelon/Apple, 3½ oz	100	0	24

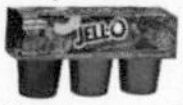

Chicken Eggs

Fresh Eggs

Raw (weight with shell):	C	F	Cb
Small, 1.4 oz	65	4	0
Medium, 1.55 oz	70	4	0
Large, 1.76 oz	75	4.5	0
Extra Large, 1.98 oz	80	5	0
Jumbo, 2.22 oz	90	5.5	0
Egg Yolk, 1 extra large	63	5	0
Egg White, 1 extra large	16	0	0

Dried Egg Powder

	C	F	Cb
Whole Egg: ¼ cup, 1 oz	170	12	0
1 Tbsp	30	2	0
Egg White, ¼ cup, 1 oz	105	0	0
Egg Yolk, ¼ cup, 1 oz	195	18	0

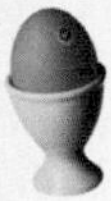

Egg Substitutes

¼ Cup (Equivalent to 1 Egg) ~ Zero Cholesterol.

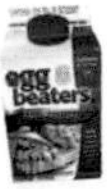

	C	F	Cb
Better 'n Eggs (*Papetti*), ¼ cup, 2 oz	30	0	1
Egg Beaters (*Fleischmann's*) Frozen/Liquid, Regular/Flavors, ¼ cup, 2.2 oz	30	0	1
Ener-G, Egg Replacer, 1½ tsp, 4 g	15	0	4
Egg Substitute (*Albertson's*), ¼ cup	30	0	1
Egg Whites, 4 Tbsp, ¼ cup, 2 oz	30	0	0
Nature Egg, Simply Egg White, ¼ cup, 2 oz	25	0	0
Second Nature, Fat-Free, ¼ cup, 2 fl.oz	35	0	1

Other Eggs

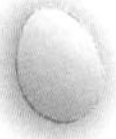

	C	F	Cb
Duck, 1 large, 2½ oz	130	9.5	0
Goose, 1 large, 5 oz	280	19	0
Quail, 3 eggs, 1 oz	42	3	0
Turkey, 1 large, 3 oz	135	9.5	0
Turtle, 1 egg, 1¾ oz	75	5	0

Omega-3 Fat Enriched

	C	F	Cb
Eggland's Best, 1 large	70	4	0
Eggs Plus (*Pilgrim's Pride*), 1 large	70	4.5	1

Note: Cholesterol content same as regular eggs, but Omega-3 fats inhibit blood cholesterol increase.
(Extra Notes ~ *See Page 259*)

Cooked Eggs

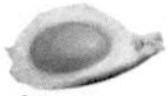

	C	F	Cb
Boiled Egg: *Same as raw egg*			
Hard-Cooked (*Egg•Lands*), Small, Peeled	65	4	0
Fried Egg:			
With fat: 1 large egg	105	9	0.5
2 small eggs	175	13	1
No fat/nonstick pan, 1 large	75	5	0.5
Deviled Egg, 2 halves	145	13	0.5
Eggs Benedict (2) on toast or English muffin	860	56	25
Eggs Florentine (2) on toast or English muffin	890	59	25
Pickled Egg, 1 large	80	5.5	0
Poached Egg, 1 large	65	4	0
Quiche (Homemade, average):			
Egg & Bacon, 1 slice, 5.3 oz	580	43	27
Ham & Cheese, 1 slice, 5.3 oz	475	33	29
Scotch Egg, 1 egg	300	21	16
Scrambled Eggs: 1 large egg:			
With 1 Tbsp milk + 1 tsp fat	120	9	1
With 1 Tbsp skim milk/no fat	85	5.5	1
2 large eggs:			
With 2 Tbsp milk + 2 tsp fat	260	20	2
With 2 Tbsp skim milk, w/o fat	180	11	2

Omelets

	C	F	Cb
1 Egg: Plain (with 1 tsp fat)	125	10	0.5
With ½ oz cheese	175	15	0.5
With ½ oz cheese + ½ oz ham	200	16	0.5
2 Eggs: Plain (with 2 tsp fat)	250	20	1
With 1 oz cheese	360	29	2
With 1 oz cheese+1 oz ham	410	32	2
3 Eggs: Plain (with 1 Tbsp fat)	360	29	1.5
With 2 oz cheese	580	47	2.5
With 2 oz cheese+2 oz ham	680	53	2.5
Extras: Tomato/Onion/Veggies	20	0	4.5
Egg Substitute (*EggBeaters*):			
2 eggs (½ cup) + 1 tsp fat	100	4	2
3 eggs (¾ cup) + 2 tsp fat	160	8	3
Extras: 1 oz Cheese	110	9	1
1 oz Ham	50	3	1
Tomato/Onion/veggies	20	0	4.5

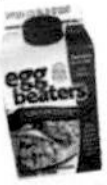

Egg Nog ~ *Per ½ Cup (4 fl.oz)*

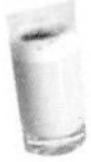

	C	F	Cb
Average all Brands, ½ cup	170	9.5	17
Regular: *Borden*	160	9	17
Hood (*Golden*)	180	9	22
Light/Low-Fat: *Horizon; Hood*	140	4	22

Breakfast Sides

	C	F	Cb
Toast: Plain, 1 thick slice	85	1	13
With 2 tsp butter/margarine	155	9	13
With 3 tsp/1 Tbsp fat	190	13	13
English Muffin: Plain, 2 oz	130	1	26
With 3 tsp fat	230	12	26
Bacon, 2 strips	70	5	0
Ham, Lean, 2 oz	100	3	0
Hash Browns:			
½ cup, 3 oz	125	6.5	14
1 cup serving, 6 oz	250	13	28
Sausages, 2 links (1 oz each)	180	16	1.5

Frozen Egg Breakfasts

	C	F	Cb
Aunt Jemima Breakfast Sandwiches: *Per Package*			
Ham, Egg & Cheese Griddlecake	240	8	33
Sausage, Egg & Cheese Biscuit	340	21	27
Sausage, Egg & Cheese Croissant	350	23	22
Jimmy Dean			
Biscuit, Sausage, Egg & Cheese (1)	440	31	27
Croissant: Sausage, Egg & Cheese (1)	430	29	30
Muffin, Sausage, Egg & Cheese	350	21	28
Omelet: 3 Cheese (1)	290	23	4
Ham & Cheese (1)	250	19	4
Pillsbury: Toaster Scrambles,			
Cheese Sauce, Egg & Bacon	180	12	16
Cheese Sauce, Egg & Sausage	180	11	16
Red Baron: Scrambles			
Bacon (1), 5 oz	410	21	36
Sausage (1), 5 oz	370	19	36
Western (1), 5 oz	350	16	36
Frozen Pancake/Waffles: *See Page 132*			

Frozen Egg Rolls

	C	F	Cb
Kahiki: Chicken (1), 3 oz	80	3.5	10
Pork & Shrimp (1), 3 oz	100	5	10
Vegetable (1), 3 oz	70	2	11
Sauce, 1 packet	10	0	3
La Choy Mini,			
Chicken (1), 3 oz	140	4.5	18
Lotus: Pork (1), 3.8 oz	180	7	18
Vegetable (1), 3.8 oz	70	1.5	13
Minh,			
Chicken (1), 3 oz	160	6	20
Pagoda Express,			
Vegetable (1), without sauce, 3 oz	130	4.5	20
TGI Friday's,			
Thai Style Chkn (1), 3 oz	150	5	19
Trader Joes,			
Vegetable (1), 3 oz	100	4	16

Fast-Foods/Restaurants

	C	F	Cb
Arby's:			
Bacon, Egg & Cheese Croissant	390	24	26
Au Bon Pain: Egg on a Bagel	430	12	58
Bob Evans			
Farmers Market Omelette	630	45	14
Ham & Cheddar Omelette	515	36	4
Three Cheese Omelette	530	40	5
Western Omelette	530	36	8
Bojangles: Egg Biscuit	400	30	26
Bacon, Egg & Cheese Biscuit	550	42	27
Bruegger's Bagels:			
Breakfast Sandwiches:			
Egg & Cheese	470	14	63
Egg, Cheese & Sausage	560	23	63
Burger King: Croissan'wich			
Bacon Egg & Cheese	340	19	26
Ham Egg & Cheese	330	17	27
Sausage & Cheese	380	24	26
Carl's Jr, Bacon & Egg Burrito	550	32	37
Chick-Fil-A			
Chicken, Egg & Cheese Bagel	480	20	49
Denny's: T-Bone Steak & Eggs	780	36	4
Omelette: Ham & Cheddar	590	44	4
Ultimate with Hash Browns	880	66	34
Veg.-Cheese with Hash Browns	700	49	36
Del Taco, Egg & Cheese Burrito	400	18	35
Dunkin Donuts			
Bacon, Egg & Cheese Croissant	510	31	39
Ham, Egg & Cheese Bagel	510	16	67
Eat 'N Park: Cheese Omelette	390	30	2.5
Western Omelette	345	21	7
Hardee's: Loaded Omelet Biscuit	610	42	36
Sausage & Egg Biscuit	590	42	36
IHOP: T-Bone Steak & Eggs	1160	n/a	70
Colorado Omelette	1890	n/a	130
Jack in the Box			
Bacon, Egg & Cheese Biscuit	420	24	36
Sausage, Egg & Cheese Biscuit	570	39	37
McDonald's: Egg McMuffin	300	12	30
Bacon, Egg & Cheese Biscuit, regular	420	23	37
Scrambled Eggs (2)	170	11	1
Whataburger			
Breakfast Platter with Bacon, 2 slices	730	45	93

Quick Guide   C   F   Cb

Butter & Margarine
Average All Brands

	C	F	Cb
Regular: 1 tsp, 0.18 oz	35	4	0
1 Pat/Single Portion, 0.18 oz	35	4	0
1 Tbsp, approximately ½ oz	100	11	0
2 Tbsp, 1 oz	205	23	0
1 Stick, ½ cup, 4 oz	815	92	0
1 Pound, 2 cups, 16 oz	3260	368	0
Light (Regular) 40% Fat:			
1 tsp, 0.18 oz	25	3	0
1 Tbsp, ½ oz	75	8.5	0
2 Tbsp, 1 oz	150	16	0
Whipped Butter (Regular):			
1 tsp, 0.14 oz	30	3	0
1 Tbsp, 0.35 oz	70	7.5	0
1 Stick, ½ cup, 2 ⅔ oz	545	62	0
Whipped Light Butter (40% Fat):			
1 tsp, 0.18 oz	25	3	0.5
1 Tbsp, 0.32 oz	45	5	1
2 Tbsp, 0.63 oz	90	10	2
Unsalted: Same as Regular			

Flavored Butter/Spreads

Average All Brands

	C	F	Cb
Honey Butter (60% Fat):			
1 Tbsp, ½ oz	90	8	4
Downey's, 1 Tbsp, ½ oz	60	1	11
Garlic Butter (80% Fat):			
1 Tbsp, ½ oz	100	11	0
Sweet Cream Butter:			
Regular, 1 Tbsp	100	11	0
Stick *(Parkay)*, 70% Fat, 1 Tbsp	90	10	0
Tub *(Land O'Lakes)*, 50% Fat, 1 Tbsp	90	10	0

Ghee (Clarified Butter)

(Example: *Purity Farms*)
Note: Ghee is 100% fat compared to regular butter (80% fat + 20% water)

	C	F	Cb
1 tsp, 0.18 oz	45	5	0
1 Tbsp, ½ oz	120	14	0
2¼ Tbsp, 1 oz	250	28	0

Light & Reduced Fat Spreads

Per 1 Tablespoon, ½ oz	C	F	Cb
Albertson's: Country (48%)	60	7	0
Butter Blend	80	9	0
Benecol: Spread	70	8	0
Light Spread	50	5	0
Blue Bonnet, Homestyle (48% Veg Oil)	60	7	0
Brummel & Brown, Spread	45	5	0
Country Crock *(Shedd's):*			
Regular	60	7	0
Light; Calcium & Vitamins	50	5	0
Spreadable Butter	80	9	0
Fleischmann's: Soft Spread	60	7	0
Original Stick	80	9	0
Light Spread	40	4.5	0
'I Can't Believe It's Not Butter': Reg.	70	8	0
Light Soft Spread	50	5	0
Imperial: Stick	80	8	0
Tub	50	5	0
Land O'Lakes: Butter	100	11	0
Honey Butter	90	8	4
Light Butter Whipped	45	5	0
Light Butter	50	6	0
Parkay: Squeeze	70	8	0
Light Stick	45	5	0
Original Spread	70	7	0
Original Stick	80	9	0
Promise: Buttery	80	8	0
Fat-Free	5	0	0
Light	45	5	0
Smart Balance: 67% Buttery	80	9	0
Heart Right	80	8	0
Light (37%)	45	5	0
Omega Plus	80	9	0
Smart Beat, Fat-Free	50	0	1
Smart Squeeze,	5	0	1

Butter Substitutes

	C	F	Cb
Butter Buds:			
1 serving, ½ tsp	5	0	2
Sprinkles, 1 tsp	5	0	1
Earth Balance, Non GMO, 1 T.	100	11	0
Molly McButter, ½ tsp	5	0	1
Shedd's Willow Run, Soy, 1 Tbsp	90	10	0
Sunsweet, Lighter Bake,			
1 Tbsp, 0.67 oz	35	0	9
(Butter/Oil Replacement)			

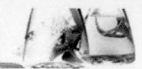

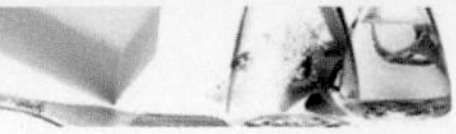

Animal Fats/Lards

Average All Types
**Beef Tallow/Drippings, Lard (Pork),
Chicken, Duck, Goose, Turkey.**

1 Tbsp, 13g	**115**	**13**	0
2¼ Tbsp, 1 oz	**255**	**28**	0
1 cup, 7¼ oz	**1850**	**205**	0
½ pound, 8 oz	**2040**	**227**	0

Ghee/Butter Oil:

1 Tbsp, ½ oz	**120**	**14**	0
2¼ Tbsp, 1 oz	**250**	**28**	0

Vegetable Shortening

Average All Types (example: Crisco)

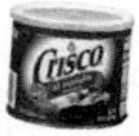

1 Tbsp, 13g	**115**	**13**	0
2¼ Tbsp, 1 oz	**250**	**28**	0
1 cup, 7¼ oz	**1810**	**205**	0

Vegetable Oils

Includes almond, avocado, canola, corn, coconut, flaxseed, grapeseed, linseed, mustard, olive, palm, peanut, rice bran, safflower, sesame, sunflower, soybean, wheat germ. Note: Oil is 100% fat.

1 tsp, 5g	**45**	**5**	0
1 Tbsp, ½ oz	**120**	**14**	0
2 Tbsp, 1 oz	**250**	**28**	0
1 cup, 7¾ oz	**1930**	**205**	0

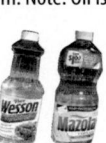

Fish Oils

Average All Types (Includes Cod Liver, Herring, Salmon, Sardines): 1 Tbsp, ½ oz   **125**   **14**   0

Cooking Sprays/Squeezes

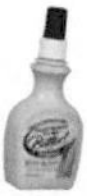

Cooking Sprays (PAM, Mazola, I Can't Believe It's Not Butter, Weight Watchers, Wesson):

Per serving	**2**	**0**	0
1-3 second spray	**6**	**1**	0
I Can't Believe It's Not Butter	**0**	**0**	0
Parkay Buttery Spray	**0**	**0**	0
Squeeze (Parkay), 1 Tbsp, ½ oz	**70**	**8**	0

Olestra (Olean)

Olestra *(Olean)*	**0**	**0**	0

Note: *Olean* is Proctor & Gamble's brand name for Olestra – a no-calorie cooking oil that gives snacks (like potato chips, tortilla chips and crackers) taste and texture without adding fat or calories.

Examples:
- *Frito-Lay* Light Products
  (Lays, Ruffles, Tostitos, Doritos)
- *Pringles* Fat-Free Potato Crisps

Quick Guide

Mayonnaise

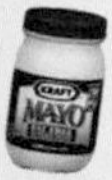

Regular

Average All Brands, 1 Tbsp	**90**	**10**	0
Best Foods; Kraft, 1 Tbsp	**90**	**10**	0
½ cup, 4 oz	**720**	**80**	0
Hain, Safflower Oil, 1 Tbsp	**100**	**11**	0
Spectrum, Canola Mayo, 1 Tbsp	**100**	**11**	0

Light/Reduced Fat

Best Foods; Hellman's, 1 Tbsp	**35**	**3.5**	1
Kraft, 1 Tbsp	**45**	**4**	2
Smart Balance, Omega, 1 Tbsp	**50**	**4.5**	2
Spectrum,			
Light Canola Mayo Eggless, 1 Tbsp	**35**	**3.5**	0

Fat Free

Kraft: 1 Tbsp	**10**	**0**	2
½ cup, 4 oz	**80**	**0**	16
Smart Beat, 1 Tbsp	**10**	**0**	3
Sugar Free: Dukes Mayo, 1 Tbsp	**100**	**12**	0

Mayonnaise Style Dressing

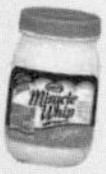

Best Foods, Sandwich Spread, 1 Tbsp	**60**	**5**	2
Kraft, Sandwich Shop Mayo, av, 1 oz	**80**	**7**	4

Miracle Whip Salad Dressing:

Regular, 1 Tbsp, ½ oz	**35**	**3**	2
Light, 1 Tbsp, ½ oz	**25**	**1.5**	3
Free, 1 Tbsp, ½ oz	**15**	**0**	3

Nayonaise *(Nasoya)*
(Tofu Base/Dairy Free/Eggless)

Regular, 1 Tbsp, ½ oz	**35**	**3.5**	1
Fat-Free, 1 Tbsp, ½ oz	**10**	**0**	2

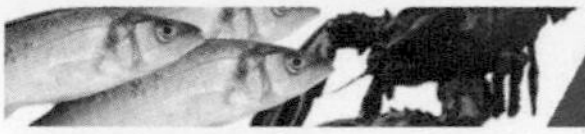

Quick Guide

Fresh Fish **C** **F** **Cb**
Low Oil (Less than 2.5% fat)
White/Lightly-colored flesh. Examples:
Cod, Flounder, Haddock, Halibut, Mahi Mahi,
Perch, Pike, Pollock, Snapper, Sole, Whiting.

Per 4 oz Edible Portion

	C	F	Cb
Raw, 4 oz (without bones)	90	1	0
Steamed, Broiled, Baked	130	1	0
Fried: Lightly Floured	210	8	3.5
Breaded	260	12	8
In Batter	320	16	27

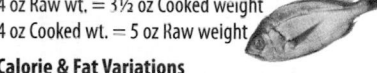

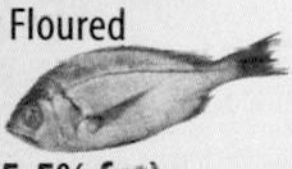

Medium Oil (2.5-5% fat)
Lightly-colored flesh. Examples: **C** **F** **Cb**
Bluefin Tuna, Catfish, Kingfish, Orange Roughy,
Salmon (Pink), Swordfish, Rainbow Trout, Yellowtail.

	C	F	Cb
Raw, 4 oz (without bones)	140	5	0
Baked, Broiled, 4 oz	175	6	0
Fried, 4 oz	230	11	8

High Oil (Over 5% fat) **C** **F** **Cb**
Darker-colored flesh. Examples:
Albacore Tuna, Bluefish, Herring, Mackerel,
Salmon (Atl./Chinook/Sockeye), Sardines, Trout,
Whitefish.

	C	F	Cb
Raw, 4 oz (without bones)	230	16	0
Baked, Broiled, 4 oz	275	17	0
Fried, 4 oz	340	23	12

Cooking Yields (Fin Fish):
4 oz Raw wt. = 3½ oz Cooked weight
4 oz Cooked wt. = 5 oz Raw weight

Calorie & Fat Variations
The amount of fat/oil in fish varies with the species,
season and locality. Within the same fish, fat/oil content
is generally higher towards the head.

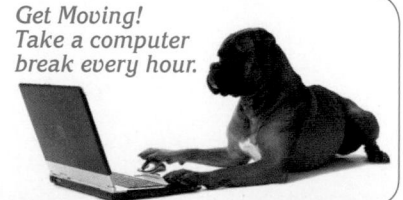

Get Moving!
Take a computer
break every hour.

Fish & Shellfish | C | F | Cb

Edible Weights: (no bones/shell)

	C	F	Cb
Abalone, Raw, 3 oz	90	0.5	5
Ahi Tuna, grilled, 6 oz fillet (w/o fat)	235	2	0
Anchovy: Paste, 1 Tbsp, ¼ oz	15	1	0.5
Canned in oil, drained, 5 only, ¾ oz	40	2	0
Pickled, 1 oz	50	3	0
Barracuda (Pacific), raw, 4 oz	130	3	0
Bass: Sea, raw, 4.6 oz fillet	125	2.5	0
Striped: Raw, 1 fillet, 5½ oz	150	3.5	0
Baked, 3 oz	105	3	0
Blue Fish: Raw, 1 fillet, 5¼ oz	185	6.5	0
Baked, 3 oz	130	5	0
Butterfish, raw, 3 oz	125	7	0
Cajun & Creole Dishes: *See Page 168*			
Calamari, breaded/fried, 7 oz	350	15	16
Carp, raw, 3 oz	110	5	0
Catfish (Wild): Raw, 4 oz	110	3	0
Fried, breaded, 1 fillet, 3 oz	200	12	7
Baked, 3 oz	90	2.5	0
Caviar, black/red, 1 Tbsp, 16g	40	3	0.5
Clams: Raw, 3 oz (4 large/9 small)	65	1	2
Fried, breaded, 6.6 oz (20 small)	380	21	20
Canned, drained, ½ cup, 2½ oz	120	1.5	4
Minced, ¼ cup, 2 oz	25	0	2
Clam Juice: (*Snow's*) 1 Tbsp	0	0	0
Cod, Atlantic/Pacific: Raw, 4 oz	95	1	0
Baked/Broiled, 1 fillet, 6¼ oz	190	2	0
Canned, 3 oz	90	1	0
Minced, ¼ cup, 2 oz	25	0	0
Smoked/Dry Heat, 3 oz	90	1	0
Crab: Alaska King, raw, 1 leg, 6 oz	145	1	0
1 leg, cooked, 4¾ oz	130	2	0
Blue: Raw, 1 crab			
(⅓ lb whole crab, ¾ oz flesh)	20	0.2	0
Steamed, 3 oz	85	1	0
Canned, drained, ½ cup, 2½ oz	65	1	0
Dungeness, 1 crab, 5¾ oz edible			
(from 1½ lb whole crab)	180	2	2
Imitation Crab Legs/Stix, 3oz	80	0.5	13
Crab Cakes (Low-fat), (1), 2 oz	95	4.5	0.5
Regular (1), 3 oz	130	6.5	0.5
Crab Legs, restaurant (*Red Lobster*)	260	4.5	0
Crayfish, raw, 4 oz (edible)	90	1	0
Croaker, raw, 3 oz	90	3	0
Cuttlefish, raw, 3 oz	70	1	1
Dolphinfish, raw, 1 fillet, 7 oz	175	1.5	0
Eel: Raw, 3 oz	155	10	0
Smoked/Dry Heat, 3 oz	200	13	0
Fish & Chips: *Arthur Treacher*	1540	101	132
Denny's, without condiments	960	54	83
Fish S'wich with Tartar Sauce, 5½ oz	430	23	41
Fish Sticks (1), frozen, breaded, 1 oz	70	3.5	6

9 5

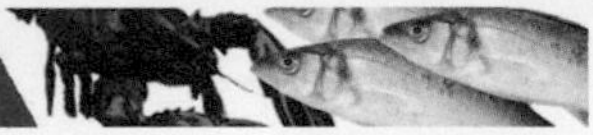

Fish & Shellfish (Cont)

Edible Weights: (no bones/shell)	C	F	Cb
Fish Oil, 1 Tbsp, ½ oz	125	14	0
Flounder/Sole: Raw, 4 oz	105	1.5	0
Baked, 1 fillet, 4½ oz	150	2	0
Frozen Fish: See Page 97			
Gefilte Fish: See Kosher/Deli Foods, Page 171			
Grouper, raw, 4 oz	105	1	0
Haddock: Raw, 4 oz	100	1	0
Broiled, 1 fillet, 5¼ oz	170	1.5	0
Smoked, 3 oz	100	1	0
Baked, 3 oz	95	1	0
Halibut: Raw, 4 oz	125	3	0
Baked, ½ fillet, 2¾ oz	225	5	0
Herring: Atlantic, raw, 4 oz	180	10	0
Pickled, 2 pieces, 1 oz	80	5	3
In Sour Cream, 1 oz	55	3	5
Party Snacks, ¼ cup, drained, 2 oz	120	5	0
Rollmops, 1½ oz	110	8	6
Canned: Plain, drained, 3 oz	130	8	0
in Tomato Sauce, 3.5 oz	140	8	2
Smoked, kippered, 4 oz	245	14	0
Jellyfish: Raw, 4 oz	30	0	0
Dried, Salted, 1 cup, 2 oz	20	1	0
King Fish, raw, 4 oz	120	2.5	0
Ling, raw, 4 oz	100	0.5	0
Lobster, Northern: Raw, 4 oz	105	1	0.5
1 Lobster, 6¼ oz			
(from 1½ lb whole lobster)	160	1.5	1
Cooked, 1 cup, 5 oz	140	1	2
Lobster Newberg, average, ¾ cup	360	20	9
Lobster Thermidor, av., 1 serving	370	22	15
Lobster Salads, average, ½ cup	220	13	5
Lobster Tail, restaurant (Red Lobster)	260	3	0
Lomi Salmon, ¼ cup, c cup	20	1	3
Lox, Regular/Nova, 2 oz	65	2.5	0
Mackerel: Atlantic, raw, 4 oz	230	16	0
Broiled, 3 oz fillet	230	16	0
Jack, canned, ½ cup, 3⅓ oz	150	6	0
King, raw, 4 oz	120	2	0
Pacific/Jack: Raw, 4 oz	180	9	0
Broiled, 3 oz	170	9	0
Spanish, raw, 4 oz	160	7	0
Mahi-Mahi, raw, 4 oz	125	1	0
Milkfish, raw, 4 oz	170	7.5	0
Monkfish: Raw, 4 oz	85	1.5	0
Baked, 3 oz	80	2	0
Mullet, striped, raw, 4 oz	135	4.5	0
Mussels: Raw, 4 oz (edible weight)	100	2.5	4
1 cup, 5¼ oz (edible weight)	130	3.5	5
Cooked, moist heat, 3 oz	150	4	6

	C	F	Cb
Ocean Perch: Raw, 4 oz	105	2	0
Baked, 3 oz	105	2	0
Octopus, common, raw, 4 oz	95	1	2.5
Orange Roughy, raw, 4 oz	85	1	0
Oysters: Common, raw, 3 oz	70	2	4
Eastern raw: 6 medium, 3 oz	50	1.5	4.5
1 cup, 8¾ oz	150	4	14
Fried/breaded, 6 medium, 3 oz	170	11	10
Pacific, raw, 1 medium, 1¾ oz	40	1	2
Oysters Rockerfeller, 3 oysters	220	13	12
Perch, average, raw, 4 oz	105	1	0
Pike: Northern, raw, 4 oz	100	1	0
Walleye, raw, 4 oz	105	1.5	0
Pollock, raw, 4 oz	105	1	0
Pout (Ocean), raw, 4 oz	90	1	0
Pompano, Florida, raw, 4 oz	185	11	0
Porgy/Scup, raw, 4 oz	150	4	0
Quahogs ~ See Clams			
Red-Snapper, raw, 4 oz	115	1.5	0
Rockfish, Pacific, raw, 4 oz	110	2	0
Roe, raw, 2 Tbsp, 1 oz	40	2	0.5
Sablefish: Raw, 4 oz	220	17	0
Smoked, 3 oz	220	17	0
Salmon:			
Raw: Chinook, 4 oz	205	12	0
Atlantic; Coho/Silver, 4 oz	210	12	0
Chum; Pink, 4 oz	135	4	0
Red/Sockeye, 4 oz	190	10	0
Baked: Atlantic/Coho, 3 oz	160	5	0
Smoked Salmon: Chinook, 3 oz	100	4	0
Pacific Supreme, 2 oz	100	4	0
Canned Salmon: *Average All Brands*			
Pink: 1 oz	40	2	0
¼ cup, 2.2 oz 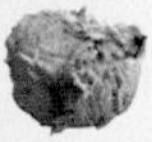	90	5	0
3¾ oz can, whole	155	8.5	0
7½ oz can, whole	300	17	0
Skinless/boneless, ¼ cup, 2 oz	70	2	0
Red Sockeye: 1 oz	50	3	0
¼ cup, 2.2 oz	110	7	0
3¾ oz can, whole	190	12	0
Atlantic, ½ cup, 3½ oz	230	14	0
Chinook/King, ½ cup 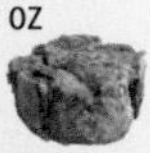	210	14	0
Chum, ½ cup, 3½ oz	140	5	0
Coho/Silver, ½ cup	155	5	0
Atlantic Steaks: Small, 8 oz	320	14	0
Medium, 12 oz 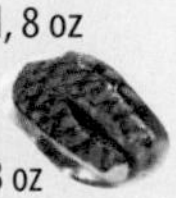	480	21	0
Large, 16 oz	640	28	0
Salmon Cake, take-out, 3 oz	240	15	6

Fish (Cont)

	C	F	Cb
Sardines (Canned): *Average All Brands*			
In Oil, undrained, 1 oz	85	7	0
Drained of oil, 1 oz	60	3	0
3¾ oz can, drained, (3¼ oz)	190	11	0
1 large/2 med. ⅗ " small, 0.8 oz	50	3	0
In Tomato/ Mustard Sauce, 1 oz	55	3	0
3¾ oz can (3 sardines)	210	12	1
Sashimi: *See Japanese Foods, Page 171*			
Scallop: Raw, 6 large/15 small, 3 oz	80	0.5	2
Breaded/fried, 6 pieces, 3½ oz	200	10	10
Sea Bass, raw, 4 oz	110	2	0
Seafood Salad, (Deli Style),			
½ cup, 3.5 oz	250	21	11
Shark: Raw, 4 oz	150	5	0
Batter-dipped, fried, 4 oz	220	13	6
Baked, 4 oz	185	7	0
Shark Fin, dried, 1 oz	30	0	0
Shrimp: Raw, in shell, ½ lb	140	2	1.5
Raw, shelled, 3 oz (12 large)	90	1.5	0.5
Breaded/fried, 3 oz (11 large)	210	11	10
Canned, 1 oz (10 shrimp)	30	0.5	0
Tiger, cooked, 1 shrimp, ½ oz	15	0.5	0
Battered, fried, 1 shrimp	60	4	3
Shrimp Cocktail, restaurant-style	140	2	1
Smelt, Rainbow, raw, 4 oz	110	3	0
Snapper: Raw, 3 oz	85	1	0
Cooked, 1 fillet, 6 oz	220	3	0
Sole, Raw, 4 oz	105	1.5	0
Squid: Raw, 4 oz	105	1.5	3.5
Fried, 3 oz	150	6	7
Surimi (Imitation Crab), 4 oz	110	0.5	17
Sweet & Sour Fish, ½ dish, 10 oz	580	29	53
Swordfish raw:			
Small Steak, 4 oz	135	4.5	0
Medium Steak, 6 oz	205	7	0
Tilapia, Rain Forest Fillets, 4 oz	110	2	0
Trout, Rainbow: Raw, 4 oz	135	4	0
Broiled, 3 oz	125	5	0
Smoked, 2 oz	110	6	0
Tuna: *Average All Brands*			
Raw: Albacore, 4 oz	190	8	0
Bluefin, 4 oz	165	5.5	0
Skipjack, Yellowfin, 4 oz	125	1	0
Broiled, 3 oz	115	1	0
Canned:			
In Water, drained:			
Chunk/Solid: 2 oz can	75	1.5	0
3 oz can	110	2.5	0
6 oz can	220	5	0

Tuna (Cont)

	C	F	Cb
In Oil, drained:			
Chunk Light: 2 oz	110	5	0
6 oz can, drained	315	14	0
Solid White, 2 oz	105	4.5	0
6.3 oz can, drained	330	14	0
Tuna Salad: Deli Style, ½ cup, 4 oz	300	24	15
Lower fat, 4 oz	210	10	11
Whitefish: Raw, 4 oz	150	6.5	0
Baked, 3 oz	145	6.5	1
Smoked, 3 oz	90	1	0
Whiting: Raw, 4 oz	100	1.5	0
Baked, 3 oz	100	1.5	0
Yellowtail: Raw, 4 oz	165	6	0
Grilled, 3 oz (from 4 oz raw)	160	6	0

Other Canned/Packaged Fish

	C	F	Cb
Bumble Bee:			
Tuna Salad Kits: *With Crackers*			
Original, 3.5 oz	300	22	18
with Mayonnaise	420	23	24
Fat-Free, 3.5 oz	150	1.5	24
Lunch on the Run, 8.2 oz	560	31	59
Seafood Salad with Crackers, 3.3 oz	180	5.5	27
Sensations Bowls:			
Spicy Thai Chili, 3 oz	160	7	9
Lemon & Cracked Pepper, 3 oz	110	4	2
Chicken of the Sea			
Albacore Tuna in Water, 3 oz pouch	100	3	0
Light Tuna in Oil, 3 oz pouch	100	4	0
Pink Salmon, skinless/boneless, 2 oz	60	2	0
Shrimp, medium, 4 oz can	90	1	2
Starkist			
Pouch: *Per 3 oz Pouch, Drained*			
Albacore Tuna, in water, 2 oz	70	1.5	1
Tuna Chunk Light, in water, 2 oz	60	0.5	1
Lunch-To-Go Kit: Chunk Light Tuna			
with Mayo & Crackers, 4.5 oz	240	9	20
Tuna Creations, av. all varieties, 2 oz	70	1	0

Frozen Fish Products

Gorton's: *Page 119*
Kroger: *Page 119*
Van De Kamp's: *Page 122*
Restaurant Chains: *Page 175*
Captain D's Seafood: *Page 187*
Long John Silver's: *Page 213*
Shoney's: *Page 239*
Southern Tsunami: *Page 242*
Wahoo's Fish Taco: *Page 254*

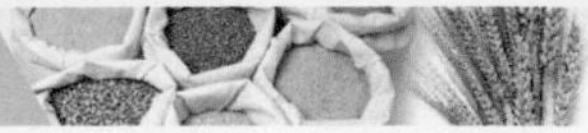

Flours & Grains	C	F	Cb
Amaranth Flour, ½ cup, 3½ oz	365	6.5	65
Arrowroot Flour, ½ cup, 2¼ oz	230	0	56
Barley: Regular, ½ cup, 2.6 oz	255	1	55
Pearled, raw, 3½ oz	350	1	78
Buckwheat: Regular, ½ cup, 3 oz	290	3	61
Groats: Roasted, dry, ½ cup, 2.9 oz	285	2	62
Roasted, cooked, 3½ oz	80	0.5	17
Flour, whole-groat, ½ cup, 2 oz	200	2	42
Bulgur: Dry, ½ cup, 2½ oz	240	1	53
Cooked, ½ cup, 3.2 oz	75	0.5	17
Carob Flour, ½ cup, 1.8 oz	115	0.5	46
Corn Kernels av., ckd, ½ cup	80	0.5	18
Corn Bran, ½ cup, 1.3 oz	85	0.5	33
Corn Flour/Masa, ½ cup, 2 oz	215	2.5	43
Corn Grits: Dry, ½ cup, 2¾ oz	290	1	62
Cooked, ½ cup, 4¼ oz	70	0.5	15
Corn Germ, toasted, ½ cup, 4 oz	100	1.5	22
Cornmeal: Average all Types,			
3 Tbsp, 1 oz	105	0.5	22
½ cup, 2½ oz	255	1	54
Mixes: same as above	230	1	48
Cornstarch: 1 Tbsp, 0.3 oz	30	0	8
½ cup, 2¼ oz	245	0	58
Couscous: Dry, 1 oz (3 oz cooked)	110	0	22
1 cup cooked, 5½ oz	175	0.5	37
Farina: Dry, ½ cup, 3.1 oz	325	0.5	69
Cooked, ½ cup, 4.1 oz	55	0	12
Flaxseed: Seeds, 1 Tbsp, 0.3 oz	45	3.5	2
Ground, 2 Tbsp, 0.3 oz	60	4.5	4
Garbanzo (Chick Pea), ½ cup, 1.6 oz	180	3	27
Kuzu Root Starch, 1 Tbsp, 0.35 oz	35	0	9
Matzo Meal, ½ cup, 2.2 oz	230	0.5	48
Millet: Raw, ½ cup, 3½ oz	380	4	73
Cooked, ½ cup, 3 oz	105	1	21
Oat Bran: Raw, ⅓ cup, 1.1 oz	75	2	21
Cooked, ½ cup, 3¾ oz	45	1	13
Oats, rolled/oatmeal:			
Dry/Groats, ½ cup, 1.5 oz	160	3	28
Cooked, ½ cup, 4.2 oz	75	1	13
Polenta: *See Cornmeal*			
Potato Flour, ½ cup, 2.8 oz	285	0.5	66
Psyllium Husks, 1 Tbsp, 0.15 oz	20	0	4
Quinoa: Dry ½ cup, 3 oz	320	5	59
Cooked, ½ cup, 3¾ oz	130	2	24
Rice Bran, ½ cup, 2 oz	180	12	28
Rice Flour, ½ cup, 2¾ oz	290	1	63

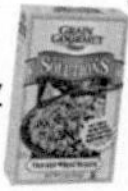

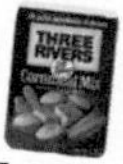

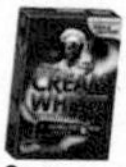

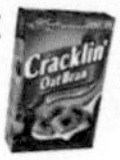

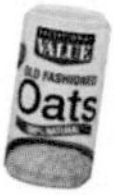

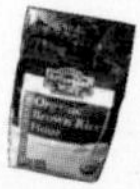

Flours & Grains (Cont)	C	F	Cb
Rice Polish, ½ cup, 3½ oz	360	0.5	80
Rye Flour: Dark, ½ cup, 2.3 oz	210	2	44
Medium, ½ cup, 1.8 oz	180	1	40
Light, ½ cup, 1.8 oz	190	1	41
Rye Grain: ½ cup, 3 oz	280	2	59
Flakes, ¼ cup, 1 oz	100	0.5	21
Semolina, ½ cup, 3 oz	300	1	61
Sorghum, ½ cup, 3.4 oz	325	3	72
Soy Flour:			
Defatted, 1 cup, 3½ oz	330	1	38
Low-Fat, 1 cup, 3 oz	325	6	33
Full-Fat, 1 cup, 3 oz	365	17	29
Soy Meal, defatted, 1 cup, 4.3 oz	415	3	49
Spelt Flour, ½ cup, 2 oz	190	1	41
Tapioca, Pearl:			
Dry, ½ cup, 2.7 oz	270	0	67
3 Tbsp, 1 oz	100	0	25
Teff (Seed) Flour, 2 oz	215	2	42
Tortilla Flour Mix, ½ cup, 2 oz	220	6	37
Triticale: ½ cup, 3.4 oz	325	2	70
Flour, wholegrain, ½ cup, 2.3 oz	220	1	48
Wheat Bran, unproc., ½ cup, 1 oz	65	1	19
Wheat Flakes, ½ cup, 1½ oz	160	1	35
Wheat Germ:			
Raw, ¼ cup, 1 oz	105	3	15
Toasted, ¼ cup, 1 oz	110	3	14
Wheat Flour:			
White, All Purpose/Self-Rising,			
1 level Tbsp, 0.28 oz	30	0	6
½ cup, 2.2 oz	230	0.5	48
1 cup, 4.4 oz	455	1.5	95
Whole Wheat, 1 cup, 4.2 oz	405	2	87

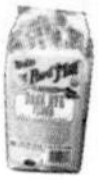

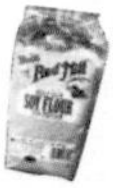

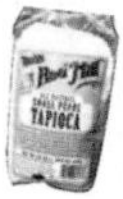

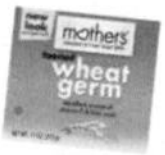

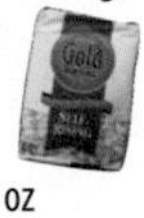

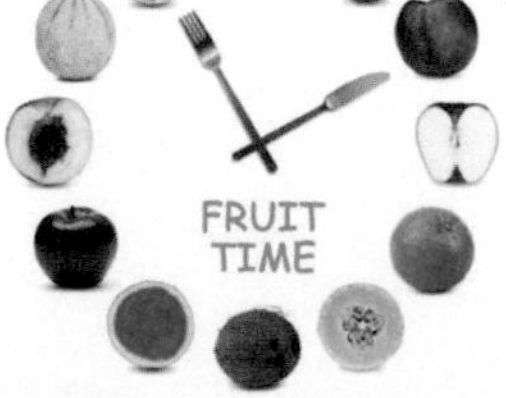

FRUIT TIME

Weights As Purchased	C	F	Cb
Acerola, 1 cup, 20 pieces, 3½ oz	30	0	7.5
Apples: Whole, average all varieties,			
1 small (4 per lb), 4 oz	55	0	13
1 medium (3 per lb), 5½ oz	70	0	17
1 large (2 per lb), 8 oz	110	0	26
1 extra large, 11 oz	150	0	36
Without skin: 1 medium, 4½ oz	60	0	14
1 cup slices, 4 oz	55	0	13
Candy/Caramel Apple, 1 med., 6½ oz	245	4	54
Nut Coated, 1 medium, 7 oz	325	11	56
Chiquita Apple Bites, 10 slices, 3½ oz	50	0	12
Apricots: 1 small (12 per lb)	17	0	4
1 medium (8 per lb), 2 oz	25	0	6
1 large (5-6 per lb), 3 oz	40	0	10
Asian Pear (Nashi Fruit), 1 medium, 7 oz	85	0	21
Avocado (without seed/skin):			
Average, ½ medium, 3½ oz	160	15	8
1 salad slice, ½ oz	25	2	1
Mashed/Puree, 2 Tbsp, 1 oz	50	4.5	2
¼ cup, 2 oz	90	9	5
Californian, ½ medium, 3 oz	160	14	8
Mashed/Puree, ½ cup, 4 oz	190	18	10
Florida, ½ medium, 5½ oz	180	15	12
Mashed/Puree, ½ cup, 4 oz	140	11	9
½ cup cubed, 3 oz	105	8	7
Banana, (weight with skin):			
1 small (6", 4 per lb), 4 oz	90	0	23
1 medium (7", 3 per lb), 5 oz	105	0	27
1 large (8"), 7 oz	120	0	30
1 extra large (9"), 9 oz	135	0	35
without skin, 1 oz	25	0	6
Black Raspberries, 1 cup, 5 oz	70	0	16
Blackberries: 1 cup, 5 oz	60	0.5	14
Blueberries: Approx. 20, 1 oz	15	0	4
1 cup, 5 oz	80	0.5	20
1 pint, 14 oz	225	1	57
Boysenberries, 1 cup, 4.5 oz	60	4.5	14
Breadfruit, ½ cup, 4 oz	115	0	30
Cactus Pear, 1 fruit, 3½ oz	40	0	9
Cantaloupe: Flesh (without rind), 1 oz	10	0	2
1 cup pieces/balls, 5.5 oz	55	0	13
½ Circle Slices (no rind):			
1 thin (¼"), 1 oz	10	0	2
1 medium (½"), 2 oz	20	0	5
1 thick (¾"), 3 oz	30	0	7
Wedges (Length cut, w/o rind):			
1 thin, 1⁄16 medium, 2 oz	20	0	5
1 thick, ⅛ medium, 4 oz	40	0	9
Whole (Weights with seeds and rind):			
½ small, 20 oz	195	1	46
½ medium, 28 oz	270	1.5	65
½ large, 2½ lb	370	2	90
Carambola (Starfruit), 1 medium, 3 oz	30	0	6
Cassava, ⅓ cup, 2½ oz	115	0	27
Cherimoya, 1 cup, 5.5 oz	115	1	27

Weights As Purchased	C	F	Cb
Cherries: Sweet (Red/White), raw,			
8 cherries, 2 oz	30	0	8
1 cup, 4½ oz	75	0	19
½ lb (30 cherries)	130	0.5	32
Sour, red, raw, 1 cup, 4 oz	50	0	12
Clementine, 1 medium, 2.6 oz	35	0	9
Coconut: Fresh,			
1 piece, 2"x2"x ½", 1 oz	100	10	4.5
Shredded, fresh, ½ cup, 1.4 oz	140	13	6
Sweetened, dried, ½ cup, 1.6 oz	235	16	22
Crabapples, ½ cup slices, 2 oz	40	0	11
Cranberries, ¼ cup, 1 oz	25	0	6.5
Currants, raw, ½ cup, 2 oz	35	0	8
Custard Apple, 4 oz, edible	115	1	28
(from 7 oz with skin/seeds)			
Dates: See Dried Fruits			
Dragon Fruit (Pitahaya),			
1 medium, 12 oz	145	0.5	39
Durian, flesh, 4 oz	165	6	31
Elderberries, ½ cup, 2½ oz	55	0.5	13
Feijoa (Pineapple Guava),			
1 medium, 2 oz	30	0.5	5.5
Figs, green/black:			
1 medium, 2 oz	40	0	10
1 large, 3 oz	60	0	15
Gooseberries, raw, ½ cup, 2½ oz	35	0	7
Grapefruit: Average all types,			
½ fruit, 10 oz (6 oz flesh)	55	0	13
1 cup sections w/ juice, 8 oz	75	0	18
Grapes: Average, 1 cup, 5½ oz	105	0	28
1 small bunch, 4 oz	80	0	20
1 medium bunch, 7 oz	140	0	36
1 large bunch, 16 oz	315	0	82
Granadilla, flesh, 3½ oz	95	0	23
Guava, 1 medium, 4 oz	80	1	16
Honeydew: 1 slice, ¾" thick, 3 oz	30	0	7
1 wedge (⅛ of 7" diam.),			
12 oz (with rind)	80	0	20
1 cup cubes/balls, 6 oz	60	0	14
½ small (4½ lb whole)	180	0.5	42
½ medium (6lb whole)	230	1	56
Honey Murcots, 1 only, 5 oz	45	0	11
Jaboticaba, flesh, 4 oz	75	2	15
Jackfruit, flesh, ⅛ average, 4 oz	105	0	27
Java-Plum, 4 plums, ½ oz	10	0	2
Jujube, 2 oz	65	0	17
Kiwifruit,: 1 Medium, 2.7 oz	45	0	11
1 Large, 3.2 oz	55	0.5	13
Kumquats, 5 medium, 3½ oz	65	1	15
Kiwano, ½ medium, 5 oz	35	0	8
Langsat, Duku, 1 medium, 2 oz	25	0	5
Lemon: 1 medium, 3 oz	25	0	8
1 wedge, 1 oz	5	0	1.5
Peel, grated, 1 Tbsp	5	0	1

Weights As Purchased

	C	F	Cb
Limes, 1 medium (2" diam.), 2.4 oz	20	0	7
Loganberries, frozen, ½ cup, 2½ oz	40	0	9
Longans, 5 fruit, ½ oz	10	0	2.5
Loquats, 4 fruit, 2¼ oz	30	0	8
Lychees, 4 fruit, 2¼ oz	30	0	7
Mamey Apple: ¼ fruit, 7 oz	100	1	25
Mandarin: 1 small, 3 oz	35	0	9
1 medium, 4 oz	45	0	11
1 large, 6 oz	50	0	13
Mango: Flesh, ½ cup slices, 3 oz	55	0	14
1 small mango, 7 oz	90	0.5	24
1 medium, 10 oz	130	0.5	34
1 cheek, 4 oz	60	0	14
1 large, 17 oz	220	1	58
1 extra large mango, 24 oz	310	1.5	82
Marionberries, 1 cup, 5 oz	75	1	15
Melon, average, 1 cup, cubes/balls, 6 oz	60	0	14
Monstera Deliciosa (Taxonia), Edible part, 4 oz	50	0	11
Mulberries, 20 fruit, 1 oz	15	0	3
Nashi Fruit (Asian Pear), 1 med. 7 oz	85	0	21
Nectarines: 1 medium, 4 oz	50	0	12
1 large, 5½ oz	70	0	16
Oheloberries, ½ cup, 2½ oz	20	0	5
Olives (Pickled): Green, 10 large, 1½ oz	60	6.5	1.5
Ripe, Greek Style, 10 medium, 1 oz	70	6	4
Ripe (Black) Californian:			
1 small/medium	5	0	0.2
1 large/extra large	6	0.5	0.5
1 jumbo	7	0.5	0.5
1 colossal	11	1	0.5
Oranges: Average all varieties (weights with skin)			
1 small, 5 oz	45	0	11
1 medium (3" diam.), 7 oz	85	0	21
1 large, 10 oz	130	0	33
Californian Valencia, 1 medium (2¾" diam.), 6 oz	60	0	14
Calif. Navels (3" diameter), 7 oz	70	0	17
Sunkist Navel, large, 14 oz	130	0	30
Florida Orange, 1 med, 7 oz	70	0	17
Flesh only, 1 cup, 6 oz	85	0	21
Peel, 1 Tbsp	0	0	0
Papaya: ½ cup, cubed, 2½ oz	30	0	7
1 medium, (5"x3" diam.), 16 oz	120	0	30
Green (unripe), ½ cup, 3½ oz	20	0	5
Passionfruit, 1 medium, 1¼ oz	35	0	8
PawPaw (see Papaya)			
Peaches: 1 small/donut, 3 oz	30	0	7.5
1 medium (4 per lb), 4 oz	45	0	11
1 large, 6 oz	65	0	16
1 extra large, 10 oz	110	0	27

Weights As Purchased

	C	F	Cb
Pears, Average all types:			
1 mini, 2½ oz	35	0	8
1 small, 5 oz	75	0	18
1 medium, 7 oz	105	0	25
1 large, 9 oz	135	0	33
1 extra large, 12 oz	175	0	42
Pepino, ½ medium, 4 oz	20	0	4
Persimmons: Native, 1 oz	35	0	9
Japanese (2½"d. x 2½"h), 7 oz	120	0	30
Seedless (Maui), 1 medium, 5 oz	100	0	25
Pineapple (wts without skin):			
1 thin slice (½"), 2 oz	25	0	6
1 thick slice (¾"), 3 oz	40	0	10
1 cup, diced, 5½ oz	75	0	19
1 medium, 1½ lb (peeled)	325	0	86
Wedges (*Del Monte*), 12 oz package	195	0	47
Canned: *See Page 102*			
Pitanga, (Surinam-Cherry) (5), 1.2 oz	10	0	2
Plaintains, ½ cup slices, 2½ oz	90	0	22
Plums: Average all types,			
Mini/Damson, (1" diameter), ½ oz	7	0	1.5
Small (2" diameter), 2¼ oz	30	0	7
Med. (2½" diam.), 3½ oz	45	0	10
Large (3" diameter), 5 oz	60	0	14
Pluot (plum-apricot), 1 medium, 5 oz	80	0	19
Pomegranate, 1 medium, 10 oz	105	0.5	25
Pummelo, flesh, ½ cup, 3½ oz	35	0	9
Prickly Pear, (Nopal):			
1 small, 2½ oz	20	0	5
1 medium, 5 oz	40	0	10
Quince, 1 medium, 3½ oz	55	0	14
Rambutan (Rambotang), Red/Yellow, 1 medium, 2 oz	15	0	4
Raspberries, ½ cup, 2 oz	30	0	7
10 Raspberries, ¾ oz	10	0	2
1 Cup, 4¼ oz	65	1	15
1 Pint, 11 oz	160	2	37
Sapodilla (Chico), 1 medium, 7½ oz	140	2	34
Sapote, ½ medium, 8 oz	150	0.5	38
Satsuma Tangerine, 1 medium, 3 oz	45	0	11
Soursop, 1 cup pulp, 8 oz	150	0.5	38
Starfruit, 1 medium, 3 oz	30	0	6
Strawberries: 1 cup, 5½ oz	50	0.5	12
6 medium/3 large, 2 oz	20	0	4
1 pint, 14 oz	115	1	27
Chocolate Dipped, 1 large	45	2.5	6
Sugar Apple (Custard Apple) ½ cup pulp, 4 oz	120	0	30
Tamarillo, 1 med., 3 oz	20	0	3
Tamarind: 1 fruit (3"x1")	5	0	1.5
Pulp, ½ cup, 2 oz	140	0.5	37

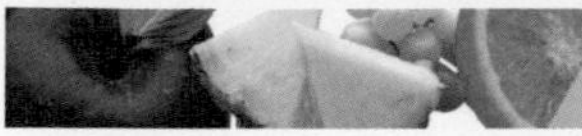

Weights as Purchased

	C	F	Cb
Tangelo: 1 small, 4 oz	55	0	13
1 medium, 5 oz	70	0	17
1 large, 7 oz	95	0	23
Tangerine, 1 medium, (2½″ diam.), 4 oz	50	0	13
Tangor, 1 medium, 4 oz	35	0	7
Tomatillos (3), 3½ oz	35	1	6
Tomatoes:			
1 small (2¼″ diameter), 3 oz	15	0	3
1 medium (2¾″ diameter), 5 oz	25	0	5
1 large (3½″ diameter), 8 oz	40	0.5	9
1 extra large (3″ diameter), 12 oz	60	0.5	14
Grape, 5 medium, 2 oz	10	0	2
Yellow Tear Drop, 3 medium, 1 oz	5	0	2
Cherry: 4 medium, 2 oz	10	0	2
1 cup, 5 oz	25	0	6
Slices (Medium Tomato):			
2 thin slices, 1 oz	5	0	1
2 thick (⅜″), 2 oz	10	0	2
Wedge, ¼ medium tomato, 1¼ oz	6	0	1
Chopped, 1 cup, 6½ oz	35	0.5	7
Fried Green Tomato, 2 slices, 2½ oz	140	11	9
Canned Tomatoes/Products: See Page 144			
Tree Tomato (Tamarillo), 3 oz	20	0	5
Ugli Fruit, Tangelo type, 5 oz	40	0	8
Watermelon: Flesh only, 1 oz	8	0	2
1 thin slice, (¼ circle, ⅜″), 2 oz	15	0	4
1 Extra			
1 cup cubes or balls, 5½ oz	45	0	11
10 balls, 4.3 oz	35	0	9
Buffet Slice, thin, 1 oz	8	0	2
Regular (Long Shape):			
1 thick (1″) slice (¼ circle, 4½″ radius)			
9 oz w. skin (5½ oz no rind)	50	0	12
1 thin (½″) slice (¼ circle)	25	0	6
1 thick (1″) slice (½ circle)			
18 oz with rind	100	1	22
1 whole melon (15″ long, 7½″diameter)			
20 lb with rind, 10 lb w/o rind	1360	7	330
Seedless (Round Shape):			
Medium size (13 lb, 8¼″ diameter)			
1 whole, 8½ lb without rind	1160	5	280
Wedge (⅛ whole melon),			
26 oz with rind	145	1	35
Flesh only, without rind, 8 oz	70	0.5	17
Mini size (6 lb, 6½″ diameter),			
1 whole, 3½ lb without rind	480	2.5	110
Wedge (⅛ whole),			
1½ lb, with rind	60	0.5	14
Xoconostle: *see Prickly Pear*			

> **FRUIT & VEGETABLE JUICES**
> *~ See Page 41*

Dried Fruit

	C	F	Cb
Apples, 5 rings, 1 oz	80	0	19
Apricots, 8 halves, 1 oz	65	0	16
Banana Chips, ½ cup, 1½ oz	220	14	25
Banana Flakes, 4 Tbsp, 1 oz	80	0	20
Cranberries *(Craisins):*			
Sweetened, ¼ cup, 1 oz	100	0	24
Unsweetened, ¼ cup, 1 oz	80	0	19
Choc-coated, 1 oz	135	7.5	18
Currants, ¼ cup, 1¼ oz	100	0	25
Dates: 5 medium dates, 1½ oz	120	0	29
Large Calif.: 1 date, 0.7 oz	55	0	13
3 dates, 2 oz	170	0	39
½ cup, chopped, 3 oz	240	0	58
Pecan Date Rolls, 1 oz	100	2.5	19
Date Crumbles *(Bob's Redmill),*			
¼ cup, 1 oz	90	0	22
Figs, 3 medium figs, 1 oz	90	0	23
Goji Berries, 3 Tbsp, 1 oz	100	1	20
Longans; Lychees, 1 oz	80	0	20
Mango Slices, 5 pieces, 1.4 oz	25	0	6
Papaya Spears, 2 pieces, 1.4 oz	120	0	30
Peaches, 2 halves, 1 oz	60	0	15
Pears, 3 halves, 2 oz	140	0.5	34
Plums *(Sunsweet)* (5), 1.4 oz	100	0	24
Prunes (dried Plums): with pits, 1 oz	70	0	17
1 medium (60/lb)	16	0	4
1 large (50/lb)	22	0	5
1 extra large (40/lb)	25	0	6
Without pits, 4 medium, 1 oz	70	0	17
Cooked: with sugar, ½ cup, 5 oz	155	0	38
without sugar, ½ cup, 4½ oz	135	0	33
Raisins, 2 Tbsp, 1 oz pack	85	0	20
½ cup, 2.8 oz	220	0.5	56

Candied/Glazed Fruit

	C	F	Cb
Apricot, 1 medium, 1 oz	70	0	17
Cherry, (Maraschino) (1)	8	0	2
Citron/Fruit Peel, 1 oz	85	0	20
Ginger, 1 oz	90	0	21
Pineapple, 1 slice, 1¼ oz	120	0	29

Fruit Leather/Rolls

	C	F	Cb
Average All Brands, 1 oz	105	1	24
Fruit By The Foot, *(Betty Crocker)*			
1 roll, ¾ oz	80	0	17
Fruit Gushers, *(Betty Crocker),* 1 oz	90	1	20
Fruit Roll-Ups, *(Betty Crocker)* 1 roll	50	1	12
Stretch Island, Leathers, 2 pieces, 1 oz	90	0	24

Canned/Bottled Fruit

Solids & Liquids: | **C** | **F** | **Cb**

Per ½ Cup, 4½ oz

	C	F	Cb
Apricots: In water/diet	35	0	8
In juice/lite	60	0	15
In syrup	105	0	28
Black/Blueberries: Heavy syrup	120	0	30
In light syrup	110	0	26
Cherries, pitted: in water	55	0	15
In light syrup	85	0	22
In heavy syrup	105	0	27
In extra heavy syrup	135	0	34
Maraschino, 1 oz	50	0	12
Pie Cherries, ⅔ cup, 5 oz	90	0	23
Fruit Salad: In water/diet	35	0	10
In light juice	60	0	16
In heavy syrup	95	0	25
Gooseberries, Light syrup	90	0	24
Grapefruit: Juice pack	45	0	12
In light syrup	75	0	20
Lychees, ½ cup, 4.5 oz	105	0	26
Mixed Fruit: In water/diet	40	0	10
In fruit juices/light syrup	70	0	18
In heavy syrup	90	0	24
Peaches (halves/slices): In water/diet	30	0	7
In juice/light	55	0	14
In light syrup	70	0	18
Drained, ½ peach	55	0	14
In heavy syrup	100	0	26
Pears: In water/diet	35	0	10
In light juice	60	0	16
In heavy syrup	100	0	26
Pineapple: All types			
In own juice	75	0	20
In heavy syrup	100	0	26
1 slice (ring), drained, 1½ oz	15	0	4
Prunes: In heavy syrup	125	0	33
In Liqueur, ½ cup, 4.4 oz	280	0	70
Stewed in Water, ½ cup	135	0	35
Tropical Fruit Salad: In light syrup	80	0	21
In heavy syrup	110	0	29

Fruit Snack Cups | C | F | Cb

	C	F	Cb
Deli/Take-Out: Small, 6 oz	70	0	16
Large, 12 oz	140	0	32
Yogurt & Fruit Cup, 15 oz	380	4.5	75
Del Monte Fruit Cups			
Fruit Cups: *Per 4 oz Cup*			
Strawberry Banana Peaches	70	0	17
Mandarin Orange Segments	70	0	17
Pineapple Tidbits	70	0	18
Tropical Fruit	70	0	18
Fruit Naturals: *Per 8 oz Cup*			
Cherry Mixed Fruit	140	0	35
Peach Chunks	140	0	34
Pineapple Chunks	140	0	36
Red Grapefruit	120	0	32
Fruit-n-Gel Cups: *Per 4½ oz Cup*			
Mixed Fruit/Peaches in Fruit Gel	90	0	23
Lite varieties in Gel, average	60	0	14
Pull Top Cans: in 100% Juice, 4 oz	80	0	20
Lite varieties, 4 oz	60	0	15
Super Fruits: *Per 6 oz cup*			
Mixed Fruit/Pear Chunks	120	0	30
Peaches in Pomeg. & Orange Juice	100	0	25
Dole Fruit Bowls			
4 oz Bowls: Diced Peaches	80	0	20
Mixed Fruit; Tropical Fruit	80	0	19
Pineapple	60	0	15
Fruit-n-Gel Bowls, Regular, 1 cup	60	0	14
Mott's: Healthy Harvest, 4 oz cup	50	0	13
Vons: Fruit Cocktail,			
In heavy syrup, ½ cup, 4.5 oz	90	0	25
In lite syrup, ½ cup	80	0	14

Apple & Fruit Sauces | C | F | Cb

	C	F	Cb
Apple Sauce:			
Regular/sweetened, 2 Tbsp, 1 oz	20	0	6
4 oz package	85	0	22
¼ cup	50	0	13
Fruit Sauces & Purees:			
Average all fruit types, 2 Tbsp, 1 oz	25	0	6
½ cup, 4 oz	100	0	24
Mott's:			
Classics, average, 4 oz	100	0	24
Apple Sauce: Original, 4 oz	100	0	24
Fruit Flavored, average, 4 oz	90	0	23
No Sugar Added, 4 oz	50	0	12
Ocean Spray: *Per ¼ Cup*			
Jellied Cranberry Sauce	110	0	25
Whole Berry Cranberry Sauce	110	0	27

Pie Fillings ~ See Page 134

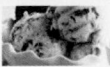 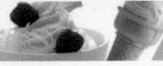

Ice Cream ◆ Frozen Yogurt

Quick Guide — C F Cb

Ice Cream
Vanilla: *Average All Brands*
Other flavors ~ See Brand Listings.
Regular Ice Cream (10% fat):
Examples: *Borden/Hood*

	C	F	Cb
3 fl.oz scoop	105	5	12
½ cup, 4 fl.oz	140	7	17
1 Pint, 16 fl.oz	560	28	68
½ Gallon (4 Pints)	2240	112	272

Rich (16% fat):
Example: *Hood (Red Sox)*

3 fl.oz scoop	135	7.5	15
½ cup, 4 fl.oz	180	10	20
1 Pint	720	40	80

Super-Rich (20% fat): *Haagen-Dazs/Ben & Jerry's*

3 fl.oz scoop	200	13	18
½ cup, 4 fl.oz	270	17	24
1 Pint	1080	68	96

Reduced-Fat/Light (6% fat):
Breyer's Light/Hood Light

3 fl.oz scoop	95	3	15
½ cup, 4 fl.oz	125	4	20
1 Pint	500	16	80

Fat-Free: *Baskin-Robbins FF/Borden FF/Breyers FF/Dreyers FF/Hood FF*

3 fl.oz scoop	70	0	16
½ cup, 4 fl.oz	90	0	21
1 Pint	360	0	84

Soft Serve: Regular, ½ cup

	190	11	19
1 cup	380	22	38
Light, ½ cup	110	2	19
1 cup	220	4	38

Quick Guide

Frozen Yogurt — C F Cb
Average All Brands

	C	F	Cb
Hard: Low-Fat, ½ cup	110	3	19
Non-Fat, ½ cup	110	0	24
Soft: Low-Fat, ½ cup	120	4	17
Non-Fat, ½ cup	100	0	30

Brands: *See Ice Cream & Ices Section*

Quick Guide — C F Cb

Gelato/Ices/Frozen Custard
Gelato: *Per ½ Cup*

	C	F	Cb
Milk base: Vanilla	160	6	25
Chocolate Hazelnut	230	15	21
Water base, ½ cup	100	0	26

Frozen Custard: *Per ½ Cup*

Chocolate	140	6	18
Orange Sherbet	105	2	21
Vanilla	130	6	16

Ice (Milk base): Average all flavors

Hard (4% fat), ½ cup	100	3	15
Soft Serve (3% fat), ½ cup	110	2	19
Shaved Ice: Average, 12 fl. oz	160	0	40
Sherbet: Average, ½ cup	110	1.5	22
Sorbet: Fruit (without fat), ½ cup	70	0	19
Fruit Ice Pops	80	0	20

Sundaes — C F Cb

Baskin Robbins:

	C	F	Cb
Banana Royale	620	28	87
Banana Split	1010	34	173
Brownie	920	47	119
Made With Snickers	1000	46	138
Oreo Outrageous	1130	55	158
Reeses Peanut Butter Cup	1220	80	109

Denny's:

Oreo Blender Blaster	890	44	113
Oreo Sundae	760	37	103
Chocolate, Topping, 2 oz	135	0.5	34
Other Toppings ~ See Page 195			

McDonald's:

Hot Caramel Sundae	340	8	60
Hot Fudge Sundae	330	10	54
Strawberry Sundae	280	6	49
Toppings: Peanuts, ¼ oz	45	3.5	2

Ice Cream, Cones & Cups

Average All Brands — C F Cb

	C	F	Cb
Wafer Cone/Cup, average	20	0	4
Sugar Cone, average	50	0	14
Waffle Cone:			
Small	50	1	10
Large	90	0.5	19
Brands:			
Oreo Chocolate Cone	50	1	10
Comet Sugar Cone	50	0	11
Keebler Sugar Cone	50	0	10

Ice Cream & Frozen Yogurt

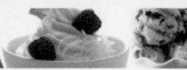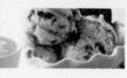

Brands | C | F | Cb

Baskin-Robbins: *See Fast-Foods Section*
Ben & Jerry's
Hand Scoop: *Per ½ Cup*

	C	F	Cb
Butter Pecan, 3 oz	260	20	17
Cake Batter, 3 ¼ oz	240	14	24
Cherry Garcia, 3 oz	200	11	23
Chocolate, 3 oz	200	12	21
Chocolate Chip Cookie Dough, 3 oz	220	12	26
Chocolate Therapy, 3 oz	210	12	25
Cinnamon Buns, 3 oz	240	12	30
Coconut Seven Layer Bar, 3¼ oz	275	17	25
Coffee, Coffee BuzzBuzzBuzz, 3 oz	230	14	23
Half Baked, 3 oz	230	11	28
Imagine Whirled Peace, 3.2 oz	250	15	26
Mint Chocolate Chunk, 3 oz	230	14	23
New York Super Fudge Chunk, 3 oz	250	17	24
One Cheesecake Brownie, 3.2 oz	235	14	23
Phish Food, 3 oz	230	11	32
Strawberry Cheesecake, 3 oz	210	11	24
Sweet Cream & Cookies, 3 oz	240	13	24
Triple Caramel Chunk, 3 oz	230	12	38
Vanilla, 3 oz	190	12	18

Original: *Per ½ Cup*

	C	F	Cb
Banana Split, 3.9 oz	270	15	30
Boston Cream Pie, 3.65 oz	250	13	29
Cake Batter, 3.7 oz	280	17	28
Cherry Garcia, 3.7 oz	240	14	27
Chocolate Chip Cookie Dough, 3.7 oz	270	14	32
Everything But The... ,3.8 oz	300	19	31
Imagine Whirled Peace	270	16	28
Karamel Sutra, 3.77 oz	270	14	32
Milk & Cookies, 3.55 oz	270	15	30
Mission To Marzipan, 3.6 oz	260	13	32
New York Super Fudge Chunk, 3¾ oz	300	19	29
One Cheesecake Brownie, 3.65 oz	250	15	26
Peanut Britle, 3.65 oz	260	15	29
Peanut Butter Cup, 3.8 oz	340	24	28
Phish Food, 3.55 oz	270	12	37
Strawberry Banana, 3.35 oz	150	1.5	32
Triple Caramel Chunk, 3.77 oz	280	16	32
Turtle Soup, 3.65 oz	280	15	30

Frozen Yogurt: *Per ½ Cup*

	C	F	Cb
Fro Yo: Half Baked, 3.5 oz	180	3	35
Cherry Garcia, 3.5 oz	160	3	31
Chocolate Fudge Brownie	170	2.5	34
Strawberry Banana, 3.35 oz	150	1.5	32
Sorbet: Average all flavors	115	0	30

Blue Bunny: *Per ½ Cup*
Fat-Free, No Added Sugar:

	C	F	Cb
Brownie Sundae, 2.6 oz	90	0	23
Caramel Toffee Crunch, 2½ oz	90	0	24
Vanilla, 2½ oz	80	0	20

Reduced-Fat, No Added Sugar:

	C	F	Cb
Banana Split, 2½ oz	120	5	20
Butter Pecan, 2½ oz	130	6	16
Rocky Road, 2½ oz	130	6	21
Turtle Sundae, 2½ oz	140	7	20
Hi Lite: Chocolate, 2.3 oz	110	3	17
Fudge Nut Sundae, 2.3 oz	120	4	19
Homemade Vanilla, 2.35 oz	110	3.5	18

Personals (Light):

	C	F	Cb
Bunny Tracks, 2.4 oz	130	6	20
Choc. Raspb. Cheesecake	100	2.5	18
Super Fudge Brownie, 2.4 oz	120	3	23

Frozen Yogurt:

	C	F	Cb
Brownie Fudge Fantasy, 2.6 oz	110	0	24
Homemade Vanilla, 2.6 oz	100	0	19
Strawberry Cheesecake, 2 6 oz	100	0	21

Bars/Pops: See Page 108
Breyers: *Per ½ Cup*
All Natural:

	C	F	Cb
Original: Butter Pecan	150	10	14
Cherry Vanilla	130	6	18
Cookies & Cream; Rocky Road	150	7	19
Vanilla; Chocolate	130	6	15
Half The Fat: Butter Pecan	130	5	16
Chocolate Chocolate Chip	140	5	21
Cookies & Cream	130	4	20
Creamy, Chocolate/Vanilla, average	110	3.5	16
Mint Chocolate Chip	130	4.5	18
Strawberry Cheesecake	120	3.5	20
Vanilla Bean; Van. Choc. Strawberry	110	3	17
CarbSmart: Chocolate	90	6	13
Vanilla	90	6	13
Fun Flavors: Brownie Mud Pie	130	3.5	23
Heath English Toffee	160	6	25
Oreo	160	8	20
Snickers	170	8	20
Overload: Fried Ice Cream	140	4.5	23
Very Chocolate Cherry	120	3	21

Smooth & Dreamy:

	C	F	Cb
Fat Free: Chocolate Cookies & Cream	110	0	25
Chocolate Fudge Brownie	110	0	25
Creamy Vanilla	90	0	21
French Chocolate	90	0	22
Strawberry	90	0	22
No Added Sugar: Butter Pecan	110	6	14
Chocolate Fudge Brownie	90	1.5	20

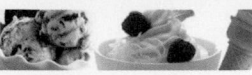

Brands (Cont)

	C	F	Cb
Brigham's: *Per ½ Cup, 4 fl.oz*			
Ice Cream: Big Dig	210	12	24
Chocolate	200	12	20
Coffee	190	12	17
Frozen Pudding	180	9	20
Just Jimmies	220	13	21
Mocha Almond; Pistachio	210	15	18
Vanilla	190	12	18
Elan Frozen Yogurt			
Average all flavors, ½ cup, 4 fl.oz	135	3	24
Bruster's			
Frozen Yogurt: *Per 3 fl.oz*			
Chocolate	150	4.5	24
Vanilla	150	4	24
Fat Free, No Added Sugar Ice Cream: *3 fl.oz*			
Chocolate	100	0	26
Chocolate Caramel Swirl	120	0	31
Cinnamon	100	0	23
Coffee	100	0	24
Fudge Ripple	110	0	30
Vanilla	100	0	23
Average other varieties	110	0	30
Carvel Ice Cream: *See Fast-Foods Section*			
Coldstone Creamery: *See Fast-Foods Section*			
CremaLita (Soft Serve)			

Calories will vary with density (air in product) and serving size.
Best to weigh product and calculate on 25 cals per 1 oz weight.

	C	F	Cb
Vanilla: Small (4 fl.oz cup),			
If 4 oz weight*	100	0.5	23
If 6 oz weight*	150	1	35
(*) Most common weights			
Medium, 8 fl.oz cup, 11 oz wt	275	1.5	63
Chocolate: Small, 6 oz weight	160	1	36
Dairy Queen/Brazier: *See Fast-Foods Section*			
Dippin' Dots			
Dots 'n Cream: *Per ½ Cup*			
Banana Split	170	10	6
Caramel Cappuccino	190	12	18
Mint Chocolate	165	10	15
Vanilla	170	10	16
Wild About Chocolate	240	14	26
Dove: *Per ½ Cup*			
Beyond Vanilla	240	15	23
Caramel Pecan Perfection	300	18	30
Chocolate & Brownie Affair	300	19	31
Chocolate & Cherry Courtship	270	16	27
Irresistibly Raspberry	240	12	30
Unconditional Chocolate	290	17	31
Vanilla with Chocolate Soul	300	18	30

	C	F	Cb
Dreyers/Edys: *Per ½ Cup, 4 fl.oz*			
Grand: Chocolate	150	8	17
Fudge Swirl	150	7	19
Mint Chocolate Chip	160	9	18
Neapolitan; Vanilla Bean, average	140	8	15
Real Strawberry	130	6	16
Vanilla	140	8	15
Average other flavors	160	9	18
Loaded, Choc. Chip Cookie Dough	130	4	21
Slow Churned: Light, Neapolitan	100	3	15
Cookie Dough	130	4.5	20
Cups ½ Fat ⅓ Calories:			
Chocolate, 1 cup	170	6	25
Mint Chocolate Chip, 1 cup	210	8	29
Yogurt Blends: Cookies & Cream	120	4	20
Average other flavors	100	2	17
Friendly's: *Per Single Scoop*			
Ice Cream: Butter Crunch	130	6	16
Chocolate	110	6	10
Chocolate Almond Chip	120	7	11
Coffee	110	6	13
Hunka Chunka PB Fudge	180	11	17
Pistachio	130	7	14
Strawberry	110	5	14
Vanilla	120	6	14
Vienna Mocha Chunk	140	8	16
Frozen Yogurt: *Per ½ Cup*			
Raspberry Swirl, Non-Fat	90	0	19
Sundaes: *Per 3 Scoops*			
Royal Banana Split	880	35	132
Jim Dandy	1080	46	156
Reese's Peanut Butter Cup	870	51	90
Friend-Z's, Reese's P'nut Butter Cup	860	45	96
Gelati-da			
Gelato: *Per ½ Cup (4 oz)*			
Amaretto Chocolate	150	4.5	23
Choc Mint Milano	120	2.5	22
Coffee Fudge Latte	130	2	22
Limoncello	120	3	20
Red Raspberry	130	1.5	25
Vanilla Marsala	120	2	21
Haagen-Dazs			
Ice Cream, Sorbet, Frozen Yogurt: *See Fast-Foods Section*			
Bars: *See Page 109*			
Hola Fruta!: *Per ½ Cup, 3.35 oz*			
Pure Fruit Sherbet: Margarita	140	1	30
Peach	130	1	30
Pina Colada	140	1.5	31
Pomegranate; Raspberry	140	1	32
Pomegranate & Blueberry	150	1	31
Strawberry	130	1	31

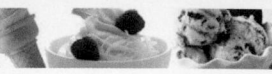
Brands (Cont)

Hood: *Per ½ Cup*

	C	F	Cb
Frozen Fat-Free Yogurt:			
Maine Blueberry & Sweet Cream	90	0	19
Mocha Fudge	100	0	22
Strawberry	80	0	18
Strawberry Banana	90	0	20
Tangy, average all flavors	110	1	24
Vanilla	90	0	19
Ice Cream: *Per ½ Cup*			
Birthday Party	150	8	19
Chocolate	140	6	18
Classic trio	140	7	17
Cookie Dough Delight	160	8	19
Cookies 'N Cream	150	8	19
Creamy Coffee	140	7	16
Fudge Twister	140	6	20
Golden Vanilla	140	7	17
Maple Walnut	150	9	17
Natural Vanilla Bean	140	7	17
Patchwork	140	7	17

New England Creamery ~ *www.CalorieKing.com*

Bars: *See Page 109*

Jerseymaid (Vons): *Per ½ Cup*

	C	F	Cb
Cookies & Cream	160	8	18
Choc Chip; Mint Choc Chip	150	9	16
Heavenly Hash; Nut Chunky Chocolate	170	10	17
Mocha Almd Fudge; Rocky Road	160	10	17
Neapolitan; Vanilla	140	8	15
Strawberry	130	6	17

Oberweis: *Per 6 oz Scoop*

	C	F	Cb
Super Premium:			
Chocolate	480	31	43
Chocolate Peanut Butter	550	39	42
Cookie Dough	500	28	56
Vanilla	460	31	40

Pinkberry Frozen Yogurt:

Original: *Without Toppings*

	C	F	Cb
Mini, 3.2 oz	90	0	19
Small, 5.3 oz	150	0	31
Medium, 8 oz	230	0	48
Large, 13½ oz	380	0	80
Cone, (with 3 oz Frozen Yogurt)	105	0	23

Other Flavors: *Per Medium Serving*

	C	F	Cb
Chocolate	275	3.5	53
Coconut	320	1	69
Green Tea; Mango; P'fruit, av.	250	0	52

Purely Decadent: *Per ½ Cup*

	C	F	Cb
Belgian Chocolate, 3.5 oz	180	7	30
Blueberry Cheesecake, 3.5 oz	180	6	33
Gluten Free: Key Lime Pie, 3.5 oz	190	7	34
Peanut Butter Zig Zag, 3.5 oz	230	13	32
With Coconut Milk: Chocolate, 3 oz	150	9	20
Coconut, 3 oz	170	10	19
Cookie Dough, 3 oz	190	9	24
Mint Chip, 3 oz	170	9	20
Vanilla Bean, 3 oz	150	8	19

Red Mango Frozen Yogurt: *No Toppings Included*

	C	F	Cb
Original/Tangomonium:			
Small	90	0	20
Regular	160	0	35
Large	225	0	50
Pomegranate: Small	100	0	22
Regular	175	0	39
Large	250	0	55

Rice Dream (Non-Dairy):
Per ½ Cup, 70g, Unless Otherwise Stated

	C	F	Cb
All Natural: Carob Almond	180	10	26
Cocoa Marble Fudge	160	7	29
Cookies & Dream; Mint Carob Chip	170	8	27
Neapolitan	160	6	26
Orange Vanilla Swirl	160	8	26
Strawberry, 2.8 oz	160	8	25
Vanilla	160	8	26
Van. Hazelnut Fudge	150	7	22
Supreme: Chocolate Caramel Chai	150	7	22
Sweet Peach Pie	150	6	23

Bars: *See Page 110*

Skinny Cow: *Per Single Serve Cup*

	C	F	Cb
Choc Fudge	150	2	29
Cookies 'N Cream	150	2	29
Caramel Cone	170	3	33
Dulce de Leche; Strawb. Cheesecake	150	1	32

Bars/Sandwiches/Cones: *See Page 110*

So Delicious Organic: *Per ½ Cup, 3 oz wt*

	C	F	Cb
Butter Pecan	160	7	22
Chocolate Velvet	130	3.5	23
Cookies 'N Cream	150	4	26
Creamy Vanilla	130	3	24
Dulce de Leche	140	3	26
Mint Marble Fudge	140	3	27
Mocha Fudge	130	3	26
Neapolitan; Strawberry	120	3	23
Purely Decadent, Cookie Dough	190	9	24

Soy Delicious: *Per ½ Cup*

	C	F	Cb
It's Soy Delicious: Choc Almond	140	4.5	23
Choc Peanut Butter	135	3.5	24
Pistachio Almond	130	4.5	23
Other flavors, average	110	1.5	25

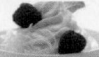

Brands (Cont)	C	F	Cb

Soy Dream (Non-Dairy): *Per ½ Cup, 70g*

	C	F	Cb
Butter Pecan	150	9	19
Chocolate	120	6	17
Choc. Fudge Brownie	130	7	18
French Vanilla; Vanilla	140	8	17
Green Tea	140	8	18
Mocha Fudge	140	7	21

Starbucks: *Per ½ Cup*

	C	F	Cb
Caramel Macchiato	240	13	27
Coffee	210	13	21
Java Chip Frappuccino	250	15	25
Mocha Frappuccino	220	13	23

Stonyfield Farm (Organic)

Premium Ice Cream: *Per ½ Cup, 100g*

	C	F	Cb
Chocolate Raspberry Swirl	230	13	25
Cookies 'N Cream	270	17	27
Creme Caramel	260	14	28
Gotta Have Java	250	16	22
Gotta Have Vanilla	250	16	21
Vanilla Chai	240	16	21

Stop & Shop: *Per ½ Cup*

	C	F	Cb
Butterscotch Ripple	140	6	20
Chocolate	150	8	18
Chocolate Chip, Regular/Chunky	150	8	18
Country Club	130	6	19
Heavenly Hash	170	8	22
Neapolitan; Vanilla	135	7	16
Vanilla Fudge Swirl	130	6	19

Tasti D-Lite (Soft Serve): *Per ½ Cup*
Calories will vary with density (air in product) and serving size
Best to weigh product and calculate on 25 cals per 1 oz weight.

	C	F	Cb
Banana	70	1.5	11
Blueberry Cheesecake	90	1.5	14
Brownie Batter	90	2	14
Buttercrunch	100	3	13
Chocolate Marshmallow	90	1.5	16
Vanilla Cream; Vanilla Marshmallow	80	1.5	12

TCBY~ *See Page 250*

Tofutti, Non-Dairy Dessert: *Per ½ Cup*

Premium Pints: Better Pecan	210	13	21
Chocolate Cookie Crunch	210	11	26
Chocolate Supreme	180	11	18
Vanilla	210	13	21
Vanilla Almond Bark	240	15	24
Vanilla Fudge; Wildberry, average	190	9	25

Turkey Hill: *Per ½ Cup*

Premium: Black Cherry	130	6	18
Butter Pecan	160	10	15
Choco Mint Chip	160	9	17
Choc. P'Nut Butter Cup	180	11	18
Cookies 'n Cream	150	8	19
Rocky Road	170	8	23
Tin Roof Sundae	150	8	19
Vanilla	140	7	16
Lite: Moose Tracks	130	6	19
Vanilla Bean	100	2.5	16
Average other flavors	130	4	19
All Natural: Average all flavors	150	8	17

No Sugar Added: *Per ½ Cup*

Cherry Fudge Ripple	80	0	22
Dutch Chocolate; Vanilla	70	0	20
Moose Tracks	120	5	22

Frozen Yogurt:

Choc. Chip Cookie Dough	120	2	23
Low-Fat, Skinny Minty	140	5	20
Fat-Free: Chocolate Marshmallow	110	0	24
Average other flavors	100	0	19
Sherbet	120	1	26

Walgreens

Premium 1 Pint Container: *Per ½ Cup*

Banana Split	150	6	22
Crème de Menthe	160	9	19
Homemade Vanilla	150	8	17
New York Cherry	130	6	17
Rocky Road	150	7	18
Strawberry Cheesecake	130	6	18
Toasted Butter Pecan	140	8	15
Waffle Cone	150	7	19

Premium 1.75 Quarts Container: *Per ½ Cup*

Banana Split	150	6	22
Homemade Vanilla	150	8	17
New York Cherry	150	7	20

Old Fashioned 1.75 Quarts (Square)

Average all flavors, ½ cup	140	7	16

Wawa

Premium 1 Pint Container: *Per ½ cup*

Chocolate; Choc. Marshmallow, av.	160	8	21
Butter Pecan; Mint Choc Chip, av	180	10	20
French Vanilla	140	8	16
Vanilla Bean	160	8	19

Whole Soy Frozen Yogurt
Average all flavors,

½ cup, 2½ oz	120	1	25

Bars & Pops

	C	**F**	**Cb**

Per Bar/Serving Unless Indicated

Barq's

	C	**F**	**Cb**
Root Beer & Ice Cream Float, 4 fl.oz cup	120	3	22

Ben & Jerry's

	C	**F**	**Cb**
Bars: Cherry Garcia	270	19	28
Half Baked	360	18	46
Vanilla	310	21	26
The Cone: Cherry Garcia	310	16	41
Vanilla Almond	440	27	47

Big Bear: *See Klondike*

Blue Bunny:

	C	**F**	**Cb**
Pops: Banana, 1.87 oz	35	0	9
Bomb Pops, average, 1.87 oz	50	0	12
Bars: Big Fudge, 2.22 oz	90	1	18
Big Star, 1.48 oz	110	7	11
Caramel Ice Cream Crunch, 1.69 oz	150	10	14
Choc. Ice Cream Sundae Crunch	170	9	21
Chocolate Raspberry, 2.82 oz	270	18	25
English Toffee, 1.38 oz	130	9	12
Milk Choc. with Almond, 3.14 oz	320	23	25
Orange Dream, 1.86 oz	70	1	15
Root Beer Float, 2 oz	80	2	14
King Size: Chocolate Eclair, 2.82 oz	220	12	27
Cookies 'n Cream, 2.47 oz	220	13	24
Crunch with Candy Center, 3 oz	340	28	24
Strawberry Shortcake, 2.78 oz	210	11	26

FrozFruit:

	C	**F**	**Cb**
Banana; Strawb. Cream, average	160	6	27
Creamy Pina Colada, 4.3 oz	190	3.5	37
Creamy Coconut	150	10	14

Champ Cones: Caramel Lovers, 3.5 oz

	C	**F**	**Cb**
Champ Cones: Caramel Lovers, 3.5 oz	320	19	34
Caramel Nut	320	19	34
Chocolate Lovers	290	15	37
Fudge Nut	330	19	35
Vanilla	310	19	31

Sandwiches: Big Bopper, 5.01 oz

	C	**F**	**Cb**
Sandwiches: Big Bopper, 5.01 oz	460	23	60
Big Double Strawberry, 3.84 oz	270	10	41
Mississippi Mud, 2.08 oz	150	4	25
Neapolitan, 2.18 oz	150	3.5	27
Chips Galore, 3.42 oz	310	16	40

Per Bar/Serving

Breyers:

	C	**F**	**Cb**
Pomegranate Blends	40	0	10

Ice Cream Poppers:

	C	**F**	**Cb**
Heath (27)	410	30	32
Hershey's Kisses: Chocolate (26)	470	31	31
Vanilla (26)	460	34	33
Oreo (27)	410	27	38
Reese's (27)	470	34	35

Double Churn Light Bars: Rocky Road

	C	**F**	**Cb**
Double Churn Light Bars: Rocky Road	180	9	23
Creamy Vanilla	160	8	21
Vanilla & Almond	170	9	21
No Sugar Added: Creamy Vanilla	150	9	18
Krunch	150	9	18

Smooth & Dreamy: Bars, av. all

	C	**F**	**Cb**
Smooth & Dreamy: Bars, av. all	125	5	18
Sandwiches, all flavors	160	4	30

Butterfinger *(Nestle):* 1.9 oz bar

	C	**F**	**Cb**
Butterfinger (Nestle): 1.9 oz bar	210	15	17
Loaded Bar, 2.8 oz	270	17	28

California Natural: Mango Sorbet

	C	**F**	**Cb**
California Natural: Mango Sorbet	130	0	33
Lemon & Strawberry Sorbet Cups	120	0	31

Cool Classics:

Arctic Blasters: Crispy Bar

	C	**F**	**Cb**
Arctic Blasters: Crispy Bar	160	11	15
Fudge Bar	80	0	20
Ice Cream Bar	150	10	13
Orange Cream	100	2.5	18

Icepix: Grape; Cherry; Orange

	C	**F**	**Cb**
Icepix: Grape; Cherry; Orange	35	0	8
Honeydew; Watermelon Cantelope	35	0	9
Sugar-Free, Banana	15	0	3

Swirl Pops, Mango-Cherry

	C	**F**	**Cb**
Swirl Pops, Mango-Cherry	80	0	21

Creamsicles: Regular

	C	**F**	**Cb**
Creamsicles: Regular	100	2	20
Sugar-Free, all flavors	25	0	5

Crunch *(Nestle):*

	C	**F**	**Cb**
Caramel	210	14	18
Vanilla Flavored	220	15	18
Reduced-Fat	140	8	15
Loaded, King Size, 2.68 oz	270	17	15

Dove: Milk Chocolate with Vanilla

	C	**F**	**Cb**
Dove: Milk Chocolate with Vanilla	330	21	31
Milk Chocolate with Almonds	340	23	28
Dark Chocolate with Vanilla	330	21	33

Dreyers/Edys

Dibs: With Chocolaty Coating (26 Pieces)

	C	**F**	**Cb**
Chocolate	360	25	30
Crunch; Mint	340	24	30
Drumstick	350	25	30

Real Fruit Bars: Orange & Cream

	C	**F**	**Cb**
Real Fruit Bars: Orange & Cream	80	1.5	16
Strawberry	80	0	21

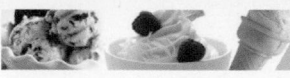

Ice Cream Bars & Pops ①

Bars & Pops (Cont)

Per Bar/Serving

	C	F	Cb
Drumstick *(Nestlé)*: Classic Vanilla	290	16	33
Vanilla Caramel	320	17	37
Vanilla Fudge	310	16	37
King Size, Triple Choc.	390	21	46
Simply Dipped: Vanilla	270	13	37
Cookies & Cream	300	14	39
Mint	290	14	38
Lil' Drums, average all flavors	120	6	16
Edy's, Fruit Bars:			
Creamy Coconut	120	3	21
Other flavors, average	80	0	21
Fat Boy:			
Sundae On A Stick:			
Casco Vanilla Nut, 3 oz	290	22	22
Chocolate	240	18	20
Peppermint, 3 oz	280	20	26
Sandwiches: Chocolate, 3 oz	210	9	31
Cookies n' Cream 3 oz	240	10	36
Raspberry Cheesecake, 2.8 oz	210	7	34
Strawberry, 3 oz	220	10	30
Vanilla, 3 oz	220	10	31
Fudge Bar *(Nestlé)*: Polar	90	2	16
Mini's	80	2	14
Fudgesicle: *(The Original Brand)*			
Fudge Bar	100	2	17
Fat-Free	60	0	13
No Added Sugar	40	1	10
Good Humor: Oreo Bar	250	15	28
Candy Center Crunch	310	23	24
Chocolate Eclair	220	10	30
Premium Vanilla	260	17	24
Reese's Peanut Butter Cups	310	21	27
Toasted Almond	240	12	30
Cones: King	250	13	30
Sundae	260	15	29
Triple Choc. Brownie	420	19	58
Vanilla Chocolate	390	21	44
Sandwiches: Choc. Chip Cookie	270	10	44
Giant Neapolitan	250	9	38
Giant Vanilla	220	4	43
Snack Pops, average all flavors	210	13	23

Per Bar/Serving

	C	F	Cb
Haagen-Dazs:			
Dark Chocolate: Chocolate	290	20	24
Vanilla	300	21	23
Milk Chocolate:			
Vanilla & Almonds	310	22	22
Vanilla	290	21	22
Snack Size: Coffee & Alm. Crunch	190	13	15
Vanilla & Almonds	190	14	14
Healthy Choice: Fudge Bar	80	1	13
Caramel Swirl S'wich	150	2	30
Mocha Swirl	90	1.5	17
Sorbet & Cream Bar	90	1	17
Vanilla Sandwich	130	2	25
Hood: Chocolate Eclair	150	10	14
Fudge Bar, Fudge Stix	70	0	14
Orange Cream	90	1.5	19
Rocket	120	5	16
Hoodsie Cups: Vanilla; Chocolate	100	5	12
Pops	60	0	16
Sundae	120	5	19
Sandwiches: Vanilla	180	6	29
Light	160	3	29
Ice Cream Sandwich *(Nestle)*: Mini	90	2.5	15
Super	260	11	39
Vanilla	160	4	29
Icee Freeze, 2.25 oz	70	0	17
Klondike			
Bars: Caramel Pretzel	260	15	29
Choco Taco	290	15	36
Dark Chocolate	250	14	29
Heath	230	15	24
Krunch	250	14	30
Neapolitan	250	14	29
Oreo	260	17	26
Original Vanilla, 3 oz	250	14	29
3.6 oz	330	23	28
Reese's	260	16	26
Triple Chocolate	230	14	26
Whitehouse Cherry	250	14	31
Cones: Nascar; Vanilla	280	14	35
Vanilla Caramel; Vanilla Fudge	290	14	37
Sandwiches			
Oreo	230	10	34
Vanilla	170	3	32
Slim-a-Bear Sandwich			
100 Calorie, Vanilla	100	1.5	21

Updated Nutrition Data ~ www.CalorieKing.com
Persons with Diabetes ~ See Disclaimer (Page 22)

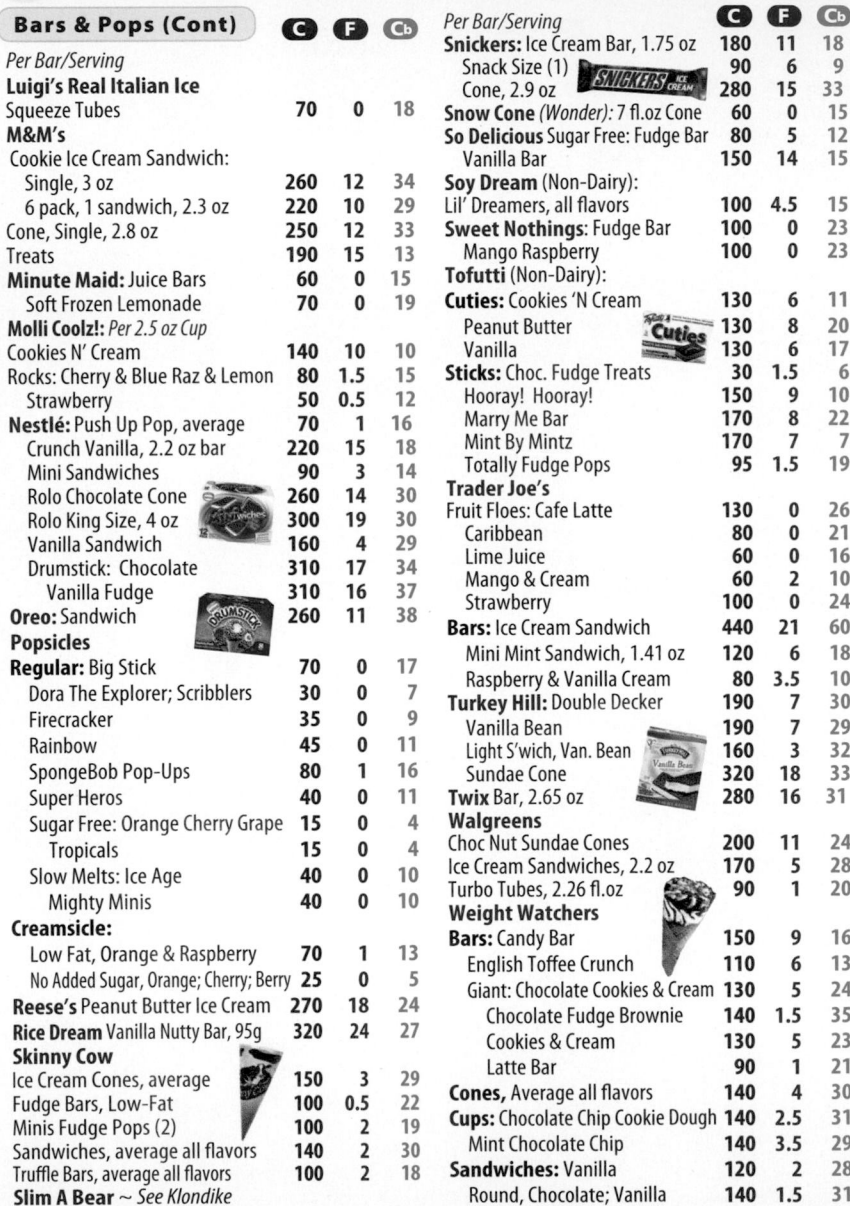

Bars & Pops (Cont)

Per Bar/Serving

	C	F	Cb
Luigi's Real Italian Ice			
Squeeze Tubes	70	0	18
M&M's			
Cookie Ice Cream Sandwich:			
Single, 3 oz	260	12	34
6 pack, 1 sandwich, 2.3 oz	220	10	29
Cone, Single, 2.8 oz	250	12	33
Treats	190	15	13
Minute Maid: Juice Bars	60	0	15
Soft Frozen Lemonade	70	0	19
Molli Coolz!: *Per 2.5 oz Cup*			
Cookies N' Cream	140	10	10
Rocks: Cherry & Blue Raz & Lemon	80	1.5	15
Strawberry	50	0.5	12
Nestlé: Push Up Pop, average	70	1	16
Crunch Vanilla, 2.2 oz bar	220	15	18
Mini Sandwiches	90	3	14
Rolo Chocolate Cone	260	14	30
Rolo King Size, 4 oz	300	19	30
Vanilla Sandwich	160	4	29
Drumstick: Chocolate	310	17	34
Vanilla Fudge	310	16	37
Oreo: Sandwich	260	11	38
Popsicles			
Regular: Big Stick	70	0	17
Dora The Explorer; Scribblers	30	0	7
Firecracker	35	0	9
Rainbow	45	0	11
SpongeBob Pop-Ups	80	1	16
Super Heros	40	0	11
Sugar Free: Orange Cherry Grape	15	0	4
Tropicals	15	0	4
Slow Melts: Ice Age	40	0	10
Mighty Minis	40	0	10
Creamsicle:			
Low Fat, Orange & Raspberry	70	1	13
No Added Sugar, Orange; Cherry; Berry	25	0	5
Reese's Peanut Butter Ice Cream	270	18	24
Rice Dream Vanilla Nutty Bar, 95g	320	24	27
Skinny Cow			
Ice Cream Cones, average	150	3	29
Fudge Bars, Low-Fat	100	0.5	22
Minis Fudge Pops (2)	100	2	19
Sandwiches, average all flavors	140	2	30
Truffle Bars, average all flavors	100	2	18
Slim A Bear ~ *See Klondike*			

Per Bar/Serving

	C	F	Cb
Snickers: Ice Cream Bar, 1.75 oz	180	11	18
Snack Size (1)	90	6	9
Cone, 2.9 oz	280	15	33
Snow Cone *(Wonder):* 7 fl.oz Cone	60	0	15
So Delicious Sugar Free: Fudge Bar	80	5	12
Vanilla Bar	150	14	15
Soy Dream (Non-Dairy):			
Lil' Dreamers, all flavors	100	4.5	15
Sweet Nothings: Fudge Bar	100	0	23
Mango Raspberry	100	0	23
Tofutti (Non-Dairy):			
Cuties: Cookies 'N Cream	130	6	11
Peanut Butter	130	8	20
Vanilla	130	6	17
Sticks: Choc. Fudge Treats	30	1.5	6
Hooray! Hooray!	150	9	10
Marry Me Bar	170	8	22
Mint By Mintz	170	7	7
Totally Fudge Pops	95	1.5	19
Trader Joe's			
Fruit Floes: Cafe Latte	130	0	26
Caribbean	80	0	21
Lime Juice	60	0	16
Mango & Cream	60	2	10
Strawberry	100	0	24
Bars: Ice Cream Sandwich	440	21	60
Mini Mint Sandwich, 1.41 oz	120	6	18
Raspberry & Vanilla Cream	80	3.5	10
Turkey Hill: Double Decker	190	7	30
Vanilla Bean	190	7	29
Light S'wich, Van. Bean	160	3	32
Sundae Cone	320	18	33
Twix Bar, 2.65 oz	280	16	31
Walgreens			
Choc Nut Sundae Cones	200	11	24
Ice Cream Sandwiches, 2.2 oz	170	5	28
Turbo Tubes, 2.26 fl.oz	90	1	20
Weight Watchers			
Bars: Candy Bar	150	9	16
English Toffee Crunch	110	6	13
Giant: Chocolate Cookies & Cream	130	5	24
Chocolate Fudge Brownie	140	1.5	35
Cookies & Cream	130	5	23
Latte Bar	90	1	21
Cones, Average all flavors	140	4	30
Cups: Chocolate Chip Cookie Dough	140	2.5	31
Mint Chocolate Chip	140	3.5	29
Sandwiches: Vanilla	120	2	28
Round, Chocolate; Vanilla	140	1.5	31

Canned & Packaged Meals

	C	F	Cb
B & M: Per ½ Cup (4½ oz)			
Baked Beans: Original	170	2	31
Barbeque	190	0.5	39
Vegetarian	160	1	28
Raisin Brown Bread, ½" slice, 2 oz	130	0.5	29

Banquet
Homestyle Bakes: Per Serving, Prepared

	C	F	Cb
Asian Style Fried Rice	240	1.5	47
Chicken & Dumplings	230	4.5	33
Country Chicken, Mashed Potato & Bisc.	360	17	43
Creamy Cheesy Chicken Alfredo	400	22	36
Creamy Chicken & Biscuits	350	17	39
Lasagna	290	11	36
Pasta & Meatballs	310	10	41

Betty Crocker
Complete Meals: Per Serving, ⅓ Package

	C	F	Cb
Cheesy Beef Taco	240	4.5	42
Chkn & Buttermilk Biscuits	280	11	37
Chkn Fettuccini Alfredo	230	6	34
Stroganoff	190	4	30
Three Cheese Chicken	240	7	36

Hamburger Helper: Per Cup, Prepared

	C	F	Cb
Beef Fried Rice	300	12	22
Beef Pasta	280	9	24
Cheeseburger Macaroni	310	10	26
Cheesy Hashbrown	400	19	39
Cheesy Jambalaya	320	13	28
Chili Macaroni	270	16	26
Crunchy Taco	340	13	33
Salisbury	280	9	24

Tuna Helper: Per Serving

	C	F	Cb
Creamy Parmesan	290	7	36
Average other varieties	310	12	37

Chicken Helper: Per Cup, Prepared

	C	F	Cb
Cheesy Chicken Enchilada	330	10	40
Chicken Fried Rice	250	7	22
Italian Fettuccini Alfredo	330	9	29

Side Dishes/Casseroles: Per Serving, Prepared

	C	F	Cb
Au Gratin, ⅔ cup	150	4	23
Cheddar & Bacon; Cheesy Scallops	140	4	25
Roasted Garlic	120	5	20
Scalloped Potatoes, ½ cup	130	5	25
Sour Cream and Chives, ⅔ cup	120	2.5	21

Deluxe Potatoes: Per ½ Cup, Prepared

	C	F	Cb
Cheesy Cheddar Au Gratin	180	8	25
Loaded Au Gratin	140	4	25
Three Cheese Mashed Potato Bake	190	9	24

Betty Crocker (Cont)

Seasoned Skillets: Prepared

	C	F	Cb
Hash Brown, ½ cup	120	3	18
Roasted Garlic & Herb, ⅔ cup	170	7	21
Traditional, ½ cup	180	7	22

Bowl Appetit: Per Bowl

	C	F	Cb
Cheddar Broccoli Rice	290	6	52
Homestyle Chicken Pasta	250	5	44
Pasta Alfredo	350	9	55
Teriyaki Rice	250	1	57
Three-Cheese Rotini	340	7	59

Bush's Best: Per ½ Cup

	C	F	Cb
Black Beans	110	0.5	23
Chili Beans	120	1	20
Dark Red Kidney Beans	105	0	22
Garbanzo Beans	105	2	20
Refried Beans: Traditional	150	3	24
Fat Free	130	0	24
Baked Beans: Vegetarian	130	0	29
Average other flavors	150	1	32

Campbell's
Beans: Per ½ Cup

	C	F	Cb
Baked Beans	160	2.5	30
Pork & Beans	140	1.5	25

Chunky Microwavable Bowls: Per Cup

	C	F	Cb
Firehouse; Roadhouse	230	8	25

Spaghetti O's: Per Cup

	C	F	Cb
Original	180	1	37
With Meat Sauce	180	2	32
With Meatballs	240	8	32

Chef Boyardee: Per Cup

	C	F	Cb
Beefaroni in Tomato Sauce	260	10	33
Beef Ravioli In Tomato & Meat Sauce	240	8	35
Cheesy Burger Macaroni	200	5	30
Pepperoni Pizzaroli	250	7	38
Spaghetti & Meatballs in Sauce	270	10	32
99% Fat-Free: Beef Ravioli in Sauce	170	1.5	33
Cheese Ravioli in Tomato Sauce	240	2.5	45

Forkables, Sports; Sealife:

	C	F	Cb
Pasta in Sauce with Meat	240	6	37

Microwaveable Big Bowls: Per ½ Bowl

	C	F	Cb
Beefaroni in Tomato Sauce	250	9	31
Lasagna	250	7	33
Mini Beef Ravioli in Sauce	240	8	33

Chef Boyardee (Cont)	C	F	Cb
Microwaveable Cups: *Per Cup*			
Beefaroni	210	8	27
Beef Ravioli	190	5	29
Macaroni & Cheese	190	8	23
Spaghetti & Meatballs	200	8	23
Mini Bites: *Per Cup*			
Beef Ravioli with Meatballs	280	12	33
Pasta Shells with Meatballs	250	10	29
Spaghetti with Meatballs	250	10	30
Overstuffed: Beef Ravioli in Sauce	270	6	44
Italian Sausage Ravioli in Sauce	240	4.5	40
Dinner Kits: *Per Serving*			
Cheese Pizza	260	4.5	45
Lasagna	270	10	36
Dennison's Chili: *Per Cup*			
Chili Con Carne W/ith Beans:			
Original	360	14	38
Chunky	300	10	32
99% Fat Free: Beef Chili with Beans	210	2	29
Turkey Chili with Beans	210	3	29
Dinty Moore *(Hormel Foods)*			
Beef Stew: 7½ oz cup	150	6	15
15 oz can, 1 cup, 8.3 oz	200	10	17
Microwave Cup: Beef Stew, 7.5 oz	150	6	15
Chicken & Dumplings, 7.5 oz	220	7	29
Noodles & Chicken, 7.5 oz	190	9	20
Average other varieties	180	8	17
Dr. McDougall's: *Per 10 oz*			
Ramen Noodles, Chicken flavor	200	1	40
Rice Pilaf, average	260	2	52
Eden Organics: *Per ½ Cup (4½ oz)*			
Baked Beans with Sorghum, Mustard	150	0	27
Black Eyed Peas	90	1	16
Black Soybeans	120	6	8
Refried: Black Beans	110	1.5	18
Pinto; Kidney Beans, av.	105	0.5	18
Farmhouse			
Pasta: *Unprepared*			
Herb & Butter, 4.7 oz	240	2	45
White Cheddar, 6.2 oz	260	2.5	47
Rice: *Unprepared*			
Chicken Flavor, 6 oz	200	1	43
Long Grain & Wild Herb & Butter	200	1.5	42
Mexican, 6 oz	190	0.5	42

French's Fried Onions	C	F	Cb
Regular: 2 Tbsp, ¼ oz	45	3.5	3
¼ cup, ½ oz	90	7	6
1 cup, 2 oz	360	28	24
Cheddar: 2 Tbsp, ¼ oz	45	3.5	3
¼ cup, ½ oz	90	7	6
1 cup, 2 oz	360	28	24
Health Valley			
Chili, average all varieties, 1 cup	150	1	31
Microwavable Chili: *Per Cup*			
Vegetarian Spicy	120	1	25
Vegetarian Spicy 3 Bean	140	1	28
Heinz			
Vegetarian Beans, ½ cup	140	0.5	27
Hormel: *Per Cup*			
Compleats: *Per 10 oz Serving*			
Beef Pot Roast	270	6	29
Beef Steak Tips	270	9	29
Chicken & Dumplings	260	8	34
Chicken & Noodles	240	8	27
Chicken & Rice	280	11	34
Chicken Alfredo	330	18	28
Chicken Breast and Dressing	270	7	29
Chicken Breast & Gravy	200	3	24
Homestyle Beef	220	6	30
Lasagne with Meat Sauce	280	7	42
Meatloaf with Potato & Gravy	310	11	34
Salisbury Steak	280	11	30
Santa Fe Style Chicken	280	4	41
Sesame Chicken	320	8	41
Spaghetti	290	9	36
Teriyaki Chicken with Rices	270	1.5	50
Turkey & Hearty Vegetables	180	3.5	24
Turkey & Dressing	290	9	31
Kid's Kitchen: Beans & Wieners	310	13	37
Cheesy Mac 'N Cheese	270	14	24
Mini Beef Ravioli	240	6	38
Noodle Rings & Chicken	140	4	18
Chili (15 oz Can):			
With Beans: *Per 8.7 oz*			
Regular; Hot; Chunky	260	7	33
99% Fat Free: Turkey	210	3	28
Vegetarian	190	1	35
Without Beans: *Per 8.3 oz*			
Regular; Hot Chili	220	9	18
Chunky	210	8	19
Turkey	190	3	16

	C	F	Cb
Hungry Jack Potatoes			
Instant Potato Flakes, ⅓ cup	80	0	19
Hunt's			
Manwich Sloppy Joe, Original, ¼ cup	30	0	7
Knorr:			
Sides: Dry Mix Only			

Note: Figures are only for package contents and not for extra ingredients added in preparation.

	C	F	Cb
Asian: Chicken Fried Rice, ½ cup, 2.3 oz	220	1.5	47
Teriyaki Noodles, ¾ cup, 2.3 oz	240	2	48
Teriyaki Rice, ½ cup, 2.1 oz	240	1.5	51
Cajun: Garlic Butter Rice, ½ cup, 2.4 oz	240	4	46
Red Beans & Rice, ½ cup, 2.8 oz	290	1	62
Fiesta: Mexican Rice, ½ cup, 2.4 oz	240	1	52
Spanish Rice, ½ cup, 2.3 oz	230	1	49
Taco Rice, ½ cup, 2.4 oz	230	1	48
Pasta: Alfredo, ⅔ cup, 2.2 oz	240	4.5	40
Alfredo Broccoli, ⅔ cup, 2.2 oz	240	4.5	41
Butter, ⅔ cup, 2.2 oz	240	4	43
Butter & Herb, ⅔ cup, 2.2 oz	230	3.5	44
Cheesy Cheddar, ¾ cup, 2.1 oz	220	2	41
Parmesan, ⅔ cup, 2.1 oz	220	4.5	37
Stroganoff, ⅔ cup, 2 oz	210	2	39
Rice: Cheddar Broccoli, ½ cup, 2.4 oz	240	1.5	49
Chicken Broccoli, ½ cup, 2.3 oz	210	1	46
Chicken Flavor, 2.3 oz	240	2.5	47
Sides Plus Veggies:			
Butter & Herb Rotini, 1 cup	260	3.5	49
Cheddar Rice, 2.4 oz	250	2	51
South Western Style Rice, 2.5 oz	250	1.5	51
Vegetable Fried Rice, ½ cup, 2.3 oz	240	1.5	50
Kraft			
Dinners: *Per Serving, Prepared*			
Macaroni & Cheese: Cheesy Alfredo	380	14	50
Pasta & Sauce	310	9	49
Scooby-Doo	290	6	50
Spirals	290	6.5	48
Thick 'N Creamy	380	15	50
Bistro Deluxe:			
Creamy Portobello Mushroom	310	11	40
Sundried Tomato Parmesan	300	11	40
Deluxe, Original; Sharp Cheddar	320	9	47
Easy Mac, average all varieties	220	5	39
Velveeta Shells & Cheese, Original	360	12	49

	C	F	Cb
Kraft (Cont)			
Velveeta Potatoes: *Per ½ Cup, Prepared*			
Cheesy: Au Gratin	190	6	26
Bacon Scalloped	200	7	26
Cheesy Mashed Potatoes	200	12	21
Kroger: *Prepared as Directed*			
Kitchen Creation Skillet Dinners: *Per Cup Prep'd*			
Cheeseburger	300	13	24
Cheesy Hashbrowns	400	20	39
Creamy Broccoli	300	12	33
Lasagna	280	12	26
Stroganoff	320	14	27
Noodles & Sauce: *Per Cup, Prepared*			
Alfredo	310	12	42
Butter; Stroganoff, average	290	11	39
Chicken & Broccoli	290	8	42
La Choy			
Beef Chow Mein, 1 cup	90	2	11
Chicken Chow Mein, 1 cup	100	3	10
Chop Suey Vegetables, ½ cup	15	0	3
Chow Mein Noodles, ½ cup	130	5	19
Creations: *Per Cup, Prepared*			
Asian Fried Rice	280	1.5	36
Sweet & Sour Chicken	340	2	51
Teriyaki Chicken	320	4	42
Lightlife			
Organic Tempeh:			
Flax; Soy, average, 4 oz	225	9	16
Garden Veggie, 4 oz	240	10	17
Three Grain; Wild Rice, 4 oz	230	9	21
Smart Tenders:			
Lemon Pepper (3)	130	3	8
Savory Chick'n (3), 3 oz	130	3.5	7
Tempehtations: Classic BBQ, 3 oz	160	6	16
Ginger Teriyaki, 3 oz	160	5	18
Zesty Lemon, 3 oz	160	8	10
Lunchables (Oscar Mayer): *Per Package*			
Cracker Stackers Ham & Cheddar	410	21	39
Mini Beef Taco Wrapz, 5.7 oz	400	10	61
Nachos Chse & Salsa, 4¾ oz	500	18	66
Maxed Out: Combo Ham & Cheddar	660	22	101
Combo Turkey & Cheddar, 5.4 oz	680	22	106
Pizza: Pepperoni, 7.1 oz	530	17	75
Extra Cheesy, 7.3 oz	510	12	77
Ultimate Nachos with Dip & Salsa	580	27	75
Lunchmakers (Armour)			
Loco Nachos	400	14	69
Cheese Pizza	360	9	53

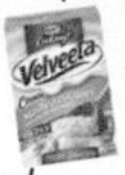

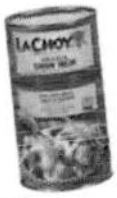

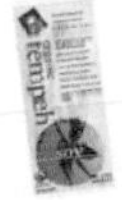

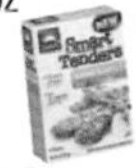

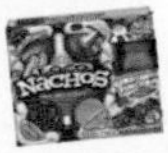

Macaroni Grill: *Per 1 Cup, Prep'd*

	C	F	Cb
Chicken Piccata	280	11	24
Chicken Alfredo/Parmesan, average	305	11	27
Chicken Marsala	330	13	30
Garlic & Herb Chicken	240	7	22

Maruchan:
Ramen Noodles: Beef/Chicken/Shrimp Flavors,

	C	F	Cb
½ block, 1½ oz	190	7	26

Noodles: Instant Lunch,

	C	F	Cb
Lime Chili with Shrimp Flavor	290	11	39
Roast Beef/Chicken Flavor	290	12	38

Yakisoba: *Per ½ Package*

	C	F	Cb
Cheddar Cheese Flavor	280	14	33
Chicken Flavor	260	11	36
Teriyaki Beef Flavor	260	10	36

Minute Rice: *1 Cup, Prepared*
Ready To Serve: *Per 4.4 oz Container, Prepared*

	C	F	Cb
Brown/Chicken Rice Mix, av.	230	3.5	40
White Rice	200	3	40
Yellow Rice Mix	190	4	35

Nissin
Chow Mein: *Per ½ Package, 2 oz*

	C	F	Cb
Chicken Flavor	240	9	35
Spicy Chicken Flavor	260	11	36
Teriyaki Beef; Thai P'nut	270	12	36
With Shrimp	280	14	32

Noodle Cups: *Per Cup*

	C	F	Cb
Beef/Shrimp Flavor	300	13	38
Beef Flavor Minestrone	270	11	37
Chicken Flavor	300	13	38

Top Ramen: *Per ½ Dry Noodle Block, w/ Seasoning*

	C	F	Cb
Beef/Chicken Flavor	190	7	27

Old El Paso
Dinner Kits: *Per Kit, Unprepared*

	C	F	Cb
Burrito	170	3.5	31
Soft Taco Bake	180	7	28

Side Dishes: *Prep'd*

	C	F	Cb
Spanish Rice, ⅓ packet	270	7	54
Cheesy Mexican Rice, ⅓ packet	280	7	55

Refried Beans: Traditional, ½ cup

	C	F	Cb
Refried Beans: Traditional, ½ cup	90	0.5	16
with Green Chili, ½ cup, 4.3 oz	90	0.5	16
Vegetarian, ½ cup, 4.16 oz	90	0.5	16
Fat-Free varieties, ½ cup, 4.37 oz	100	0	18

Pasta Roni: *Per Cup (Prepared)*

	C	F	Cb
Angel Hair Pasta varieties, average	310	13	41
Butter & Herb Italiano	300	12	40
Chicken & Broccoli	360	15	49
Chicken Flavor	300	12	39
Fettuccine Alfredo	450	25	47
Four Cheese Corkscrew	370	16	49

Pasta Roni (Cont): *Per Cup, Prep'd*

	C	F	Cb
Shells & White Cheddar	290	12	38
Tomato Parmesan	270	9	40

Nature's Way: Creamy Parmesan

	C	F	Cb
Nature's Way: Creamy Parmesan	280	9	41
Mushroom in Cream Sauce	280	10	39
Olive Oil & Italian Herb	250	8	38

Rice-A-Roni
Classic Favorites: *Per Cup, Prepared*

	C	F	Cb
Beef; Herb & Butter; Rice Pilaf, av.	310	9	51
Broccoli Au Gratin	350	16	46
Chicken	300	9	50
Lower Sodium	270	5	51
Chicken & Broccoli	220	5	40
Chicken & Garlic	250	8	41
Fried Rice	310	10	50
Spanish Rice	260	8	44

(Reduced Fat Recipe: If only 1 Tbsp fat is used instead of 2 Tbsp, deduct 35 calories and 0.15 oz fat.)

Nature's Way: Parmesan & Romano

	C	F	Cb
Nature's Way: Parmesan & Romano	280	9	42
Italian Cheese & Herb	340	12	52
Long Grain & Wild Rice	250	7	43

Savory Whole Grains:

	C	F	Cb
Chicken & Herb Classico	260	8	41
Roasted Garlic Italiano	270	9	41
Spanish	250	8	42

Rosarita
Refried Beans: *Per ½ Cup*

	C	F	Cb
Traditional	120	2	18
Vegetarian; Spicy	120	2	19
Non-Fat: Black Bean	110	0	19
Traditional	100	0	19

S & W: *Per ½ Cup*

	C	F	Cb
Baked Beans: Original, 4.6 oz	160	1	32
With Maple Sugar, 4.6 oz	140	0.5	28
Black Beans, 4.5 oz	100	1	17
Chili Beans with Chipotle, 4.55 oz	110	1	23
Kidney Beans, 4.66 oz	120	1	20
White Beans, 4.48 oz	110	0.5	19

Shedd's
Country Crock Side Dishes

	C	F	Cb
Garlic Mashed Potato, ⅔ cup, 5 oz	160	7	22
Homestyle Mashed Potato, ⅔ cup	180	9	23

Deluxe: Cheddar Broccoli Rice, 1 cup

	C	F	Cb
Deluxe: Cheddar Broccoli Rice, 1 cup	270	11	35
Elbow Macaroni & Cheese, 1 cup	370	17	40
Four Cheese Pasta, 1 cup, 8.11 oz	380	17	41
Loaded Mashed Potatoes, ⅔ cup	200	11	23

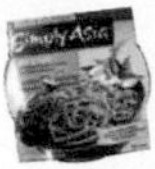
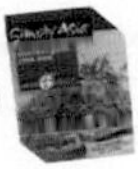
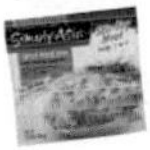
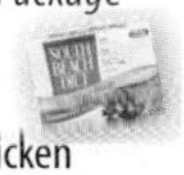
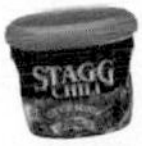

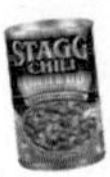

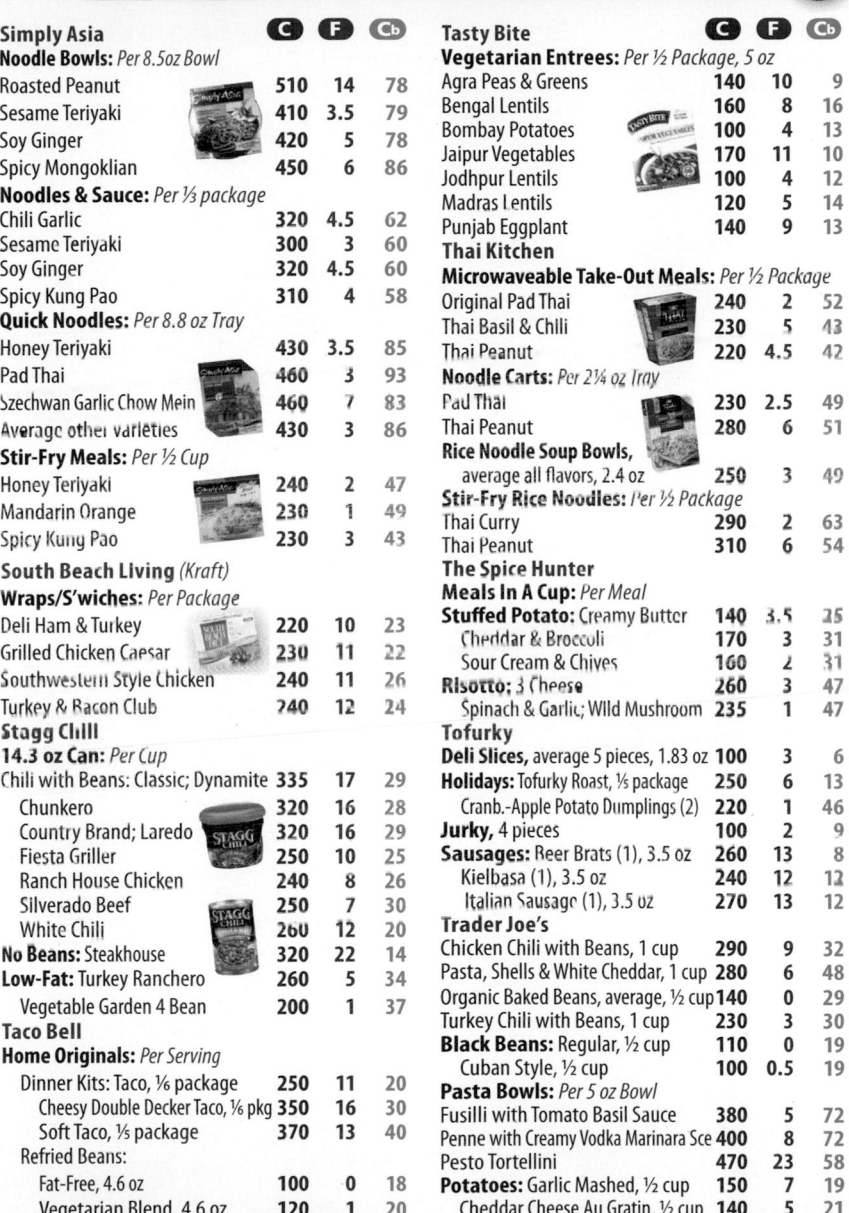

Simply Asia	C	F	Cb
Noodle Bowls: *Per 8.5oz Bowl*			
Roasted Peanut	510	14	78
Sesame Teriyaki	410	3.5	79
Soy Ginger	420	5	78
Spicy Mongoklian	450	6	86
Noodles & Sauce: *Per ⅓ package*			
Chili Garlic	320	4.5	62
Sesame Teriyaki	300	3	60
Soy Ginger	320	4.5	60
Spicy Kung Pao	310	4	58
Quick Noodles: *Per 8.8 oz Tray*			
Honey Teriyaki	430	3.5	85
Pad Thai	460	3	93
Szechwan Garlic Chow Mein	460	7	83
Average other varieties	430	3	86
Stir-Fry Meals: *Per ½ Cup*			
Honey Teriyaki	240	2	47
Mandarin Orange	230	1	49
Spicy Kung Pao	230	3	43
South Beach Living *(Kraft)*			
Wraps/S'wiches: *Per Package*			
Deli Ham & Turkey	220	10	23
Grilled Chicken Caesar	230	11	22
Southwestern Style Chicken	240	11	26
Turkey & Bacon Club	240	12	24
Stagg Chili			
14.3 oz Can: *Per Cup*			
Chili with Beans: Classic; Dynamite	335	17	29
Chunkero	320	16	28
Country Brand; Laredo	320	16	29
Fiesta Griller	250	10	25
Ranch House Chicken	240	8	26
Silverado Beef	250	7	30
White Chili	260	12	20
No Beans: Steakhouse	320	22	14
Low-Fat: Turkey Ranchero	260	5	34
Vegetable Garden 4 Bean	200	1	37
Taco Bell			
Home Originals: *Per Serving*			
Dinner Kits: Taco, ⅙ package	250	11	20
Cheesy Double Decker Taco, ⅙ pkg	350	16	30
Soft Taco, ⅕ package	370	13	40
Refried Beans:			
Fat-Free, 4.6 oz	100	0	18
Vegetarian Blend, 4.6 oz	120	1	20

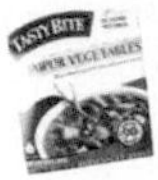
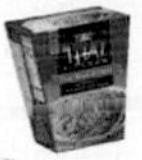
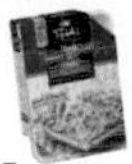

Tasty Bite	C	F	Cb
Vegetarian Entrees: *Per ½ Package, 5 oz*			
Agra Peas & Greens	140	10	9
Bengal Lentils	160	8	16
Bombay Potatoes	100	4	13
Jaipur Vegetables	170	11	10
Jodhpur Lentils	100	4	12
Madras Lentils	120	5	14
Punjab Eggplant	140	9	13
Thai Kitchen			
Microwaveable Take-Out Meals: *Per ½ Package*			
Original Pad Thai	240	2	52
Thai Basil & Chili	230	5	43
Thai Peanut	220	4.5	42
Noodle Carts: *Per 2¼ oz Tray*			
Pad Thai	230	2.5	49
Thai Peanut	280	6	51
Rice Noodle Soup Bowls,			
average all flavors, 2.4 oz	250	3	49
Stir-Fry Rice Noodles: *Per ½ Package*			
Thai Curry	290	2	63
Thai Peanut	310	6	54
The Spice Hunter			
Meals In A Cup: *Per Meal*			
Stuffed Potato: Creamy Butter	140	3.5	25
Cheddar & Broccoli	170	3	31
Sour Cream & Chives	160	2	31
Risotto: 3 Cheese	260	3	47
Spinach & Garlic; Wild Mushroom	235	1	47
Tofurky			
Deli Slices, average 5 pieces, 1.83 oz	100	3	6
Holidays: Tofurky Roast, ⅕ package	250	6	13
Cranb.-Apple Potato Dumplings (2)	220	1	46
Jurky, 4 pieces	100	2	9
Sausages: Beer Brats (1), 3.5 oz	260	13	8
Kielbasa (1), 3.5 oz	240	12	12
Italian Sausage (1), 3.5 oz	270	13	12
Trader Joe's			
Chicken Chili with Beans, 1 cup	290	9	32
Pasta, Shells & White Cheddar, 1 cup	280	6	48
Organic Baked Beans, average, ½ cup	140	0	29
Turkey Chili with Beans, 1 cup	230	3	30
Black Beans: Regular, ½ cup	110	0	19
Cuban Style, ½ cup	100	0.5	19
Pasta Bowls: *Per 5 oz Bowl*			
Fusilli with Tomato Basil Sauce	380	5	72
Penne with Creamy Vodka Marinara Sce	400	8	72
Pesto Tortellini	470	23	58
Potatoes: Garlic Mashed, ½ cup	150	7	19
Cheddar Cheese Au Gratin, ½ cup	140	5	21

Uncle Ben's	C	F	Cb
Country Inn: *Per Cup, Prepared w/o Margarine*			
Broccoli Rice Au Gratin	200	2	43
Chicken & Vegetable Rice	200	1.5	41
Mexican Fiesta Rice	200	1	42
Oriental Fried Rice	200	1	42
Ready Rice: *Per 1 Cup, Prepared*			
Butter & Garlic Flavored Rice	220	4	41
Roasted Chicken	220	3.5	41
Teriyaki	220	3	42
Whole Grain Brown	240	3	39
Ready Whole Grain Medley: *Per 1 Cup, Prepared*			
Brown & Wild	220	3.5	42
Chicken Medley	210	3.5	41
Roasted Garlic	200	3	38
Santa Fe	220	3	42
Vegetable Harvest	220	3	34
Valley Fresh			
Chicken: *Per 2 oz*			
Premium White	80	3	0
White & Dark	80	3.5	0
Turkey, Premium White	80	3	0
Van Camps			
Pork & Beans, ½ cup	110	1	23
Original Baked Beans, ½ cup	140	1	30
Beanee Weenee Original, 10½ oz	340	11	39
White Wave			
Seitan: Chicken with Broth, 5 oz	110	2	4
Traditional, 3 oz	90	1	3
Worthington/Loma Linda			
Big Franks: 1 link, 1.8 oz	110	6	3
Low-fat, 1 link, 1.8 oz	80	2.5	3
Chili, 1 cup, 8.10 oz	280	10	25
Choplets, 2 slices, 3.2 oz	90	1	4
Diced Chik, 2 oz	50	0	2
Linketts, (1), 1¼ oz	70	4	1
Little Links (2), 1.6 oz	90	5	3
Low-Fat Veja-Links (1), 1 oz	45	1.5	3
Multigrain Cutlets, 2 slices, 3¼ oz	100	1	5
Prime Stakes (1) 3¼ oz	120	6	7
Redi-Burger, ⅝" slice, 3 oz	120	2.5	7
Saucettes (1), 1 oz	90	6	1
Super Links (1), 1.7 oz	110	8	2
Tender Bits (6), 2.8 oz	120	4	7
Tender Rounds (6), 2.8 oz	120	4.5	6

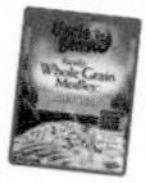

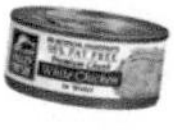

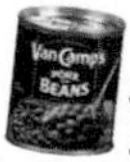

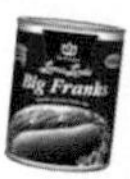

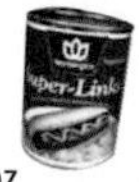

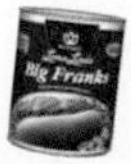

Worthington/Loma Linda (Cont)	C	F	Cb
Veja-Links (1), 1 oz	50	3	1
Vege-Burger, ¼ cup, 2 oz	60	0.5	2
Vegetable Skallops, ½ cup, 3 oz	90	1	4
Vegetarian Burger, ¼ cup, 1.9 oz	70	1.5	3
Yves Veggie Cuisine (*Vegetarian*)			
Breakfast: Patties (2), 1.8 oz	80	2	4
Canadian Bacon, 3 slices	80	0.5	2
Burgers: Meatless Beef Burger (1)	110	4	8
Meatless Chicken (1)	100	3	5
Deli: Bologna, 4 slices	80	2.5	2
Ham, 4 slices	100	2	5
Pepperoni, 6 slices	60	1	4
Roast Beef, 4 slices	110	2.5	4
Salami, 4 slices	80	0	4
Smoked Chicken, 4 slices	100	1.5	5
Turkey, 4 slices	100	1.5	5
Hot Dogs & Brats:			
Jumbo Dog (1), 2.7 oz	110	3	5
Good Dog (1), 2 oz	70	3.5	1
Hot Dog (1), 1.6 oz	50	0.5	2
Tofu Dog (1), 1.3 oz	45	1	2
Brats: Veggie Classic (1), 3.3 oz	160	5	9
Zesty Italian (1), 3.3 oz	150	5	9
Skewers:			
Lemon Herb Chicken (1), 2.8 oz	100	1	7
Meatless:			
Ground: Turkey, ⅓ cup, 1.95 oz	60	1	4
Taco Stuffers, ⅓ cup, 1.95 oz	90	2.5	5
Rounds: Original, ⅓ cup, 1.95 oz	60	0.5	5
Asian Lettuce Wrap, ⅓ cup, 1.95 oz	60	0.5	8
Strips: Beef, 3 oz	120	1	4
Chicken, 3 oz	110	1	3
Zatarain's			
Beans & Rice Mix: *Per ⅓, Cup Dry Mix Only*			
Black Beans & Rice	220	0.5	47
Blackeyed Peas & Rice	220	0.5	46
Caribbean Rice	160	1.5	34
Chicken Creole Rice	130	0.5	28
Chicken Flavor Rice	210	1	44
Fire Roasted Vegetables & Rice	170	0	38
Garlic & Herb & Rice	150	0	33
Gravy & Rice	200	0.5	45
Rice Pilaf	200	0	45
Smothered Chicken Rice	130	0	28
Yellow Rice	190	0	43

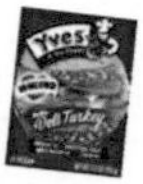

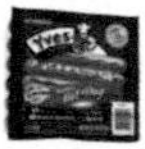

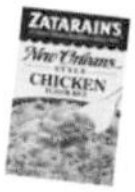

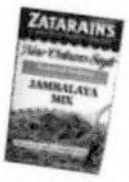

Amy's (Vegetarian) | C | F | Cb

Per Serving

	C	F	Cb
Asian Meals: Thai Stir Fry, 9.5 oz	310	11	45
Asian Noodle Stir Fry, 10 oz	290	7	50
Bowls: Brown Rice & Veges, 10 oz	260	9	36
Santa Fe Enchilada, 10 oz	350	11	47
Burritos: Bean & Cheese, 6 oz	300	9	43
Bean & Rice, 6 oz	300	8	48
Breakfast Burrito, 6 oz	250	7	38
Entrees: Cheese Enchilada, 4.9 oz	240	14	18
Cheese Lasagna, 10.3 oz	380	14	44
Macaroni & Cheese, 9 oz	410	16	47
Macaroni & Soy Cheeze, 9 oz	370	15	42
Roasted Vegetable Lasagna, 9.8 oz	350	11	47
Tofu Vegetable Lasagna, 9.5 oz	330	11	41
Whole Meals: Cheese Enchilada, 9 oz	350	15	38
Black Bean Enchilada, 10 oz	330	8	53
Bl. Bean Tamale Verde, 10.3 oz	330	10	55
Enchilada Verde, 10 oz	390	13	54
Veggie Loaf, 10 oz	290	8	47
Pot Pies: Broccoli	430	22	46
Mex. Tamale; Shepherd's Pie	155	4	27
Vegetable, 7½ oz	420	19	54
Snacks: Nacho, 5-6 pieces	210	8	26
Cheese Pizza, 5-6 pieces	190	7	22
Veggie Burgers,			
Californian Veggie (1), 2½ oz	140	5	19
Wraps: Breakfast Scramble, 5.5 oz	380	19	30
Indian Samosa, 5 oz	250	9	34
Indian Spinach Tofu, 5.5 oz	310	14	35
Teriyaki, 5.5 oz	310	7	51

Extra Product Listings ~ www.CalorieKing.com

Bagel Bites

	C	F	Cb
Three Cheese, 4 pieces, 3 oz	210	6	30
Cheese Sausage & Pepperoni, 4 pieces	210	7	30

Banquet

	C	F	Cb
Breaded Chicken: Breast Patties (1)	160	9	11
Chicken Breast Nuggets (6), 3 oz	240	16	12
Crispy Chicken, Skinless, 4.2 oz	360	23	13
Popcorn Chicken, 11 pieces	180	9	18
Wings: Hot & Spicy, 3 oz	270	18	11
Honey Barbecue, 3 oz	270	18	11
Crock Pot Classics			
Chicken & Dumplings, ⅔ cup	200	8	21
Hearty Beef & Veggies, ⅔ cup	140	6	15
Meatballs in Stroganoff Sauce, ⅔ cup	300	14	29

Banquet (Cont) | C | F | Cb

	C	F	Cb
Dinners:			
Boneless Pork Rib, 10 oz	320	11	42
Chicken Fingers, 7.1 oz	480	21	56
Fettuccine Alfredo, 8 oz	290	12	34
Lasagna with Meat Sauce, 8 oz	270	8	35
Mac & Cheese, 8 oz	260	6	39
Macaroni & Beef, 8 oz	210	4.5	32
Meatloaf Meal, 9.5 oz	280	13	28
Pepperoni Pizza, 5.75	340	12	47
Salisbury Steak Meal, 9.5 oz	290	16	25
Spaghetti & Meatballs, 9 oz	380	16	42
Swedish Meatballs, 10.25 oz	440	18	51
Turkey, 9.25 oz	250	7	32
Hearty One Dinners:			
Chicken Fried Beef Steak	750	42	66
Chicken Fried Chicken	660	40	48
Select Recipe: Chicken Parmesan	360	16	37
Corn Dog Meal, 7.5 oz	460	16	68
Fried Chicken Meal, 9 oz	440	26	30
Homestyle Pot Roast, 9.6 oz	170	5	19
Pot Pies: Beef, 7 oz	390	22	36
Chicken; Turkey, average, 7 oz	3880	21	36

Birds Eye – Voila!

Per 1 Cup, Cooked

	C	F	Cb
Voila!: Beef & Broccoli Stir Fry	210	6	27
Chicken Parmesan	240	8	31
Creamy Tomato Penne with Chicken	210	4.5	29
Garlic Chicken	240	8	29
Garlic Shrimp	230	9	27
Shrimp Scampi	190	2.5	31
Sweet & Sour Chicken	200	1	38
Family Skillets: Alfredo Chicken	280	12	27
Cheesy Chicken	250	6	35
Garlic Chicken	240	8	29
Three Cheese Chicken	210	8	21

Boca (Vegetarian)

	C	F	Cb
Burger: Cheeseburger, 2.5 oz	100	4.5	6
All American Classic, 2.5 oz	140	5	9
Vegan, Original, 2.5 oz	70	0.5	6
Organic Burgers: Vegan, Original	100	2.5	9
Grilled Vegetables, 2.5 oz	80	1	7
Chik'n: Orig Nuggets (4)	180	7	17
Patties (1), 2.5 oz	160	6	15
Veggie Patties, Bruschetta	90	1.5	9

Boston Market

	C	F	Cb
Dinners: Beef Steak & Noodles, 14 oz	460	12	58
Chicken Parmesan	620	24	69
Salisbury Steak	710	40	53
Swedish Meatballs	760	43	57
Turkey Breast Medallions with Potato	360	14	35
Entrees: Chicken Pot Pie, 8 oz	560	36	43
Honey Roasted Chicken, 9.2 oz	410	17	46

Claim Jumper

	C	F	Cb
Beef Pot Roast, 8 oz	270	11	27
Chicken Alfredo, 8 oz	320	13	33
Chicken Fried Beef Steak, 16¼ oz	720	39	71
Country Fried Chicken, 17¼ oz	700	34	75
Creamy Fettuccine Bake, 8 oz	320	16	28
Lasagna with Meat Sauce, 8 oz	310	14	30
Meatloaf Dinner, 15¼ oz	520	31	36
Roased Turkey Breast with Brocc., 14 oz	430	17	49
Salisbury Steak, 16 oz	640	35	48
Family Meal, Chicken & Noodle, 8 oz	300	15	34
Pot Pies: Beef, 1 cup, 8 oz	590	42	39
Chicken, 1 cup	550	37	39

Contessa

	C	F	Cb
On The Stove: *Per Serving, Unprepared*			
Beef/Chicken Stir Fry, average, 7 oz	180	2	24
Cashew Chicken with Sauce, 1½ cups	260	5	39
Jambalaya with Sauce, 1½ cups	240	7	29
Mongolian Beef with Sauce, 1¾ cups	310	7	47
Shrimp Stir-Fry with Sauce, 2 cups	180	0.5	29
Microsteam: *Per 1 Cup Prepared*			
Chicken Alfredo	270	13	27
Italian Sausage Rigatoni	310	11	43
Spaghetti Bolognese	250	11	27

GardenBurger

	C	F	Cb
Veggie Burgers: *Per Patty*			
Portabella	100	2.5	17
Sun-Dried Tomato Basil	100	2.5	17
The Original	100	3	18

Gorton's

	C	F	Cb
Fish Fillets:			
Battered:			
Beer Battered (2), 3.63 oz	250	18	16
Crispy Battered (2), 3.81	230	12	22
Lemon Peppered Battered (2), 2.7 oz	270	18	20

Gorton's (Cont)

	C	F	Cb
Fish Fillets:			
Breaded: Classic Crunchy Golden (2)	240	12	23
Crunchy Tilapia (2), 3.8 oz	250	12	23
Garlic & Herb (2)	230	12	22
Lemon Herb (2)	240	13	21
Potato Crunch (2)	240	14	20
Grilled: Garlic Lemon Butter (1)	100	3	1
Salmon (1), 3.15 oz	100	3	2
Tilapia (1), 3.15 oz	80	2.5	1
Shrimp:			
Butterfly (5)	250	11	27
Shrimp Scampi, 4 oz	120	6	8
Grilled: Classic, 4 oz	110	1.5	5
Shrimp Scampi, 4oz	130	4.5	3

Healthy Choice

	C	F	Cb
All Natural Entrees:			
Portabella Spinach Parmesan, 9.4 oz	270	7	40
Ravioli: Lobster Cheese, 9 oz	250	6	37
Pumpkin Squash, 9.2 oz	300	6	52
Sweet Asian Potstickers, 10 oz	380	4.5	75
Tortellini Primavera Parmesan, 9 oz	220	4.5	35
Asian/Cafe/Mediterranean Steamers:			
5-Spice Veef & Vegetables, 10.2 oz	290	4.5	48
Chicken Margherita, 10 oz	320	7	45
Chicken Pad Thai, 10 oz	270	3.5	40
Chicken Pesto Classico, 10.6 oz	320	9	39
Grilled Whiskey Steak	250	4	34
Lemon Garlic Chicken & Shrimp, 10 oz	260	6	35
Complete Meals:			
Beef Pot Roast, 11 oz	260	5	40
Chicken Parmigiana, 11½ oz	340	9	49
Homestyle Salisbury Steak, 12.5 oz	290	6	42
Lemon Pepper Fish	310	4.5	53
Sweet & Sour Chicken	400	10	61
Select Entrees:			
Bacon & Smokey Cheddar Chicken	260	6	32
Ravioli Florentine, 8.5 oz	240	4	38
Spicy Caribbean Chicken, 8.5 oz	310	2	56

Hot Pockets

	C	F	Cb
Calzones: *Per ½ Calzone, 4.2 oz*			
4 Meat & 4 Cheese	290	12	33
Pepperoni & 3 Cheese	330	16	34
Supreme	280	12	33

Hot Pockets (Cont'l)

	L	F	Cb
Mexican Style: *Per Sandwich*			
Beef Taco	290	12	34
Three Cheese & Chicken Quesadilla	280	11	34
Paninis: *Per ½ Panini*			
Bruschetta Chicken	220	7	28
Deli Style Ham & Swiss	220	8	26
Steak & Cheddar	220	8	25
Pizzeria: Four Cheese Pizza	330	13	39
Sausage & Pepperoni Pizza	340	16	39
SideShots, Cheeseburger, Mini, (2)	300	10	40
Soft Baked Subs: *Per Sub*			
Ham & Three Cheese	260	9	34
Meatballs & Mozzarella	330	16	34
Philly Steak & Cheese	310	13	33
Spicy Pepperoni Pizza	360	18	34
Stuffed Sandwiches: *Per 4 oz Sandwich*			
Barbecue Recipe Beef	340	14	44
Cheeseburger	310	12	38
Meatballs & Mozzarella	340	16	36
Philly Steak & Cheese	310	13	37

Hungry-Man

Hungry-Man Dinners:			
Boneless Fried Chkn	860	39	85
Boneless Pork Rib	840	36	105
Buffalo Chicken Strips	860	50	57
Classic Fried Chicken	1050	65	62
Meatloaf	690	29	74
Mexican Style Fiesta	590	22	87
Roasted Carved Turkey	570	18	80
Rotisserie Chicken	460	36	31
Salisbury Steak	580	31	50
Hungry-Man XXL Dinners: *Per ½ Package*			
Backyard BBQ, 12 oz	570	28	52
Carved Turkey Breast	430	18	47
Gr. Beef Steak Strips	620	14	94
Meatloaf	690	27	86
Roasted Carved Turkey Dinner	1360	70	114
Southern Fried Boneless Chicken	500	26	44
XXL Sandwiches: *Per 8 oz Sandwich*			
Angus Beef Charbroil	700	41	55
Buffalo Fried Chicken	660	27	70
BBQ Pork Ribs	750	45	60
Country Fried Pork	660	33	70
Chili Cheese Dogs	300	15	31
Crispy Fried Chicken	670	30	68

José Olé

	C	F	Cb
Breakfast Burrito			
Egg & Bacon, 4 oz	250	9	32
Egg & Ham, 4 oz	250	8	34
Egg & Sausage, 4 oz	270	10	34
Burrito: Steak & Cheese (1)	310	10	40
Chicken Monterey (1)	270	7	41
Chimichangas:			
Premium: Chicken & Cheese (1), 5 oz	330	11	45
Steak & Cheese (1), 5 oz	350	14	41
Snacks:			
Chimichangas, Steak & Ched. Mini (3)	370	20	37
Quesadillas: Grilled Chkn & 3 Cheese (1)	270	9	31
Grilled Steak & 3 Cheese (1)	260	9	32
Tacos, Beef & Cheese Mini, (4)	230	12	23
Taquitos: Chicken, Corn Tortillas, (3)	200	8	26
Steak & Cheese, Flour Tortillas, (2)	250	12	26

Kid Cuisine

All American Fried Chicken	470	20	48
All Star Chicken Breast Nuggets	400	15	51
Cheese Blaster Mac & Cheese Meal	410	9	69
Magical Cheese Stuffed Crust Pizza	410	10	63
Popstar Popcorn Chicken	420	13	62
Twist & Twirl Spaghetti with Meatballs	430	13	61

Kroger

Meals Made Simple			
Chicken Alfredo, 1¾ cups, 7.4 oz	410	16	47
Chicken Florentine, 2¼ cups, 6.9 oz	330	19	25
Shrimp Fried Rice, 1¼ cups, 8 oz	190	0.5	36
Shrimp Linguini, 1⅓ cups, 8 oz	340	8	51
Oven Ready			
Breaded Calamari Rings (13), 3 oz	230	14	18
Coconut Shrimp with Dipping Sauce	310	18	24
Shrimp Scampi, 1 cup, 4 oz	80	2.5	2
Pot Pies: Beef, (1), 7 oz	450	27	36
Chicken (1), 7 oz	380	22	36
Turkey (1), 7 oz	370	20	38

Lean Cuisine

Cafe Cuisine: *Per Complete Meal*			
Beef & Broccoli	260	5	39
Beef Chow Fun	320	5	54
Beef Portabello	220	6	25
Chicken with Almonds	250	4	38
Sun Dried Tomato Pesto Chicken	290	9	34
Thai Style Chicken	220	4	28

Lean Cuisine (Cont) | C | F | Cb

Comfort Cuisine: *Per Complete Meal*

	C	F	Cb
Baked Chicken	240	5	32
Beef Pot Roast	210	6	26
Roasted Turkey & Vegetables	150	5	12

Dinnertime Selects:

	C	F	Cb
Chicken Fettuccini	400	8	48
Lemon Garlic Shrimp	350	7	54
Salisbury Steak	270	8	27

Market Creations:

	C	F	Cb
Asiago Cheese Tortellini	270	7	39
Chicken Margherita	300	8	37
Shanghai Style Shrimp	250	3	41
Sweet & Spicy Ginger Chicken	280	2	43

Simple Favorites:

	C	F	Cb
Asian Style Pot Stickers	260	4	47
Cheese Ravioli	220	5	33
Macaroni and Cheese	290	7	41

Spa Cuisine:

	C	F	Cb
Butternut Squash Ravioli	280	7	43
Lemongrass Chicken	260	6	33
Salmon with Basil	220	6	26

Pizzas ~ *See Page 136*

Lean Pockets *Per Single Pocket*

	C	F	Cb
Original: Cheeseburger	290	8	41
Meatballs & Mozzarella	290	9	40
Philly Steak & Cheese	270	8	39
Culinary Creations, av., 1 piece	260	7	39
Mexican Style, average all flavors	250	7	35
Pizzeria: Four Cheese	280	6	41
Sausage; Pepperoni	280	8	40
Quesadillas: Average	360	9	48
Breakfast	240	7	33
Whole Grain: Chicken Brocc. & Chedd.	250	6	39
Garlic Chicken White Pizza	260	8	38
Grilled Chicken Mushroom & Spinach	250	6	37
Ham & Cheddar	270	8	39
Meatball & Mozzarella	240	7	22
Supreme Pizza	220	6	33
Turkey, Broccoli & Cheese	260	8	38
Soft Baked Subs, average	250	7	36

Macaroni Grill

Restaurant Favorites: *As Prepared*

	C	F	Cb
Basil Parmesan Chicken, 1½ cups	480	21	44
Chicken Alfredo/Marsala, av, 1 cup	320	12	29
Creamy Basil Parm. Chicken, 1 cup	300	11	26
Garlic Herb & Chkn Penne, 1 cup	240	7	22
Italian Sausage Pomodora, 1½ cups	460	21	48

Marie Callender's | C | F | Cb

Complete Dinners: *Per Meal*

	C	F	Cb
Country Fried Chicken & Gravy	560	26	61
Golden Battered Fish Fillet	410	12	60
Grilled Chicken Breast	400	17	32
Honey Roasted Chicken	340	12	37
Honey Roasted Turkey	320	10	31
Meatloaf & Gravy with Potatoes	450	18	41
Old Fashioned Beef Pot Roast	260	6	31
Salisbury Steak & Gravy	370	15	35
Spaghetti with Meat Sauce	490	14	67
Swedish Meatballs	540	28	48

Pasta Al Dente:

	C	F	Cb
Cavatappi Genovese, 11 oz	400	16	40
Fettuccine Chicken Balsamic, 10.5 oz	440	18	46
Penne Chicken Piccata, 10 oz	360	14	35
Rigatoni: Con Pesce, 10.5 oz	340	12	44
Marinara Classico, 10.5 oz	460	24	41
Tortellini Romano, 10 oz	430	14	59
Pot Pies: Chicken	640	38	56
Grilled Chicken Alfredo	680	39	58
Savory Herb Turkey, 10 oz	660	36	64

Michael Angelo's *Per Single Serve Package*

	C	F	Cb
Baked Ziti & Meatballs, 12 oz	480	15	60
Chicken Alfredo, 12 oz	470	14	57
Chicken Cacciatore, 10 oz	260	8	26
Chicken w/ Creamy Garlic, 10 oz	310	9	31
Chicken Piccata, 10 oz	510	24	52
Chicken Toscana, 12 oz	490	15	58
Eggplant & Chkn, 12 oz	360	16	28
Eggplant Parmesan, 12 oz	480	28	16
Four Cheese Lasagna, 12 oz	600	33	42
Lasagna with Meat Sauce, 12 oz	450	16	45
Manicotti with Sauce, 12 oz	460	24	22
Shrimp Scampi, 10 oz	570	30	53
Vegetable Lasagna, 12 oz	345	11	35

Morningstar Farms

Burgers: *Made with Organic Soy*

	C	F	Cb
Mushroom Lovers (1)	110	6	8
Spicy Black Bean (1)	120	4	13
Grillers: Original Veggie Burger (1)	130	6	5
Prime Veggie Burger (1)	170	9	4
Vegan Burger (1)	100	2.5	7

Morningstar (Cont) | C | F | Cb

	C	F	Cb
Chik'n: Buffalo Wings (5)	200	8	20
Chik'n Nuggets (4)	190	9	19
Patties: Breakfast Pattie (1)	80	3	4
Chik Patties, Original (1)	140	5	16
Garden Veggie Pattie (1)	110	3.5	9
Italian Herb Chik Pattie (1)	170	5	22

Safeway Select

	C	F	Cb
Beef Salisbury Steak, 9.35 oz	400	25	23
Bow Tie Pasta Pepperoni, 9.5 oz	340	14	36
Chicken Parmesan, 9.25 oz	350	11	48
Classic Lasagna, 11 oz	280	9	35
Fettucini Alfredo, 11.5 oz	480	15	75
Five Vegetable Lasagna, 10.6 oz	330	7	58
Orange Chicken, 9 oz	450	15	64
Pasta Primavera, 9 oz	300	11	41
Penne Pasta, 8 oz	340	12	53
Pot Roast, 9 oz	280	14	26
Spaghetti with Meat Sauce, 12 oz	450	16	61
Swedish Meat Balls, 11.5 oz	470	24	43
Triple Rich Macaroni & Cheese, 7.95 oz	360	18	37

Stouffer's

	C	F	Cb
Corner Bistro: *Per Single Serve Packet*			
Flatbread Melts:			
Chicken Quesadilla, 6 oz	370	15	41
Steak, Mushroom & Cheddar	390	17	40
Stromboli: Italian-Style Supreme	430	19	45
Pepperoni & Provolone, 6 oz	430	17	45
Toasted Subs: Meatball Italiano, / oz	400	18	42
Philly-Style Steak & Cheese, 6 oz	370	16	39
Craveable Classics: *Per Serving*			
Creamed Chipped Beef, 4.4 oz	140	7	11
Macaroni & Cheese, 8 oz	340	16	36
Easy Express Skillets: *Per Serving*			
Broccoli & Beef, 12.5 oz	350	6	57
Chicken & Pasta Parmesan, 12.5 oz	480	15	60
Teriyaki Chicken, 12.5 oz	310	4.5	44
Yankee Pot Roast, 12 oz	300	8	39
Homestyle Classics: *Per Single Serve Packet*			
Beef Pot Roast	240	8	27
Fish Fillet	400	16	36
Meatloaf	340	19	20
Roast Turkey Breast	290	12	30
Homestyle Recipe: *Per Package*			
Chicken Pot Pie	660	37	62
Turkey Pot Pie	710	41	61
Homestyle Selects: *Per Serving*			
Five Cheese Lasagna, 9 oz	330	14	33
Meatloaf, 8 oz	600	31	45
Salisbury Steak, 8 oz	710	39	48

Stouffer's (Cont) | C | F | Cb

	C	F	Cb
Restaurant Classics: *Per Package*			
Cheese Ravioli	380	13	47
Chicken Parmigiana	410	14	47
Green Pepper Steak	240	4	32
Veal Parmigiana	460	22	46
Restaurant Selects: *Per Package*			
Bourbon Steak Tips	490	17	61
Chicken Fettuccini Alfredo	840	38	94
Monterey Chicken	530	21	54
Sesame Chicken	590	16	87
Shrimp Scampi	400	12	56

Swanson

	C	F	Cb
Classics: *Per Complete Meal*			
Breaded Fish Fillet, 7.3 oz	370	14	45
Boneless Fried Chicken, 7.5 oz	240	13	21
Fried Chicken Strips 6¾ oz	290	14	28
Macaroni & Cheese, 10.25oz	450	17	61
Meatloaf, 9.5 oz	230	9	22
Mexican Style Fiesta	380	15	51
Roasted Carved Turkey	250	11	29
Salisbury Steak, 9.5 oz	230	12	19
Pot Pies: Beef (1), 7 oz	390	24	33
Chicken/Turkey (1), 7 oz	380	22	34

TGI Friday's

	C	F	Cb
Beer Battered Onion Rings (3)	180	8	26
Buffalo Wings (3)	180	11	4
Chicken Quesadilla (3)	260	11	28
Honey BBQ Wings (3)	150	9	6
Mozzarella Sticks & Sauce, 1 oz	80	4.5	7
Popcorn Chicken, 3 pieces, 2.6 oz	250	8	29
Potato Skins, Cheddar & Bacon, 3 pieces	210	12	17

Trader Joe's

	C	F	Cb
Meals: *Per Serving*			
Asian Style Chkn Stir Fry w/ Sauce, 8 oz	190	1	30
Chicken Chow Mein, ⅓ package, 6.35 oz	210	2	35
Chicken Fried Rice, 1 cup, 5 oz	200	3.5	33
Chicken Quesadilla (1), 6 oz	320	16	26
Citrus Glazed Chicken with rice, 8 oz	270	5	40
Macaroni & Cheese, 1 cup, 6.98 oz	360	15	42
Rice Bowls, average, 11 oz bowl	390	3.5	55
Shrimp Stir Fry, 8 oz	220	1	29
Sweet & Sour Shrimp with Rice, ⅓ pkg	190	0	39
Turkey Sausage Stromboli, ¼ loaf, 4.5 oz	250	7	31
Pies: Chicken Pot Pie, ½ Pie, 8 oz	360	22	28
Spinach Pie, ¼ pie, 6 oz	240	4	37

Tyson

	C	F	Cb
Any'tizers:			
Buffalo Style: Chicken Wyngs, 3 pieces	150	7	8
Hot Wings (Bagged), 3 pieces	230	15	1
Stuffed Chicken Peperoni Minis (3)	200	11	10
Stuffed Chicken Cordon Bleu Minis (3)	180	10	9
Popcorn Chicken (Boxed), 6 pieces	220	10	19
Popcorn Chicken Bites (Bag), 7 pces	180	9	11
Fully Cooked Chicken: *Per Serving*			
Buffalo Style Chicken Strips (2)	230	10	21
Fajita Chicken Strips, 3 oz	110	4	1
Grilled Chicken Breast Strips, 3 oz	100	2	1
Honey BBQ Chicken Strips (1)	180	8	18
Southwestern Style Chkn Brst Strips	120	3	3
100% All Natural Breaded Chicken			
Breast: Fillets (1), 4.5 oz	240	9	20
Patties (1), 2.57 oz	180	11	12
Southern Style Tenderloins (1)	150	7	9
Tenders (5)	240	14	15
Crispy Strips (2)	200	10	13
Nuggets (5), 3.2 oz	270	17	15
Skillet Creations: *Per Serving*			
Asian Style Orange Chicken, ½ package	340	5	50
Chicken Tuscany & Penne, ½ package	320	6	44
Grilled Chicken Fajitas (2)	250	7	32

Van De Kamp's

	C	F	Cb
Crispy Battered Halibut (3), 4 oz	280	13	24
Crunchy Fish Sticks (6), 4 oz	240	11	22
Fish Shaped Nuggets (4), 4.25 oz	280	13	25
Fried: Beer Battered Fillets (2)	240	13	18
Breaded: Butterfly Shrimp, 7 pieces	330	16	31
Popcorn Fish, 8 pieces, 4.13 oz	270	13	25

Weight Watchers

	C	F	Cb
Smart Ones			
Anytime Selection:: *Per Meal*			
Calzone Italiano, 10 oz	290	6	47
Chicken & Cheese Quesadilla, 8 oz	220	7	26
Entrees: *Per Meal*			
Angel Hair Marinara	230	4	40
Broccoli & Cheddar Roasted Potato	240	7	35
Chicken Carbonara	250	4.5	32
Chicken Enchiladas Suiza	290	5	49
Chicken Fettuccini	340	6	47
Chicken Parmesan	290	5	35
Cranberry Turkey Medallions	250	2	43
Honey Mango BBQ Chicken	240	3.5	34
Lasagna Bake with Meat Sauce	270	4	43

Weight Watchers (Cont)

	C	F	Cb
Entrees cont: *Per Meal*			
Lemon Herb Chicken Piccata	230	1.5	41
Macaroni & Cheese	270	2	52
Meatloaf with Mashed Potatoes	250	8	23
Orange Sesame Chicken	320	8	48
Pasta Primavera	280	6	44
Picate Chicken & Pasta	260	4	32
Pineapple Beef Teriyaki	260	4.5	38
Roasted Chicken with Potato	180	4	20
Roast Turkey Medallions	220	1.5	38
Salisbury Steak, 9.5 oz	280	3.5	33
Shrimp Marinara	180	1.5	31
Sirloin Beef Asian Vegetables	220	1.5	27
Spaghetti with Meat Sauce	310	6	48
Spicy Szechuan Style Vege. & Chicken	240	5	36
Stuffed Turkey Breast	290	6	42
Swedish Meatballs	270	5	35
Sweet & Sour Chicken	210	2	31
Teriyaki Chicken & Vegetables	230	2.5	39
Thai Style Chicken & Rice Noodles	26	4	43
Three Cheese Mcaroni	300	6	48
Traditional Lasagna with Meat Sauce	300	6	43
Tuna Noodle Gratin	240	4.5	37
Morning Express: *Per Meal*			
Breakfast Quesadilla	220	6	28
Canadian Style Bacon English Muffin	210	6	27
English Muffin Sandwich	210	5	27
Stuffed Breakfast Sandwich	240	7	28

Worthington/Loma Linda

	C	F	Cb
Chic-ketts, 2 slices	110	5	3
Dinner Roast, ¾" slice	180	11	6
Fried Chik'n with Gravy, 2 pieces	150	10	5
FriPats, 1 pattie, 2¼ oz	130	6	5
Leanies, 1 link, 1.4 oz	100	7	2
Meatless: Chicken Style Roll, ⅜" slice	90	4.5	2
Smoked Turkey Roll, ⅜" slice	130	8	4
Prosage Links (2), 1.6 oz	80	3	3
Stakelets, 2.5 oz piece	150	7	7
Stripples, 2 slices	60	4.5	2
Swiss Stake, 1 piece	130	6	9

Zatarains

Per 12oz Package Unless Indicated

	C	F	Cb
Blackened Chicken Alfredo, 10.5 oz	500	25	46
Jambalaya seasoned with Chicken	400	5	69
Jambalaya seasoned with Sausage	480	14	77
Red Beans & Rice with Sausage	510	20	68

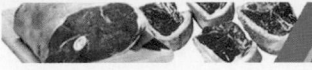

Note: Cooking reduces weight of meat by 20-45% due to water and fat losses. Average weight loss is 30%. Actual loss depends on cooking method and cooking time. Examples:

4 oz raw weight = approx. 3 oz cooked weight
4 oz cooked weight = approx. 5½ oz raw weight

What 3 oz Cooked Meat Looks Like

• Half the size of this book (4¼" x 3" x ³⁄₈" thick)
• Rectangular piece (4" x 2½" x ½" thick)
• Deck of cards (3½" x 2½" x ⁵⁄₈" thick)

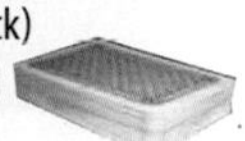

STEAK QUICK GUIDE

Sirloin (Choice Grade)
External fat trimmed to ¼"
Broiled, Edible Portion (no bone)

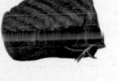

C F Cb

Small/Regular Serving, 3 oz (cooked)
(from 4-4½ oz raw)

	C	F	Cb
Lean + external fat (¼"), 3 oz	225	13	0
Lean + marbling, 3 oz	195	10	0
Lean only, 3 oz	160	6	0
(No external fat or marbling)			

Medium Serving, 5 oz (cooked wt)
(from approximately 7 oz raw)

Lean + external fat (¼"), 5 oz	350	21	0
Lean + marbling, 5 oz	325	17	0
Lean only, 5 oz	265	10	0

Large Serving, 8 oz (cooked wt)
(from 11-12 oz raw)

Lean + external fat, 8 oz	600	36	0
Lean + marbling, 8 oz	520	27	0
Lean only, 8 oz	425	15	0

Extra Large Serving, 12 oz (cooked wt)
(from approximately 16-17 oz raw)

Lean + external fat (¼"), 12 oz	900	52	0
Lean + marbling, 12 oz	740	40	0
Lean only, 12 oz	640	23	0

Pan Fried
Sirloin (choice), medium serving:

Lean + external fat (¼"), 5 oz	460	33	0
Lean only, 5 oz	340	16	0

Other Steaks   C F Cb

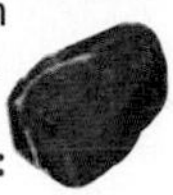

Filet Mignon (Tenderloin):
1 Medium steak (6 oz raw weight)
Broiled, with ¼" fat trim

	C	F	Cb
Lean + fat (¼"), 4 oz	360	27	0
Lean only, 3½ oz	230	12	0

New York/Club Steak:
Top Loin/Short Loin
1 steak, regular (9¼ oz raw, ¼" fat)

Broiled: Lean + fat (¼"), 6¼ oz	580	43	0
Lean + marbling, 5½ oz	400	25	0
Lean only, 5¼ oz	360	20	0

Porterhouse Steak:
1 Medium, 6 oz raw weight (no bone), broiled

Lean + fat (¼"), 4¼ oz	410	33	0
Lean only, 3½ oz	210	11	0

1 Large ,12 oz raw weight (no bone), broiled

Lean + fat (¼") 8½ oz cooked	820	66	0
Lean only, 7 oz cooked	420	22	0

T-Bone Steak: *Broiled or Grilled*
Medium Size: *8 oz raw weight*
(Approximately 6 oz cooked)

Lean + Fat (¼"), 5 oz (no bone)	400	28	0
Lean only, 4 oz (no bone)	265	12	0

Large Size: *12 oz raw weight*
(Approximately 9 oz cooked)

Lean + fat (¼"), 7 oz (no bone)	560	39	0
Lean only, 6 oz (no bone)	400	18	0

Extra Large Size: *20 oz raw weight*
(Approximately 16 oz cooked)

Lean + Fat (¼"), 12 oz (no bone)	960	66	0
Lean Only, 10 oz (no bone)	660	30	0

Also See Fast-Foods & Restaurants Section ~
Lone Star Steakhouse
Outback Steakhouse

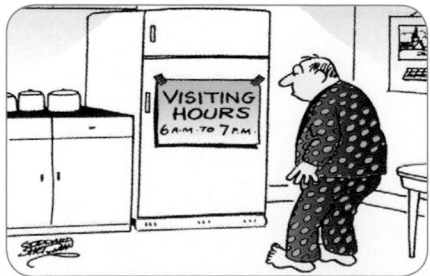

VISITING HOURS 6 A.M. TO 7 P.M.

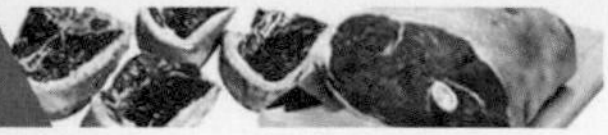

Beef – Individual Cuts

	C	F	Cb
Average All Grades			
Edible Weight (no bone)			
Brisket, whole, braised:			
Lean + fat (¼" trim), 3 oz	330	27	0
Lean + marbling, 3 oz	250	17	0
Lean only, 3 oz	185	9	0
Chuck blade, braised:			
Lean + fat (¼"), 3 oz	310	24	0
Lean + marbling, 3 oz	295	22	0
Lean only, 3 oz	245	13	0
Flank: Raw, 4 oz	175	8	0
Braised, 3 oz	225	14	0
Broiled, 3 oz	155	6	0
Round, bottom, braised:			
Lean + marbling, 3 oz	190	7.5	0
Lean only, 3 oz	185	6.5	0
Round, eye/tip, roasted:			
Lean + fat (¼"), 3 oz	205	11	0
Lean (with marbling), 3 oz	150	5	0
Round, top: Per 3 oz (cooked wt)			
Braised, Lean + fat	210	10	0
Lean only	170	4	0
Broiled, Lean + fat	180	8	0
Lean only	160	5	0
Pan-fried, Lean + fat	235	13	0
Lean only	195	7	0

Beef Ribs

	C	F	Cb
Back Ribs (7" long, visible fat trimmed to ¼")			
10.3 oz raw (with bone) or 3½ oz cooked (braised, no bone)			
1 average rib	410	34	0
3 ribs	1230	102	0
Short Ribs (2½" long, visible fat trimmed to ¼")			
6 oz raw (with bone) or 2½ oz cooked (braised, no bone)			
1 average rib	320	28	0
3 ribs	960	85	0

Ground Beef

	C	F	Cb
Ground Beef, Raw: Per 4 oz			
70% lean (30% fat)	380	34	0
75% lean (25% fat)	335	29	0
80% lean (20% fat)	290	23	0
85% lean (15% fat)	245	17	0
90% lean (10% fat)	200	12	0
95% lean (5% fat)	155	6	0
Baked/Broiled: Reg. (70%), 3 oz	230	16	0
Lean (80%), 3 oz	215	14	0
Extra lean (90%), 3 oz	185	10	0
Pan-Broiled: Reg. (70%), 3 oz	230	15	0
Lean (80%), 3 oz	210	14	0
Extra lean (90%), 3 oz	195	10	0
Ground Beef Patties: Average (23% Fat)			
Raw, 4 oz	330	25	0
Broiled, 3 oz (from 4 oz raw)	250	19	0

Quick Guide

	C	F	Cb
Roast Beef (Roasted)			
Round (Eye/Tip, average) Average All Cuts			
Small/Regular Serving, 3 oz			
(2 thin slices/1 thick slice)			
Lean + fat (¼")	200	11	0
Lean only	150	5	0
Medium Serving, 5 oz			
(3-4 thin slices)			
Lean + fat	330	19	0
Lean only	245	9	0
Large Serving, 8 oz (3 thick slices)			
Lean + fat	525	30	0
Lean only	390	14	0

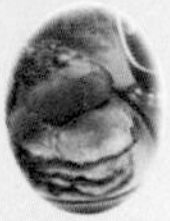

Roast Dinner Extras

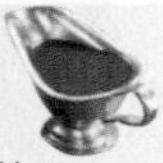

	C	F	Cb
Gravy: Thin, 2 Tbsp	20	0.5	3.5
Thick, 2 Tbsp	50	2	0.5
1 Ladle/4 Tbsp	100	4	1
Veggies: Beans, green, ½ cup	20	0	5
Cauliflower with cheese sauce, 4 oz	135	9	15
Corn, kernels, ¼ cup	35	0	9
Carrots, ¼ cup	20	0	3
Peas, ¼ cup	35	0	6
Potato: Roasted with fat, 1 small	155	8	30
Baked in Jacket, 1 large	280	0	63
with 1 Tbsp whipped butter	350	8	63
with Sour Cream, 2 Tbsp	270	5	64
Sweet Potato/Yam, 1 medium	105	1	24

	C	F	Cb
Beef Kebob (Cooked):			
Beef & Veggies, 2 oz	160	10	4
If very lean meat	100	4	4

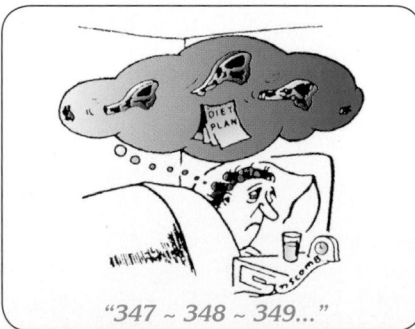

"347 ~ 348 ~ 349..."

Updated Nutrition Data ~ www.CalorieKing.com
Persons with Diabetes ~ See Disclaimer (Page 22)

Lamb

	C	F	Cb
Choice Grade			
Leg (Whole), roasted:			
Lean + fat, 3 oz	220	14	0
Lean only, 3 oz	160	7	0
Leg (Sirloin Half), roasted:			
Lean + fat, 3 oz	250	18	0
Lean only, 3 oz	175	8	0
Leg (Shank Half), roasted:			
Lean + fat, 3 oz	190	11	0
Lean only, 3 oz	155	6	0
Loin Chop, broiled:			
1 chop (raw weight, 4¼ oz):	250	17	0
Lean + fat (2¼ oz edible)	180	12	0
Lean only (1.6 oz edible)	85	3.5	0
Rib Chop, broiled/roasted:			
1 chop (raw wt., 3½ oz)			
Lean + fat (2½ oz edible)	255	21	0
Lean only (1¾ oz edible)	105	6	0
Shoulder (Arm/Blade):			
Braised: Lean + fat, 3 oz	295	21	0
Lean only, 3 oz	240	12	0
Broiled: Lean + fat, 3 oz	240	17	0
Lean only, 3 oz	170	8	0
Roasted: Similar to Broiled			
Cubed Lamb (Leg/Shoulder):			
For stew or kabob			
Braised, lean only, 3 oz	190	8	0
Broiled, lean only, 3 oz	160	6	0

Veal

	C	F	Cb
Edible Weights			
Leg (Top Round):			
Braised: Lean + fat, 3 oz	180	6	0
Lean only, 3 oz	175	5	0
Pan-fried, breaded:			
Lean + fat, 3 oz	195	8	9
Lean only, 3 oz	185	6	9
Pan-fried, not breaded:			
Lean + fat, 3 oz	180	7	0
Lean only, 3 oz	155	4	0
Roasted: Lean + fat, 3 oz	135	4	0
Lean only, 3 oz	130	3	0

Veal (Cont)

	C	F	Cb
Loin Chop: 1 chop, (7 oz raw weight)			
Braised: Lean + fat, 3 oz	240	15	0
Lean only, 3 oz	190	8	0
Roasted: Lean + fat, 3 oz	185	11	0
Lean only, 3 oz	150	6	0
Rib, roasted: Lean + fat, 3 oz	195	12	0
Lean only, 3 oz	150	7	0
Shoulder, Arm/Blade, roasted:			
Lean + fat, 3 oz	155	7	0
Lean only, 3 oz	140	5	0
Sirloin, roasted:			
Lean + fat, 3 oz	170	9	0
Lean only, 3 oz	145	6	0
Cubed for Stew, braised:			
Leg/Shoulder, lean only, 3 oz	160	4	0
(1 lb raw yields approx. 9¼ oz cooked)			

Pork

	C	F	Cb
Fresh Pork (Cooked Weight, no bone)			
(4 oz raw weight = approx. 3 oz cooked weight)			
Blade Steak, broiled:			
Lean + fat, 3 oz	220	15	0
Lean only, 3 oz	190	11	0
Country Style Ribs, broiled/roasted:			
Lean + fat, 3 oz	280	22	0
Lean only, 3 oz	210	13	0
Spareribs, braised: lean & fat, 6 oz			
(from 1 lb raw weight)	675	52	0
Leg (Ham), whole, roasted:			
Lean + fat, 3 oz	230	15	0
Lean only, 3 oz	180	8	0
(Ham, cured ~ See Cold Meats)			
Loin Chops, broiled: Average			
(From 1 chop: 5 oz raw weight with bone			
or 4 oz raw weight, without bone)			
Lean + fat, 3 oz	200	11	0
Lean only, 3 oz	165	7	0
Loin Roast, roasted:			
Lean + fat, 3 oz	210	13	0
Lean only, 3 oz	180	8	0
Rib Chops, (Boneless), broiled:			
Lean + fat, 3 oz	220	14	0
Lean only, 3 oz	185	9	0
Rib Roast, roasted:			
Lean + fat, 3 oz	215	13	0
Lean only, 3 oz	180	9	0

Pork (Cont)

	C	F	Cb
Sirloin Chop, broiled:			
Lean + fat, 3 oz	180	8	0
Lean only, 3 oz	165	6	0
Sirloin Roast, roasted:			
Lean + fat, 3 oz	175	8	0
Lean only, 3 oz	170	7	0
Tenderloin (Boneless), roasted:			
Lean + fat, 3 oz	125	4	0
Lean only, 3 oz	120	3	0
Ground Pork			
Raw: Average, ¼ lb, 4 oz	300	24	0
Broiled, 3 oz	250	18	0
Pan-fried, drained, 3 oz	260	19	0

Bacon

	C	F	Cb
Raw: 1 medium slice (20 lb), ¾ oz	95	9	0
1 thick slice (12 lb), 1⅓ oz	175	17	0
(1 lb raw yields approximately 5 oz cooked)			
Broiled/Pan-Fried:			
1 medium slice., 0.3 oz	40	3	0
3 medium slices, 0.8	125	10	0
2 thin slices, ½ oz	75	6	0
1 thick slice, 0.85 oz	65	5	0
Canadian Bacon: Cooked, 1 slice, 1 oz	45	2	0.5
Packaged, 3 slices, 2 oz	90	4	1
Bacon Bits, 1 Tbsp, ¼ oz	35	2	0
Breakfast Strips, Broiled, 1 sl.,, 0.42 oz	50	4	0

Ham

	C	F	Cb
Boneless Ham, cooked:			
Regular, (approximately 13% fat):			
Roasted, 3 oz	150	8	0
Extra Lean (5% fat),			
Roasted, 3 oz	125	5	0
Whole Ham, cooked:			
Lean + fat (as purchased)			
Roasted, 3 oz	210	15	0
Lean only, Roasted, 3 oz	135	5	0
Canned Ham: Similar to boneless ham			
Chopped, canned, 3 oz	200	16	0
Ham Patties, cooked, 1 pattie, 2¼ oz	220	20	1
Ham Steak, extra lean, 2 oz	70	2.5	0
Lunch Slices: See Deli Meats, Page 128			

Game & Other Meats

	C	F	Cb
Bison Steak,			
lean, 6 oz (raw)	205	4	0
Boar (wild), roasted, 3 oz	140	4	0
Buffalo Steak: New West Foods, 4 oz	70	3	0
Trader Joe's, 1 pattie	430	30	1
Caribou, roasted, 3 oz	140	4	0
Deer/Venison, roasted 3 oz	135	3	0
Goat (Capretto): Raw, 3 oz	95	2	0
Roasted, 3 oz	120	2.5	0
Ostrich: Blackwing Ostrich Meats,			
Sport Jerky, ½ oz piece	25	0	0
Sausage Patties (2) 2 oz	60	0.5	0
New West Foods:			
Ground Ostrich, 4 oz	165	7	0
Ostrich Steak, 4 oz steak	130	2.5	0
Rabbit: Roasted, 3 oz	165	7	0
Stewed, 1 cup, diced, 5 oz	290	12	0

Variety & Organ Meats

	C	F	Cb
Brain (Lamb): Braised, 3 oz	125	9	0
Pan-fried, 3 oz	230	19	0
Chitterlings, pork, simmered, 3 oz	260	25	0
Ears, pork, simmered, 1 ear, 4 oz	185	12	0
Feet, pork: Simmered, 3 oz	200	14	0
Cured, pickled, 3 oz	170	14	0
Hormel, 2 oz	80	6	0
Head Cheese (Pork Snouts/Ears/Vinegar/Spices):			
1 oz slice	50	4	0
Heart, Beef, braised, 3 oz	140	4	0
Jowl, pork, raw, 4 oz	750	80	0
Kidneys, braised, 3 oz	140	5	0
Liver (beef): Raw, 4 oz	150	4	4
Braised, 3 oz	140	4	3
Pan-fried, 3 oz	185	7	7
Pancreas, pork, braised, 3 oz	185	8	0
Pork Cracklins, 0.5 oz	80	6	0
Pork Hocks, 1 piece, 6 oz	340	23	0
Scrapple, pork, 2 oz	120	8	8
Spleen, pork, braised, 3 oz	130	3	0
Stomach, pork, raw, 4 oz	185	12	0
Sweetbreads: Beef, cooked, 3 oz	125	9	0
Lamb, cooked, 3 oz	125	9	0
Tail, pork, simmered, 3 oz	340	31	0
Tongue, braised: Veal, 3 oz	170	9	0
Beef/Lamb/Pork, average, 3 oz	235	17	0
Tripe, beef, raw, 3 oz	85	3.5	0

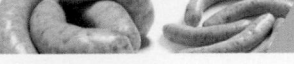

Meat ~ Sausages ◇ Franks (M)

Quick Guide

Franks & Weiners
Average All Brands

	C	F	Cb
Regular/Smoked: *Per Frank*			
Regular, 1.5oz (10/16 oz package)	140	13	1
Jumbo, 2 oz (8/16 oz package)	170	16	0
Bun Length, 2 oz	180	17	2
Extra Long, 2.75 oz	240	21	2
Small/Cocktail (50/lb) each	30	3	0.5
Beef Franks: *Per Frank*			
Regular, 1.6 oz (10/16 oz package)	140	13	2
Jumbo, 2 oz (8/16 oz package)	170	15	2
Bun Length, 2 oz	180	16	2
¼ lb Dog, 4 oz	300	24	4

Franks & Weiners

	C	F	Cb
Ball Park			
Franks & Wieners: *Per Frank*			
Angus Beef Franks	170	15	3
Cheese	180	15	4
Turkey Franks	110	7	6
GrillMaster: Deli Style Beef; Beef	250	21	3
Lite Franks, Beef	100	7	3
Foster Farms			
Chicken/Turkey Franks (1), 2 oz	140	12	1
Hebrew National			
Beef: 1.72 oz link	150	14	1
¼ Pound	360	33	3
Jumbo, 3 oz link	270	25	2
97% Fat-Free, 1.6 oz link	40	1	3
Beef Frank in a Blanket, 5 pces, 3 oz	290	23	12
Jennie-O			
Turkey Franks:			
1.2 oz link	70	5	1
Jumbo, 2 oz link	120	9	2
Oscar Mayer			
Beef, Light, 1.6 oz	90	7	2
Cheese Dogs, 1.6 oz	140	13	1
Turkey Frank: 1.6 oz	100	8	2
Bun Length, 2 oz link	120	10	3
Shelton's			
Chicken Franks, 1.2 oz link	70	6	0
Turkey Franks, 1.2 oz link	70	6	0
Zacky Farms			
Turkey Franks, 2 oz link	160	12	1

Quick Guide

Fresh Sausages
Pork/Beef: *Average All Types*

	C	F	Cb
Small: Raw, 4" link, 1 oz	85	7.5	0
Broiled/Pan-fried	80	7	0
Medium: Raw, 2 oz	170	15	0
Broiled/Pan-fried	165	14	0
Large: Raw, 3 oz	255	22	0
Broiled/Pan-fried	245	21	0
Italian: Raw, 3.2 oz	315	28	0.5
Cooked, 2.4 oz	230	18	3
Chorizo: Beef Chorizo, 2.5 oz piece	250	23	5
Pork Chorizo, 2 oz piece	250	23	5

Note: Fat is lost in broiling/pan frying.
(Cooked weight = approx. 60-70% raw weight)

Smoked Sausage

	C	F	Cb
Average All Brands: 2 oz link	170	15	0
3 oz link	255	22	0
Ball Park, Turkey, Bun Size, 1.75 oz	45	0	5
Butterball			
Turkey, 1.8 oz	100	6	4
Eckrich, Grillers, 2 oz	180	16	2
Hillshire Farm, Beef/Pork/Trky, 2 oz	190	16	3
Hardwood Smoked Chicken, 2 oz	90	5	3
Italian, 2 oz	190	16	4
Turkey, 2 oz	90	5	3

Breakfast Sausages/Patties

	C	F	Cb
Armour, Sizzle 'n Serve			
Beef Sausage, 3 links, 2 oz	230	22	1
Pork/Turkey, 3 links, 2.1 oz	210	19	2
Lite Original, 3 links, 1.8 oz	90	7	1
Butterball: Turkey Burger Pattie (1)	150	8	0
Turkey Breakfast Links (3)	130	7	0
Jennie-O			
Fully Cooked: Sausage Links, 2 oz	110	7	0
Sausage Patties, 1 oz	65	4	0
Maple Turkey Sausage (1)	140	11	3
Jimmy Dean, *Heat 'N Serve*			
Sausage Links (3)	210	19	1
Sausage Patties (2)	200	17	1
Maple Sausage Links (3)	170	14	2
Breakfast Sandwiches: *See Page 92*			
Jones *Golden Brown:*			
All Natural:			
Beef Sausage Links (3)	200	18	2
Maple Sausage (3)	240	22	2
Sausage Patties, Maple Pork (1)	130	12	1
Vegetarian Patties:			
Boca: *See Page 117*			
Garden Burger: *See Page 118*			

Bagel, Corn & Hot Dogs

Hot Dogs, Ready-To-Go

(Includes Ketchup/Relish; w/o Mayo)

	C	F	Cb
Regular (1.5 oz frank, 1.5 oz bun)	260	15	22
Bun Length (2 oz frank, 1.5 oz bun)	290	18	21
Jumbo Dog (2 oz frank, 2 oz bun)	360	20	36
¼ lb Beef Dog (¼ lb dog, 2 oz bun)	480	15	36
Mile Long Dog (2.6 oz dog, 1.5 oz bun)	360	24	23

Corn Dogs

	C	F	Cb
Beef/Pork Frank: Average, 2.6 oz	170	10	16

Foster Farms

	C	F	Cb
Chili Cheese Dog (1), 2.7 oz	200	9	24
Honey Crunchy Dog (1), 2.7 oz	180	10	15
Mini (4), 2.7 oz	210	12	18

State Fair with Ball Park Franks,

	C	F	Cb
Beef Corn Dogs (1), 2.7 oz	220	10	25
Mini Beef Corn Dogs (6)	260	15	24

Bagel Dogs

	C	F	Cb
Vienna Beef: Bageldog (1), 5 oz	420	17	33
Mini (1), 2.8 oz	150	4	20

Hot Dog Toppings/Extras:

	C	F	Cb
American Cheese, 1 slice, 1 oz	110	9	1
Chili (w. Beans), ¼ cup	70	3.5	9
Ketchup, 1 Tbsp	15	0	4
Mustard, 1 Tbsp	20	0	1
Onions, Chopped, 1 Tbsp	5	0	1
Pickle Relish, 1 Tbsp	20	0	5
Sauerkraut, ½ cup	20	0	5

Deli & Lunch Meats

Beef Jerky/Meat Snacks:

	C	F	Cb
Bridgford: Beef Jerky, 1 oz	100	0.5	5
Beef Stick (5.5 oz stick), 1 oz	150	13	2
Beef Steak, 1 oz	70	0.5	2
Beef & Cheese (Giant Size), ½ package, 1.5 oz	170	14	1
Pepperoni Sticks (2), 1 oz	160	13	2
Teriyaki, 1 oz package	80	0.5	4
Original; Hot 'n Spicy	70	1	5
Berliner (pork/beef), 1 oz	65	5	1

Beerwurst (Beef):

	C	F	Cb
Small (2.75"diam), ¹⁄₁₆" slice	20	2	0
Large (4"diam), ⅛" slice	75	7	0.5
Slim Jim: Original, 0.28 oz	40	3.5	0
Super Original, 0.64 oz	90	8	1
Monster Original, 1.94 oz	290	25	3

Deli & Lunch Meats

Beerwurst (Pork):

	C	F	Cb
Small (2.75"diameter), ¹⁄₁₆" slice	15	1	0
Large (4"diameter), ⅛" Slice	55	4	0.5
Bologna: 1 Slice, 1 oz	65	6	1
Fat-Free, 1 slice, 1 oz	20	0	2
Beef Bologna: 1 slice, 1 oz	90	8	1
Light, 1 slice, 1 oz	60	4	2
Light *(Oscar Mayer),* 1 slice, 1 oz	60	4	2
98% Fat Free *(Oscar Mayer),* 1 oz	25	0.5	3
Ring *(Boar's Head),* 2 oz	150	13	1
Turkey, average, 1 oz	60	5	0.5
Blood Sausage, 1 oz	100	9	0.5
Bratwurst: Average, 1 oz	80	7	1
Boar's Head, cooked, 1 wurst, 4 oz	300	25	0
Bob Evan's, Beer, 2.6 oz link	270	21	1
Braunschweiger (Pork/Liver/Sausage),			
Oscar Mayer, 1 oz slice	110	10	1
Chicken, *Average All Brands*			
1 thick or 2 thin slices, 1 oz	30	1	1
Hillshire Farm, Rstd/Smkd, av.,2 oz	60	1	2
Corned Beef: Average, full fat, 1 oz	60	5	0.5
Hillshire Farm, 2 oz	60	1	0.5

Ham, Sliced:

	C	F	Cb
Baked/Boiled, sliced, 1 oz	30	1	0.5
Chopped, *Eckrich* (97% FF), 1 oz	25	1	1
Armour: Canned, 1 oz	35	1.5	0.5
97% Fat Free, 1 oz	25	1	1.5
Oscar Mayer, 1 oz slice	60	2	0.5
Honey/Brown Sugar, Average, 1 oz	30	1	1
Prosciutto, average, 1 oz	70	5	0
Ham & Cheese Loaf, average, 1 oz	70	5	1
Italian Sausage, 2.6 oz	250	20	3
Kielbasa (Polish Sausage), 2 oz	65	5	1
Beef, 2 oz link	190	17	1
Boar's Head, 1 oz	60	5	0
Hillshire Farm, 2.68 oz	250	22	4
Knockwurst, 1 oz	90	8	0.5
Linguica *(Gaspar's),* 2 oz	180	8	1
Liverwurst, 1 oz	65	5	2
Liver Pate, fresh, average, 1 oz	90	8	1
Luncheon Loaf *(Foods Co),* 1 oz	65	5	2
Mortadella, 1 oz	105	9	0
Olive Loaf: Average, 1 oz	70	5	3
Oscar Mayer, 1 oz	75	6	2
Pancetta, (Boars Head), 1 slice	50	4.5	0

Updated Nutrition Data ~ www.CalorieKing.com
Persons with Diabetes ~ See Disclaimer (Page 22)

Deli & Lunch Meats (Cont)

	C	F	Cb
Pastrami (Beef):			
Healthy Deli, 2 oz	70	2	1
Hillshire (DeliSelect), 6 slice, 2 oz	60	1	0
Boar's Head, Round, 2 oz	80	3.5	1
Peppered Beef, 1 oz slice	40	2	1
Pepperoni, 5 slices, 1 oz	140	13	0
Pickle Loaf, av., 1 oz	70	5	5
Pickle & Pimento Loaf			
Oscar Mayer, 1 oz	75	6	3
Proscuitto/Proscuitti: Average, 1 oz	70	5	1
Hormel, 1 oz	90	7	1
Roast Beef: Lean, 1 oz	40	2	0
Healthy Choice, all types, 2 oz	60	1.5	1
Salami: Beef, average, 1 oz	80	7	1
Beer Salami, average, 1 oz	50	4	0.5
Cotto: Oscar Mayer, 1 slice, 1 oz	70	6	1
Dry: Hard, average, 4 slices, 1 oz	110	10	3
Oscar Mayer, 2 slices, 1.6 oz	100	8	1
Genoa: Average, 1 oz	120	9	1
Stick (Best's Kosher), 2, 1.75 oz	180	15	2
Italian (Bridgeford), 1 oz	120	11	0
Turkey, average, 1 oz	55	4	1
SPAM (Hormel): Per 2 oz Serving			
Classic: 2 oz serving	180	16	2
7 oz can	630	56	3
12 oz can	1030	96	6
Spam Lite: 2 oz	110	8	1
12 oz can	660	48	6
Other Spam Products:			
Hickory Smoked, 2 oz	170	15	2
Hot & Spicy, 2 oz	180	16	2
Oven Roastd Turkey, 2 oz	80	4	2
Spam with Bacon, 2 oz	180	16	1
Spam with Cheese, 2 oz	170	15	2
Spam Spread, 2 oz	140	12	1
25% Less Sodium	180	16	1
Spam Singles:			
Classic, 3 oz package	250	22	2
Lite, 3 oz package	160	11	2
Summer Sausage:			
Bridgford, 1 oz	100	9	1
Hillshire Farm, 2 oz	190	16	0.5
Oscar Mayer, 1 slice, 1 oz	90	7	1

Deli & Lunch Meats (Cont)

	C	F	Cb
Treet (Armour), canned, 2 oz	140	3.5	4
Turkey: Average, 1 oz slice	30	1	0.5
¾ oz slice	22	0.5	0.5
Turkey Breast:			
Butterball Fat Free, 3 slice, 2 oz	60	0	4
Hillshire Deli Select, 6 slice, 2 oz	50	0.5	3
Healthy Choice: Deli Thin: Per 4 Slices, (1.8 oz)			
Oven-Roasted	60	1.5	2
Smoked/Rotisserie Seasoned	60	1.5	3
Honey Roasted & Smoked	60	1.5	4
Hearty Deli Sliced,			
Oven Rsted Turkey Brst, 1 sl., 1 oz	30	1	1
Turkey Ham, 1 slice, 1 oz	35	1.5	0.5
Turkey Pastrami, 1 oz	35	1.5	1
Turkey Roll, 1 oz	40	2	0.5
Turkey Loaf, 1 oz	50	1	0.5
Vegetarian Deli (Worthington): See Page 118			

Meat Spreads

	C	F	Cb
Average All Brands: Per ¼ Cup (2 oz)			
Chicken	90	10	2
Ham, Deviled	140	11	0
Liverwurst	190	16	2
Roast Beef	130	10	2
Sandwich Spread	140	10	9
Turkey	110	7	2
Underwood: Per 2 oz			
BBQ Chicken	130	8	2
Chicken, White Meat	130	8	2
Deviled Ham	180	15	1
Liverwurst	160	13	4
Roast Beef	130	10	2
Turkey, White Meat	140	9	2

Paté

	C	F	Cb
Boar's Head Liverwurst Pate, 2 oz	145	12	0
Les Trois Petit Cochons: Per 2 oz			
Black Peppercorn	240	24	1
Chicken Livers & Black Truffle	140	11	2
Country Pate	220	25	1
Duck Liver with Port Wine	130	11	2
Smoked Salmon	110	9	2
Marcel Henri			
Pate de Champagne	210	19	1
Chicken Liver with Port Wine, 2 oz	200	19	1
Duck Truffle with Port Wine, 2 oz	240	24	1
Old Wisconsin Pate			
All types, 2 oz	210	18	3

Nuts

Per 1 oz Unless Indicated

	C	F	Cb
Acorns, raw 1 oz	110	7	12
Almonds, dried/dry roasted:			
Whole, 24-28 medium, 1 oz	170	15	5.5
½ cup, 2½ oz	420	37	13
Chopped,½ cup, 2¼ oz	380	34	12
Sliced, ½ cup, 1⅔ oz	280	25	9
Choc. coated (5-6), 1 oz	150	10	15
Oil Roastd *(Blue Diamond)*, 1 oz	170	16	5
Honey Roasted, 1 oz	170	14	8
Almond Meal (partially defatted)			
1 cup (not packed), 2¼ oz	260	11	11
Brazil Nuts, 8 medium, 1 oz	185	19	3.5
Cashews, dry or oil roasted:			
14 large/18 medium/26 small, 1 oz	165	14	9
½ cup, 2.4 oz	375	31	20
Honey Roasted, 1 oz	165	13	10
Chestnuts, av. all: Dried, 1 oz	105	1	22
Raw/Fresh, 5-6 nuts, 1 oz	60	0	13
Canned, water chestnuts,			
sliced/whole/drained, 1 oz	30	0	7
Coconut, fresh:			
1 piece, 2"x2"x ½", 1 oz	100	10	4.5
Shredded, fresh, ½ cup, 1.4 oz	140	13	6
Dried (Desiccated):			
Unsweetened, 1 oz	185	18	7
Sweetened: Shredded, 1 oz	140	10	13
Grated, ½ cup, 1.3 oz	185	12	18
Cream (canned), ½ cup, 5.2 oz	285	26	12
Milk (canned), ½ cup, 4 oz	225	24	3
Water (center liquid), ½ cup, 4¼ oz	25	0	4.5
Filberts or Hazelnuts:			
Shelled, 18-20 nuts	180	17	4.5
Chopped, ¼ cup, 1 oz	180	18	5
Ground, ¼ cup, 0.6 oz	120	12	3
Ginkgo Nuts, canned, 14 medium, 1 oz	32	0.5	6.5
Hickory, 30 small nuts, 1 oz	200	18	5
Macadamia Nuts, shelled:			
Raw, 7 medium/14 small, 1 oz	200	21	4
½ cup, 2.3 oz	480	51	10
Dry Roasted, 1 oz	205	22	4
½ cup, 2.4 oz	480	51	9
Choc. coated, 2-3 pieces, 1 oz	170	12	14
Mixed Nuts: 18-22 nuts, 1 oz	170	15	7
Planters: Dry Roasted/Honey	160	12	9
Oil Roasted, all types	170	16	6
Sweet Roasts, 26 pieces, 1 oz	160	12	10
Nut Toppings, chopped, 1 Tbsp, ¼ cup	40	4	1.5

Per 1 oz Unless Indicated

	C	F	Cb
Peanuts:			
Raw/Dried:			
In shell, 1 oz	117	10	3
Shelled, 1 oz	160	14	4.5
Boiled, shelled, ½ cup, 3.1 oz	285	20	19
Roasted: 30 large/60 small, 1 oz	165	14	6
1 cup, 5.1 oz	860	76	22
Chopped, 3 Tbsp, 1 oz	165	14	6
Planters: Cocktail, 1 oz	170	14	6
Rich Roasted in Chocolate, 2½ oz	220	14	19
Roasted in Shell, Salted, 1 oz	160	14	5
Dry Roasted, 1oz	160	13	6
Honey/ & Dry Roasted, 1 oz	160	13	8
Spanish Raw, 1 oz	150	13	6
Spanish Redskin, 1 oz	180	14	5
Sweet N' Crunchy, 1 oz	140	7	16
Pecans: Kernel halves, 1 oz	195	20	4
(20 jumbo or 31 large halves)			
1 cup halves, 3.8 oz	755	78	15
Chopped, ½ cup, 2 oz	380	39	7.5
Oil Roasted, 15 halves, 1 oz	205	20	4
Honey Roasted, 1 oz	200	21	4
Pilinuts, dried, ¼ cup, 1 oz	215	24	1
Pine Nuts, dried, 1 Tbsp, 0.3 oz	70	7	1.5
Pistachios: Unshelled, ½ cup, 2 oz	165	14	7
Shelled, ¼ cup, 45 nuts, 1 oz	170	14	8.5
Lance, 1.1 oz package	95	7	4
Sesame Nut Mix: *Planters,* 1 oz	160	13	9
Soy Nuts: Dry Roasted, 1 oz	130	6	9
½ cup, 3 oz	390	18	28
Dr Soy: Chocolate coated, 1 oz pkg	140	7	13
Average other flavors, 1 oz	150	8	8
Trail Mix *(Planters):* Fruit & Nut, 1 oz	140	9	14
Golden Nut Crunch, 1 oz	160	11	12
Honey Nut & Caramel, 1 oz	160	10	16
Mixed Nuts & Raisins, 1 oz	150	11	10
Nut & Chocolate, 1 oz	160	10	16
Nuts, Seeds & Raisins, 1 oz	160	12	11
Spicy Nuts & Cajun Sticks, 1 oz	150	10	13
Sweet & Nutty, 1 oz	150	10	14
Walnuts:			
Black: 15-20 halves, 1 oz	175	17	3
Chopped, ¼ cup, 1.1 oz	195	18	3
English/Persian:			
14 halves, 1 oz	185	18	4
Chopped, ¼ cup, 1 oz	190	19	4
Ground, ¼ cup, 0.7 oz	130	13	3

Updated Nutrition Data ~ www.CalorieKing.com
Persons with Diabetes ~ See Disclaimer (Page 22)

Quick Guide | C | F | Cb

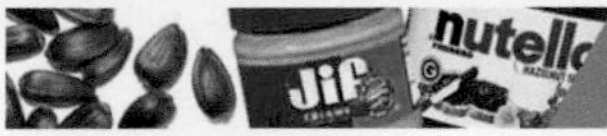

Peanut Butter: *Average All Brands*

	C	F	Cb
1 level tsp, 0.2 oz	35	3	1.5
1 level Tbsp, 0.6 oz	105	8.5	3.5
2 level Tbsp, 1.2 oz	210	17	7
1 oz Quantity	170	14	6
½ cup, 5 oz	850	70	30
Jif: Reduced Fat, 2 Tbsp	190	12	15
Creamy; Crunchy; Simply, 2 Tbsp	190	16	7
Peanut Butter & Honey, 2 Tbsp	180	14	10
Laura Scudder's:			
Smooth; Crunchy, 2 Tbsp	210	16	6
Reduced-Fat, 2 Tbsp, 1¼ oz	200	12	12
Peanut Wonder, Original, 2 Tbsp	100	2	13
Peter Pan: Creamy; Crunch, 2 Tbsp	200	16	6
Whipped, 2 Tbsp	150	12	5
Smucker's Goober,			
Grape/Strawberry 3 Tbsp	240	13	24
Skippy: Reduced Fat, 2 Tbsp	180	12	15
Roasted Honey Nut Creamy, 2 Tbsp	190	16	7

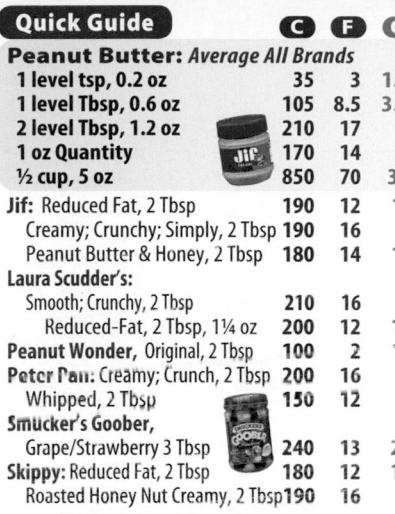

Peanut Butter & Jelly Sandwich

1 sandwich, with 2 oz Bread:			
Light Spread:	310	10	48
(1 Tbsp Peanut Butter + 1 Tbsp Jelly)			
Thick Spread:	480	19	67
(2 Tbsp Peanut Butter + 2 Tbsp Jelly)			
With **Goober Grape**, 3 Tbsp, 2 oz	380	15	52

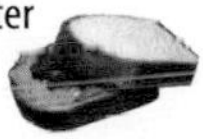

Nutella | C | F | Cb

Nut & Chocolate Spread

	C	F	Cb
1 Tbsp, 0.7 oz	100	5.5	11
2 Tbsp, 1.3 oz	200	11	22

Note: *Nutella* contains approximately 50% sugar and only 13% hazelnuts

Other Nut & Seed Butters

Almond Butter, 1 Tbsp, ½ oz	100	10	3.5
Almond Butter Honey Roasted, 1 Tbsp	90	7	5.5
Beanut Butter, 1 Tbsp, ½ oz	90	5.5	7
Cashew Butter, 1 Tbsp, ½ oz	95	8	4.5
Hazelnut Butter, 1 Tbsp, ½ oz	105	10	2.5
Pecan Butter, 1 Tbsp, ½ oz	110	10	2
Pistachio Butter, 1 Tbsp, ½ oz	90	6.5	4.5
Sesame Butter (Tahini), 1 Tbsp, ½ oz	90	8	3
Soy Nut Butter, 1 Tbsp, ½ oz	75	5	4
Tahini ~ *See Sesame Butter*			

Seeds | C | F | Cb

	C	F	Cb
Alfalfa Seeds,			
sprouted, ½ cup, ½ oz	5	0	1
Caraway, Fennel, 1 tsp	7	0.5	1
Cottonseed Kernels,			
roasted, 1 Tbsp	50	3.5	2
Flax Seeds,			
3 Tbsp, 1 oz	140	9	9
Lotus Seeds,			
dried, ½ cup, ½ oz	55	0.5	10
Poppy Seeds, 1 tsp	15	1	1
Pumpkin & Squash Seeds, whole:			
Roasted/Tamari, 1 oz	150	12	4
½ cup, 4 oz	590	48	15
Dried, (hulled), ¼ cup, 1 oz	155	13	5
Safflower Kernels,			
dried, 1 oz	150	11	10
Sesame Seeds:			
Dried, 1 Tbsp, 0.3 oz	50	4.5	2
Roasted/Toasted, 1 oz	160	14	7.5
Sunflower Kernels/Seed:			
Dried, ¼ cup without hulls, ¼ oz	200	18	7
Dry Roasted, 1 Tbsp, 0.3 oz	45	4	2
¼ cup, 1 oz	165	14	7
Oil Roasted, ⅓ cup, 1 oz	170	14	6.5
Watermelon Seeds, dried.			
¼ cup, 1 oz	150	13	4

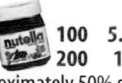

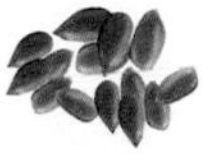

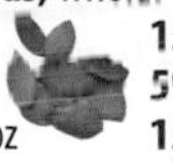

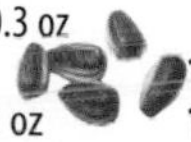

*N**ut eaters are healthier and live longer, say scientists.*

Nuts are a nutritious source of protein, vitamins, minerals, fiber, healthy fats, and antioxidants.

The fat and fiber of nuts can help reduce blood cholesterol. Their protein and fiber also promotes meal satiety (fullness) and reduces hunger levels – of benefit in weight control.

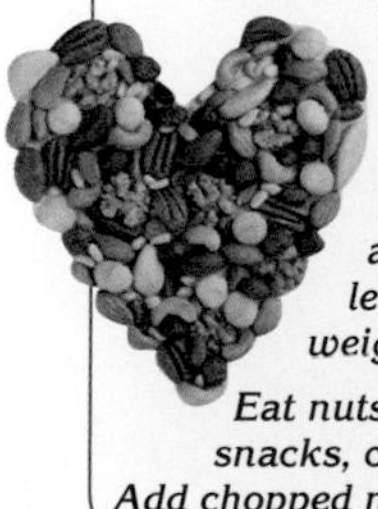

Eat nuts instead of high-sugar snacks, candy and soft drinks. Add chopped nuts to breakfast cereals.

Quick Guide   C   F   Cb

Pancakes

	C	F	Cb
Plain: *Average All Types*			
Small (3" diameter), ¾ oz	50	2	6
Medium (4" diameter), 1¼ oz	85	3.5	11
Large (5" diameter), 2½ oz	175	7.5	22
Add Extra for Syrups/Butter			
Pancake Syrup: Regular, 1 Tbsp	50	0	13
¼ cup, 4 Tbsp	210	0	52
Lite, 1 Tbsp	25	0	6
¼ cup, 4 Tbsp	100	0	26
Butter/Margarine: Regular, 1 Tbsp	100	11	0
Whipped, 1 Tbsp	70	7.5	0

Waffles

	C	F	Cb
Homemade: 7" waffle, 2½ oz	245	13	26
From Mix: 7" waffle, 2½ oz	205	8	28

Frozen Breakfasts

	C	F	Cb
Aunt Jemima			
Pancakes: Buttermilk (3)	240	6	41
Homestyle (3)	240	6	41
Low-Fat (3)	200	3	39
Whole Grain (3)	240	6	42
Mini Pancakes (11)	240	4.5	44
Frozen Breakfasts:			
French Toast: Cinnamon, 2 slices	220	4.5	37
Homestyle, 2 slices	220	4.5	37
Sticks (5)	360	12	58
Eggo *(Kellogg's)*			
Bake Shop Swirlz, Cinnamon (1), 2.2 oz	150	3	28
French Toast: Toaster Swirlz, (4)	120	3	20
French Toaster Sticks, average, (2)	225	6	37
Stuffed French Toaster Sticks (2)	300	7	54
Pancakes: Buttermilk (3)	280	9	44
Minis (11)	260	8	31
Krusteaz			
Pancakes: Mini (8)	160	2	30
Buttermilk (3)	270	4	52
French Toast: Homestyle; Thick, 1 sl.	170	3.5	28
Sticks, Griddled (4)	230	5	41
Pillsbury			
Pancakes: Buttermilk (3)	240	4	47
Mini (11)	240	4	45
Chocolate Burst (3)	280	7	51
Toaster Strudel, av. all flavors (1)	190	6	26

Pancake Brands   C   F   Cb

	C	F	Cb
Aunt Jemima Mixes: *Prepared as Directed*			
Buttermilk, 4 x 4"	180	5	23
Original Complete, 2 x 4"	160	1.5	32
Original, 4 x 4"	250	6	33
Whole Wheat Blend, 3 x 4"	200	5	30
Betty Crocker Pancake Mixes			
Complete Orig./Buttermilk (3)	200	2.5	40
Bisquick (Shake 'N Pour), (3)	220	3	42
Hungry Jack Pancakes			
Mixes: *Per ⅓ Cup, Prepared as Directed*			
Complete: Buttermilk, 3 x 4"	150	1.5	31
Extra Light & Fluffy, 3 x 4"	150	2	30
Original, with 2% Milk, Oil, Egg	250	8	37
With Skim Milk, Oil, Egg Whites	180	1	37
Easy Packs: *Per ⅓ Cup Dry Mix, Prepared*			
Blueberry Wheat	160	2.5	32
Buttermilk	150	1.5	31
Northern Pines: (3), 3 x 4", 3.5 oz	200	3.5	38

Frozen Waffles

	C	F	Cb
Aunt Jemima: Buttermilk (2)	200	6	33
Homestyle; Blueberry (2)	190	6	32
Low-Fat (2)	160	3	31
Eggo *(Kellogg's):* Blueberry (2)	190	6	29
Chocolate Chip (2)	210	7	32
French Toast (1)	140	6	19
Homestyle	190	7	27
Nutri-Grain: (2), av.	170	4.5	27
Low-Fat (2)	140	2.5	27
GO-LEAN *(Kashi):* Average (1)	170	3	33
Nature's Path: Flax Plus (2), average	185	7	24
Homestyle (2)	270	10	44
Mesa Sunrise (2)	200	7	34
Van's: Belgian Homestyle (2)	220	9	31
Hearty Oats: Berry Boost (2)	190	8	26
Maple Fusion (2)	190	9	26
Mini: Chocolate Chip (12)	240	9	35
Homestyle (12)	210	8	32
Wheat Free Minis (12)	210	7	35
97% Fat Free, Original (2)	140	2	26

- Pasta includes all shapes and sizes; (e.g. spaghetti, fettuccini, elbows, shells, twists, sheets, cannelloni, tubes, ziti).
- All regular pasta products have the same cals/fat/carbs on a weight basis.
- 1 oz Dry = approximately 2½ -3 oz cooked.

Dry Spaghetti/Pasta

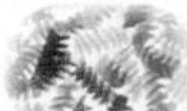

	C	F	Cb
1 oz quantity	105	0.5	21
1lb box/package, 16 oz	1685	7	339
Elbows, 1 cup, 3¾ oz	380	2	80
Shells, small, 1 cup, 3¼ oz	330	1.5	69
Spirals, 1 cup, 3 oz	305	1.5	64

Cooked Spaghetti/Pasta

Plain, All Types (no added fat):			
Firm/Al Dente (8-10 minutes), 1 oz	42	0.5	8.5
Medium (11-13 minutes), 1 oz	37	0.5	7.5
Tender (14 20 minutes), 1 oz	32	0.5	7
(Longer cooking increases water absorbed)			
Spaghetti, ½ cup, 2 ½ oz	90	0.5	18
Medium serving, 1 cup, 5 oz	225	1.5	44
Large Serving, 2 cups, 10 oz	450	3	88
Extra Large, 3 cups, 15 oz	675	5	132
Elbows/Spirals, 1 cup, 5 oz	220	1.5	43
Small Shells, 1 cup, 4 oz	180	1	36
Protein-fortified: Dry, 1 cup, 3⅓ oz	350	2	63
Cooked, 1 cup, 5 oz	230	0.5	45
Spinach/Vegetable: Dry, 1 cup, 3 oz	310	1	61
Cooked, 1 cup, 5 oz	180	0.5	38
Whole-wheat: Dry, 1 cup, 3¾ oz	365	1.5	79
Cooked, 1 cup, 5 oz	175	1	37

Fresh Pasta (Refrigerated)

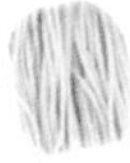

Plain/Spinach/Tomato, average:			
As purchased, 4.5 oz	370	3	70
Cooked, 1 cup, 5 oz	185	1.5	35
Home-made, without egg:			
Cooked, 1 cup, 5 oz	175	1	35
Buitoni			
Cut Pasta: Per ⅓ of 9 oz Pkg			
Angel Hair	230	2.5	43
Fettuccine	260	3	46
Linguine	240	2.5	45
Whole Wheat Linguine	240	3	41
Ravioletti, Three Cheese, 1 cup, 3.2 oz	270	5	43

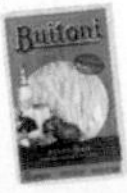

Buitoni (Cont):	C	F	Cb
Ravioli: Four Cheese, 1¼ cups	330	10	45
Light Four Cheese, 1¼ cups	260	4.5	41
Whole Wheat Four Chse, 1¼ cups	320	11	40
Tortellini: Herb Chicken, 1 c., 4 oz	350	10	52
Spinach Cheese, 1 cup, 3.7 oz	320	7	49
Three Cheese, 1 cup, 3.7 oz	320	7	50
Tortelloni: Cheese & Rstd Garlic, 1 c.	270	8	37
Other varieties, average, 1 cup	330	10	47
Pasta Sauces: See Page 148			

Macaroni & Cheese

Packaged: Hormel/Kraft ~ See Page 112			
Restaurant, average: Side, 6 oz	265	13	26
Medium serving, 1 cup, 9 oz	350	17	34
Large serving, 2 cups, 18 oz	700	34	68

Noodles

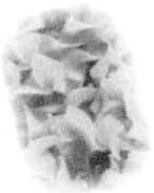

Plain/Egg: Dry, 1 oz	110	1.5	20
1 cup, 1⅓ oz	145	1.5	27
Cooked: 1 oz	40	0.5	7
½ cup, 2¾ oz	110	1.5	20
1 cup, 5½ oz	220	3.5	40
Stir-Fried: 1 cup, 5½ oz	270	9	40
2 cup serving, 11 oz	540	18	80
Yolk Free (Cooked): Per Cup			
'No Yolks' (Foulds), 2 oz	210	0.5	41
Passover Gold (Manischewitz)	200	0	41
Chinese: Cellophane/Rice, dry, 1 oz	100	0	25
Chow Mein/hard, dry, 1 oz	150	9	16
Japanese: Soba, dry, 1 oz	95	0.5	21
Cooked, 1 cup, 4 oz	115	0.5	24
Somen, dry, 1 oz	100	0.5	21
Cooked, 1 cup, 6 oz	230	0.5	49
Japanese Style Pan Fried:			
Maruchan's Yaki-Sobu, 5.6 oz cup	260	3	50
Ramen Noodles (Maruchan/Nissin): See Page 114			
Rice Noodles: Dry, 3.5 oz	365	0.5	83
Cooked, 1 cup, 6.2 oz	190	0.5	44
Stir Fry (Yakisoba), 3.5 oz serving	430	6	52
Tofu Shirataki (House Foods), 4 oz	20	0.5	3
Udon (Chikara), average, 7.5 oz pkt	250	1	52
Simply Asia/Thai Kitchen ~ Page 115			

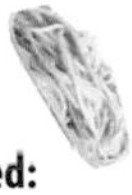

Egg Roll/Won Ton Wrappers

Egg/Spring Roll (1), 0.8 oz	65	0	15
Won Ton Wrapper (1), ¼ oz	20	0	4

Quick Guide

	C	**F**	**Cb**
Fruit Pies: *Average All Brands (9")*			
Apple; Blueberry; Cherry:			
Small, 1/8 pie, 4¾ oz	320	15	46
Medium, 1/6 pie, 6⅓ oz	425	20	61
Large, ¼ pie, 9½ oz	640	30	92
Whole Pie (9"), 38oz	2560	120	368
Other Pies: *Per Serving (⅙ of 8" Pie)*			
Chocolate Cream Pie	345	22	38
Custard; Coconut Custard	270	14	31
Lemon Chiffon Pie	360	14	50
Lemon Meringue	360	13	57
Pecan Pie	440	23	57
Pumpkin Pie	300	12	42
Strawberry Pie	230	9	37

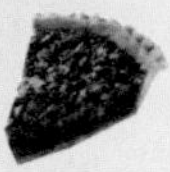

Brands ~ *Per Serving*

	C	**F**	**Cb**
Denny's: Apple Pie, 7 oz	510	23	72
French Silk Pie, 7 oz	770	57	59
Hostess: Fruit; Cherry Pie, 4.5 oz	480	20	68
Lemon Pie, 4.5 oz	490	22	69
Long John Silver's:			
Chocolate Cream Pie	280	17	28
Pineapple Cream Pie	300	17	35
Turtle Pie	290	16	34
Marie Callender's			
Cobbler, 1/8 pie, average	330	17	44
Mrs Smith's:			
Classic Pies: Apple, 1/6 pie	320	14	47
Dutch Apple Crumb, 1/6 pie	340	14	52
Peach, 1/6 pie	310	14	42
Deep Dish, Apple, 1/10 pie	290	13	41
Peach Cobbler, 1/8 cobbler	210	6	39
Sara Lee			
Pies: Choc Dream Pie, 1/8 pie	420	24	47
Choc Mint Creme Pie, 1/8 pie	420	27	44
Key West Lime Pie, 1/8 pie	380	18	50
Peach Pie, 1/8 pie	310	15	42
Southern Pecan Pie, 1/8 pie	470	23	62
Oven Fresh Pies (9", 37 oz Box): *Per Slice (4.6 oz)*			
Apple Pie, 1/8	340	16	47
Cherry Pie, 1/8	340	16	45
Mince Pie; Blueberry Pie, av., 1/8	380	17	53
Pumpkin Pie, 1/8	260	10	39
Southern Sweet Potato Pie, 1/8	280	9	45
Simple Sweets: Apple Pie, ¼ pie	290	15	37
Cherry Pie, ¼ pie	330	16	45
Tastykake: Apple Pie	270	11	40
Coconut Cream Pie	370	20	42
Lemon Pie	300	14	44
Strawberry Pie	340	12	55

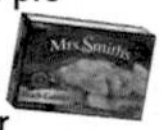

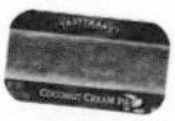

Croissants

Average all Brands

	C	**F**	**Cb**
Plain/Butter/Cheese: Mini, 1 oz	115	6	13
Small, 1½ oz	170	9	19
Medium, 2 oz	230	12	26
Large, 2½ oz	290	15	32
Extra Large, 3 oz	330	19	37
Sweet Croissants:			
Almond Filled, 3 oz	330	18	39
Chocolate Filled, 3 oz	360	19	43
Dunkin' Donuts: Plain Croissant	310	16	35
Sara Lee: French Style Petite, 2 oz	230	11	26
French Style Original, 1½ oz	170	8	20
Croissant Sandwiches: *See Page 165*			

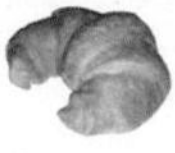

Pastry & Pie Crust

	C	**F**	**Cb**
Pie Crust: Baked, 9" diameter shell			
1 Pie Shell, 6½ oz	970	64	87
2-crust Pie, 9", 11¼ oz	1660	109	150
Filo Pastry: 4 sheets, 2½ oz	210	2.5	40
Athens, 14"x18", 2½ sheets, 2 oz	180	1.5	37
Puff *(Pepp.Farm)*, ½ sheet, 4.5 oz	510	33	42
Bake & Fill Shell, 1.7 oz	190	13	16
Arrowhead Mills, Pie Crust, 1/8 of 9"	110	5	14
Bisquick: Baking Mix,			
Original, ⅓ cup, 1½ oz	160	4.5	26
Heart Smart, ⅓ cup, 1½ oz	140	2.5	27
Keebler:			
Ready Crust: *Per 1/8 of 9" Crust*			
Chocolate	100	4.5	14
Graham	110	5	14
Reduced Fat	100	3.5	15
Shortbread Crust	110	5	14
Graham Crackers Minis (1), 0.8 oz	110	5	15
Marie Callenders, Deep Dish Pie Shell,			
1/8 pie, 1 oz	140	10	11
Mrs Smith's, Homestyle			
Deep Dish, 9", 1/8	130	7	15
Nabisco:			
Honey Maid Graham, 1/6 of 9", 1 oz	150	8	18
Nilla Pie Crust, 1/6 of 9", 1 oz	140	8	18
Pillsbury (All Ready Rolled), 1/8,1 oz	110	6	12
Trader Joe's, Pie Crust, 1/8 pie, 1.2 oz	170	12	12

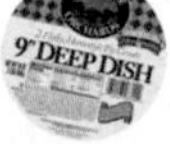

Pie Fillings (Canned)

Fruit: *Average all Fruits*
(Apple/Blueberry/Cherry/Strawberry)

	C	**F**	**Cb**
Sweetened: ⅓ cup, 3.2oz	90	0	22
1 cup, 9½ oz	270	0	66
1 can, 21 oz	600	0	150
Light/Lite, ⅓ cup, 3.2 oz	60	0	15
Unsweetened, ⅓ cup, 3.2 oz	35	0	8
Lemon Cream/Creme, ⅓ cup, 3.2 oz	130	1.5	28

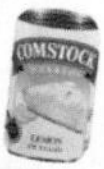

Updated Nutrition Data ~ www.CalorieKing.com
Persons with Diabetes ~ See Disclaimer (Page 22)

Pizzas ~ Ready-To-Eat **C F Cb**

Average All Retail Outlets/Restaurants

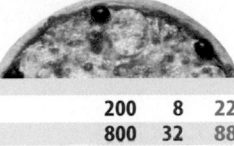

Cheese Pizza
Medium Size (12"):

Thin Crust:

	C	F	Cb
⅛ Pizza (1 slice)	200	8	22
½ Pizza (4 slices)	800	32	88
Whole Pizza (8 slices)	1600	64	172

Deep Dish/Pan:

	C	F	Cb
⅛ Pizza (1 slice)	270	13	27
½ Pizza (4 slices)	1080	52	108
Whole Pizza (8 slices)	2160	104	216

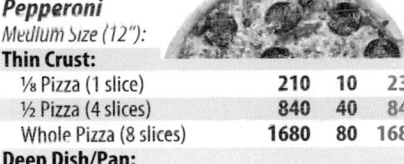

Pepperoni
Medium Size (12"):

Thin Crust:

	C	F	Cb
⅛ Pizza (1 slice)	210	10	23
½ Pizza (4 slices)	840	40	84
Whole Pizza (8 slices)	1680	80	168

Deep Dish/Pan:

	C	F	Cb
⅛ Pizza (1 slice)	280	15	27
½ Pizza (4 slices)	1120	60	108
Whole Pizza (8 slices)	2240	120	216

Supreme:
Medium Size (12"):

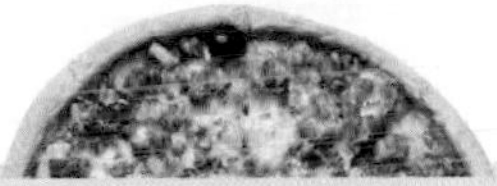

Thin Crust:

	C	F	Cb
⅛ Pizza (1 slice)	240	11	23
½ Pizza (4 slices)	960	44	92
Whole Pizza (8 slices)	1920	88	184

Deep Dish/Pan:

	C	F	Cb
⅛ Pizza (1 slice)	310	16	28
½ Pizza (4 slices)	1240	64	112
Whole Pizza (8 slices)	2480	128	224

Meat Deluxe
Medium Size (12"):

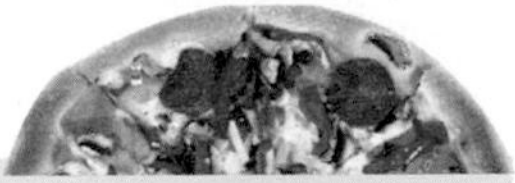

Thin Crust:

	C	F	Cb
⅛ Pizza (1 slice)	310	18	23
½ Pizza (4 slices)	1240	72	92
Whole Pizza (8 slices)	2480	144	184

Deep Dish/Pan:

	C	F	Cb
⅛ Pizza (1 slice)	380	22	28
½ Pizza (4 slices)	1520	88	112
Whole Pizza (8 slices)	3040	176	224

Hawaiian *(Ham & Pineapple)*
Medium Size (12"):

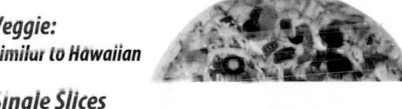

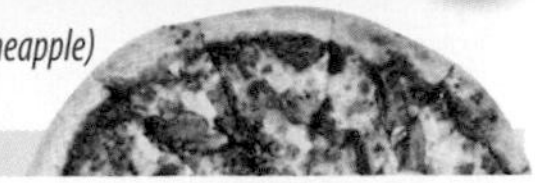

Thin Crust:

	C	F	Cb
⅛ Pizza (1 slice)	190	7	23
½ Pizza (4 slices)	760	28	92
Whole Pizza (8 slices)	1520	56	184

Deep Dish/Pan:

	C	F	Cb
⅛ Pizza (1 slice)	250	11	28
½ Pizza (4 slices)	1000	44	112
Whole Pizza (8 slices)	2000	88	224

Veggie:
Similar to Hawaiian

Single Slices
(Extra Large): **C F Cb**
(Example: Sbarro's)

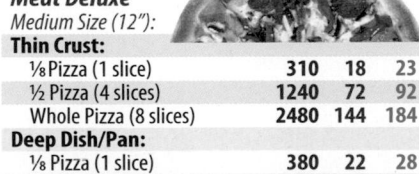

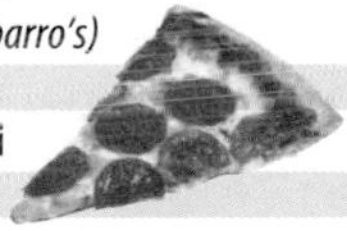

	C	F	Cb
Cheese	460	13	60
Pepperoni	730	37	61
Sausage	670	31	60
Supreme	630	27	63

Individual Pizza (6")
Deep Dish/Pan
(Approx. 9 oz weight):

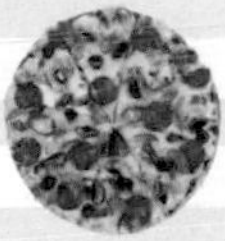

	C	F	Cb
Cheese	600	24	69
Hawaiian	570	21	70
Meat Deluxe	900	50	70
Pepperoni	650	30	67
Veggie	560	22	70

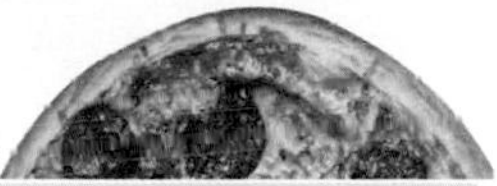

Large (14") Thin Crust

	C	F	Cb
Cheese: ⅛ Pizza	290	12	30
½ Pizza	1160	48	120
Hawaiian: ⅛ pizza	260	9	33
½ Pizza	1040	36	132
Pepperoni: ⅛ Pizza	310	15	30
½ Pizza	1240	60	120
Supreme: ⅛ Pizza	340	17	32
½ Pizza	1360	68	128
Meat Deluxe: ⅛ Pizza	440	26	31
½ Pizza	1760	104	124
Veggie: ⅛ Pizza	260	10	32
½ Pizza	1040	40	128

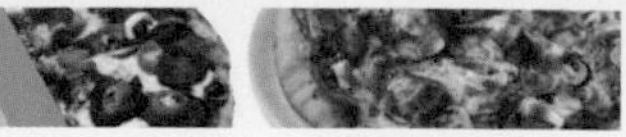

Frozen Pizzas

	C	F	Cb
Amy's: *Per ⅓ Pizza*			
Cheese Pesto	360	18	37
Cheese Pizza	290	12	33
Mushroom & Olive	250	9	33
Pesto	310	12	39
Roasted Vegetable	270	9	42
California Pizza Kitchen			
Crispy Thin Crust: *Per ⅓ Pizza*			
Margherita	290	13	31
Sicilian Recipe	310	14	30
White	290	12	31
For One:			
Four Cheese, 6.9 oz	510	17	69
Margherita, 6 oz	420	18	45
Sicilian, 5.5 oz	450	22	42
Self Rising Crust: *Per ⅓ Pizza*			
BBQ Chicken, 4.3 oz	270	9	33
Five Cheese & Tomato, 4.3 oz	330	11	41
Garlic Chicken, 4.3 oz	260	9	31
Celeste			
Pizza For One: Original, 1 pizza	350	16	39
Deluxe; Pepperoni; Cheeseburger	410	21	42
Meatball	420	22	40
Sausage & Pepperoni; Suprema	420	23	39
Zesty 4 Cheese	350	16	38
DiGiorno			
Crispy Flatbread Pizza: *Per Slice*			
Italian Sausage & Onion, 5.5 oz	400	26	27
Mushroom Medley, 4.3 oz	320	19	26
Pepperoni & Roasted Peppers, 4.5 oz	340	20	26
Tuscan Style Chicken, 4.7 oz	280	14	25
For One: *Per Pizza*			
Garlic Bread Crust:			
Pepperoni	840	44	81
Thin Crust Supreme	590	24	63
Classic Crust: Pepperoni	770	35	83
Supreme	790	36	85
Microwave: *Per ½ Pizza*			
Rising Crust: Four Cheese	370	15	44
Supreme	410	18	45
Three Meat	420	19	44
Thin Crispy Crust, Four Cheese	320	12	38
Rising Crust: *Per ⅙ Pizza*			
Four Cheese	310	11	40
Pepperoni	330	13	40
Thin Crispy Crust: *Per ⅕ Pizza*			
Four Meat	320	14	32
Grilled Chicken Tomato & Spinach	260	8	33

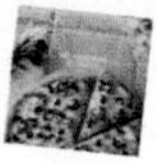

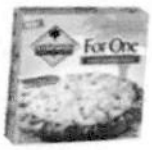

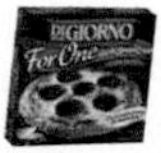

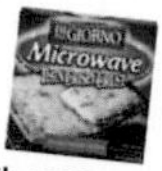

	C	F	Cb
DiGiorno (Cont)			
Ultimate Thin Crust: *Per ⅕ Pizza*			
Four Cheese	330	14	33
Four Meat; Pepperoni, average	390	20	33
Ultimate Toppings: *Per ⅕ Pizza*			
Cheese	320	13	34
Pepperoni; Supreme, average	365	19	33
Four Meat; Pepperoni, average	390	20	33
Freschetta			
Naturally Rising: *Per ⅕ of Large Pizza*			
4 Cheese	360	13	43
4 Meat	380	14	44
Can. Bacon P'apple	310	9	44
Pepperoni	360	14	44
Supreme	320	13	37
PizzAmore:			
6 Cheese, ¼ pizza	380	14	47
Meat Medley, ⅕ pizza	340	14	38
Pepperoni Duo, ¼ pizza	340	15	38
Supreme, ⅕ pizza	340	14	38
Stuffed Breadsticks: Garlic (1)	110	3	19
Cinnamon with Cream Cheese (1)	140	4	23
Healthy Choice: *Per Pizza, 6 oz*			
French Bread Pizza	345	4.5	54
Jeno's: *Per Pizza , 7 oz*			
Crispy 'N Tasty: Cheese	450	21	51
Sausage; Pepperoni, average	485	25	50
Home Run Inn (Chicago): *Per ⅙ Pizza*			
Classic Large 12": Cheese, 4.5 oz	340	18	30
Sausage, 5 oz	360	19	29
Sausage & Pepperoni, 5.15 oz	380	20	30
Signature, Sausage Supreme, 5½ oz	360	18	31
Kashi, Original Crust, av., ⅓ pizza	290	9	38
Lean Cuisine:			
Casual Eating: *Per Pizza, 6 oz*			
Deep Dish: Roasted Vegetable	320	5	52
Spinach & Mushroom	340	7	52
French Bread: Cheese	340	7	53
Deluxe	340	10	46
Traditional: Four Cheese	340	6	51
Pepperoni	350	8	50
Wood Fired: Margherita	300	7	43
Roast Garlic Chicken	330	8	42
Private Selection			
Flat Bread: *Per Pizza*			
Chicken	550	16	77
Margherita	600	22	70
Thin Crust: BBQ Chicken, ⅓ pizza	360	15	36
Extra Pepperoni, ⅓ pizza	440	24	32
Grilled Chicken Caesar, ⅓ pizza	350	15	35
Margherita, ⅓ pizza	310	13	32

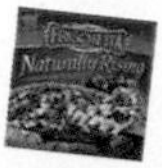

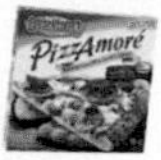

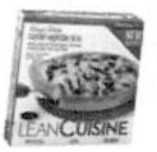

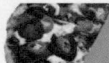

Frozen Pizzas (Cont)

	C	F	Cb
Red Baron			
Classic (Large):			
4 Cheese, ¼ pizza	380	17	41
Pepperoni, ¼ pizza	370	16	40
Sausage & Pepperoni, ¼ pizza	400	19	41
Supreme, ⅕ pizza	310	14	33
Fire Baked Singles: *Per Pizza*			
Original Crust: 4-Cheese	550	22	67
Pepperoni	570	24	67
Fire Baked Thin Crust: *Per ⅓ Pizza*			
5 Cheese	360	16	40
Pepperoni	400	19	40
Pan: 4 Cheese, ⅕ pizza	390	18	40
Meat Trio; Supreme, ⅙ pizza, av	355	18	35
Pepperoni, ⅕ pizza	400	19	41
Pizza By The Slice: *Per Slice*			
4 Cheese	340	13	41
Meat Trio	380	19	41
Pepperoni; Supreme, average	355	15	41
Singles: *Per Pizza*			
Deep Dish: 4 Cheese; Meat Trio, av	410	18	45
Pepperoni; Supreme, averagei	420	19	45
French Bread: Extra Cheese	360	12	43
5 Cheese & Garlic	410	22	39
Pepperoni	360	15	42
Supreme	310	10	42
Reggio's			
Deep Dish: Cheese, ⅙ pizza	350	16	39
Sausage, ⅙ pizza	410	20	39
Dinner Size: Cheese, ¼ pizza	330	12	41
Pepperoni & Sausage, ¼ pizza	400	18	41
Sausage; Supreme, av., ¼ pizza	380	16	41
Safeway Select			
Thin and Crispy:			
Four Cheese, ⅙ pizza	310	11	37
Pepperoni, ⅕ pizza	350	16	37
Ultra Thin Crust: *Per ⅓ Pizza Unless Indicated*			
BBQ Chicken ¼ pizza	250	10	23
Margherita	330	17	28
Primo Italiano Meat	330	17	28
Stouffer's: *Per ½ Pizza*			
French Bread Pizzas: Deluxe	430	21	45
Extra Cheese	400	18	44
Pepperoni	430	21	44
Sausage & Pepperoni	460	24	43

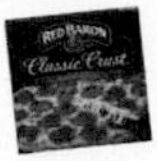

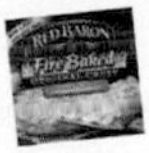

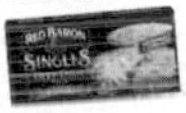

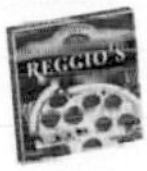

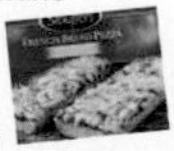

	C	F	Cb
Tombstone			
Original: *Per ⅕ of Large 12" Pizza Unless Indicated*			
4 Meat	310	14	30
Canadian Style Bacon, ¼ pizza	320	12	37
Deluxe	290	12	31
Extra Cheese, ¼ pizza	350	15	37
Pepperoni, ⅓ pizza	280	14	28
Pepperoni & Sausage	370	17	37
Sausage & Mushroom	290	13	30
Supreme	300	14	31
Double Top: Sausage, ⅙ pizza	310	16	27
Sausage & Pepperoni, ⅙ pizza	330	18	26
Harvest Wheat Thin Crust:			
Cheese, ⅓ pizza	300	10	37
Pepperoni, ¼ pizza	260	10	29
Supreme, ¼ pizza	260	10	29
Light Vegetable	230	6	31
Thin Crust: Three Cheese, ¼ pizza	310	15	28
Pepperoni; Sausage, av., ¼ pizza	325	18	29
Brick Oven Style, Cheese, ⅓ pizza	350	15	38
Pepperoni; Supreme, av., ¼ pizza	315	16	29
Tony's			
Original Crust: Cheese, ⅓ pizza	290	12	37
Pepperoni, ⅓ pizza	310	14	36
Ssg & Pepperoni; Supreme, av., ⅓	340	17	37
Deep Dish (Individual):			
Cheese (1)	400	16	47
Pepperoni (1)	470	24	49
Totino's			
Crisp Crust Party Pizza: *Per ½ Pizza*			
Cheese	320	15	34
Classic Pepperoni	370	20	35
Pizza Rolls: Cheese (6), 3 oz	180	5	26
Pepperoni (6), 3 oz	210	10	24
Trader Joe's:			
3 Cheese, ⅓ pizza	310	9	42
Parlanno, ¼ pizza	340	16	34
Spinach, ⅓ pizza	300	12	38
Weight Watchers (Smart Ones): *Per Pizza*			
Fajita Chicken	380	7	58
Four Cheese	370	7	57
Pepperoni	390	8	58
Wolfgang Puck			
All Natural Pizzas: *Per ⅓ Pizza*			
4 Cheese Tomato & Pesto	330	17	30
BBQ Chicken	360	15	40
Cheese	340	16	33
Margherita	330	16	33
Uncured Pepperoni	360	19	32

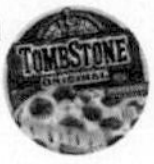

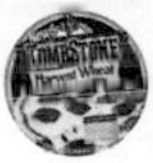

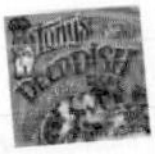

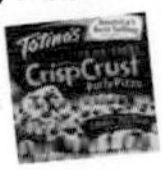

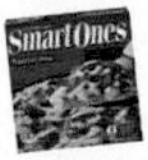

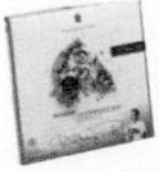

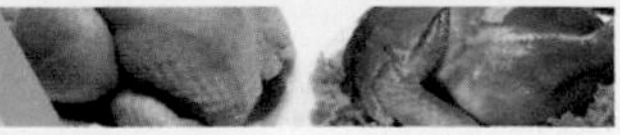

Quick Guide

Chicken	C	F	Cb
From 3lb ready-to-cook chicken			
Breast/Wing Quarter			
Roasted: With skin	300	15	0
Without skin	185	5	0
Fried, batter dipped	530	30	17
Leg Quarter:			
Thigh & Drumstick			
Roasted: With skin, 4 oz	265	15	0
Without skin, 3.35 oz	180	8	0
Fried, batter dipped	430	25	14
(**KFC:** *See Fast-Foods Section*)			

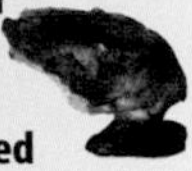

Per 4 oz Edible Portion

	C	F	Cb
Average of Light Meat: *Per 4 oz (no bone)*			
Roasted: With skin	250	12	0
Without skin	175	4.5	0
Stewed: With skin	230	12	0
Without skin	180	4.5	0
Fried: Batter-dipped, 4 oz	315	17	11
Flour-coated, 4 oz	280	14	2
Average of Dark Meat: *Per 4 oz (no bone)*			
Roasted: With skin	290	18	0
Without skin	235	11	0
Stewed: With skin	265	17	0
Without skin	220	10	0
Fried: Batter-dipped, 4 oz	340	21	11
Flour-coated, 4 oz	325	19	5

Chicken Parts

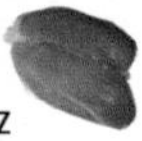

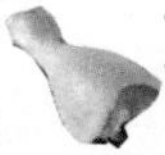

	C	F	Cb
Broilers or Fryers: Edible Weights (no bone)			
Breast: *Per ½ Breast*			
Raw: With skin, 5 oz	250	14	0
Without skin, 4¼ oz	130	1.5	0
Roasted: With skin, 3½ oz	195	8	0
Without skin, 3 oz	140	3	0
Stewed: With skin, 4 oz	200	8	0
Without skin, 3¼ oz	145	3	0
Fried: Batter-dipped, 5 oz	365	19	13
Flour-coated, with skin, 3½ oz	220	9	2
Drumstick: *Per Drumstick*			
Roasted: With skin, 2 oz	115	6	0
Without skin, 1½ oz	75	2.5	0
Fried: Batter-dipped, 2½ oz	195	11	6
Flour-coated, 1¾ oz	120	7	1
Stewed: With skin, 2 oz	115	6	0
Without skin, 1½ oz	80	3	0

Chicken Parts (Cont)

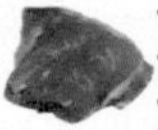

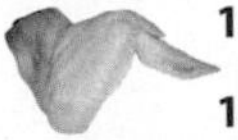

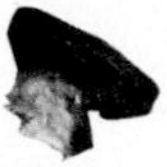

	C	F	Cb
Thigh Portion: Edible Weight (no bone)			
Raw: With skin, 3.3 oz			
(4¼ oz with bone)	200	14	0
Without skin, 2.4 oz	80	3	0
Roasted: With skin, 2¼ oz	155	10	0
Without skin, 2 oz	110	6	0
Stewed: With skin, 2½ oz	160	10	0
Without skin, 2 oz	105	5	0
Fried: Batter-dipped, 3 oz	240	14	8
Flour-coated, 2¼ oz	165	9	2
Wing: *Per Wing*			
Raw Weight 3.2 oz (with bone)			
Raw: With skin	110	8	0
Without skin	35	1	0
Roasted: With skin	100	7	0
Without skin	45	2	0
Fried: Batter-dipped	160	11	5
Flour-coated	105	7	1
Stewed: With skin, 4 oz	100	7	0
Buffalo Wings: *See Fast-Foods Section*			
Neck: Simmered, with skin	95	7	0
Without skin	30	2	0
Skin Only: *Skin from ½ Chicken*			
Raw skin, 2¾ oz	275	26	0
Roasted skin, 2 oz	255	23	0
Stewed skin, 2½ oz	260	24	0
Fried, Flour-coated, 2 oz	280	24	5
Fried, Batter-dipped, 6¾ oz	750	55	44
Roasters			
Average of Light & Dark Meat:			
Roasted: With skin, 4 oz	250	15	0
Without skin, 4 oz	190	8	0
Light Meat: Without skin, roasted	175	5	0
Dark Meat: Without skin, roasted	200	10	0
Stewing Chicken			
Average of Light & Dark Meat: *Per 4 oz Stewed*			
With skin	325	22	0
Without skin	270	14	0
Light Meat: Without skin	240	9	0
Dark Meat: Without skin	290	17	0
Capon Chicken			
Roasted: With skin, 4 oz	260	13	0
½ Chicken, with skin	1460	74	0
Chicken Offal & Stuffing			
Giblets: Simmered, 1 cup	230	7	0.5
Fried, flour-coated, 1 cup	400	20	6
Gizzard, simmered, 1 cup	210	4	0
Heart, simmered, 1 cup	270	12	0.2
Liver: Raw, 4 oz	130	5.5	0
Simmered, 1 cup	215	8.5	1
Liver Pate Fresh, 1 Tbsp, ½ oz	30	2	1
Stuffing: Average, ½ cup	180	9	22

Updated Nutrition Data ~ www.CalorieKing.com
Persons with Diabetes ~ See Disclaimer (Page 22)

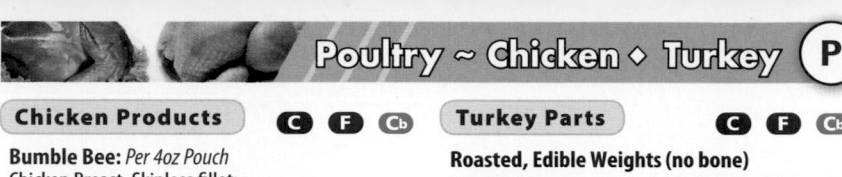

Chicken Products C F Cb

Bumble Bee: *Per 4oz Pouch*
Chicken Breast, Skinless fillet:

	C	F	Cb
Garlic & Herb	110	1.5	1
With Barbeque Sauce	170	1.5	10
With Southwest Seasoning	120	1	0

Foster Farms

	C	F	Cb
Grilled Chicken Breast Strips, 3 oz	100	1.5	2
Wings: Chipotle, 4 wings, 2.9 oz	190	14	1
Honey BBQ, 4 wings, 2.9 oz	170	10	5
Hot & Spicy, 4 wings, 2.9 oz	170	13	1

Tyson:
Any'tizers:

	C	F	Cb
BBQ Style Wings (3)	200	13	7
Buffalo Style Hot Wings (3)	230	15	1
Breaded Nuggets (5)	270	17	15
Breast Nuggets (5)	220	13	15
Southern Style Nuggets (6)	270	21	11
Breast Patties: Southern Style (1)	260	20	11

Duck, Goose, Quail

Duck: Roasted,

	C	F	Cb
With skin, 3 oz	290	24	0
Without skin, 3 oz	170	10	0
½ whole duck, with skin	1290	108	0
Goose: Roast, with skin, 3 oz	260	19	0
Without skin, 3 oz	200	11	0
Pheasant, cooked, 3 oz	210	10	0
Quail, cooked, 1 whole, 6 oz	400	24	0

Turkey

Fryer-Roasters: *Per 3 oz Serving*

	C	F	Cb
Roasted: Light Meat, with skin	140	4	0
Without skin	120	1	0
Dark Meat: With skin	155	6	0
Without skin	140	4	0

½ of Whole Turkey: (Approx. 3¼ lbs raw weight
Without neck and giblets; 1.8 lbs cooked weight)

	C	F	Cb
Roasted: With skin	1650	74	0
Without skin	1125	31	0

Ground Turkey, Raw: (4 oz raw wt. = 3 oz ckd wt.)

	C	F	Cb
Regular (85% lean), 4 oz	170	10	0
Lean (93% lean), average, 4 oz	160	8	0
Foster Farms (94% lean), 4 oz	150	7	0
Jennie-O (93% lean), 4 oz	170	8	0
Trader Joe's (93% lean), 4 oz	150	8	0
Breast, no skin, 4 oz	115	1	0
Patties: Small, 3 oz	130	7	0
Medium, 4 oz	170	10	0
Large, 5.3 oz	225	13	0

Turkey Parts C F Cb

Roasted, Edible Weights (no bone)
Breast (½): (from 17¼ oz raw weight with bone)

	C	F	Cb
With skin, 12 oz (no bone)	525	11	0
Without skin, 10¾ oz	415	2	0
Back (½): With skin, 4½ oz	265	13	0
Without skin, 3½ oz	165	6	0

Leg (Thigh & Drumstick):
(from 1 lb raw weight with bone)

	C	F	Cb
With skin, 8½ oz (without bone)	410	13	0
Without skin, 7¾ oz	355	8.5	0

Wing: (from 7¼ oz raw weight)

	C	F	Cb
With skin, 3 oz (without bone)	185	9	0
Without skin, 2 oz (with bone)	100	2	0

Neck: Simmered, 1 neck,

	C	F	Cb
(9 oz with bone)	275	11	0
Giblets, simmered, 1 cup, 5 oz	240	7	3

Young Hens (Roasted)

	C	F	Cb
Light Meat: With skin, 3 oz	175	8	0
Without skin, 3 oz	135	3	0
Dark Meat: With skin, 3 oz	200	11	0
Without skin, 3 oz	165	7	0

Young Toms – Similar to Young Hens

Turkey Products

Banquet: *See Frozen Meals, Page 117*
Foster Farms:

	C	F	Cb
Homestyle Meatballs (3)	160	9	3

Hormel: Turkey Chunks (canned), cooked:

	C	F	Cb
Chunk Turkey, 2 oz	70	2.5	0
White & Dark Turkey, 2 oz	60	1.5	0

Jennie-O:

	C	F	Cb
All Natural: Lean Meatloaf, 4 oz	250	20	1
White Burgers, 5.25 oz	180	7	0
Fully Cooked: Italian Meatballs, 3 oz	170	11	1
Home Style Meatballs, 3 oz	180	12	2
Turkey Bacon, 1 slice	35	3	1
Turkey Bratwurst, lean, 4 oz	170	10	2

John Morrell: Off the Bone,

	C	F	Cb
Oven Roasted Turkey Strips, 4 oz	140	5	10
Spam, Oven Roasted Turkey, 2 oz	80	4	2

Swanson: *Frozen Meals, Page 121*

	C	F	Cb
Trader Joe's, Ital. Turkey Meatloaf, 3 oz	140	8	5

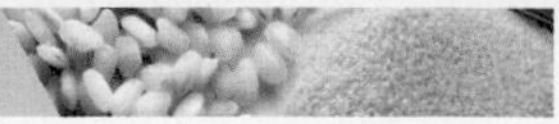

White Rice

	C	F	Cb
Raw: Short/Med. Grain, 1 cup, 7 oz	715	1	158
Long Grain, 1 cup, 6½ oz	675	1	148
Glutinous, 1 cup, 6½ oz	685	1	151
Cooked Rice (Boiled/Steamed):			
Short/Medium Grain:			
½ cup, 3¼ oz	135	0	30
1 cup (½ Pint), 7.2 oz	270	0.5	59
2 cups (1 Pint), 13 oz	480	1	106
Long Grain: ½ cup, 2¾ oz	105	0	22
1 cup, 5½ oz	205	0.5	44
Glutinous/Sticky, cooked, 1 c., 6 oz	170	0.5	37
Parboiled, cooked, ½ cup, 3 oz	105	0.5	22
Precook./Instant: Dry, ½ cup, 3½ oz	370	0	80
Cooked, ½ cup, 3 oz	90	0	20
Wild Rice: Raw, 1 cup, 5½ oz	570	2	120
Cooked, 1 cup, 5¾ oz	165	0.5	35

Brown Rice

	C	F	Cb
Average of Short or Long Grain			
Raw/Dry: ½ cup, 3¼ oz	340	2.5	71
1 cup, 6½ oz	685	5.5	143
Cooked: ½ cup, 3½ oz	110	1	22
1 cup, 7 oz	220	2	46

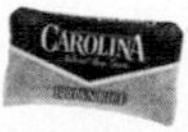

Rice Dishes

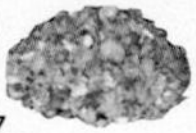

	C	F	Cb
Chinese Fried Rice:			
½ cup, 2½ oz	140	4.5	21
1 cup, (½ Pint), 5 oz	280	9	42
2 cups, (1 Pint), 10 oz	565	18	84
Mexican Rice: 1 cup	500	12	90
Taco John's, 1 serving (6 oz)	250	5	45
Taco Time, 1 serving (4 oz)	160	2	30
Rice-A-Roni: *See Page 114*			
Rice with Raisins/Pinenuts, 1 cup	400	11	60
Rice Pilaf: Restaurant, 1 cup	275	7.5	46
O'Charley's, 1 order	190	5	30
Rice Pudding (*Kozy Shack*),			
Original, ½ cup	130	3	22
Risotto, 1 cup	420	12	70
Saffron Rice, 4 oz	175	7	25
Spanish Rice: 1 cup	390	9	72
El Pollo Loco, small, 5 oz	160	1	35
Taco Cabana, 4 oz	180	5	30
Sticky Rice, 5 oz	155	0.5	34
Sushi Rice: 1 Tbsp	25	0	5
1 cup, 5.2 oz	390	0	77

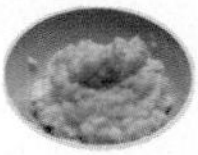

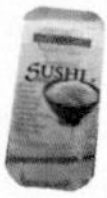

Other Packaged Rice Products:
Uncle Ben's / Zatarain's: See Page 116

CalorieKing.com Recipes

See the CalorieKing website for a salubrious selection of healthy recipes — all analysed for calories, fat, protein, carbohydrate, fiber and sodium.

Choose from:
- Starters/Appetizers
- Salads
- Entrees: Meat, Fish and Chicken
- Vegetarian
- Desserts
- Cakes, Cookies
- Drinks

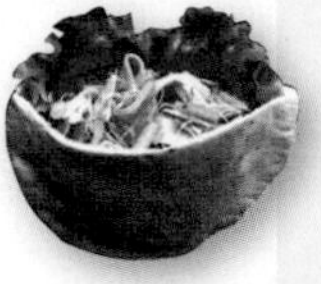

www.Calorieking.com/recipes

HEALTHY RECIPE TIPS

- **Use non-fat milk** in place of whole or 2% milk

- **Use low-fat yogurt** in place of sour cream
- **Skim fat** from surface of soups and casseroles after cooling
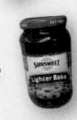
- **Add extra vegetables** to soups and hot entrees
- **Cakes/cookies/muffins:** Replace most or all the fat/oil with applesauce and/or prune puree (Example: *Sunsweet Lighter Bake*)

- **Drinks:** Replace sugar with no-calorie sweeteners such as *Equal, Stevia, Splenda and Sweet 'N Low*

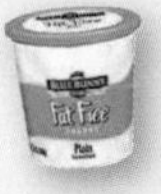

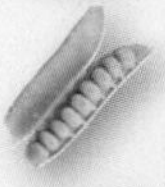

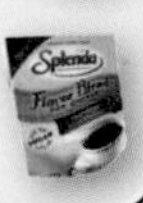

Deli Salads

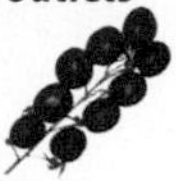

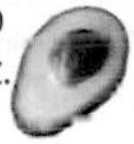

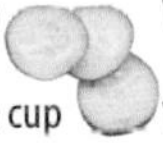

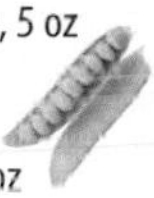

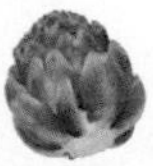

General Average, All Outlets

	C	F	Cb
Antipasto Salad, ½ cup	135	8	13
3-Bean Salad, ½ cup	110	4	17
Bulgur Salad, ½ cup	70	2	12
Caesar Salad, Classic, 1 cup	200	14	15
Side Salad, without Dressing	25	0	6
Carrot Raisin: w/o Dressing, ½ cup	20	0	5
With Dressing, ½ cup	135	12	6
Chef's Salad: Regular, w/o Dressing	620	37	8
With 2 oz 1000 Island	860	61	8
Chicken Salad, ½ cup/scoop, 4 oz	280	21	2
Coleslaw: Traditional, ½ cup	150	8	18
With Low Cal Dressing, ½ c.	50	2	8
Corn, Mexican, ⅓ cup	240	12	33
Cucumber: Non-Oil Dressing, ½ c.	60	0	14
With Oil Dressing, ½ cup	140	12	8
Eggplant Salad, ½ cup	75	5	7
Fettucini with veges, ½ cup	135	6	16
Garden Salad, without Dressing, 1 c.	10	0	2
Greek Salad, 1 cup	105	8	7
Greek Vegetables, 1 cup	110	8	6
Lettuce, hearts, ½ head	15	0	2.5
Lobster Salad, ½ cup, 4 oz	250	21	11
Macaroni Salad, ½ cup, 5 oz	360	26	26
Nicoise, 1 cup	450	32	18
Pasta Salad, ½ cup	200	11	19
Potato Salad: Dijon, 3 oz	120	7	13
With Mayonnaise, ½ cup, 4 oz	215	15	17
Lowfat, ½ cup	110	1.5	21
Rice Salad, ½ cup	150	10	13
Saffron Rice, 4 oz	175	7	25
Spinach Salad, 1 cup	180	13	13
Tabouli, ½ cup	125	7	13
Three Bean Salad, ½ cup	90	4.5	12
Tomato & Mozzarella, ½ cup	180	14	10
Tortellini with Basil Pesto, ½ cup	150	9	15
Waldorf with Mayo, ½ cup	110	7	12

Signature Salads: *Per 6 oz Serving*
(Supplied to Deli's and Institutions)

	C	F	Cb
Antipasto Salad, 6 oz	510	50	4
Artichoke Salad, marinated	400	41	8
California Medley	120	7	15
Cheese Agnolotti	250	8	23
Chicken Salad	420	33	11
Crabmeat Flavored	450	38	20

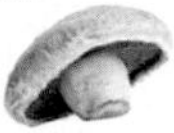

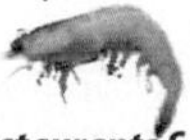

Signature Salads (Cont): *Per 6 oz Serving*

	C	F	Cb
Egg Salad	300	23	14
Fresh Button Mushroom	190	16	6
Garden Olive	630	67	3
Ham Salad	400	32	14
Prima Pasta Salad	360	30	18
Seafood Pasta Del Mar	170	10	21
Seafood with Crab & Shrimp	420	34	20
Shrimp Salad	360	32	8
Tuna Salad	450	36	14

See Fast-Foods & Restaurants Section

Fresh Salad Packs

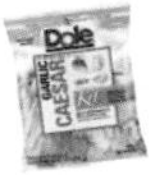

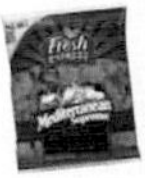

Pre-Packaged (Supermarkets)

Dole:

Kits: *Per 3½ oz, Includes Dressing*

	C	F	Cb
Asian Island Crunch	140	7	17
Caesar	140	11	8
Hearty Italians	180	13	10
Perfect Harvest	160	12	11
Southwest Salad	150	11	10

Salad Blends: *Without Dressing*

	C	F	Cb
American; Mediterranean, 3 oz	15	0	3
Baby Arugula with Spinach, 3 oz	40	1	8

Fresh Express

Complete Salad Kits: *Per Serving, Prepared*

	C	F	Cb
Asian Supreme, ¼ bag	120	5	17
B.L.T. Caesar, ⅓ bag	170	14	8
Caesar: Classic, ⅓ bag	150	13	8
Lite, ⅓ bag	100	7	8
Supreme, ⅓ bag	140	12	7
Mediterranean Supreme, ⅓ bag	150	10	16
Pacifica! Veggie Supreme, ½ bag	220	15	18
Salsa! Ensalada Supreme, ¼ bag	120	8	10

Salad Toppings

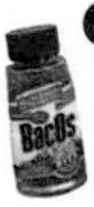

	C	F	Cb
Bacon Bits: Bacos, 1 Tbsp	30	1.5	2
Hormel, 1 Tbsp	25	1.5	0
Chow Mein Noodles, dry, ½ c.	120	7	13
Croutons, 2 Tbsp, 0.3 oz	40	1	7
Olives, 5 medium	25	2	0
Sunflower Seeds, 1 T., 0.3 oz	45	4	1.5
Toasted Sliced Almonds, 2 T., ½ oz	85	7	3
Tortilla Chips, 12 chips, 1 oz	140	7	19

S Salad Dressings

Quick Guide

Salad Dressings
Average All Brands
Per 2 Tbsp (Approx 1 fl.oz)

	C	F	Cb
Balsamic Vinaigrette: Regular	90	9	3
Light, 2 Tbsp	45	4	2
Fat Free, 2 Tbsp	25	0	6
Blue Cheese: Regular, 2 Tbsp	150	16	2
Regular, ¼ cup, 2 oz	300	32	4
Light, 2 Tbsp	30	1	4
Caesar: Regular, 2 Tbsp	155	17	1
Regular, ¼ cup, 2 oz	310	34	2
Light, 2 Tbsp	70	8	5
Coleslaw: Regular, 2 Tbsp	125	11	8
Regular, ¼ cup, 2 oz	245	21	15
Light, 2 Tbsp	110	7	14
French/Italian: Regular	150	14	5
Regular, ¼ cup, 2 oz	290	28	10
Light, 2 Tbsp	65	4	9
Fat/Oil-Free, 2 Tbsp	40	0	10
Ranch: Regular, 2 Tbsp	145	16	2
Regular, ¼ cup, 2 oz	290	31	4
Light, 2 Tbsp	80	3	7
Fat-Free, 2 Tbsp	50	0.5	11
Thousand Island: Regular	120	11	5
Regular, ¼ cup, 2 oz	230	22	9
Light, 2 Tbsp	60	4	7
Fat-Free, 2 Tbsp	40	0.5	10

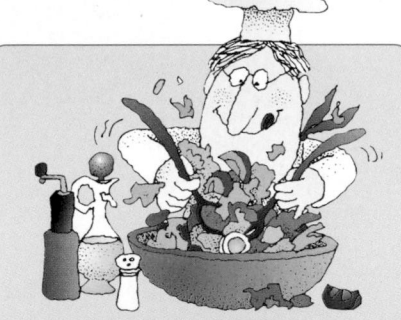

Enjoy a healthy salad but don't drown it in high-fat salad dressings.
Use 'light' dressings to halve the fat and calories.

Brands ~ Salad Dressings

	C	F	Cb
Annie's Naturals: *Per 2 Tbsp*			
Buttermilk	70	7	1
French	110	11	3
Green Garlic	80	8	2
Oil & Vinegar	120	13	1
Papaya & Poppyseed	90	8	5
Pomegranate Vinaigrette	80	7	2
Red Wine & Olive Oil	130	14	0
Roasted Garlic	110	11	3
Sesame Ginger	70	8	4
Shitake Sesame	120	13	1
Thousand Island	80	7	4
Bernstein's: *Per 2 Tbsp*			
Creamy Caesar	120	13	1
Herb Garden French	130	12	6
Italian	110	12	1
Restaurant Recipe Italian	120	12	1
Sweet Herb Italian	130	11	8
Fat-Free Cheese & Garlic Italian	10	0	2
Light Fantastic: Cheese Fantastico	25	1.5	3
Roasted Garlic Balsamic	45	3.5	3
Best Foods: Dijonnaise, 1 tsp	5	0	1
Mayonnaise: *Per 1 Tbsp*			
Canola	45	4.5	0
Low-Fat	15	1	2
Light	35	3.5	1
Real Mayonnaise	90	10	0
Tartar Sauce, 2 Tbsp	80	7	4
Cardini's: *Per 2 Tbsp*			
Caesar	160	17	1
Fat-Free Caesar	40	0	9
Light Caesar	80	7	5
Honey Mustard	140	13	5
Italian	100	8	7
Parmesan Ranch	150	16	1
Roasted Asian Sesame	120	10	7
Vinaigrette Dressing:			
Balsamic	100	8	5
Lite: Balsamic	50	3	5
Caesar	80	7	5
Hidden Valley: *Per 2 Tbsp*			
Regular Ranch: Italian Ranch	140	14	2
Old-Fashioned Buttermilk Ranch	140	14	2
Bacon Ranch	140	14	1
Cracked Peppercorn Ranch	120	12	2
Cole Slaw	150	15	5
Light, Original Ranch	80	7	3
Fat-Free, Original Ranch	30	0	6

Updated Nutrition Data ~ www.CalorieKing.com
Persons with Diabetes ~ See Disclaimer (Page 22)

Brands ~ Salad Dressings (Cont)

Kraft

	C	F	Cb
Regular Dressings: *Per 2 Tbsp*			
Caesar Vinaigrette with Parmesan	70	5	3
Coleslaw Maker	110	9	7
Creamy Italian	100	11	2
Greek Vinaigrette	110	12	2
Honey Dijon	100	9	6
Light Raspb. Vinaigrette	60	4	5
Ranch	120	12	3
Roka Blue Cheese	120	13	1
Sundried Tomato Vinaigrette	60	5	4
Sweet Honey Catalina	130	10	8
Tangy Tomato Bacon	100	6	10
Thousand Island with Bacon	100	8	7
Tuscan House Italian	130	13	3
Kraft Free (Fat-Free): Italian	20	0	4
Classic Caesar	50	0	11
Honey Dijon	50	0	12
Light Done Right!:			
Red Wine Vinaigrette	45	4	3
Seven Seas: Viva Robust Italian	90	9	2
Red Wine Vinegar & Oil	90	9	2
Special Collection:			
Parmesan Romano	140	14	2
Marie's: *Per 2 Tbsp*			
Caesar; Creamy Ranch	170	19	1
Chunky Blue Cheese	160	17	0
Honey Dijon	130	12	5
Poppy Seed	150	13	8
Potato Salad Dressing:			
Classic	170	19	0
Dijon Herb	140	15	1
German Style	110	11	3
Sesame Ginger	100	8	7
Thousand Island	150	15	4
Premium, Spinach Salad	70	1.5	13

Marzetti's

	C	F	Cb
Asiago Peppercorn	160	16	1
Asian Ginger	120	12	4
Bistro Blue Cheese	180	19	1
Chunky Blue Cheese	150	15	1
Honey Balsamic	120	11	4
Original Slaw	160	15	6
Ranch	160	17	1

Nasoya: *Per 2 Tbsp*
Vegi-Dressing (Tofu Base/Dairy Free):

	C	F	Cb
Thousand Island	60	5	2
Other flavors	60	7	1

Newman's Own: *Per 2 Tbsp*

	C	F	Cb
Balsamic Vinaigrette	90	9	3
Creamy Caesar	170	18	1
Family Recipe Italian	120	13	1
Olive Oil & Vinegar	150	16	1
Parmesan Roasted Garlic	110	11	2
Ranch	150	16	2
Lighten Up: Light Italian	60	6	0
Light Raspberry & Walnut	70	5	7
Light Balsamic Vinaigrette	45	4	2
Seven Seas:			
Green Goddess	130	13	2
Viva Robust Italian	90	9	2
Spectrum: *Per 2 Tbsp*			
Organic Omega-3:			
Asian Ginger	140	14	3
Creamy Garlic Ranch	120	13	1
Golden Balsamic Vin,	110	11	3
Pomegranate Chipotle	130	13	2
Vegan Caesar	90	9	2

Wishbone

	C	F	Cb
Creamy: Chunky Blue Cheese	150	15	2
Creamy Caesar	170	18	1
Creamy Italian	110	10	4
Deluxe French	120	11	5
Garlic Ranch	140	15	2
Ranch	120	13	2
Russian	120	6	14
Sweet 'n Spicy	130	12	6
Thousand Island	130	12	6
Light: Blue Cheese	50	2	6
Creamy Caesar	50	2	7
Country Italian	30	1.5	3
Honey Dijon	50	2	8
Italian	35	2	4
Parmesan Peppercorn Ranch	50	2	7
Ranch	40	2	5
Thousand Island	50	2	9
Fat-Free:			
Chunky Blue Cheese	35	0	7
Italian	20	0	4
Ranch	30	0	7
Oil & Vinegar: Balsamic Vinaigrette	50	5	3
House Italian	100	10	3
Red Wine Vinaigrette	80	5	9
Robusto Italian	80	7	4
Light Vinaigrette: Balsamic & Basil	60	5	3
Asian with Sesame & Ginger	70	5	6
Raspberry Walnut	80	5	7
Salad Spritzers: Average all flavors, 10 sprays (¼ fl.oz) for 1 cup salad	10	1	1

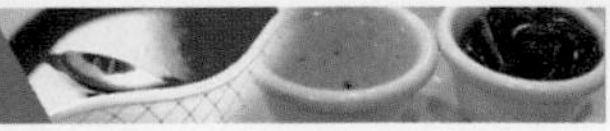

Gravy

	C	F	Cb
Homemade Gravy, average:			
Thin, little fat, 2 Tbsp, 1 oz	20	1	3
Thick, 2 Tbsp, 1¼ oz	50	2	9
¼ cup, 2½ oz	100	4	18
Pillsbury (Gravy Mixes): *Prepared*			
Brown; Homestyle, ¼ cup, 2 oz	15	0	3
Chicken, ¼ cup, 2 oz	20	0	4

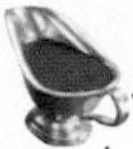

Gravy-In-Jars-Homestyle

	C	F	Cb
Boston Market, ¼ cup, 2 oz	40	2	3
Franco-American (In Jars):			
99% Fat Free, ¼ cup, 2 oz	25	0.5	3
Heinz, Regular, all flavors, ¼ cup, 2 oz	25	0	4
Fat Free Roast Turkey, ¼ cup, 2 oz	20	0	4
Vons, all flavors, ¼ cup, 2 oz	20	0.5	4

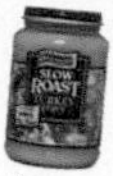

Tomato Products

	C	F	Cb
Whole/Chopped/Crushed/Diced			
1 cup, 8½ oz	50	0	10
In Aspic, ½ cup	50	0	12
With Green Chili, 1 cup, 8½ oz	60	0	16
Stewed, ½ cup, 1.7 oz	40	1.5	6.5
Wedges in Tomato Juice, 1 cup	70	0.5	18
Salsa, average, 1 Tbsp	15	0	3.5
Tomato Ketchup:			
Regular: 1 Tbsp, ½ oz	15	0	4
Single Serve, 1 packet	10	0	3
One-Carb (*Heinz*), 1 Tbsp, ½ oz	5	0	1
Tomato Paste, 2 Tbsp, 1 oz	25	0	6
Regular, ¾ cup, 6 oz	140	1	32
Tomato Puree, ½ cup, 4½ oz	50	0	10
Tomato Sauce:			
Regular, ½ cup, 4.4 oz	50	0	11
Spanish Style, ½ cup, 4.3 oz	40	0	9
With Mushr., ½ cup, 4.3 oz	45	0	10
With Onions, ½ cup, 4.3 oz	50	0	12
Tomato Seasoning, 3 tsp	20	0	4
Sundried Tomatoes:			
Natural, 5-6 pieces, 0.4 oz	22	0	5
In Oil, drained, 6 pieces, ½ oz	40	2.5	4

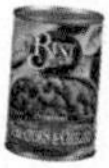

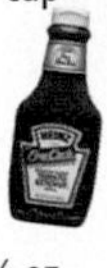

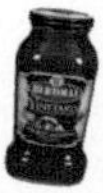

Sauces ~ Brands

	C	F	Cb
A-1			
Steak & Marinades Sauce: *Per Tablespoon (½ oz)*			
Bold & Spicy; Teriyaki; New York	20	0	5
Carb Well Steak Sauce	5	0	1
Chicago	20	1	3
Jamaican Jerk	25	0.5	5
New Orleans Cajun	25	0	5
Steak Sauce	15	0	3
Barilla: *Per ½ Cup*			
Green & Black Olives	80	3	10
Roasted Garlic	60	1	12
Average other varieties	70	2.5	12
Bertolli: *Per ½ Cup*			
Italian Sausage	100	3	15
Olive Oil & Garlic	90	3	14
Marinara; Roast Pepper, av.	80	2	13
Portobello with Merlot	80	2.5	12
Tomato & Basil	80	2	13
Vineyard Selection, Marinara	80	2	14
Best Foods/Hellmann's: *Per 2 Tbsp*			
Tartar Sauce	80	7	4
Buitoni			
Pasta Sauces: *Per ½ Cup Serving, 4½ oz*			
Alfredo	130	11	4
Light Alfredo	90	6	5
Marinara	70	3	10
With Roasted Garlic	60	1.5	10
Pesto: With Basil	300	28	6
Reduced Fat	240	14	9
Tomato Herb Parmesan	130	8	10
Vodka	100	7	7
Bull's Eye: *Per 2 Tbsp*			
Original BBQ Sauce	50	0	13
Sweet & Tangy	60	0	13
Catelli			
Garden Select Pizza Sauce, av.,1 fl.oz	65	0.5	1
Meat Sauce, ½ cup, 4 oz	85	2.5	11
Garden Select 6 Vege Recipe Sauce: *Per ½ Cup*			
Parmesan & Romano	80	2.5	12
Thick & Chunky, Diced Tomato & Basil	70	1.5	12
Other varieties, average	80	1.5	13

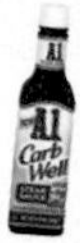

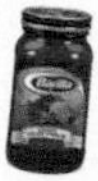

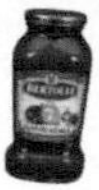

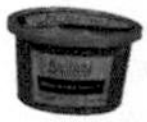

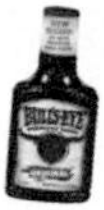

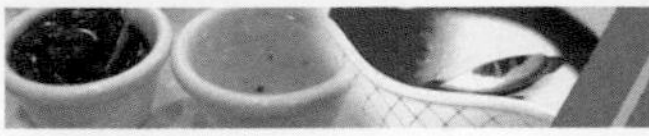

Brands (Cont)

	C	F	Cb
Cento: *Per ½ Cup*			
Sauces: Passata Tomatoes	30	0	5
All Natural: Pasta	50	3	3
Pizza	40	1.5	6
Tomato: Arrabbiata	140	9	12
Marinara	120	9	9
Puttanesca	140	9	12
White Clam	170	15	4
Classico: *Per ½ Cup Unless Indicated*			
Organic Spinach & Garlic	70	2	11
Rsted Red Pepper Alfredo, ¼ cup	60	5	3
Spicy Tomato & Basil	90	3.5	12
Signature Recipes Sauce:			
Basil Pesto, ¼ cup	230	21	6
Cabernet Marinara with Herbs	70	2	11
Caramelized Onion & Roasted Garlic	85	3	13
Creamy Alfredo, ¼ cup	100	9	3
Fire Roasted Tomato & Garlic	50	1	8
Florentine Spinach & Cheese	80	4	9
Mushrooms & Ripe Olives	60	2	10
Spicy Red Pepper	60	2.5	8
Spicy Tomato & Pesto	90	5	10
Sun-Dried Tomato	80	4	11
Traditional Favorites Sauce: *Per ½ Cup*			
Four Cheese	80	3	12
Italian Sausage with Peppers & Onions	80	3	10
Roasted Garlic	50	1	9
Colgin, Liquid Smoke	0	0	0
Contadina: *Per ¼ Cup*			
Pizza Sauce: Flavored w/ Pepperoni	35	1	5
Original; Four Cheese, average	30	0.5	6
Cooking Sauce: Sweet & Sour, 1 Tbsp	40	1	8
Tomato Sauce, average, ¼ cup	20	0	4
Crosse & Blackwell: *Per 1 Tbsp*			
Ham Glaze	25	0	7
Mint Sauce	5	0	1
Del Monte			
Spaghetti Sauces: *Per ½ Cup*			
with Four Cheeses	70	1.5	15
with Meat/Mushrooms, av.	60	1	14
Other varieties, average	75	1	16
Chunky Sauce: Garlic & Herb	60	1.5	11
Italian Herb	60	1	12
Sloppy Joe Sauce, Original, ¼ cup	50	0	11

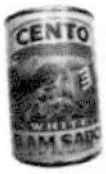

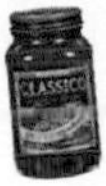

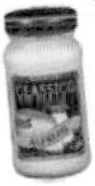

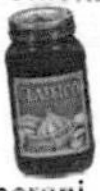

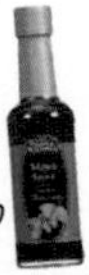

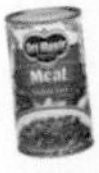

	C	F	Cb
Emiril's			
Pasta Sauces: *Per ½ Cup*			
Homestyle Marinara	90	3	14
Kicked Up Tomato	80	3.5	11
Puttanesca	80	5	9
Roasted Gaaahlic	80	3.5	12
Roasted Red Pepper	70	3.5	9
Vodka Sauce	110	7	12
Francesco Rinaldi: *Per ½ Cup*			
Traditional: Original	80	3.5	12
Meat/Mushroom	80	3	12
Average other varieties	70	2.5	12
French's			
Worcestershire Sauce, 1 tsp	60	0	1
Heinz: *Per 1 Tbsp*			
57	20	0	4
Barbecue Sauces, all flavors	35	0	9
Chili Sauce	20	0	5
Horseradish Sauce	75	6	2
Tomato Ketchup: Regular	15	0	4
Reduced Sugar	5	0	1
Worcestershire Sauce, 1 Tbsp	10	0	1
Original Cocktail Sauce,			
¼ cup, 2.2 oz	60	0	15
House of Tsang: *Per 1 Tbsp (Approx. ½ oz)*			
Bangkok Peanut	45	2.5	4
Classic Stir Fry	25	1	4
Ginger Soy	20	0	4
General Tsao	45	0.5	10
Hibachi Grill: Kobe Steak	50	4	3
Hunan Smokehut	40	1	8
Sweet Ginger Sesame	40	1	8
Thai Peanut	50	3	5
Tokyo Teriyaki	40	0	10
Hoisin, 1 tsp	15	0	4
Imperial Citrus Stir-Fry	25	0	5
Korean Teriyaki Stir-Fry	35	1.5	5
Mandarin Marinade	25	0	6
Oyster	30	0	7
Saigon Sizzle Stir-Fry	45	2	7
Sweet & Sour Stir-Fry	35	0	9
Szechuan Spicy Stir-Fry	25	1	4
Hunt's			
BBQ Sauce: Original, 2 Tbsp	60	0	15
Hickory & Brown Sugar, 2 Tbsp	70	0	18
Manwich Sloppy Joe Sauce, ¼ cup	40	0	9
Spaghetti Sauce: *Per ½ Cup*			
Classic Italian: Four Cheese	50	1	10
Garlic & Herb	40	1	8
Zesty & Spicy	60	2	10
Original Style: Traditional	50	1	10
Meat Flavor	60	1	11

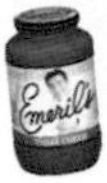

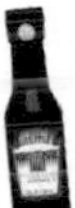

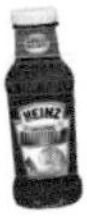

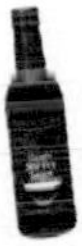

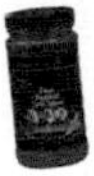

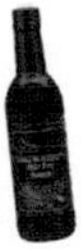

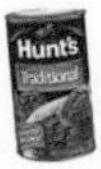

Brands (Cont)

	C	F	Cb
Kikkoman Marinades			
Black Bean Sauce, 2 Tbsp	50	1	6
Hoisin Sauce, 2 Tbsp	80	1.5	17
Honey Mustard, 1Tbsp	30	0	6
Roasted Garlic & Herbs, 1 Tbsp	20	0	4
Teriyaki, 1 Tbsp	15	0	2
Teriyaki Roasted Garlic, 1 Tbsp	25	0	4
Knorr			
Classic Sauce: *Per 2 Tbsp*			
Bernaise:			
Prepared with Whole Milk	65	5.5	3
Prepared with Non-Fat Milk	60	4.5	3
Hollandaise:			
Prepared with Whole Milk	65	5.5	3
Prepared with Non-Fat Milk	60	4.5	3
Classic Brown Gravy, av., ¼ cup	20	0.5	3
Kraft			
Specialty Sauce: Cocktail, 2 Tbsp	60	0.5	11
Coleslaw Maker, 1 oz	110	9	7
Horseradish, 1 tsp	15	1.5	1
Sandwich Spread, 1 Tbsp	35	2.5	3
Sweet 'n Sour, 2 Tbsp	60	0	13
Tartar: Original, 1 Tbsp	60	4.5	4
Fat-Free, 1 Tbsp	25	0	5
Hot & Spicy, 1 Tbsp	70	6	4
Barbecue Sauces, average, 2 Tbsp	50	0.5	12
Las Palmas			
Red Chile Sauce, ¼ cup, 2 oz	15	0.5	2
Enchilada Sauce: Green Chile	25	1.5	3
Hot Red Original, ¼ cup, 2 oz	15	0.5	2
Lawry's 30 Minute Marinade: *Per Tbsp*			
Caribbean Jerk; Teriyaki, av.	25	0	5
Herb & Garlic	10	0	2
Lemon Pepper	10	0	2
Mesquite; Steak & Chop	5	0	1
Sesame Ginger	30	0	7
Packet Seasonings: *Per 2 teaspoons (Dry)*			
Fajitas; Taco, average	10	0	3
Average other flavors	20	0	4
Lea & Perrins			
Worcestershire Sauce: 1 tsp	5	0	1
Thick, 2 Tbsp	30	0	8
McCormicks			
Seafood Sauces: *Per ¼ Cup*			
Cajun Seafood Sauce, 2 Tbsp, 1.1 oz	15	0	3
Cocktail Sauce, Original/Extra Hot	90	0.5	19
Tartar Sauce, Fat Free, 2 T., 1 oz	30	0	7
Scampi Seafood Sauce, 2 Tbsp, 1 oz	160	17	2

	C	F	Cb
Mrs. Dash:			
Marinades (Salt-Free)			
Garlic Lime, 1 Tbsp	30	1.5	4
Lemon Herb Peppercorn, 1 Tbsp	25	2	2
Southwestern Chipotle, 1 T.	20	1.5	2
Spicy Teriyaki, 1 Tbsp	25	1	5
Newman's Own: *Per ½ Cup*			
Bombolina (Tomato & Basil)	90	4.5	13
Five Cheese	80	3	10
Fra Diavolo	70	3	10
Marinara; Sockarooni	70	2	12
Roasted Garlic & Peppers	70	2.5	11
Vodka	110	5	11
Old El Paso			
Enchilada Sauce:			
Green Chile, ¼ cup	25	1.5	4
Other varieties, ¼ cup	25	1	3
Sauce Mixes, 2 tsp	10	0	2
Picante Sauce, 2 Tbsp	10	0	2
Taco Sauce, 1 Tbsp	5	0	1
Salsas, Thick & Chunky:			
Medium, 2 Tbsp	10	0	2
Mild, 2 Tbsp	10	0	2
Pace: *Per 2 Tbsp*			
Chunky Salsa	10	0	2
Picante Sauce	10	0	2
Mexican Four Cheese,			
Salsa Con Queso	90	7	5
Prego: *Per ½ Cup*			
Classic Italian Sauce: Marinara	80	3	10
Flavored with Meat	80	2.5	13
Fresh Mushroom	70	1.5	13
Italian Sausage & Garlic	90	3	13
Mini Meatball	100	3	13
Mushroom & Garlic	80	2.5	13
Roasted Garlic Parmesan	70	1	13
Three Cheese; Tom. Basil & Garlic, av.	80	2	13
Traditional	70	1.5	13
Chunky Garden:			
Combo	70	1.5	13
Mushroom Supreme	90	3	13
Other varieties, average	90	3	13
Heart Smart: Traditional Italian	70	1.5	13
Mushroom Italian	70	1.5	13
Premier Japan			
Hoisin	15	0	3
Tamari; Ginger; Wasabi	5	0	1

Updated Nutrition Data ~ www.CalorieKing.com
Persons with Diabetes ~ See Disclaimer (Page 22)

Brands (Cont)

Ragu: *Per ½ cup Unless Indicated*

	C	F	Cb
Pizza Quick Sauce, *Per ¼ Cup*			
Traditional	40	2	6
Pizza Sauce, Homemade Style, ¼ cup	30	1	5
Cheesy: *Per ¼ Cup*			
Classic Alfredo	110	10	2
Light Parmesan	70	5	3
Roasted Garlic Parmesan	110	10	3
Per ½ Cup (Unless Indicated)			
Chunky:			
Mushroom & Green Pepper	80	2.5	12
Average other varieties	80	2.5	12
Light varieties, average	50	0	10
Old World Style: Margherita	70	2	10
Meat Flavor	70	3	9
Mushroom; Traditional	70	2.5	10
Organic: Garden Veggie	80	2.5	12
Traditional	80	3	11
Robusto: 7 Herb Tomato	80	3	12
Chopped Tomato, Olive Oil & Garlic	95	5	10
Roasted Garlic	80	2.5	13
Sauteed Onion & Garlic	90	3.5	12
Six Cheese	90	3	12

Safeway Select

	C	F	Cb
Salsa, average all flavors, 2 Tbsp	15	0	3
Select Sauces: *Per ½ Cup*			
Arrabbiata	110	8	10
Artichoke Pesto	60	2	9
Four Cheese	70	3	10
Garlic Basil	70	4	9
Marinara	60	2	10
Spicy Red Bell Pepper	50	1	9
Sundried Tomato & Olive	70	0	12
Tomato Alfredo	130	10	9
Vodka	130	10	9
Tony Roma's			
Wing Sauce, 1 Tbsp	15	1	0
Trader Joe's, BBQ Sauce,			
Kansas City Style, 2 Tbsp	60	0	15
Walnut Acres: *Per ½ Cup, 125g*			
Marinara & Zinfandel	50	1	9
Tomato & Basil	50	1	9
Low Sodium	40	0	9
Tomato & Mushroom	50	1	9

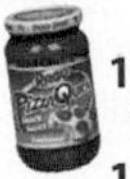

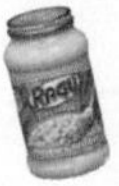

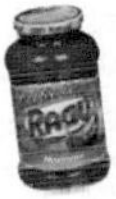

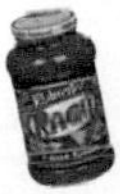

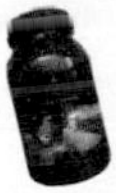

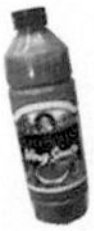

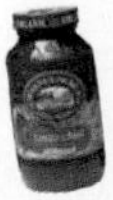

Seasonings & Flavorings

	C	F	Cb
Accent, Flavor Enhancer, 1 tsp	0	0	0
Angostura Bitters, 1 tsp	15	0	4
Bacon Bits, average, 1 Tbsp	35	2	2
Bacon Chips (Durkee), 1 Tbsp	30	1	2
Bac-Os (Betty Crocker),			
1½ Tbsp	20	1	1.5
Bragg Liquid Aminos, 1 tsp	0	0	0
Butter Buds, 1 tsp	5	0	2
Garlic Bread Sprinkle, 1 tsp	8	0.5	1
Garlic Salt, 1 tsp	2	0	0
Italian Seasoning, 1 tsp	4	0	1
Lemon Pepper Seasoning, 1 tsp	7	0	1
Meat Tenderizer, average, 1 tsp	7	0	1
Molly McButter, 1 tsp	5	1	1
Mrs Dash, Blends, 1 tsp	0	0	0
Old Bay, Seasoning, ¼ tsp	0	0	0
Salad Crunchies (McCormick), 1 tsp	10	0.5	2
Salt: Regular, Sea Salt, Lite Salt	0	0	0
Seasoning Mixes, av., ¼ package	70	1	9
Taco Seasoning, av., ¼ package	30	0.5	4
Old El Paso: Chili Season. Mix, 1 T.	8	0.5	1.5
Cheesy Taco Seasoning Mix, 1 Tbsp	10	0.5	2
Taco/Burrito Seasoning Mix, 2 tsp	15	0	4
Fajita Seasoning Mix, 1 tsp	5	0	1.5
Vegit Seasoning Mix, ¼ tsp	0	0	0

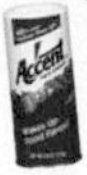

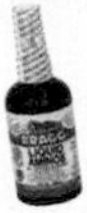

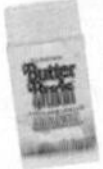

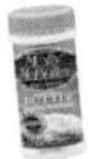

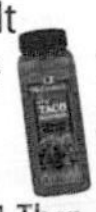

Spices & Herbs

	C	F	Cb
Per Teaspoon: Average all types	5	0	1
All Purpose, 1 tsp	0	0	0
Allspice, ground	5	0	1
Chili Powder	8	0	1
Cinnamon, ground	6	0	2
Curry Powder	6	0	1
Garlic Powder	9	0	2
Nutmeg, ground	12	0	1
Onion Powder	7	0	2
Parsley, dried	4	0	1
Pepper, average	6	0	1
Saffron	2	0	0
Salt-Free Blends, 1 tsp	0	0	0
Tumeric, ground	8	0	1
Seeds: Fenugreek	12	1	2
Mustard, Poppyseed	15	1	1
Other types, average	7	0	1

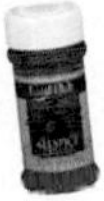

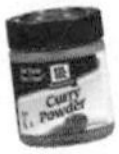

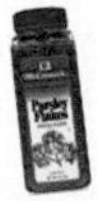

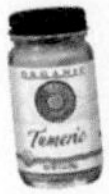

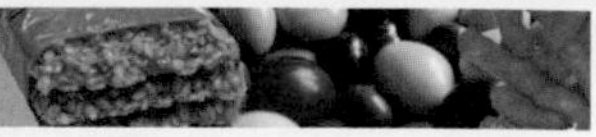

Home-Popped Popcorn

	C	F	Cb
Popping Corn Kernels:			
2 Tbsp, 1 oz	110	1	26
(makes approximately 5 cups)			
Air-popped (without oil), plain, 1 oz	110	1	22
1 cup, 0.2 oz	20	0	5
Oil-popped, plain, 1 oz	145	8	16
1 cup, 0.4 oz	55	3	6
Popcorn Oil, 1 Tbsp	120	14	0

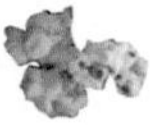

Microwave Popcorn

Average all Brands: Per 1 Cup Popped, Unless Indicated

	C	F	Cb
Butter: Regular	35	2	4
Light	25	1	4
Act II Popcorn:			
Butter, 0.3 oz	30	2	4
5 cups, 1 oz	160	10	18
Light Butter, 0.2 oz	25	1	4
5 cups, 1 oz	110	4.5	19
Butter Lovers, 0.3 oz	35	2.5	4
4½ cups, 1 oz	170	12	16
94% Fat-Free Butter	30	1.5	4.5
4½ cups, 1 oz	130	2.5	28
American Fare (K-Mart):			
Butter, 0.3 oz	40	2	5
3 cups, 1 oz	120	2	23
Theater Butter, 1 cup	40	2	5
3½ cups	140	8	15
Jolly Time:			
America's Best	20	0	4
Blast O Butter: Reg.	45	3	5
Light	30	1.5	4
Healthy Pop: Butter Flavor	20	0	4
Caramel Apple	20	0	5
Newman's Own: Butter Flavor, 3½ c.	130	5	18
Light Butter Flavor, 3½ cups	140	4.5	22
Orville Redenbacher's:			
Movie Theater Butter	35	2	3
4½ cups, popped	170	12	16
Smart Pop!:			
Butter, 6½ cups	110	2	24
100 Calorie Mini Bags (1)	100	2	24
Tender White	40	3	3
Pop Secret:			
1-Step, Cheddar	40	2.5	3
100 Calorie Pop, Butter	15	0.5	3
Butter	40	2.5	3
Extra Butter	40	2.5	3
Homestyle	20	1	3
Light Butter	20	1	3
Movie Theater Butter	40	2.5	4
94% Fat-Free: Butter	20	0	4
Kettle Corn	15	0	4
Smart Balance, Light Butter, 1 cup	25	1	3

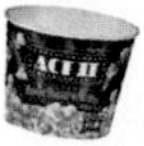

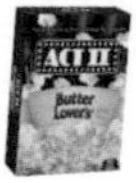

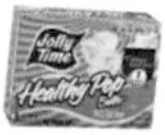

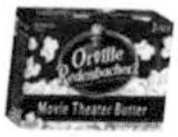

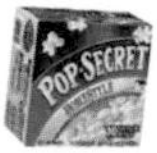

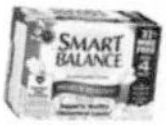

Bagged Popcorn

Average All Brands (Ready-to-Eat)

	C	F	Cb
Regular/Plain: ½ oz package	80	5	8
1 oz package	160	10	16
4 oz package	640	40	64
2 oz Box (store/airport)	320	16	32
3 oz Bag (9" high x 5" wide)	480	24	48
Caramel Popcorn,			
without nuts, 1 cup, 2 oz	240	4	46

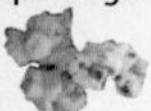

Brands ~ Bagged Popcorn

7-Select (7-11): Popcorn, 1.5 oz pkg	230	16	21
Boston's: Lite, 3½ cups, 1 oz	130	4.5	20
Homestyle, 2½ cups, 1 oz	160	9	18
Cracker Jack: Original,			
½ cup, 1 oz	120	2	23
1 cup, 2 oz	240	4	46
99-Cents Package, 3⅜ oz	410	7	78
Crunch 'N Munch			
Caramel			
⅔ cup, 1 oz	85	4	11
1 cup, 2 oz	170	8	22
4 oz box	335	17	42
7.5 oz box	630	32	70
10 oz box	840	42	105
Fiddle Faddle:			
Butter Toffee/Caramel			
1 oz	120	3.5	22
1 cup, 2 oz	240	7	44
8 oz box	960	28	176
Jay's: Fat Free Caramel Corn, ¾ cup	110	0	26
Korn Krunch: (Kornfections & Treasures):			
Almond Pecan (Sugar Free), 1 oz	150	8	19
Orville Redenbacher's:			
Popcorn Cakes, Minis, average, (8)	60	1	12
PopCorners, Butter/Kettle, 1 oz	120	3.5	21
Poppycock: Pecan Delight, ½ cup	150	8	20
Original Clusters, ½ cup, 1 oz	160	8	20

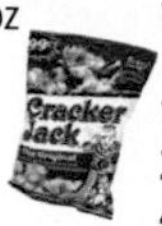

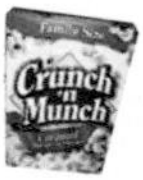

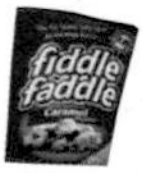

Movie Theater Popcorn

Small (7 cups): Plain	385	21	44
With Butter (3 pumps, ¾ oz)	570	42	44
Medium (15 cups): Plain	825	45	94
With Butter (4 pumps, 1 oz)	1075	73	94
Large (20 cups): Plain	1100	60	124
With Butter (6 pumps, 1½ oz)	1485	102	124
Butter: 1 Pump, ¼ oz	65	7	0
4 Pumps (2 Tbsp), 1 oz	250	28	0

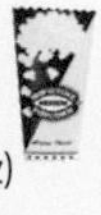

Updated Nutrition Data ~ www.CalorieKing.com
Persons with Diabetes ~ See Disclaimer (Page 22)

Corn & Tortilla Chips

Average All Brands	C	F	Cb
Corn Chips:			
Average all types, 1 oz	150	8	18
8 oz bag	1200	64	144
Fritos, Original, 32 chips, 1 oz	160	10	15
Tortilla Chips: Average, 1 oz	140	7	18
(1 oz = approx. 12 chips or 13 strips)			
Doritos: 13 chips, 1 oz	140	7	18
White Nacho Cheese, 1 oz	150	8	17
Reduced Fat (13), 1 oz	130	5	19
Baked! Nacho Cheese (15), 1 oz	120	3.5	21
Snyder's, Multigrain, 1 oz	130	5	20
Stacy's,			
Simply Naked Pita Chips (14), 1 oz	130	5	19
Utz Reduced-Fat Baked,			
10 chips, 1 oz	140	7	18
Tostitos:			
Crispy Rounds, 1 oz	140	7	19
Multigrain, 1 oz	140	7	19

Potato Chips/Crisps

Average All Brands	C	F	Cb
Regular:			
Plain or flavored, (2 chips)	15	1	1.5
1 oz package (20 chips)	150	10	15
4 oz quantity	600	40	60
14 oz package	2100	140	210
Brands:			
Lay's Classic, 1 oz	150	10	15
Lay's Stax, av. all, 1 oz	150	10	15
Pringles: Original (16)	150	9	15
Large, 6.41 oz can	960	58	96
Minis, 1 bag, 0.8 oz	140	9	16
Snack Stack, 0.8 oz tub	120	8	12
Extreme, av., (15), 1 oz	150	9	15
Multi Grain, all flavors, 1 oz	140	8	16
Ruffles, 12 chips, 1 oz	160	10	14
Reduced Fat:			
Pringles, 16 Chips, 1 oz	140	7	17
Sun Chips, Original			
16 chips, 1 oz	140	6	18
Low-Fat/Baked:			
Lay's Baked!, Original (15), 1 oz	120	2	23
Ruffles Baked!: Original (9),1 oz	120	3	21
Cheddar Sour Cream (10), 1 oz	120	3	22
Baked! Tostitos Scoops (15) 1 oz	120	3	22
Fat Free: *Lay's Light,* Original, 1 oz	75	0	17
Pringles (Fat-Free) (15). 1 oz	70	0	15

Pretzels

Average All Brands	C	F	Cb
Hard-Baked Pretzels: *Each*			
1 oz quantity	100	0	22
Sticks, thin, 2¼" (9/oz)	12	0	3
Twists, thin, ¼" thick, (5/oz)	25	0	5
Dutch (2¾"x 2⅝") ½ oz	55	1	11
Sourdough *(Snyder's)*, ¾ oz	100	0	22
Soft Pretzels (Twists) average: *Each*			
Plain: Regular, 2.2 oz	210	2	43
King Size, 5.1 oz	485	4.5	99
New York Street Vendors, 7 oz	660	6	135
Big Cheese, 1.76 oz	130	3	22
Peanut Butter filled *(Tr. Joe's)* 1 oz	150	8	14
Choc-Coated *(Snyders)*, 1 oz	140	6	18
White Choc covered, 7 pieces, 1 oz	140	6	19

Brands ~ Pretzels

	C	F	Cb
7-Select:			
Choc Covered Pretzels			
10 pieces, 2 oz	265	13	35
1 pkg (4 oz), actual weight, 4.75 oz	630	30	84
Rold Gold *(Frito-Lay)*			
Braided Twists,			
Honey Wheat (8), 1 oz	110	1	23
Classic: Pretzel Sticks, 1 oz	100	0	23
Rods; Tiny Twists, 1 oz	110	1	23
Fat-Free, Tiny Twists, 1 oz	100	0	23
Snyder's of Hanover Pretzels			
100 Calorie Pack, Snaps, 0.9 oz	100	0.5	22
Multigrain:			
Pretzel Sticks, 1 oz	120	2	23
Pretzel Nibblers,			
Honey Mustard, 1 oz	130	3	23
Homestyle (15), 1 oz	120	1	25
Mini (20), 1 oz	110	0	25
Nibblers, all flavors (16), 1 oz	130	3	24
Rods (3), 1 oz	120	1	24
Thins, 1 oz	110	0	23
SuperPretzel: Soft Pretzels (1)	160	1	34
Softstix (2)	130	3	22
Soft Pretzel Bites (5)	150	0.5	32
Pretzelfils: Pizza (2)	120	2	20
Pepperjack; Mozzarella, (2)	130	4.5	19
Utz: Pretzels, average, 1 oz	110	1	21
Real Choc-covered Pretzels (2)	120	8	17

Snacks | C | F | Cb

Note: Actual weight of packaged snacks is usually 5-10% more than label Net Wt. For accuracy, weigh snack and allow extra calories, fat and carbs for any extra weight.

	C	F	Cb
Apple Chips *(Seneca)*, 1 oz	150	9	18
Bagel Crisps *(N.Y. Style)* 6 crisps, 1 oz	130	5	17
Banana Chips, ¼ cup, 13 chips, 1 oz	150	7	21
Beef Jerky *(Lance)*, average, 1 oz	70	1	4
Bugles, Original, 1⅓ cup, 1 oz	160	9	18
Cheese Balls *(Utz)*, 1 oz package	130	7	16
Cheese Crackers *(Lance)* (6), 1.4 oz	190	9	25
Cheese Curls: 1 cup, 1 oz	150	8	16
Cheese Nips, 1.25 oz package	170	7	22
Cheese Puffs: Average, 1 oz	160	10	15
American Fare, 1½ cup, 1 oz	160	11	13
Snyder's Multigrain, 1 oz	130	6	19
Cheese Twists (Snyders),1 oz	140	8	15
Cheerios, Snack Mix,			
average, ⅔ cup, 1.1 oz	125	3.5	22
Cheetos: Average all flavors, 1 oz	160	10	15
4 oz package	640	40	60
Baked!, 1 oz	130	5	19
Cheez Balls, 27 balls, 1 oz	150	9	11
Cheez-It Crackers:			
Average all flavors, 1 oz	150	7	18
1.25 oz package	190	9	24
3 oz package	420	21	57
Reduced Fat, 1 oz	130	4.5	20
Party Mix, ½ cup, 1 oz	130	4.5	20
Chex *(General Mills)*:			
100 Calorie Pouch, average	100	3	18
Mix, Bold Party Blend, ½ cup, 1 oz	120	4	18
Chips Ahoy! Choc Chip Cookies,			
1.4 oz package	190	9	27
Mini: 3 oz package	410	20	57
Go-Pak!, 4 oz cup	550	27	77
Snak-Saks, 8 oz pkg	1100	51	154
Churros *(Mex. Pastry)* 10", 1 oz	100	5	12
Combos *(Oven Baked)*:			
Crackers, ⅓ cup, 1 oz	140	6	18
1 cup, 3 oz	420	18	54
Pretzels, ⅓ cup, 1 oz	130	4.5	19
1 cup, 3 oz	390	14	57
Cookies: *See Pages 81*			
Cool Cuts, Carrot & Ranch, 2.3 oz	70	5	5
Corn Chips: *See Page 149*			
Corn Crunchies/Spirals, 1 oz	95	0	22
Corn Nuts: ⅓ cup, 1 oz	130	4.5	20
1.7 oz bag	220	7.5	34
Corn Puffs: *(Pirate's Booty)*, 1 oz	130	5	18
Wotsits *(Walker)*, ¾ oz package	105	6.5	11
Dunkin Stixs *(Hostess)*, 3, 4oz	490	25	63

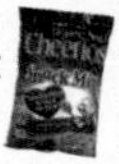

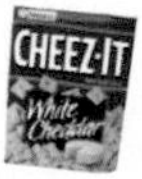

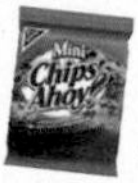

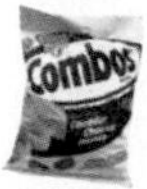

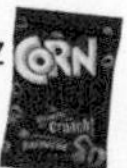

Snacks (Cont) | C | F | Cb

	C	F	Cb
Fig Newtons: Regular, 2 oz package	200	4	39
Fat-Free, 2.1 oz package	180	0	44
Minis, Fig/Strawb., av., 1.34 oz pkg	130	3	27
Flavor Twists *(Fritos)*, 1 oz	160	10	16
French's Potato Sticks ¾ cup, 1 oz	180	12	16
Genisoy Soy Crisps, average, 1 oz	120	3	17
Garden Harvest Tst'd Chips, av., 1 oz	120	3.5	20
Goldfish *(Pepperidge Farm)* 1 oz	140	5	20
Gold-N-Chees *(Lance)*, 1 oz	150	8	17
Hot Peanuts *(Lays)*, 3½ oz	310	25	10
Jerky (Beef), 1 oz stick	70	1	4
Lance S'wich Crackers, av., 1.4 oz	180	9	23
Munchies Snack Mix *(Frito-Lay)*:			
Cheese Fix, ¾ cup	140	7	18
Flaming; Totally Ranch, ¾ c.	140	6	19
Munchos, 16 pieces, 1 oz	160	10	16
Nibblers: Garlic Bread (13), 1 oz	130	3	24
Fat Free, Sourdough (16), 1 oz	120	0	25
Nutter Butter: Sandwich Cookies			
Singles, 1.9 oz package	250	10	37
Bites: 1.25 oz package	170	7	24
Milk Choc-Covered, 2.54 oz pkg	350	17	48
Onion Rings *(T.G.I. Friday)*, 1 oz	130	6	19
Oreo: 100 Calorie Pack, 0.84 oz	100	3	16
2 Go! (4 cookies), 2 oz	270	11	41
Double Stuf, 1.5 oz package	210	10	30
Mini Bite Size: (9 cookies), 1.25 oz	170	7	25
Go-Pak, 4 oz cup	530	22	81
Snak-Saks, 8 oz package	1040	48	168
Oreo Cakesters, 2 oz pkg	250	12	36
Oriental Mix *(Rice Snacks)*, 1 oz	125	3.5	21
Oyster Crackers *(Sunshine)*, 1 oz	60	1.5	11
Peanut Butter Nuggets (10), 1 oz	140	6	15
Pirate's Booty:			
1 oz bag	130	5	19
4 oz bag	520	20	76
With Caramel, 2.75 oz bag	330	5.5	63
Pirate's Cannon Balls: 1 oz bag	130	5	18
5 oz bag	715	27	99
Pita Chips, average, (9) 1 oz	130	4	18
PopCorners, Butter/Kettle, 1 oz	120	3.5	21
Popcorn: *See Page 148*			
Pork Cracklins, 1 oz	180	14	0
Pork Skins/Rinds, 1 oz	160	10	0
Baken-ets, 99c pkg, 1¼ oz	200	13	0
Mission, 3 oz package	480	27	0
Potato Chips: *See Page 149*			
Potato Skins *(TGI Friday)* (16), 1 oz	130	9	24
Pretzels *(Snyder's)*, 2 oz, average	280	14	36

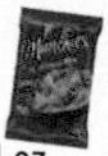

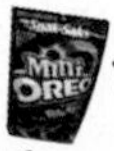

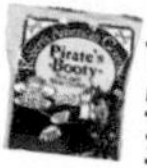

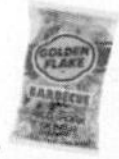

Snacks (Cont)

	C	F	Cb
Quakes Rice Snacks, average, 1 oz	130	4	26
Quaker Mini Delights, av.,1 bag, 0.7 oz	90	3.5	16
Rice Chips, Bar-B-Q/Onion, 1 oz	140	7	18
Ritz Bits S'wiches:			
Cheese: 1.5 oz package	220	13	24
Carry Me Pack, 2 oz	290	17	33
Go-Pak, 1 oz	150	9	17
P'nut Butter: 1.25 oz package	170	10	20
Big Bag (99cents), 3 oz	420	23	48
Sandwich Crackers *(Austin):* Per Pkg			
Cheese Cracker w/ Cheddar, 1.38 oz	190	10	23
Cheese Cracker w/ Pnut Butter, 1.38 oz	190	10	23
PB & J Flavored, 1.38 oz	190	8	26
Sesame Sticks *(Cityfarm),* 1 oz	160	9	13
Smart Puffs *(Pirates Booty),* 1.37 oz	180	8	23
Snack Mix *(Quaker):*			
Baked Cheddar, 1 oz	130	4.5	19
Kids Mix, 1 oz	130	4.5	20
Snackwells Cookies, Pack 2 Go!, 1.7oz	210	5	38
Soy Crisps, average,1 oz	120	3	17
Soy Nuts: Dry Roasted, ¼ cup, 1 oz	130	6	9
Choc-coated, 1 oz	140	7	13
Sunflower Chips: *(Snyders)*			
100 Calorie Snack Pack (1)	100	4.5	14
Multigrain, all flavors, 1 oz	140	6	20
Takis Fajitas (12), 1 oz	140	7	17
4 oz package	560	28	68
TastyKake:			
Koffee Kake Jr., 2½ oz	280	10	45
Chocolate Jr., 3.3 oz	340	12	65
Creme Filled Koffee Kakes (2)	230	10	25
Tings *(Robert's),* 2 oz bag	300	14	36
Toasted Cheese Crackers, 1 package	220	11	23
Tortilla Chips: *Page 149*			
Tostitos:			
Blue; Yellow; Scoops,			
average, 1 oz	140	7	19
Multigrain, 1 oz	150	8	18
Trader Joe's, Cheese Crunchies, 1 oz	130	6	19
7 oz package	910	42	133
Trail Mix (Nuts/Seeds/Dried Fruit):			
Regular, 3 Tbsp, 1 oz	140	9	13
Tropical, 3 Tbsp, 1 oz	130	7	16
Turkey Jerky: Teriyaki *(Oberto),* 1 oz	70	1	8
BBQ Beef; Hot & Spicy, average, 1 oz	90	1	6
Veggie Crisps, *(Snyder's),* 1 oz	140	7	20
Wasabi Peas, ¼ cup, 1 oz	120	3	19
Yogurt Pretzels (7), 1.5 oz	190	7	30
Yogurt Raisins *(Sun-Maid),* 1 oz	120	4.5	20

Fruit Snacks

	C	F	Cb
Betty Crocker: Fruit Gushers, 0.9 oz	90	1	20
Fruit by the Foot, 1 roll, 0.75 oz	80	1	17
Fruit Roll Ups: 1 roll, ½ oz	50	1	12
Scooby Doo; G-Force, 0.9 oz	90	0	21
General Mills:			
Dora the Explora , 0.9 oz	90	0	21
Other varieties	90	0	21
Kellogg's: Disney Fruit Snacks, 0.9 oz	80	0	19
Fruit Streamers, 1 Roll	80	1	17
Rolls,1 pouch, 0.63 oz	70	1.5	14
Yogos Bits, av., 0.7 oz	80	1.5	16
Sunkist: Fruit Snacks, 1 pouch	90	0	21
Fruit Smoothie Blitz, 1.3 oz	140	1	32

Vending Machines

	C	F	Cb
Cheese Balls *(Utz),* 1 oz	130	7	16
Chips Ahoy, Choc Chip Cookies 1.4 oz	190	9	27
Choc Milk, 8 fl.oz	260	9	36
Coca-Cola Classic, 12 fl.oz	145	0	40
Diet Coke, 12 fl oz	0	0	0
Corn Chips, 1 oz	160	10	16
Hostess Sweet Roll, 4¼ oz	400	12	69
Donut, plain, 1.4 oz	160	9	18
Fruit Pie *(Hostess),* 4½ oz	480	20	68
Granola/Cereal Bars *HERSHEY'S*	140	3	26
Hershey's, **1.55 oz bar**	210	13	26
Hot Fries *(Andy Capp),* 1 oz	150	7	17
Rice Krispies Treat	90	2.5	17
Lance Captain's Wafers, 1 package	200	9	27
M & M's: Milk Chocolate, 1.7 oz	240	10	34
Peanuts, 1.7 oz	250	13	30
Milk: Whole, 8 fl.oz	160	9	13
Reduced Fat, 2%, 8 fl.oz	140	5	14
Milky Way, 2 oz	260	10	41
Orange Juice, 8 fl.oz	190	14	6
Popcorn, plain, 1 oz	160	10	16
Pork Skins, 1 oz	160	10	0
Potato Chips: 1 oz	150	10	15
Reduced Fat, 1 oz	120	3	21
Pretzels, 1 oz	110	1	23
Raisins, ½ oz package	45	0	11
Reese's Peanut Butter Cups, 1½ oz	230	13	23
Snickers, 2.1 oz bar	280	14	35
Tortilla Chips, 1 oz	140	7	18

Homemade & Restaurant

Restaurant & Take-Out
Average All Preparations, Per 8 fl.oz

	C	F	Cb
Bean Medley	200	3	34
Beef Consomme	30	0	2
Borscht (with Sour Cream)	130	8	14
Bouillabaisse	400	15	10
Chicken & Corn	290	14	20
Chicken & Wild Rice	80	4	9
Chicken Consomme	50	0	2
Chicken Curry	180	8	18
Chicken Jambalaya	160	7	8
Chicken Noodle	80	2	12
with Chicken	160	4	12
Chicken Soup	80	2	6
Chili with Beans	250	12	25
Clam Chowder	240	15	17
Corn & Crab	120	3	18
Corn Chowder	150	8	16
Cream of Broccoli	200	12	20
Cream of Potato	150	6.5	17
Cream of Mushroom	200	13	15
Fish Chowder	220	15	6
French Onion	420	15	25
Gazpacho	50	0	5
Lentil Soup	250	9	28
Lobster Bisque	320	15	10
Matzo Ball (with 1 large ball)	180	7	24
Minestrone	125	2.5	20
Mulligatawny	300	15	8
Pea & Ham	240	10	25
Potato & Bacon	170	7	19
Pumpkin, Creamy	210	10	26
Shark Fin Soup	100	4	8
Spicy Shrimp Soup, 1 bowl	160	7	10
Split Pea Soup	180	2.5	30
Vegetable (Fat Free)	75	0	18
Vegetable Beef	80	2	10
Vichyssoise	200	9	15
Watercress	90	4	13

Other Soups: *See International & Fast-Foods Sections (Arby's, Au Bon Pain, Boston Market, Dunkin' Donuts, Denny's, Schlotzsky's, Sizzler, Souplantation, Sweet Tomatoes, Zoup!)*

Homemade Soups: Calculate calories, fat and carbohydrates from recipe ingredients.

Bouillon Cubes & Powders

	C	F	Cb
Bouillon Cubes: *Average all Types*			
Regular, 1 cube	5	0	1
Low Sodium (LiteLine)	12	0	1
Powders: Average, 1 tsp	10	0	1
Herb-Ox:			
Instant Broth & Seasoning,			
Beef, 1 envelope	5	0	1
Chicken; Vegetarian	5	0	1

Amy's (Organic)

Per ½ Can, 1 Cup, Unless Indicated

	C	F	Cb
Alphabet, Fat-Free	80	0	16
Black Bean Vegetable	140	1.5	26
Chunky Vegetable	60	0	13
Cream of Mushroom, ¾ cup	150	9	13
Cream of Tomato	100	2	17
Curried Lentil	230	8	30
Lentil Vegetable	150	4	23
Roasted Southwestern Vegetable	140	4	21
Split Pea	100	0	19
Thai Coconut	140	10	9
Tuscan Bean & Rice	160	4.5	25
Vegetable Barley	70	1	13

Andersen's   ~ Per Cup

	C	F	Cb
Lentil	110	2	19
Split Pea	130	0	24
Split Pea with Bacon	140	1	23
Tomato	130	3.5	22

Campbell's

Condensed Soup: *Per ½ Cup*

	C	F	Cb
Bean with Bacon	160	3	25
Beef w/ Vegs & Barley; Minestrone, av.	90	1.5	15
Cheddar Cheese	100	5	11
Chicken & Dumplings	70	2.5	10
Chicken Won Ton	60	1	8
Cream of Broccoli	90	3.5	12
Cream of Chicken & Mushroom	80	6	7
Cream of Mushroom	70	2	10
Cream of Potato	90	2	15
Cream of Shrimp	100	6	8
French Onion	45	1.5	6
Manhattan Clam Chowder	60	0.5	12
New England Clam Chowder	90	2.5	13
Old Fashioned Vegetable	80	1.5	14
Split Pea with Ham & Bacon	180	3.5	27
Tomato	90	0	20

Updated Nutrition Data ~ www.CalorieKing.com
Persons with Diabetes ~ See Disclaimer (Page 22)

Campbell's (Cont)   **C** **F** **Cb**

Healthy Request Condensed: *Per ½ Cup*

	C	F	Cb
Chicken Rice	70	1.5	13
Vegetable Beef	90	1	15

Kids Condensed Soup: *Per ½ Cup*

	C	F	Cb
Dora; Jimmy Neutron	80	2	13
Chicken Alphabet	70	2.5	12
Chicken & Stars	70	2.5	12
Curly Noodle	80	2	11
Goldfish Pasta & Meatballs	90	3	11

Chunky: *Per 8 fl.oz Cup*

	C	F	Cb
Baked Potato with Cheddar & Bacon Bits	160	6	23
Chicken Corn Chowder	200	10	20
Classic Chicken Noodle	120	3	14
Fajita Chkn with Rice & Beans	130	1.5	23
Gr. Chicken & Sausage Gumbo	140	3	21

Select Harvest: *Per 8 fl.oz Cup*

	C	F	Cb
Beef w. Roasted Barley	130	1	21
Carmelized French Onion	80	2	12
Chicken Vegetable Medley	120	1	20
Chicken w. Egg Noodles	100	3	11
Creamy Chicken Alfredo	220	13	15
Creamy Potato with Rstd Garlic	180	10	20
Italian-Style Wedding	130	5	13
New England Clam Chowder	170	10	15
Potato Broccoli Cheese	150	9	15
Split Pea with Roasted Ham	150	1	29

Select Harvest Bowls: *Per Cup*

	C	F	Cb
Mexican-Style Chkn Tortilla	130	2.5	19
Minestrone	100	1	19
Savory Chicken & Rice	110	0.5	20
98% Fat-Free, New Eng. Clam Chowder	110	2.5	17

Soup at Hand: *Per Container*

	C	F	Cb
Chicken & Stars	70	2	10
Chicken with Mini Noodles	80	2	11
Creamy Chicken	130	9	13
Cream of Broccoli	150	7	17
Creamy Tomato	190	4	34
New England Clam Chowder	160	10	13
Vegetable Beef	70	1	11

Dr McDougall's

Big Cup Soups/Meals: *Per Cup*

	C	F	Cb
Black Bean & Lime	340	2	60
Hot & Sour Noodle	320	1	34
Minestrone & Pasta	200	1	40
Pad Thai Noodle, average	200	1	42
Split Pea with Barley	240	1	42
Tamale/Tortilla with Baked Chips	200	2	35

Dr McDougall's (Cont)   **C** **F** **Cb**

Ready To Serve: *Per Cup, 8.6 fl.oz*

	C	F	Cb
Black Bean	120	1	23
Lentil	115	0.5	21
Minestrone	70	0.5	14
Roasted Pepper Tomato	80	0	19
Split Pea	100	0	19

Health Valley

Per Cup, Prepared

Broths:

	C	F	Cb
Chicken: Fat-Free	20	0	0
Low-Fat	35	1.5	0
Vegetable, Fat-Free	20	0	5

Fat-Free Soup:

	C	F	Cb
Chicken Flavored Noodles w/ Veggie	110	0	24
Lentil with Couscous	130	0	28
Zesty Black Bean with Rice	100	0	22

Low-Sodium:

	C	F	Cb
14 Garden Vegetable	80	0	18
Corn & Vegetable	80	0	24
Lentil & Carrot	110	0	24
Vegetable Barley	80	0	20

Organic Microwaveable:

	C	F	Cb
Black Bean	130	1.5	26
Garden Vegetable	100	2	17
Lentil	110	0	24
Minestrone	110	0	26
Split Pea	120	10	26
Tomato Bisque	110	3.5	17

Healthy Choice

Canned: *Per Cup*

	C	F	Cb
Chicken & Dumplings	140	2.5	21
Chicken Tortilla Style	160	2	25
Country Vegetable	110	1	19
New England Clam Chowder	110	1	19
Old Fashioned Chicken Noodle	100	1.5	13

Microwavable Containers: *Per 14 oz Container*

	C	F	Cb
Hearty Vegetable Barley	245	2	53
Tomato & Basil	225	1	49

Imagine

Per Cup

Bistro:

	C	F	Cb
Corn Chipotle	100	1	22
Cuban Black Bean	170	3.5	30
Fire Roasted Tomato	120	2.5	24

Canned Organic: *Per Cup*

	C	F	Cb
Chicken Pot Pie	160	4.5	22
Classic Minestrone	120	3.5	20
Country Split Pea	180	2.5	30

Imagine (Cont)   C F Cb

Garden Natural Soup, Creamy:

	C	F	Cb
Acorn Squash & Mango; Chicken	70	1.5	13
Portobello Mushroom	80	3	10
Potato Leek	110	3	18
Sweet Corn	120	3	20
Sweet Pea	80	1.5	14
Tomato	80	1	15

Knorr

Recipe Mix: *Dry Mix*

	C	F	Cb
Cream of Spinach, 2 Tbsp	60	1.5	11
French Onion, 2 Tbsp	45	1	8
Vegetable, 2 Tbsp, 0.3 oz	25	0	6

Bouillon Cubes: *Per ½ Cube, 1 Cup, Prepared*

	C	F	Cb
Beef; Chicken, average	15	0.5	1

Lipton

Cup-a-Soup: *Per Envelope*

	C	F	Cb
Cream of Chicken	70	1.5	14
Chicken Noodle	80	0.5	17

Recipe Secrets: *Per Dry Mix*

	C	F	Cb
Beefy Onion, 1 Tbsp	25	0.5	5
Onion, 1 Tbsp	20	0	4
Onion Mushroom, 1⅔ Tbsp	25	0	7

Manischewitz

Condensed: *Per ½ Cup*

	C	F	Cb
Chicken Broth, Clear	15	0	2
Chicken with Kreplach	40	1	6
Chicken with Matzo Balls	80	3.5	9

Quart Jars: *Per 6 fl.oz, Prepared*

	C	F	Cb
Borscht with Beets	50	0	13
Borscht, Low Calorie	15	0	4

Ready To Serve: Matzo Balls in Broth

	C	F	Cb
	220	9	27

Maruchan

	C	F	Cb
Instant Lunch, Av. all flavors, 1 pkg	290	12	38
Ramen, all flavors: ½ pkg, 1½ oz	190	7	26
1 pkg, 3 oz	380	14	52

Nile Spice   ~ *Per Cup*

	C	F	Cb
Black Bean; Lentil	195	1.5	35
Couscous Lentil Curry	200	1	39
Potato Leek	120	3	17
Low-Fat: Split Pea	190	1	33
Chicken Flavored Vegetable	110	2.5	21

Nissin   C F Cb

Souper Meal: *Per ½ Container*

	C	F	Cb
Chicken	290	13	38
Picante Shrimp	270	11	37
Top Ramen: Beef Flavor	380	14	54
Chicken Flavor	380	14	52

Pacific Foods   ~ *Per Cup*

Creamy Organic:

	C	F	Cb
French Onion	30	1	5
Butternut Squash	90	2	17
Cashew Carrot Ginger	120	5	19
Curried Red Lentil	140	4.5	19
Tomato	100	2	16

Hearty Artisan Soups:

	C	F	Cb
Chicken Fajita	160	2.5	26
Savory White Beans with Bacon	220	7	27

Progresso

Rich & Hearty: *Per Cup*

	C	F	Cb
Chicken & Homestyle Noodles	110	2.5	14
Chicken Corn Chowder	200	9	23
Chicken Pot Pie Style	140	4	19
New England Clam Chowder	180	8	22
Savory Beef Barley Vegetable	130	2.5	17
Steak & Homestyle Noodles	110	2.5	14
Other varieties, average	125	2	21

Traditional: *Per Cup*

	C	F	Cb
Chicken & Herb Dumpling	100	2.5	13
Homestyle Chicken with Vege & Pasta	100	2	14
Italian-Style Wedding	120	4	11
Roasted Garlic Chicken	100	2	13
Southwestern Style Chkn Chowder	120	2	18
Split Pea with Ham	140	1	24

Vegetable Classic: *Per Cup*

	C	F	Cb
French Onion	50	1	9
Green Split Pea with Bacon	160	2	28
Garden Vegetable	90	0	20
Lentil; Tomato Basil, average	155	2.5	29
Minestrone	100	2	20
Tomato Rotini	130	0.5	28

Light, Low-Fat/Low-Carb:

	C	F	Cb
Beef Pot Roast	80	1	12
Southwestern-Style Vegetable, 8.5 oz	60	0.5	12
Vegetable & Noodle, 8.75 oz	60	0.5	13

World Recipes: *Per Cup*

	C	F	Cb
Ablondigas	130	4.5	18
Frijoles Negros	130	1	30
Tortillay y Pollo	110	2.5	17

Shelton's

	C	F	Cb
Broth, Chicken, Regular	35	2.5	0

Signature (Safeway)

Signature Soups: *Per Cup*

	C	F	Cb
Baked Potato	420	33	20
Bistro Mushroom Trio	170	11	14
Broccoli & Cheesy Cheddar	280	21	14
Chunky Chicken Noodle	130	3.5	13
Fiesta Chicken Tortilla	100	3	11
Italian-Style Wedding	160	7	17
Pacific Coast Clam Chowder	330	24	19
Stompin' Steakhouse Chili	260	8	22
Tuscan Tomato & Basil Bisque	310	26	17

Swanson

Per Cup

	C	F	Cb
Vegetable Broth	15	0	3
99% Fat Free, Chicken Broth	10	0.5	1
Organic: Beef Broth	15	0.5	1
Chicken Broth	15	0.5	1

Tabatchnick

	C	F	Cb
Dairy: *Per Pouch*			
Corn Chowder	130	4.5	21
Cream of Broccoli	90	4	12
New England Potato	140	4	24
Gluten Free: *Per Pouch*			
Old Fashioned Potato	100	1.5	21
Split Pea	140	0	34
Southwest Bean	220	5	35
Vegetarian Chili	180	3.5	28
Low Sodium: *Per Pouch*			
Barley Mushroom	80	1	17
Pea	140	0	34
Vegetable	90	1.5	17
Meat: *Per Pouch*			
Frenchman's Onion	60	1.5	11
Wilderness Wild Rice	80	0.5	16
Parve: *Per Pouch*			
Balsamic Tomato & Rice	110	3.5	18
Black Bean	230	2.5	39
Minestrone	100	1.5	18
Vegetable	90	1.5	17

Thai Kitchen

Rice Noodle Soup Bowls: *Per Bowl*

	C	F	Cb
Hot & Sour	250	3	52
Lemongrass & Chili	250	2.5	52
Thai Ginger	260	3	52

Trader Joe's

	C	F	Cb
Organic: Black Bean	130	1.5	25
Lentil Vegetable, ½ can	130	3.5	19
Split Pea	100	0	19
Light Sodium, Tomato Bisque	130	4	21
Low Sodium: Minestrone, 10¾ can	200	4	37
Chkn & Mafalde Pasta, 10¾ can	110	3	19
Low Fat, Chicken Noodle	90	1	14
Cartons, 32 fl.oz:			
Butternut Squash	90	2	16
Carrot Ginger	80	1	17
Creamy Corn & Roasted Pepper	110	2	23
Garden Patch Veggie	60	0	14
Latin Style Black Bean	70	1	12
Sweet Potato Bisque	130	1	28
Organic: Butternut Squash	70	0	17
Creamy Tomato	90	3.5	15
Tomato & Roasted Red Pepper	100	3.5	15

Whole Foods

Per Cup

	C	F	Cb
Canned: Chicken Noodle	110	3	16
Chicken with Wild & Red Rice	110	2.5	17
Italian Style Wedding	150	6	19
Vegetable	90	1	21
Vegetable Beef	130	3.5	21
365 Organic: Black Bean	150	1	25
Chicken Noodle	90	2	11
Cream of Mushroom	100	6	11
Minestrone	120	2	21
Tomato	90	3.5	11
Vegetable	70	1	11

Wolfgang Puck

Per Cup

	C	F	Cb
Original: Chicken & Egg Noodles	130	6	11
Chicken and Dumpling	220	13	17
Chicken with Broccoli	180	10	14
Chicken with Sweetcorn	200	10	20
Chicken Tortilla	140	5	17
New England Clam Chowder	170	7	18
Old Fashioned Beef Barley	120	3.5	17
Organic: Butternut Squash	200	11	22
Chicken with Egg Noodle	110	5	11
Corn Chowder	210	13	20
Classic Tomato with Basil	130	6	18
Creamy Tomato	250	16	23
Old Fashioned Potato	200	14	17
Thick & Hearty Lentil & Vegetable	140	0	28

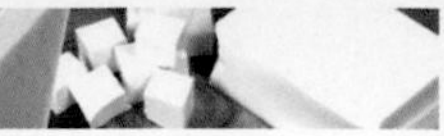

S Soy Products & Tofu

## Soybean Products	C	F	Cb
Cheeses (Soy): *See Page 78*			
Miso Soy Bean Paste			
Cold Mountain: Light Yellow, 1 tsp	10	0	1
Mellow Red, 1 tsp	15	0	3
Red, 1 tsp	10	0	3
Miso Soup (dry mix), av.			
1 Tbsp., dry mix	35	1	5
1 cup, prepared	35	1	5
Natto, ½ cup, 3 oz	160	7	14
Okara (Tofu fiber residue), ½ c., 2 oz	47	1	8
Tempeh: 1 piece, 3 oz	180	8	12
Fried, 3 oz	250	14	14
Seitan *(White Wave)*, Traditional, 3 oz	90	1	3
Soybean Protein *(TVP)*, 1 oz	95	0	8
Soy Bean Paste, 1 tsp	10	0	2
Soy Beans: *See Page 160*			
Soy Drinks: *See Page 49*			

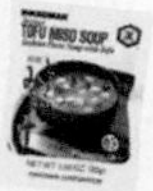

## Tofu ~ Packaged	C	F	Cb
House Foods (Cont)			
Organic Tofu: Firm, 3 oz	60	3.5	0
Extra Firm, 3 oz	70	4	0
House Tofu: Tokusen Kinugoshi, 3 oz	90	4	3
Sukui; Soon (Extra Soft), 3 oz	45	2	2
Yaki Tofu (Broiled), 3 oz	90	5	2
Seasoned Tofu Steak: Grilled, 3 oz	90	5	2
Garlic & Pepper, 3 oz	90	4	1
Mori-Nu Tofu (Silken)			
Soft, 3 oz, 1" slice	45	2.5	2
Firm, 3 oz, 1" slice	50	2.5	2
Extra Firm, 3 oz, 1" slice	45	1.5	2
Organic Firm 3 oz, 1" slice	60	2.5	2
Lite, Firm, 3 oz, 1" slice	30	0.5	1
Nasoya: Soft, ⅕ package, 2.8 oz	60	3	1
Silken, 3.2 oz	45	2	1
Firm, ⅕ package, 3.2 oz	70	3	2
Extra Firm, ⅕ pkg, 2.8 oz	80	4	2
Silken Style Creations: *Per ½ Cup*			
Chocolate; Vanilla, average	120	1.5	24
Strawberry	110	1	22
WestSoy, Firm, 2.8 oz	95	5	3

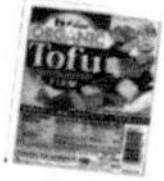

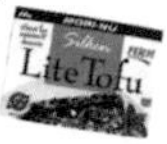

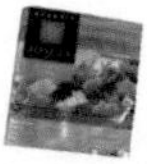

## Supplements	C	F	Cb
Aloe Vera Juice, undiluted, 2 fl.oz	5	0	1
Brewer's Yeast: Tablets, 2 tabs	4	0	0.5
Flakes, 1 heaping Tbsp, ⅓ oz	30	0.5	4
Powder, 1 heaping Tbsp, ½ oz	50	0.5	6
Calcium Chews: *CVS*, 1 chew	20	0	3
Trader Joe's, Choc., 1 chew	20	1	3
Cod Liver Oil, 1 Tbsp	125	13	0
Fiber Choice, 2 tabs	15	0	4
Fibersure, 1 heaping tsp	25	0	6
Fish Oil Capsules, av., 1	10	1	0
Flax Oil: Capsules, 2	10	1	0
Barlean's, 3 softgels	110	11	0
Garlic Tablets/Capsules, each	3	0	0
Glowelle:			
Beauty Drink, 8 fl.oz	100	0	24
Powder Stick (1)	50	0	12
Lecithin Granules, 1 Tbsp	55	4	0.5
Metamucil **Powder**:			
Orange (Smooth Texture)			
1 rounded Tbsp	45	0	12
Sugar-Free, 1 rounded tsp	20	0	5
Pink Lemonade, Sugar-Free,			
1 rounded tsp	20	0	5
Fiber Wafers (2)	120	5	17
Capsules:			
Heart & Digestive (6)	10	0	3
Strong Bones (5)	10	0	3
Protein, Powders, average, 1 oz	100	0.5	0
Seaweed: Dried, 1 oz	85	0.5	22
Soaked; drained, 1 oz	15	0.5	3
Spirulina, 1 tablet	2	0	0.5
Vitamins/Minerals: Tabs/Caps, 1	2	0	0
Vitamin E Capsules, each	5	0.5	0
Viactiv **Chews** (1)	20	0.5	4

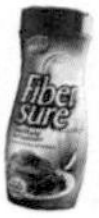

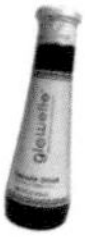

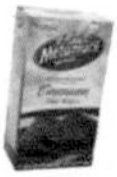

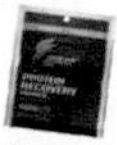

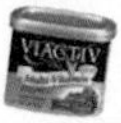

Cough & Pharmaceutical | | |
|---|---|---|---|
| **Antacids**: Av., 1 tablet | 4 | 0 | 1 |
| Liquid, 1 Tbsp | 6 | 0 | 1 |
| *(Antacid Sodium Counts ~ See Page 280)* | | | |
| **Cough/Cold Syrups**: | | | |
| Regular: With sugar, 1 Tbsp | 35 | 0 | 9 |
| With alcohol, 1 Tbsp | 46 | 0 | 9 |
| Sugar-Free *(Diabetic Tussin)*, 1 T. | 0 | 0 | 0 |
| **Cough Drops/Lozenges**: *See Page 75* | | | |
| **Sudafed** Syrup, 1 tsp | 14 | 0 | 3 |
| **Tylenol** Liquid: Child, 1 tsp | 17 | 0 | 4 |
| Extra Strength, 1 tsp | 11 | 0 | 3 |

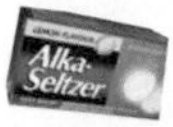

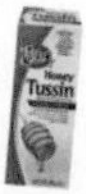

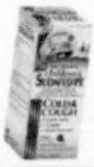

Sugar | C | F | Cb

White Sugar, granulated:

	C	F	Cb
1 level teaspoon	15	0	4
1 heaping teaspoon	25	0	6
Single portion, 1 packet	10	0	3
1 Tablespoon	50	0	12
1 ounce, 1 oz	110	0	28
1 cup, 7 oz	770	0	200
1 pound	1760	0	464
Single Portion Packages:			
1 stick	15	0	4
Square Package	25	0	6
Starbucks, 0.3 oz	30	0	8
1 cube, ½"	25	0	6
Brown Sugar: 1 Tbsp	50	0	13
1 ounce, 1 oz	110	0	28
1 cup, not packed, 5 oz	540	0	140
1 cup, packed, 7¾ oz	845	0	218
Powdered/Confectioners:			
Sifted, 1 cup, 3½ oz	385	0	98
Unsifted, 1 cup, 4¼ oz	460	0	117
Cinnamon Sugar, 1 tsp	15	0	4
Dextrose, 1¼ tsp	15	0	4
Fructose: Dry, 1 tsp	15	0	4
Liquid, 1 oz	80	0	21
Glucose, 1 oz	110	0	27
Glucose Tablets (1)	20	0	5
Palm Sugar, 3 Tbsp	45	0	11
Piloncillo (Brown Sugar), 3oz cone	325	0	81
Turbinado Sugar, 2 Tbsp, 1 oz	110	0	27
Unrefined Cane Sugar, 1 oz	110	0	27

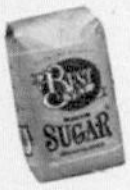

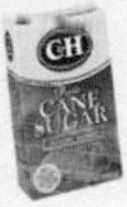

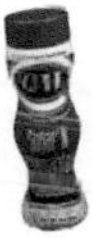

Sugar Substitutes | C | F | Cb

	C	F	Cb
DiabetiSweet, 1 teaspoon	9	0	4
(Carbohydrate as Sugar Alcohol)			
Equal: Tablet (2)	4	0	0.5
Granular, 1 tsp	4	0	0.5
Packet (1)	4	0	0.5
Flavored, 1 stick	4	0	0.5
Natra Taste; Sweet One, 1 packet	4	0	1
NutraSweet, 1 tsp	4	0	0
Splenda:			
Granular: 1 tsp	5	0	0.5
1 cup	95	0	24
Packet, all flavors	5	0	0.5
Sugar Blend,Orig/Brown, ½ cup	385	0	96
Stevia, Single Serving	0	0	0
Sugar Twin: 1 packet	3	0	0.5
Sweet 'N Low, 1 packet	2	0	0.5
Walgreens Wal-Sweet, 1 packet	0	0	0
Weight Watchers, 1 packet	4	0	1
Whey Low, 1 tsp	3	0	3

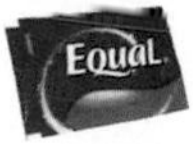

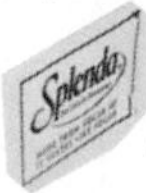

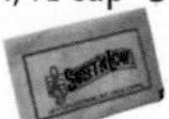

Syrups, Molasses, Agave

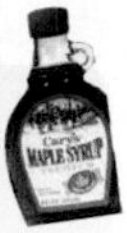

Syrups: *Average All Brands*
(Corn/Rice/Maple/Pancake/Sundae/Waffle)
Includes Aunt Jemima, Cary's, Karo, Hershey's,
Hungry Jack, Log Cabin, Mrs Butterworth's

Regular/Dark/Light Color:	C	F	Cb
1 Tbsp, ½ fl.oz	55	0	14
¼ cup (4 Tbsp)	220	0	55
Single Portion: 1½ oz package	170	0	42
Lite: 1Tbsp	25	0	6
¼ cup (4 Tbsp)	100	0	25
Sugar-Free: Cary's, 2 Tbsp, 1 oz	18	0	5
Cozy Cottage, 2 Tbsp, 1 oz	10	0	3
Da Vinci, 2 Tbsp, 1 oz	5	0	1
Honey Cream Syrup, ¼ c., 2 oz	220	0	55
Molasses: Dark/Light: 1 T., ¾ oz	55	0	14
1 cup, 11½ oz	880	0	224
Blackstrap, 1 Tbsp, ¾ oz	47	0	13
Agave Nectar, average, 1 T., ¾ oz	60	0	15

Ice Cream Toppings | C | F | Cb

Average All Types & Brands: Per 2 Tbsp
(Hershey's, Smuckers)

	C	F	Cb
Butterscotch; Caramel	140	1	30
Chocolate: Hot Fudge	140	4	22
Fat Free Chocolate	100	0	23
Pineapple, Strawberry	110	0	28
Smuckers: Lite	90	0	23
Magic Shell	210	15	18
Milky Way	130	4	23

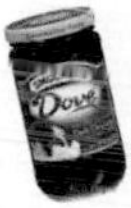

Honey, Jam, Preserves

Average All Brands	C	F	Cb
Honey: 1 tsp, ¼ oz	22	0	5.5
1 Tbsp, ¾ oz	65	0	17
1 ounce, 1 oz	85	0	23
1 cup, 12 oz	1030	0	269
Single Portion, ½ oz package	45	0	11
Jams/Jellies/Marmalade/Preserves:			
Regular, 1 tsp, ¼ oz	20	0	5
1 Tbsp, ¾ oz	55	0	14
1 ounce, 1 oz	80	0	20
Single Portion, ½ oz pkg	40	0	11
Apple/Fruit Butters, 1 T., 0.6 oz	20	0	6
Fruit Spreads: Regular, 1 tsp	15	0	4
Low Sugar, 1 tsp	8	0	2
Low Calorie *(Featherweight),* 1 tsp	8	0	2
Jelly: Regular, average, 1 tsp	18	0	4.5
Imitation, Low Calorie, 1 tsp	4	0	1

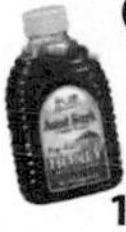

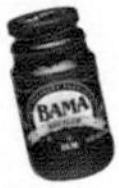

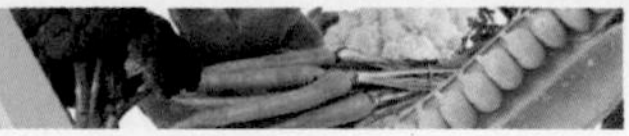

Vegetables

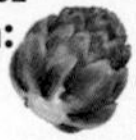
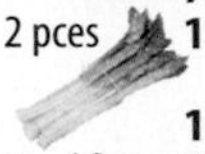
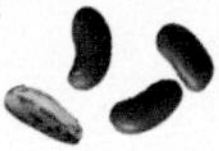
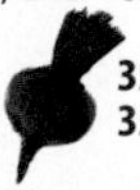
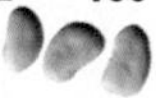
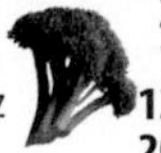
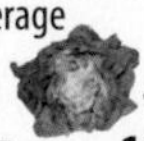

Vegetables	C	F	Cb
Alfalfa Sprouts, ½ cup, ½ oz	5	0	0.5
Artichokes, Globe/French:			
1 medium, 4½ oz	60	0	13
1 large, 5.7 oz	75	0	17
Artichoke Heart, plain, 2 pces	15	0	3
Asparagus, raw/frozen:			
3 medium spears	10	0	2
Cuts & Tips *(Del Monte)*, ½ cup, 4.3 oz	20	0	3
Bamboo Shoots, cooked, ½ c., 2 oz	7	0	1
Beans: Green/Snap/String, ½ ., 2 oz	20	0	4
10 beans (4" long), 2 oz	20	0	4
Dried Beans, *average all types:*			
(Kidney, Brown, Lima, Navy, Pinto, White)			
Raw: 2 Tbsp, 1 oz	95	0.5	18
1 cup, 7 oz	665	3	126
Cooked: 1 oz	35	0	7
½ cup, 3 oz	105	0	21
Bean Sprouts, average, ½ c., 2 oz	15	0	3.5
Beets (Beetroot):			
Raw, 1 beet (2" diam), 4 oz	35	0	8
Cooked, 1 cup, slices, 3 oz	35	0	8
Canned ~ *See Page 168*			
Beet Greens, cooked, ½ cup, 2½ oz	20	0	4
Bell Pepper: *See Peppers*			
Bitter Melon/Gourd, 1 cup, 1½ oz	15	0	1.5
Blackeye Peas, cooked, ½ cup, 3 oz	100	0.5	18
Bok Choy (Chinese Chard), ckd, 3 oz	10	0	1.5
Breadfruit, ¼ small fruit, 3 oz	100	0	26
Broadbeans (Fava Beans):			
Green (in pod), raw: 4 pods			
(3½ oz w/ shells; 1.2 oz beans)	30	0	6
1 cup beans (w/o shell), 4½ oz	110	1	22
Mature Seeds: Raw, 1 cup, 5.3 oz	510	2.5	87
Cooked, ½ cup, 3 oz	95	0	17
Broccoflower, ⅕ head, 3½ oz	35	0	7
Broccoli: Raw, chopped, 1 cup, 3 oz	30	0	6
3 Florets, 2½ oz	25	0	5
1 Spear (5" long), 1.1 oz	10	0	2
1 Whole: Medium size, 14 oz	135	1.5	26
Large, 21 oz	205	2	40
1 Head (no stalk), 11 oz	105	1	21
1 Stalk, small (5" long), 5.3 oz	50	0.5	10
Brocco Sprouts, ½ cup, 1 oz	15	0	2
Brussels Sprouts: cooked, ½ c., 2.8 oz	30	0.5	6
2 Sprouts, 1½ oz	15	0	3
Butterbeans, cooked, ½ cup, 3 oz	90	0	16
Cabbage, all types/colors, average			
Raw: 1 Leaf, large, 1 oz	5	0	2
Shredded, 1 cup, 2½ oz	15	0	4
½ Large Head (7" diam), 22 oz	150	1	35
Cooked, shredded, ½ cup, 2½ oz	15	0.5	3.5

Vegetables (Cont)

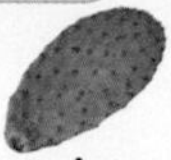
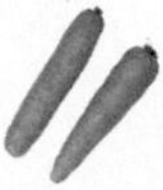
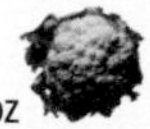
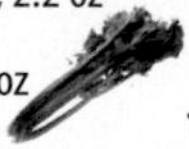
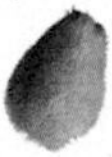

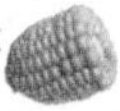
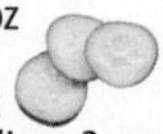

Vegetables (Cont)	C	F	Cb
Cactus Leaf (Nopales)			
1 leaf, 4½ oz	20	0	4
1 cup (slices), 3 oz	15	0	3
Carrots, Regular thick variety,			
1 small, 4 oz	45	0	11
1 medium, 6 oz	70	0	16
1 large, 8 oz	95	0	22
Chopped, 1 cup, 4½ oz	50	0	12
Grated, 1 cup, 4 oz	45	0	11
Slices, 1 cup, 4½ oz	50	0	12
Sticks (4"), 4-5, 1½ oz	20	0	4
Long thin variety, 1 medium, 2.2 oz	25	0	6
Baby: Snack size, 3 medium, 1 oz	10	0	2.5
Snack Pack, 3 oz	30	0	7
Cauliflower, Raw: 1 cup (pieces), 3½ oz	25	0	5
½ medium head, 10 oz	70	0	15
Cooked, 3 florets, 2 oz	10	0	2
Celeriac, ½ cup, raw, 2¾ oz	35	0	7
Celery: 1 large stalk, 11", 2.2 oz	10	0	2
1 small stalk, 5", ½ oz	2	0	0.5
4 Strips, thin sticks, ½ oz	5	0	1
Chopped, 1 cup, 3½ oz	15	0	3
Chard (Swiss), ½ cup, cooked, 3 oz	20	0	3.5
Chayote Squash: 1 medium, 7 oz	40	0	9
1 cup (pieces), 4½ oz	25	0	6
Chick Peas			
Dry, 1 cup, 7 oz	730	12	121
Cooked, 1 cup, 6 oz	270	4	45
Chicory Greens, 1 cup, 1 oz	7	0	1.5
Chili Peppers: *See Peppers*			
Chinese Long Bean, sl., 1 cup, 3.2 oz	45	0	8
Chives, chopped, 1 Tbsp	1	0	0
Choy Sum, 3 oz	15	0	3
Cilantro (Coriander), 1 cup	5	0	0.5
Collards, cooked, ½ cup, 3 oz	25	0	5
Corn, yellow/white:			
Raw: Kernels, ½ cup, 3 oz	80	0.5	19
Ear (5"x 1¾"), 5½ oz	155	1	37
Cooked, Kernels, ½ cup, 3 oz	77	0.5	18
Cob, cooked: Small, 2¼ oz	60	0.5	14
Large ear, 5½ oz	120	1	28
Courgette: *See Zucchini*			
Cowpeas: *See Blackeye Peas*			
Cress, garden, raw, 1 cup, 1¾ oz	15	0	3
Cucumber: 1 whole, 11 oz	45	0.5	11
½ cup slices, 2 oz	10	0	2
Mini/Lebanese (1), 3 oz	15	0	3
Daikon Radish, ½ cup, slices, 2 oz	9	0	2
Dandelion Greens, raw, ½ cup, 1 oz	10	0	2.5
Edamame *(Immature green soybeans):*			
Shelled, ½ cup, 2.6 oz	110	5	8
With shells, 10 pods, 1¼ oz	30	1	3

Updated Nutrition Data ~ www.CalorieKing.com
Persons with Diabetes ~ See Disclaimer (Page 22)

Vegetables (Cont)

	C	F	Cb
Eggplant: Raw, ¼ medium, 4 oz	30	0	7
Raw, ½ cup, 1" pieces, 1½ oz	10	0	2
1 slice, fried, 1 oz	75	4	10
Endive, Belgian/French: Raw,			
1 medium head (6"), 2½ oz	12	0	3
Fennel, 1 cup, sliced, 3 oz	25	0	7
Gai Choy Cabbage, cooked, 1 cup, 6 oz	20	0	3
Gai Lan (Chinese Kale), cooked, 1 cup	35	0.5	7
Garlic, 1 clove	4	0	1
Ginger: ¼ cup slices, 1 oz	20	0	5
Crystallized (sugared), 7 pieces, 1½ oz	130	0	35
Horseradish, raw, 1 pod, ½ oz	5	0	1
Jerusalem Artichoke, raw, ½ cup	55	0	13
Jicama, raw, sliced, ½ cup, 2¼ oz	25	0	6
Kale, 1 cup, chopped, 2½ oz	35	0.5	7
Kohlrabi, ½ cup, cooked, 1¾ oz	17	0	5
Leek, cooked, 1 whole, 4½ oz	40	0	9
Lentils, green/brown: Dry, 1 oz	100	0.5	17
Dry, 1 cup, 6¾ oz	680	2	115
Cooked, ½ cup, 3½ oz	115	0.5	20
Lettuce: 1 cup, chopped/shredded, 2 oz	7	0	1
Butterhead, 2 leaves, ½ oz	2	0	0.5
Cos/Romaine, shredded, 1 c.	10	0	2
Iceberg: 1 outer leaf, ½ oz	2	0	0.5
1 med. head, 16 oz	75	1	16
Lima Beans, baby, cooked, ½ c., 3 oz	105	0	20
Lotus Root, 10 slices, cooked, 3 oz	60	0	14
Mung Bean Sprouts, ½ cup, 2 oz	15	0	3
Mushrooms: Raw, 1 medium, 0.6 oz	4	0	0.5
Raw, 1 large, sliced, ¾ oz	5	0	1
Raw, ½ cup pieces, 1¼ oz	8	0	1
Cooked, ½ cup pieces, 2½ oz	20	0.5	4
Fried/Sauteed, 6 oz	220	16	11
Mustard Greens, Raw, ½ cup, 1 oz	7	0	2
Nopales: *See Cactus Leaf*			
Okra: Raw, 8 pods, 4 oz	30	0	7
Cooked, ½ cup, 2¾ oz	20	0	4
Onions: Raw: 1 small, 2½ oz	30	0	7
1 medium, 4 oz	50	0	11
1 large, 5½ oz	65	0	15
1 jumbo, 16 oz	190	0.5	46
Chopped: Raw, ½ cup, 3 oz	35	0	8
1 Tbsp, 0.4 oz	5	0	1
Slices: 1 cup, 4 oz	50	0	12
1 medium slice (⅛"), ½ oz	5	0	1
1 large slice (¼"), 1⅓ oz	15	0	4
Dehydrated flakes, ¼ cup, ½ oz	50	0	12
Rings, breaded & fried, 2 rings	80	5	9
Scallions, ½ cup, 2 oz	15	0	3
Spring, ½ cup, chopped, 2 oz	15	0	3
(*French's* Fried Onions: See Page 112)			
Blossom/Blooming: See Fast-Foods (Chili's/Outback)			

Vegetables (Cont)

	C	F	Cb
Parsley, chopped, ½ cup, 1 oz	10	0	2
Parsnip: 1 medium, 4 oz	85	0	20
Cooked, ½ cup slices, 2¾ oz	55	0	13
Peas: Raw, Green, ¼ cup, 1½ oz	30	0	5
Raw, with pods, ½ lb	70	0	13
Snow Peas, 10 pods, 1.2 oz	15	0	3
Split: Dry, hulled, 1 oz	100	0.5	17
Cooked, 1 cup, 7 oz	230	1	42
Peppers: Sweet, 1 medium, 4.2 oz	30	0	7
Bell: 1 medium, 4.2 oz	30	0	7
½ cup, chopped, raw, 2½ oz	20	0	5
2 rings (5" diam. x ¼" thick)	3	0	1
Chili: Green/Red, 1½ oz	20	0	5
Halluneno, 1 only, 0.3 oz	10	0	2
Pigeon Peas, cooked, ½ cup, 3 oz	95	1	17
Pimientos, 3 medium, 3½ oz	25	0	5
Poi, ½ cup, 4.2 oz	135	0	33
Potatoes: Raw (with skin)			
1 Baby, 2 oz	45	0	10
1 Small, 6 oz	135	0	30
1 Medium, 8 oz	180	0	40
1 Large, 12 oz	270	0	60
1 Extra large, 16 oz	360	0	80
Baked (no added fat): large, 10 oz (raw wt):			
Plain: With skin, 7 oz (ckd wt)	185	0	42
Without skin, 5½ oz (ckd wt)	145	0	34
With Skin/Toppings:			
+ 2 tsp fat	270	8	58
+ Sour Cream & Chives, 2 Tbsp	320	6	60
+ Plain Yogurt, 2 Tbsp	260	1	60
+ Grated Cheese, 1 oz	370	9	58
Mashed:			
With milk plus fat, ½ cup, 4 oz	120	4.5	18
KFC Style without gravy, 4 oz	100	3	16
Loaded (fat/cream/cheese/bacon):			
Side serving, 6 oz	180	9	22
Large serving, 12 oz	360	18	44
Potato Skins: (Baked with cheese topping),			
½ whole, 4 oz	240	13	22
French Fries: Small serving, 2.6 oz	250	13	30
Medium serving, 4 oz	380	20	47
Frozen, uncooked, 18 fries, 4 oz	165	5.5	28
Oven-heated, 18 fries, 4 oz	165	5.5	28
Take-Out, 1 cup, 5 oz	440	25	60
McDonald's ~ See Page 215			
Fried, 4 oz	165	5.5	28
Au Gratin, ½ c., 4.3 oz	160	9	14
Pancakes, 2 small, 2 oz	120	6.5	12
Puffs, fried, 4 puffs, 1 oz	55	2.5	8
Scalloped: 1 cup, 8½ oz	220	9	26
Ore-Ida Frozen Potatoes: See Page 168			

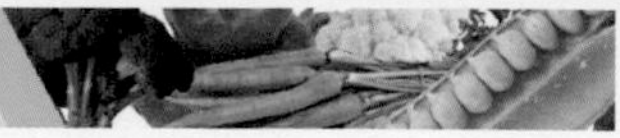

Vegetables (Cont)

	C	F	Cb
Potato Salad, ½ cup, 4½ oz	180	10	14
Pumpkin:			
Raw, 1″ cubes, 1 cup, 4 oz	30	0	7
Cooked:			
Mashed: 1 scoop, 2 oz	10	0	2
½ cup, 4⅓ oz	25	0	6
Baked, without fat, 4 oz	90	7	9
Pumpkin Flowers, 1 cup, 1.2 oz	5	0	1
Purslane: Cooked, ½ cup, 2 oz	10	0	2
Raw, 1″ cubes, 1 cup, 1.5 oz	5	0	1.5
Radicchio: 2 leaves, ½ oz	5	0	1
Shredded, 1 cup, 1½ oz	20	0	4
Radishes: 1 small	0	0	0
10 medium/5 large, 1.6 oz	5	0	1
½ cup (slices), 2 oz	10	0	2
Rhubarb, raw, ½ cup, 2 oz	15	0	3
Rutabaga, cooked, ½ c., (cubes), 3 oz	30	0	7
Salsify, ckd, ½ cup, (slices), 2½ oz	50	0	11
Sauerkraut, ½ cup, 2½ oz	15	0	3
Seaweed: Dried, 1 oz	5	0	2
Soaked, drained, 1 oz	15	0	4
Nori/Laver, dried, 6 sheets, ½ oz	35	0	5
Shallots, 1 Tbsp, (Chopped), ½ oz	5	0	1
Sorrel, raw, ½ cup, 4 oz	20	0	4
Soybeans: Mature, dry, 1 oz	120	5.5	9
Dry, ½ cup, 3.3 oz	390	18	28
Cooked, ½ cup, 3 oz	150	7.5	8
(Soy Products/Tofu/Tempeh: See Page 156)			
Spinach: Cooked, ½ cup, 3 oz	20	0	4
Raw: 3 leaves/1 cup, 1 oz	7	0	1
1 Bunch, 12 oz	80	1.5	12
Creamed, average, ½ cup, 4½ oz	190	15	8
Squash: Summer, raw, ½ cup, 2½ oz	10	0	2
Cooked, ½ cup slices, 3 oz	15	0	3
Winter, cooked,			
Acorn, ½ cup cubes, 3½ oz	35	0	9
½ medium (10 oz raw weight)	115	0	30
Butternut, ½ cup, (cubes), 3½ oz	40	0	10
¼ medium (9 oz raw weight)	115	0	30
Spaghetti, ½ cup, 1¾ oz	15	0	3
Succotash, cooked, ½ cup, 3⅓ oz	110	1	23
Sweetcorn: *See Corn*			
Sweet Potatoes:			
Cooked with skin (w/o fat)			
1 medium, 4 oz	105	0	24
Without skin, mashed, ½ c., 5½ oz	125	0	29

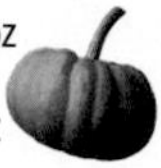
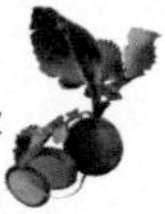
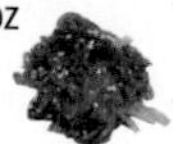
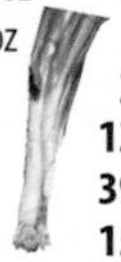
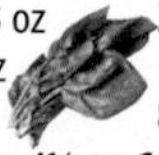
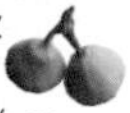
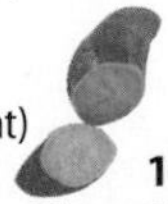

Vegetables (Cont)

	C	F	Cb
Swiss Chard, ckd, chopped, 1 c., 6 oz	35	0	7
Taro, cooked, ½ cup, 2⅓ oz	95	0	23
Tomatoes: 1 small (2¼″ diameter), 3 oz	15	0	3
1 medium (2¾″ diameter), 5 oz	25	0	5
1 large (3½″ diameter), 8 oz	40	0.5	9
1 extra large (3″ diam.), 12 oz	60	0.5	14
Chopped, 1 cup, 6½ oz	35	0.5	7
Tomatillo, 1 medium, 1.2 oz	10	0	2
Turnip: cooked, ½ cup, 2¾ oz	15	0	4
Greens, cooked, ½ cup, 2½ oz	15	0	3
Water Chestnuts: 5-6 nuts, 1 oz	56	0.5	13
½ cup, (slices), 2¼ oz, raw	60	0	15
Canned, 1 oz	15	0	3
Watercress, 10 sprigs, 1 oz	3	0	0.5
Yams: Cooked, ½ cup, 2½ oz	80	0	19
Baked, 1 medium (6″) 8 oz	265	0.5	63
1 large (9″) 12 oz	400	0.5	94
Yardlong Bean, 1 pod, ½ oz	5	0	1
Yucca Root, ½ cup, 3½ oz	165	0.5	39
Zucchini: 1 medium, 7 oz, raw	30	0.5	7
Cooked, ½ cup, (slices), 3 oz	15	0	4

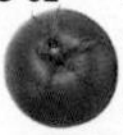
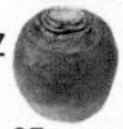
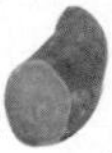
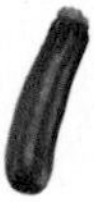

Frozen Vegetables

	C	F	Cb
Birds Eye			
Baby Varieties:			
Peas: ⅔ cup, 3 oz	70	0	12
with Pearl Onions, ⅔ cup	60	0	12
Gold & White Corn, ⅔ cup, 3.2 oz	100	1	20
Brussels Sprouts, (10), 3 oz	45	0	8
White Pearl Onions, ⅔ cup, 3 oz	30	0	6
Whole Green Beans, 1 cup, 3 oz	35	0	5
Steamfresh:			
Mixtures: Brocc & Cauliflower, 1 cup	30	0	4
with Carrots, ¾ cup, 3 oz	30	0	5
Brocc., Crts., Peas, Water Ches., ¾ cup	35	0	6
Premium Selects:			
Sugar Snap Peas, ⅔ cup	40	0	7
Whole Green Beans, 1 cup, 3 oz	35	0	5
Singles: *Per 3.25 oz Bag*			
Baby Brussels Sprouts	50	0	9
Super Sweet Corn	80	1	14
Sweet Peas	70	0	13
Specially Seasoned:			
Asian Medley, 1 cup, 3.3 oz	50	2	6
Garlic Baby Peas & Mushroom, ¾ cup	80	2	12
Lightly Sauced: Broccoli w/ Cheese	60	2	7
Roasted Red Potato w/ Chive Butter	140	1.5	29

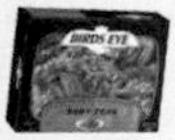

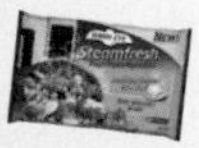

Updated Nutrition Data ~ www.CalorieKing.com
Persons with Diabetes ~ See Disclaimer (Page 22)

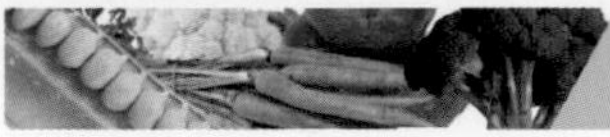

Frozen Vegetables (Cont) — C | F | Cb

Item	C	F	Cb
Green Giant			
Just for One,			
Broccoli & Cheese Sauce, 4.25 oz	40	1	7
Vegetables: Asparagus Cuts, ⅔ cup	20	0	3
Corn: Nibblers, ½ ear, 2.2 oz	80	1.5	15
Extra Sweet Niblets, ⅔ cup	70	1	13
Shoepeg, without sauce, ½ cup	80	0.5	17
Honey-Glazed Carrots, 1 cup	90	3	15
Spinach, w/o sauce, ½ cup, 3½ oz	25	0	3
Rice & Vegetables: Per ½ Package, Prepared			
Cheesy Rice & Broccoli	150	2.5	28
Rice Medley	125	2	24
Rice Pilaf	105	1.5	20
White & Wild Rice	140	3	25
Valley Fresh: Per ½ Cup, Prepared			
Rsted Red Pot., Green Beans w/ Sce	80	1	16
Ore-Ida: As Purchased			
Fries: Per 3 oz			
Classic: Golden Crinkles	120	3.5	20
Golden; Shoestring, average	135	4	22
Steak	110	3	19
Easy,			
Extra Crispy: Crinkles, Golden	180	8	25
Extra Crispy: Fast Food Fries	160	6	23
Golden Crinkles	170	7	24
Seasoned Crinkles	150	6	22
Premium: Cottage; Country Style	130	4.5	21
Crispers	220	13	23
Golden Twirls	160	6	24
Pixie Crinkles; Texas Crispers, av.	145	5	21
Hash Browns: Golden Patties (1)	170	8	15
Potatoes O'Brien, ¾ cup, 3 oz	60	0	14
Southern Style, ⅔ cup, 3 oz	70	0	16
Toaster Patties (2), 3.65 oz	220	12	25
Onion Rings: Gourmet, 2.7 oz	180	8	25
Onion Ringers (6), 3 oz	180	10	21
Steam n' Mash: Cut Russet, ¾ cup	80	0	17
Garlic Seasoned Potatoes, ¾ cup	110	4	17
Three Cheese Potatoes, ¾ cup	80	0.5	16
Tater Tots: 9 pieces, 3 oz	170	8	20
ABC (9), 3 oz	160	8	22
Extra Crispy, 12 pieces, 3 oz	170	9	20
Ultimate Bake: With Butter, 5 oz	170	5	27
With Cheese, 5 oz	190	6	28

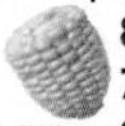

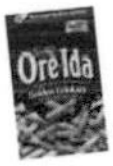

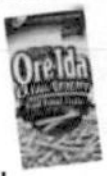

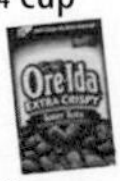

Canned/Bottled — C | F | Cb

Item	C	F	Cb
Solids & Liquid			
Artichoke Hearts (Fanci Foods):			
Plain, 1 oz (1)	8	0	1
Marinated, ¼ bottle, 1 oz	25	1.5	2
Asparagus: Drained, 3 spears	10	0	1.5
Pieces, ½ cup, 4.3 oz	25	0.5	3
Bamboo Shoots, 1 cup, 4½ oz	25	0	4
Bean Salad, ½ cup, 4⅓ oz	90	0	20
Beans: Green, ½ cup, 2½ oz	15	0	3
Baked Beans, ½ cup, 4½ oz	120	0.5	27
Butter Beans, ½ c., 4½ oz	90	0	16
Italian, ½ cup, 4½ oz	30	0	6
Kidney Beans, ½ cup 3½ oz	105	0.5	19
Lima Beans, ½ cup, 4½ oz	80	0	15
Pinto Beans, ½ cup, 4½ oz	105	1	18
Beets: Sliced, ½ cup, 3 oz	25	0	6
Crinkle/Pickled (Del Monte) ½ c.	80	0	20
Carrots: Sliced, ½ cup, 2½ oz	20	0	4
Honey Glazed (Del Monte) ½ cup	75	0	18
Corn: Kernels, ½ cup, 4½ oz	80	0.5	18
Creamed style, ½ cup, 4½ oz	90	0.5	23
Garbanzo/Chick Peas, ½ cup, 4.2 oz	145	1.5	27
Green Chilies, diced, 2 Tbsp, 1 oz	6	0	1.5
Hearts of Palm (1), 1.2 oz	7	0	1
Mushrooms: ½ cup, 2½ oz	20	0	4
in Butter Sauce, 2 oz	20	1	2
Onions: Pickled, 1 medium, ½ oz	10	0	2
Cocktail, 1 onion	0	0	0
French's Fried Onions: See Page 112			
Peas, ½ cup, 3 oz	60	0.5	10
Peppers: Hot Chili, Jalapeno, (1), 1 oz	5	0	1
Sweet, undrained, 2½ oz	13	0	3
Jalapeno, with liquid,			
½ cup chopped	20	0.5	3
Fried, drained, 2 Tbsp, 1 oz	60	5	3
Salsa, average all types, 2 Tbsp	10	0	2
Sauerkraut, drained, 1 cup, 5 oz	25	0	6
Spinach, ½ cup, 3½ oz	25	0.5	3.5
Succotash: Cream Style, ½ cup	100	0.5	23
w/ whole kernels, undrained, ½ cup	80	0.5	18
Sweetcorn: See Corn			
Sweet Potato: ½ cup, 3½ oz	90	0	24
Tomatoes, Sundr.: Natural, 5-6 pces	20	0	5
In Oil, drained, 6 pieces, ½ oz	40	2.5	4
Tomato Products: See Page 144			
Vegetables, mixed, ½ cup, 4 oz	45	0	8
Yams: in Light Syrup, ½ cup, 4 oz	105	0	25
Candied, ½ cup, 5 oz	170	0	46
Zucchini in Tomato Sauce, ½ c., 4 oz	30	0	8

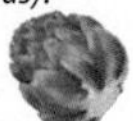

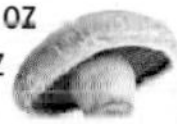

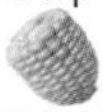

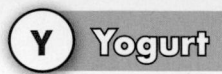
Quick Guide   **C**   **F**   **Cb**

Yogurt
***Average All Brands:** Per 8 oz Cup*

	C	F	Cb
Plain Yogurt: Whole	140	8	10
Low-Fat	145	3.5	16
Fat-Free	125	0.5	17
Fruit Flavored: Whole, 8 oz	225	8	32
Low-Fat	230	3	43
Fat-Free, regular	215	0.5	43
Fat-Free, no sugar added	80	0	15

Yogurt Parfait/Deli Cups
With Fruit Pieces:
(⅔ Yogurt + ⅓ Fruit)

	C	F	Cb
Small, 8 oz cup	140	3	20
Large, 12 oz cup	210	4.5	30
With Fruit + Granola:			
Small, 8 oz cup (+ ¾ oz Granola)	235	7	30
Large, 12 oz cup (+ 1½ oz Granola)	400	13	58

Yogurt ~ Brands   **C**   **F**   **Cb**

	C	F	Cb
Alta Dena: Low-Fat: Plain, 8 oz	170	4.5	20
All Natural, average all flavors	215	2	41
Non-Fat: Fruit, average all flavors	185	0	38
Plain, 8 oz	110	0	16
Vanilla, 8 oz	160	0	30
America's Choice, Nonfat, av., 6 oz	90	0	15
Axelrod's, fat free, av. all flavos, 6 oz	90	0	17
Blue Bunny:			
Light, average fruit flavors, 6 oz	85	0	14
Breyers:			
Creme Savers, av. all flavors, 6 oz	165	1.5	31
Fruit On The Bottom, av. all flav., 6 oz	160	1.5	32
Inspirations: Choc Chip/Mint, 6 oz	140	3.5	23
Strawberry; Vanilla Bean, 4 oz	110	1	22
Light, average all flavors, 6 oz	80	0	12
Smooth & Creamy, av. all flav., 6 oz	170	1.5	34
YoCrunch: Light, av. all flavors, 6 oz	120	1	22
Low-Fat w/ Granola, fruit, average	190	2	38
M&M's; Reese's, average	200	4.5	35
100 Calorie: Strawb.	100	0.5	23
Vanilla, Cheesecake	100	2	21
Brown Cow:			
Cream Top: Plain, 6 oz	130	7	9
Fruit Flavors, average, 6 oz	175	6	27
Low-Fat: Plain, 8 oz cup	130	3	15
Flavors, average, 6 oz	150	2	27
Non-Fat: Plain, 8 oz cup	110	0	16
Fruit Flavors, av., 6 oz	135	0	26
Greek: Plain, 5.3 oz cup	80	0	6
Strawberry, 5.3 oz cup	130	0	18

	C	F	Cb
Cabot:			
Non-Fat: Plain, 8 oz	100	0	19
Fruit flavors, 6 oz	120	0	23
Greek Style: Plain, 8 oz	290	23	12
Low-Fat (2%), 6 oz	160	3	25
Cascade Fresh:			
Low-Fat, all flavors, 6 oz	140	2	23
Fat-Free, all flavors, 6 oz	110	0	20
Whole Milk: Plain, 8 oz	170	8	12
Flavors, average, 8 oz	200	7	24
Chobani:			
Greek Yogurt:			
Non-Fat: Vanilla	120	0	13
Blueberry; Peach	140	0	20
Low-Fat, fruit, average	160	3	19
Colombo:			
Light, all flavors, 6 oz	90	0	16
Classic: Banana Strawb.	180	0	39
Vanilla, 6 oz	130	0	25
Fat-Free, Plain, 8 oz	100	0	15
Dannon:			
Activia Yogurt:			
Plain, 8 oz	170	4.5	20
Light, av. all flav., 4 oz	70	0	13
Fiber, all flavors., 4 oz cup	110	2	19
Drinks, all flavors 5.75 fl.oz	160	3	27
All Natural:			
Average all flavors, 6 oz	150	2.5	25
Low-Fat, Plain, 6 oz	100	2.5	12
Non-Fat, Plain, 6 oz	80	0	12
Danimals: Crush Cups, all flav., 4 oz	100	1.5	17
Drinkables, 3.1 fl.oz	70	0.5	15
Desserts: Blueb. Cheesecake, 4 oz	150	4	23
Average other flavors	140	4	21
Fruit On The Bottom,			
average, 6 oz	150	1.5	28
Light & Fit: All flavors, 6 oz	80	0	16
Quarts, Strawb.; Vanilla,			
8 oz serving	110	0	21
Smoothies, 7 fl.oz	70	0	14
Carb & Sugar Control: 4 oz cup	50	1.5	3
Emmi Swiss (Low-Fat): *Per 6 oz cup*			
Berry Pomegranate	180	3	30
Coffee	170	3	27
Muesli	110	2.5	10
Pink Grapefruit; Van. Bean	110	2.5	10
Fage			
Classic: Peach; Cherry; Strawb., 5.3 oz	210	12	18
Honey, 5.3 oz	250	12	28
0%, 8 oz	120	0	9
2%: Plain 8 oz	150	4.5	9
Fruit, 5.3 oz	130	2.5	18
Honey, 5.3 oz	180	2.5	29

Brands (Cont)

	C	F	Cb
Greenway Org., Lowfat, av, 6 oz	150	1.5	29
Horizon Organic: *Per 6 oz ctn*			
Fruit on Bottom, all flavors	140	0	27
Low-Fat: Blended, av. all flavors	150	1.5	27
Yogurt Tuberz (1)	60	0.5	11
Jewel: *6 oz Carton (Lowfat)*			
Blended, av. all flavors	150	1.5	30
Fruit On The Bottom, av.	180	2	33
Light, average all flavors	110	0	20
Fat-Free, Plain	90	0	14
32 oz Tubs: *Per 8 oz*			
Lowfat, average fruit flav.	205	2	39
Plain, Non-Fat	120	0	18
Kemps:			
'Light' 80 Calories', 6 oz ctn	80	0	16
Yo-J Drink, average, 8.3 fl.oz	150	0	35
Kirkland, Low-Fat:			
Blueberry; Peach; Strawberry, 8 oz	240	2	48
Kroger: *Per 6 oz carton*			
Blended, all flavors	190	2	35
Carb Master, av. all flav.	80	1.5	4
Fruit On The Bottom,			
average all flavors	170	2	30
Lite, average all flavors	80	0	13
La Yogurt: *Per 6 oz ctn*			
Original, average all flavors	150	2.5	27
Light, average all flavors	90	0	15
Rich & Creamy, av. all flav.	190	2	35
Enriched, average all flav.	170	1.5	32
Sabor Latino:			
Dulche De Leche, 6 oz	190	1.5	36
Fruit Flavors, average, 6 oz	190	1.5	37
LALA, Blended			
Fruit Flavors, average,	200	4	35
Smoothies, average, 9 fl.oz	200	4	37
Lucerne: *Per 6 oz ctn*			
Low-Fat:			
Fruit flavors, average	170	2	32
Vanilla	170	2	33
Fat-Free: Plain	80	0	13
Light Fat-Free, fruit, 6 oz	90	0	17
Mountain High			
Original Style: Plain, 8 oz	180	8	17
Strawb./Vanilla, 8 oz	210	7	28
Low-Fat: Plain, 8 oz	140	2.5	18
Lemon; Raspberry, 8 oz	190	2	33
Strawberry; Vanilla, average, 8 oz	175	2.5	29
Fat-Free: Plain, 8 oz	120	0	18
StrawberryVanilla, average, 8 oz	160	0	30

	C	F	Cb
Nancy's: *Per 8 oz ctn*			
Whole Milk:			
With Honey	170	8	17
With Fruit on Top, average	230	5	41
Low Fat:			
Plain/Lemon, average	150	3	16
Average other flavors	175	3	27
Non-Fat:			
Plain	120	0	17
Vanilla (32 oz carton)	220	0	40
Soy Cultured:			
Plain, 6 oz	150	3	25
Berry flavors, average	140	3.5	24
O Organics, (Safeway),			
Low-fat, average, 6 oz	140	2.5	23
Oikos, Greek Yogurt:			
Plain, 5.3 oz cup	80	0	6
1 cup, 8 oz	130	0	9
Blueberry, 5.3 oz cup	120	0	16
Honey, 5.3 oz cup	120	0	18
Vanilla, 5.3 oz cup	110	0	12
Publix: Fat-Free, Plain, 8 oz	140	0	23
Swiss Style, Low-Fat, 8 oz	240	2.5	41
Ralphs: *Same as Kroger*			
Roberts: *Per 6 oz ctn*			
Low-Fat, average all flavors	165	1.5	32
Fat-Free, all flavors	90	0	14
Silk (Soy): Plain, 8 oz	150	4	22
Vanilla, 6 oz	150	3	25
Average other flavors, 6 oz	155	2	30
So Delicious: *Per 6 oz ctn*			
(Made with Coconut Milk):			
Plain	130	7	16
Fruit Flavors, average	140	6	2
Chocolate	170	6	28
Vanilla	150	6	22
Stater Bros: *Per 6 oz ctn*			
Plain	105	1.5	14
Fruit on the Bottom, Strawberry	170	1.5	34
Blended Low-Fat, Strawberry	150	1.5	29
Stonyfield Farm, (Organic): *Per 6 oz ctn*			
Fat-Free:			
Plain	80	0	11
Chocolate Underground	180	0	37
Fruit Flavors, average	120	0	24
Lowfat Smooth & Creamy:			
Apple Pie	130	1.5	21
Other fruit flavors, average,	130	1.5	22
Plain	90	1.5	11

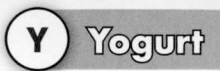

Brands (Cont)   C   F   Cb

	C	F	Cb
Stonyfield Farm (Cont):			
O'Soy Smooth & Creamy			
Chocolate; Vanilla, 6 oz	155	3	25
Fruit On The Bottom, av. all flav, 6 oz	170	2.5	29
Trader Joe's:			
French Village: Non-Fat, all flav., 6 oz	130	0	24
32 oz Containers: Plain, 8 oz	120	0	17
French Vanilla, 8 oz	180	0	34
Greek Style: *Per 8 oz Container Unless Indicated*			
Plain, 8 oz	260	18	14
Apricot Mango; Honey, average	300	15	28
Non-Fat: Plain, 8 oz	120	0	7
Blueberry, 5.3 oz	120	0	16
Honey, 5.3 oz	120	0	17
Pomegranate, 5.3 oz	110	0	12
Low-Fat Pre-Stirred,			
Fruit Flavors, 8 oz	220	3	40
Organic Lowfat,			
Fruit flavors, av., 6 oz	140	2.5	23
Organic Low-Fat Parfait: *Per 6 oz*			
Chocolate	170	5	7
Mango; Mixed Berry, average	145	2	26
Wallaby Organic:			
Crml Apple; Mango Tangrne., av., 6 oz	150	2	27
Dark Chocolate, 6 oz	170	5	27
Wawa: *Per 8 oz Cup*			
Fruit On The Bottom, average	220	2	42
Blended: Lowfat, all flavors	210	2.5	41
Nonfat, all flavors	120	0	20
Weight Watchers:			
Average all flavors	100	0.5	17
Whole Foods (365)			
365: Non-Fat, Plain, 6 oz	90	0	13
Fruit flavors, average 6 oz	145	0	30
Vanilla, 6 oz	130	0	23
Whole Soy: Plain, 6 oz	150	3.5	27
Berry; Strawb. Banana, 6 oz	180	3.5	35
Other flavors, average, 6 oz	160	3.5	30
YoCrunch: *Low-Fat, 6oz Cup*			
Cookies n' Cream	180	3.5	33
With Granola, all flavors	190	2	38
Yoplait:			
Original, av. all flav., 6 oz	170	1.5	33
Light, Fruit Flavors, 6 oz	100	0	19
Fiber One, average all flavors, 4 oz	50	0	13
Delights, av., all flavors, 4 oz ctn	100	1.5	16
Greek: Plain, 6 oz	100	0	10
Strawberry, 6 oz	130	0	19

Brands (Cont)   C   F   Cb

	C	F	Cb
Yoplait (Cont):			
Thick & Creamy, all flavors, 6 oz	190	3.5	32
Light, 6 oz	100	0	20
Large 2lb Container, 99% Fat-Free,			
1 cup, 8 oz	200	1.5	39
Whips!: Chocolate flavors, 4 oz	160	4	26
Fruit flavors, 4 oz	140	2.5	25
Yo-Plus, av. all flav., 4 oz	110	1.5	21
Yoplait Kids: 4 oz cup	80	1	13
Go-Gurt!, 2.25 oz tube	70	0.5	13
Splitz, all flavors, 1 ctn	90	1	17
Squeezers, 2 oz	60	1	11
Trix, Fruit Flavors, 4 oz	115	0.5	18

Yogurt Drinks & Probiotics

	C	F	Cb
BioKult:			
Cultured,			
All flavors, 2.1 oz bottle	35	0	8
Cacique:			
Yonique, all flavors, av.			
7 fl.oz ctn	200	1.5	35
Dannon: Activa, all flavors, 3.1 fl oz	160	3	27
Danimals, all flavors, 3.1 fl.oz	70	0.5	15
DanActive,			
average all flav., 3.1 fl.oz	80	1.5	13
Light 'n Fit Smoothies,			
Non-Fat, all flavors, 7 fl.oz	70	0	14
Glen Oaks, average all flavors, 8 fl.oz	190	3.5	35
Good Belly Probiotic,			
2.7 fl.oz bottle	50	0	12
Kemps, Yo-J Drink,			
All flavors, 8.3 fl.oz	150	0	34
LaLa, Yogurt Smoothies:			
Peach, 9 fl.oz bottle	200	4	37
Pecan & Cereal	200	4.5	36
Strawberry & Cereal	210	4	39
Ralphs, Smoothies:			
Peach, 7 fl.oz	200	2.5	37
Raspberry, 7 fl.oz	210	2.5	40
Strawberry, 7 fl.oz	190	2.5	35
Stonyfield Farm:			
Smoothies, average, 10 oz	230	3	40
Wildwood, average, 8 fl.oz	185	2.5	32
Trader Joe's: *6 fl.oz*			
Lowfat Smoothie, Strawb.	140	2	23
Yoplait Smoothies,			
All Flavors, 8 fl.oz	220	3	43

Updated Nutrition Data ~ www.CalorieKing.com
Persons with Diabetes ~ See Disclaimer (Page 22)

Cafeteria-Style Foods C F Cb

Average All Preperations

	C	F	Cb
Beef Stroganoff, 5 oz	195	13	7
Beef Stroganoff with 4 oz noodles	350	14	36
Chicken Lasagna, 1 piece	300	11	32
Chicken Chop Suey with 4 oz rice	245	4	37
Deep Dish Burrito, 7 oz	265	13	20
Grnd Beef Casserole, 2 scps, 6 oz	245	13	17
Italian Meat Sauce for Spaghetti, 5 oz	150	9	9
with 5 oz Spaghetti	350	10	49
Lasagna, 1 piece	275	11	25
Meatloaf, 3 oz	205	13	4
Ranch Beans, 2 scoops, 6 oz	350	11	45
Red Beans & Rice, 7 oz	280	9	37
Scalloped Potato/Ham, 2 scps, 6 oz	160	6	20
Stuffed Shells in Sauce (1)	105	3	17
Swedish Meatballs (3)	205	12	9
Sweet & Sour Pork/Rice, 9 oz	240	3	40
Swiss Steak w/ Mushr. Gravy, 6 oz	280	11	4
Tator Tot Casserole, 2 scoops, 6 oz	260	15	20
Tenderloin Tips/Mushroom Gravy, 5 oz	210	13	3
with 5 oz noodles	395	15	38
Tuna Noodle Casserole, 2 scps, 6 oz	180	6	17
Turkey Tetrazzini, 2 scoops, 6 oz	195	7	17
Vegetable Lasagna, 1 piece	250	13	21

Croissants

	C	F	Cb
Unfilled: Medium 1½ oz	180	10	21
Filled: With Ham (2 oz), garnish	280	14	24
With Ham (2 oz), Cheese (2 oz)	470	30	20
With Chick (2 oz) Cheese (2 oz)	470	30	20
With Turkey/Ham/Cheese (2 oz ea.)	580	36	20
Au Bon Pain. Ham & Cheese	340	10	46
Spinach & Cheese	250	9	32

7-Eleven: *Page 236*

Bagels

	C	F	Cb
Plain: Large, 4 oz (without filling)	320	2	65
With 2 oz Cream Cheese	500	27	54
With 2 oz Lox (Smoked Salmon)	400	4	65

Also see Bagels Section: *Page 54*
Fast-Foods Restaurants: *Page 176*
Au Bon Pain: *Page 179*
Bruegger's: *Page 185*
Einstein Bros Bagels: *Page 199*

Sandwiches C F Cb

No Spreads Unless Indicated
(Includes 2 Slices Bread ~ 3 oz)

	C	F	Cb
BLT (5 strips Bacon, 2 Tbsp Mayo)	600	40	46
Breaded Chicken & Garnish	540	28	46
Chicken Salad with Mayo., 5 oz	580	30	49
Chopped Liver, Egg, Mayonnaise	630	25	44
Corned Beef with Mustard, 5 oz	560	28	44
Egg Salad with Mayonnaise	570	29	49
Egg Salad Club w/ Bacon & Mayo.	780	53	49
Grilled Cheese (3 oz)	540	30	44
Ham (4 oz); Cheese (4 oz), & Mayo.	910	56	44
Lobster Salad (4 oz) w/ Mayonnaise	530	25	45
Overstuffed Tuna Salad (7 oz)	870	39	75
Philadelphia Cheese Steak Sandwich	550	23	42
Reuben (6 oz Beef/Pastrami,			
2 oz Cheese, 2 Tbsp Dressing)	920	60	28
Roast Beef (4 oz) with Mustard	460	12	45
Roast Pork (4 oz) with Apple Sauce	500	16	55
Shrimp Salad Club w/ Bacon & Mayo.	800	57	48
Sloppy Joe with Sauce (7 oz)	600	30	45
Steak Sandwich (5 oz cooked)	680	32	41
Triple Cheese Melt (4 oz)	720	45	46
Tuna Salad with Mayonnaise, 5 oz	610	30	49
Turkey Breast (5 oz) w/ Mayonnaise	460	18	44
Turkey Breast (5 oz) w/ Mustard	360	7	44
Turkey Club with Bacon, Mayonnaise	830	38	31
Vegetarian with Avocado & Cheese	820	49	72

7-Eleven: *Page 236*

Schlotzsky's: *Page 237*

Subway: *Page 245*

Wraps & Roll-Ups C F Cb

Average All Types
(Meat/Chicken/Fish/Veggie)

	C	F	Cb
Small size, approximately 9 oz	500	25	48
Regular, approximately 15 oz	830	40	80
Large, approximately 22 oz	1400	70	134

Fast-Foods Restaurants: *Page 175*

Au Bon Pain: *Page 179*

Sonic Drive-In: *Page 241*

Subway: *Page 245*

WAWA: *Page 254*

Fair & Carnival Foods

	C	F	Cb
Mexican			
Burrito with Bean/Beef, 17 oz	1100	41	104
Carne Asada, 14.5 oz	820	44	58
Chicken Taco, 3.3 oz	210	12	16
Fish Taco, 5 oz	270	13	31
Nachos with Cheese, 9" plate	860	59	70
Tamale (1), 3.5 oz	180	8	21
Taquito, 5 oz	370	17	43
Greek			
Baklava, 2" square	245	13	32
Falafel, 11.6 oz	660	27	85
Greek Salad, 14 oz	520	48	17
Gyro, 7.5", 12 oz	680	40	55
Spanakopita, 8 oz	200	7.5	23
Italian			
Garlic Bread, ½ loaf, 10 oz	1135	40	147
Pizza Bread, Pepperoni, ½ loaf, 12 oz	1115	32	151
Pizza on a Stick, 1 piece	535	28	55
Personal Pizza, 7":			
Cheese (1)	670	24	80
Pepperoni (1)	795	35	80
Ham & Pineapple (1)	800	31	87
Low Carb			
Beef Patty, wrapped in lettuce, 4 oz	480	33	0
Sandwiches: *Per 7½" Roll*			
Ham, 11 oz	645	39	47
Hot Pastrami, 9 oz	760	17	62
Roast Beef, 11 oz	620	36	46
Philadelphia Cheese Steak, 13 oz	680	36	49
Tuna, 12 oz	830	60	46
Turkey, 11 oz	665	24	65
Veggie, 11 oz	490	23	49
Oriental: Fried Egg Roll, 6 oz	400	19	44
Rice Bowl: Beef, 6" Bowl	880	13	136
Chicken, 6" Bowl	870	15	135
Hamburgers			
⅓ Pound Burger, 7.5 oz	670	41	26
Cheeseburger, 6 oz	550	36	25
Hot Dogs/Franks: *With Bun*			
Hot Dog: Regular, (1)	215	14	28
with Chili, 6 oz	450	32	32
with Chili & Cheese, 7.3 oz	500	36	31
⅓ Pound Hot Dog	550	41	31
Foot Long Hot Dog	470	26	41
Corn Dog: Regular, 4 oz	250	14	23
Jumbo, 6 oz	375	21	36
Jumbo Franks with Bun:			
Bratwurst; Sausage; Kielbasa, av.	800	60	28

Fair & Carnival Foods (Cont)

	C	F	Cb
Barbeque *(Weights with Bone)*:			
Chicken, 15 oz	740	24	34
Corn on the Cob, 8" (1), 16 oz	200	1	42
Pork Ribs, 18 oz	1360	68	21
Smoked Turkey Legs (w/ skin), 19 oz	1135	54	0
Beef Stew over Rice, 2 cups	440	14	61
Cheese Curds,			
Breaded & Fried, *(Culver's)*, 6.7 oz	670	38	54
Potatoes & Fries			
Australian Battered Potato, 12 oz	1290	66	155
Baked Potato, 14 oz	435	0.5	100
Fries: French, 7 oz	560	24	70
Cheese Fries, 10 oz	645	38	62
Chili Fries, 10 oz	700	36	83
Curly Fries, 7 oz	620	30	78
Tasti Chips, 40 chips, 6.5 oz	780	33	117
Sweet Potato, 14 oz	405	0.5	97
Ranch Dip, 3 oz	165	14	9
Finger Foods			
Artichoke: Steamed, 6 pieces	65	0	16
Fried, 9 pieces	250	14	24
Chicken Nuggets (6)	340	17	26
Chicken Strips (4), 4.5 oz	445	21	33
Finger Steaks (2), 4 oz	400	20	26
Mushrooms, Fried, 10-12 pieces	395	26	34
Onion Rings, 3 rings	310	13	40
Onion Flower	1320	72	140
Shrimp, Fried, 10-12 pieces, 5 oz	555	30	36
Sweet Potato Strips, Fried, 4 pces	750	30	106
Zucchini, Fried, 4 slices	620	40	42
Salads/Sides			
Baked Beans, 4 oz	140	2	38
Chili, 1 cup	280	11	24
Cole Slaw, 5 oz	350	21	37
Pickle, whole (6")	30	0	8
Potato Salad, 5 oz	290	15	35
Candied Apple, 7 oz	330	0	80
Cotton Candy, 5½ oz	625	0	156
Popcorn:			
Plain: Small, 3 oz	450	24	48
Large, 6 oz	900	48	96
Kettle Corn:			
Small, 5 oz	600	15	110
Large, 10 oz	1200	30	220

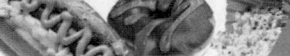

Fair & Carnival Foods (Cont)

Cakes, Donuts, Cookies

	C	F	Cb
Funnel Cake: Plain (1)	760	44	80
Toppings:			
Apple Cinn., 2 oz	85	3	36
Cinn. & Sugar, 2 tsp	40	0	10
Strawberry & Cream, 2 oz	70	0	16
Cheesecake on a Stick, 6 oz	655	47	56
Churro (1), 1½ oz	165	8	21
Cinnamon Roll, large (1)	730	24	114
Cobbler, 5 oz	350	10	62
Cream Puff, 4.3 oz	500	43	22
Donuts, Jumbo Twist, (1), 7.5 oz	905	49	109
Fried Snicker Bar, 5 oz	445	29	42
Fried Twinkie, 1	420	34	45
Fudge, 1.5 oz	200	11	25
Key Lime Pie Bar, 6 oz	635	40	59
Puff on a Stick (4), 8.6 oz	995	86	44
Strawberry Crepe, 4.3 oz	280	14	36
Soft Pretzel, 4.5 oz	340	2	70
Twinkie Dog (Sundae)	500	14	89
Fried Dough:			
Plain (1), 4½ oz	470	23	56
Toppings: Cinnamon Sugar, 2 tsp	40	0	10
Cheese Powder, 2 tsp	70	3	2

Ice Cream & Frozen Treats

Dippin' Dots Ice Cream: Small, 4 oz	150	7	17
Medium, 8 oz	305	14	35
Frozen Banana, chocolate coated, 5 oz	240	4	53
Frozen Yogurt in sugar cone, 14 oz	475	2	94
Ice Cream: Small, sugar cone, 10 oz	775	42	83
Large, sugar cone, 14 oz	935	54	96
Sherbet, 8 oz	270	4	59
Snow Cone (includes 3 oz syrup)	270	0	68
Strawberry, Choc. Dipped, 1 piece	125	7	15

Drinks, *Slushies*

Lemonade, 18 fl.oz	210	0	52
Orange Julius, 20 fl.oz	490	10	96
Strawberry Julius, 20 fl.oz	430	0	98
Icee, 16 fl.oz	235	0	59
Malt, 16 fl.oz	690	33	85
Slushies, 16 fl.oz	260	0	65
Soft Frozen Lemonade, 12 fl.oz	300	0	78
Smoothies: Berry Flavors, 16 fl.oz	350	1	80

Stadium Foods

Sandwiches

	C	F	Cb
Bacon Burger, 8.3 oz	470	25	34
Cheeseburger, 8.3 oz	450	23	33
Chicken Sandwich: w/Cheese, 8.3 oz	510	29	40
Without Cheese, 7.7 oz	460	25	40
With Bacon, 8.3 oz	530	31	41
Hamburger, 7.8 oz	400	19	33
Polish Sausage S'wich, 7 oz	565	33	46
French Fries, 6.4 oz	470	34	39
Fruit Cup, 6 oz	80	0	20

Hot Dogs

Chili Dog, 7.7 oz	520	29	45
Hot Dog, 6.4 oz	465	21	50
Jumbo Dog, 6 oz	440	25	38
Kraut Dog with Sauerkraut, 7.8 oz	490	27	41
Nachos, 40 chips w/4 oz cheese	1100	59	132

Individual Pan Pizza (6"): *Per 10 oz Pizza*

BBQ Chicken	630	24	71
Cheese	630	27	71
Pepperoni	660	30	70

Snacks

Brownie, 2.5" x 4.5"	360	18	44
Cheese Sauce, 1.25 oz	100	8	4
Cheetos, 2.75 oz package	440	28	42
Chocolate Chip Cookie, 2.3 oz	280	12	40
Churros, 8", 3 oz	325	15	42
Doritos, Nacho, 2.75 oz package	390	20	48
King Size Candy:			
Butterfinger, 3.75 oz	485	18	75
Nestle Crunch, 2.75 oz	390	21	85
Lays Chips, 2.75 oz package	440	28	42
Peanuts in shell, 8 oz	930	80	24
Popcorn: Small (9 cup size)	575	35	56
Large (15 cup size)	950	58	93
Red Vines, 5.5 oz box	560	0	136
Snow Cone, (includes 3 oz syrup)	270	0	68
Soft Pretzel: Reg., 5.5 oz	490	3.5	101
Giant, 8 oz	710	5	147
Beverages: Orange Juice, 12 fl.oz	180	0	2
Beer: Heineken, 16 fl.oz	200	0	16
Light Miller, 16 fl.oz	165	0	10
Miller Draft, 16 fl.oz	205	0	18
Jack Daniels Punch, 12 fl.oz	235	0	34
Wine, White, 9 fl.oz	190	0	6
Soda (with ½ ice), average: 20 fl.oz	160	0	40
32 fl.oz	260	0	65
Starbuck's Frappuccino, 12 fl.oz	195	2.5	39

Restaurant & International Foods

Chinese & Asian Dishes

Appetizers	C	F	Cb
Crab Cake, 2¼ oz	125	10	1
Dumplings: Pork, steamed, 1	80	4.5	5
Pork, fried, 1 dumpling	90	6	5
Vegetable, steamed, 1	35	1	5
Egg Rolls, mini, 3 rolls	100	3	11
Spring Roll:			
Small, 1½ oz	85	4	9
Medium, 3 oz	170	8	17
Large, 5 oz	290	15	29
Wonton, 1 only	75	4	5
Soup: Egg Flower, bowl 12 oz	90	2	16
Hot & Sour Soup, bowl 12 oz	110	3.5	14
Rice: Plain, 1 cup (½ Pint), 6½ oz	320	2	66
2 cups (1 Pint), 13 oz	640	4	132
Fried: 1 cup, 5 oz	365	11	55
Large dish, 16 oz	950	28	67
Noodles: Chinese Egg, ckd, 1 cup	200	4	37
Entrees & Mains: *Per Serving*			
Almond Chicken, 6 oz	270	10	21
BBQ Pork, 5.5oz	440	23	15
Beef in Black Bean Sauce, 8.5 oz	390	17	17
Broccoli Beef, 6 oz	370	21	13
Chicken & Broccoli, 5.5 oz	160	8	10
Chicken Skewers, 3 oz	210	9	18
Chop Suey:			
Chicken, 5 oz	140	9	2
Pork, 5 oz	170	12	3
Chow Mein, Beef/Chicken, 8 oz	390	12	59
Crab Puff/Rangoon, 1 dumpling	190	11	13
Crispy Fried Chicken, 8 oz	485	33	12
Egg Drop Soup: W/ Noodles, 1 cup	110	3	16
Without Noodles, 1 cup	60	3	4
Egg Foo Yung with Sauce, 1 cup	270	15	16
Kung Pao Chicken, 5.5 oz	240	15	12
Lemon Chicken, 5 oz	525	21	57
Lo Mein (stir-fried) 8 oz	705	42	49
Moo Shu Chicken (2)	360	19	25
Omelet, Chicken/Shrimp, 16 oz	990	82	16
Orange Chicken, 5.5 oz	500	27	42
Steamed Whole Fish, ½ Sockeye Salmon	646	36	23
Sweet & Sour:			
Fish, 20 oz	1160	58	106
Pork, 5.5 oz	400	23	35
Vegetable Combination, w/ oil, 6 oz	367	5	66
Vegetables, Steamed, without oil, 6 oz	137	1	29
Sauces: Mandarin Sauce 1.5 oz	70	0	17
Potsticker Sauce 1.5 oz	35	0	8
Bubble Tea, average, 12 fl oz	280	0.5	68
Fortune Cookie: Each	32	0.5	7

Cajun & Creole

	C	F	Cb
Alligator, 4 oz cooked	160	2	0
Baked Herb Chicken, 1 serving	850	53	2
Bouillabaisse	400	15	10
Cajun Fried Turkey, 1 serving	630	25	0
Cocktail Sauce, 2 Tbsp	30	0	6
Couche-couche, ½ cup	80	0	17
Crawfish Bisque, 1 serving	500	10	10
Crawfish, cooked, 2 oz	45	0.5	0
Creole Jambalaya, 1 serving	550	30	15
Frog Legs, steamed (2)	45	0	0
Guinea Fowl, flesh, 4 oz, cooked	160	4	0
Hogshead Cheese, ¼ cup	80	5.5	0
Jambalaya, Shrimp & Crabmeat	520	14	12
Red Beans & Rice, 1 serving	400	17	52
Roasted Quail, w/ Bacon on Toast	550	25	15
Remoulade Sauce, 2 Tbsp, 1 oz	110	11	2
Shrimp Creole, 1 serving	450	20	10
Stuffed Smothered Steak, with 1 cup Rice	890	50	50
Turtle, cooked, 3 oz	120	3	0

Cuban

	C	F	Cb
Bl. Beans w/ Rice (Moros con Cristianos)	510	22	76
Black-Eyed Pea Fritters (Bollitos de Carita)	80	5	6
Casserole Corn Tamale	445	20	55
Chicken w/ Yellow Rice (Arroz con Pollo)	925	49	87
Cuban Bread (Pan Cubano)	80	1.5	15
Donuts in Syrup (Bunuelos)	170	5	10
with Melado	100	5	10
Grilled Plantains	145	0	40
Gypsy's Arm Cake (Brazo Gitano)	260	18	42
Roast Pork S'wich (Pan con Lechon)	640	30	62
Seasoned Beef with Olives & Raisins (Picadillo)	435	36	10
Shredded Beef (Ropa Vieja)	550	35	10
Taro Root Mash (Pure de Malanga)	315	3	69
Yuca with Citrus Garlic Dressing (Yuca con Mojo)	190	9	25

French Foods

	C	F	Cb
Blanquette d'Agneau (Lamb Stew)	800	30	17
Brioche, 1 cake	280	14	34
Bouillabaisse	400	15	10
Coq au Vin	800	30	16
Coquilles St. Jacques	320	13	36
Crème Brulée, 1 serving	460	40	21

Updated Nutrition Data ~ www.CalorieKing.com
Persons with Diabetes ~ See Disclaimer (Page 22)

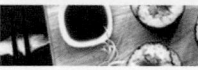

French Foods (Cont)

	C	F	Cb
Baguette, 3 slices, 2.2 oz	150	1	35
Creme Caramel (Caramel Custard)	260	10	38
Crepe Suzette, 1x6" crepe with sauce	220	10	13
Duck a l'Orange	780	35	47
Escargot (Snails), garlic butter (6)	200	10	4
Frog Legs, fried, 4 med. pairs	400	20	10
Lamb Noisettes, fried, 2 chops	500	40	1
Potage Creme Crecy (Carrot Soup)	360	18	14
Salade Nicoise (Tuna/Olives/Vegs)	450	13	14
Veal Cordon Bleu (Veal/Ham)	650	25	18
Vichyssoise (Potato /Leek Soup), 1 c.	200	9	15
Baguette & French Stick: *Page 54*			
Croissants: *Pages 135, 165*			

German

	C	F	Cb
Bavarian Bread Dumpling, 3 small	330	10	28
Beef Goulash with Veggies	520	20	46
Black Forest Cake, 1 slice	380	16	30
Bratwurst, grilled, 1 medium, 6 oz	450	37	2
Chicken: Fried, Viennese-style	530	20	28
Livers with Apple/Onion, 6 oz	460	28	10
Herring, Pickled: Rollmops, 4 oz	260	16	3
With Sour Cream, 4 oz	310	20	3
Hot Sausage Curry	300	7	6
Kugelhupf Cake, 1 large slice, 4 oz	400	23	40
Sauerbraten Pork (Pot Roast)	650	35	15
Torte: Linzer (Almond/Raspb. Jam)	430	18	58
Sacher (Chocolate/Apricot Jam)	260	12	23
Weiner Schnitzel, 1 medium	750	35	38

Greek

	C	F	Cb
Baklava Pastry: Small	240	13	32
Large, 3¾ oz	400	21	45
Calamari, deep fried, 1 cup	300	13	17
Chicken Kebob Plate	345	13	8
Dolmades (Stuffed Grape Leaves)			
2 rolls, 6 oz	200	5	13
Galactobureko, 1 only			
(Filo, Custard, Pastry in Syrup)	360	15	48
Greek Chicken Salad	400	18	9
Gyros: 6" Pita, 8 oz	475	32	35
7½" Pita, 12 oz	680	40	55
Hummus & Pita, 4 oz	260	12	30
Kataifi, (Filo, Nut, Pastry in Syrup)	350	11	56
Moussaka: Small serving, 8 oz	350	22	22
Large serving, 16 oz	700	44	44
Soup: Avgolemono (Egg Lem. Soup			
with Chicken & Rice), 1 cup	85	6	5
Souvlaki (Lamb), each, 2 oz	120	6	1

Greek (Cont)

	C	F	Cb
Stuffed Tomatoes, 2	250	12	17
Taramosalata, 1 T., ½ oz	40	3	2
Tyropita (Filo/Egg/Cheese Pastry)	350	26	31
Daphne's Greek Cafe: *See Fast-Foods Section*			

Hawaiian

	C	F	Cb
Ahi Tuna, grilled w/o fat, (6 oz fillet)	220	2	0
Chicken Long Rice, 1 cup, 7 oz	240	14	12
Gyoza, 1 only	55	2	6
Haupia (Coconut Pudd.), 1 pce (4"x 2½")	120	6	17
Hawaiian Sweet Bread, ½" sl., 2 oz	180	4.5	29
Kalua Chicken, 4 oz	280	16	0
Pork, 4 oz	350	24	0
Kim Chee (pickled cabbage), ½ c., 4 oz	20	0	5
Kulolo (Taro Pudding), 1 slice	125	5	19
Lau Lau:			
Chicken (1) 7 oz	280	21	3
Pork (1) 7 oz	320	26	5
Loco Moco (rice/burger/egg/gravy)	650	27	63
Lomi Salmon, ¼ cup, 4 oz	20	1	2
Malasadas (Donut), 2 oz	240	13	26
Manapua (Char Siu Pork Bun), 2.3 oz	180	8	25
Poi (mashed cooked taro), 1 c., 8½ oz	270	0.5	65
Poke, average all types, 3 oz	90	1	0
Portuguese Sausage, 2 oz	180	15	2
Potato Salad, ½ cup, 5 oz	170	10	17
Shave Ice *(Matsumoto),*			
all flavors:			
With Icecream, 1 large	300	4	64
With Beans, 1 large	290	0	72
Spam Musubi:			
with Regular Spam	265	11	34
(4 oz rice+1.3 oz Spam/7-Eleven Hawaii)			
Homemade: w/ Lite Spam (50% less fat)	220	5	34
Taro Pancake Mix, ⅓ cup (makes 2)	140	2	26
Plate Lunches:			
Chicken Katsu (9 oz) with 2 scps Rice	1110	48	108
+ Macaroni Salad, ¾ cup	1360	68	123
or Tossed Salad + Fr. Dress. (2 T.)	1240	61	111
Hamburger (5 oz) w/ 2 scoops Rice	710	24	81
Gravy + Macaroni Salad	1135	49	112
MahiMahi (7 oz) with 2 scps Rice	650	12	90
+ Macaroni Salad + Tartar Sce	1150	58	109
or Macaroni Salad, w/o Tartar ce	935	34	108
or Tossed Salad + Fr. Dress. (3 T.)	815	27	96
or Tossed Salad, without dressing	670	12	93
Teri Beef (5 oz) with 2 scps Rice	790	23	94
+ Macaroni Salad, ¾ cup	1095	47	113
or Tossed Salad, without dressing	800	23	95

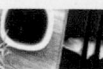

Indian & Pakistani | C | F | Cb

Per Serving
(Meat dishes allow 4 oz meat/serving)

	C	F	Cb
Aloo Samosa, each	155	12	12
Alu Gosht Kari (Meat/Potato Curry)	600	40	23
Chicken Korma	500	35	6
Chicken Pilaf (Murgh Biriyani)	700	53	50
Chicken Tikka	260	16	2
Chicken Vindaloo	400	20	8
Chapati/Roti, 7" diameter, 1 piece	60	0.5	11
Dahl (Lentil Puree): 1 cup, without oil	230	1	37
1 Tbsp Tadka (oil topping)	120	13	0
Dhakla (Lentil Dish), 1" square, 1 oz	105	5	13
Dhansak, ½ cup	105	3.5	11
Gosht Kari (Meat Curry/Tomato/Pot.)	460	25	17
Lamb Pilaf	520	35	40
Lassi (Sweet or Mango), 1 cup, 8 oz	160	4	24
Masala Gosht (Beef/Tomato/Gravy)	400	25	18
Mulligatawney Soup, average	300	15	8
Murgh Tikka, 1 cup	300	4	7
Naan Flatbread, ½, 2 oz	160	3.5	29
Pappadum, 1 large/2 small	50	3	5
Pesrattu (Lentil Crepe), 9", 2.6 oz	130	5	15
Pork Vindaloo Curry without Rice	620	47	3
Rajmah (Kidney Bean Curry), 1 cup	225	5	35
Rogan Josh (Lamb/Yogurt Sauce), without Rice/Potatoes	500	30	3
Shahi Korma (Braised Lamb)	430	28	3
Tandoori Chicken: Breast	260	13	5
Leg/Thigh portion	300	17	6

Italian Dishes | C | F | Cb

	C	F	Cb
Baked Ziti: Small	370	27	32
Regular	575	42	49
Breadstick (1), 2 oz	120	2.5	25
Broccoli Fettucine Alfredo, regular	815	23	125
Bruschetta, 2 slices	380	17	53
Calzones, average, all types	840	34	101
Cannelloni, 1 tube, 6 oz	280	15	18
Cheese Breadstick (1), 2.4 oz	180	8	20
Cheese Ravioli with Sauce	495	17	65
Chicken Alfredo	775	29	82
Chicken Parmigiana, 11 oz	520	22	16
Chicken Scallopine, dinner	1110	71	68
Eggplant Parmigiana	900	39	78
Fettucine Alfredo: Small	525	15	80
Lunch	775	22	119
Dinner	1130	81	68
Linquine & Seafood, dinner	1130	71	79
Manicotti Formaggio	800	38	57
Meat Lasagne: Small, 10 oz	440	23	39
Large, 16 oz	700	36	60
Meat Ravioli	725	22	102
Minestrone Soup, 1 bowl	110	2	18
Penne Rustica: Lunch	1300	71	76
Dinner	1540	80	101
Ravioli, over-stuffed, average	990	67	57
Spaghetti & Meatballs:			
With Tomato Sauce: Kids	500	20	58
Medium/Lunch	1080	63	89
Large/Dinner	1430	81	119
With Meat Sauce: Kids	550	25	56
Medium/Lunch	1300	79	84
Large/Dinner	1700	103	110
Veal Marsala, dinner	1320	66	132
Veal Parmigiana, dinner	1270	65	116
Vegetable Primavera	610	8	116
Macaroni & Cheese ~ *Page 133*			
Panini S'wich (Restaurant):			
Chicken, 16 oz	900	38	81
Meats, average, 18 oz	940	39	81
Vegetarian, 15 oz	750	31	83
Pizza: Ready-To-Eat ~ *Page 135*			
Gourmet Deep Dish (*Gino's East*) ~ *Page 202*			
Desserts: Lemon Ice	180	0	45
Gelato: Vanilla (Milk Base), ½ cup	200	15	18
Choc. Hazelnut (Milk), ½ cup	370	29	26
Water Base, ½ cup	100	0	25
Tiramisu, 1 piece, 5 oz	400	29	30

For more listings see Fast-Foods Section

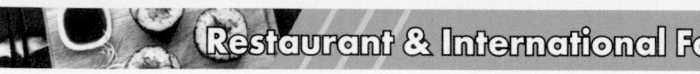

Japanese

	C	F	Cb
Sushi Rice: cooked, 1 Tbsp	25	0	5
1 cup, 5¼ oz	380	3	82
Sushi (Maki) Rolls: *Per Piece*			
Average all types (California Rolls; Cream Cheese with Crab; Eel; Salmon; Shrimp; Tuna; Yellowtail; Vegetable)			
Small (1⅛" diameter x 1⅛" high), 0.8 oz	25	0.5	3.5
Medium (1¾" diam. x 1¾" high), 1.6 oz	50	1	7
Large (2¼" diameter x ⅞" high), 2 oz	60	1.5	9
Sushi Packs: *Per Pack*			
Average all types: 6 large pieces	370	5	55
9 medium pieces	360	6	60
12 small pieces	265	3	45
Futomaki (thick roll), 6 pieces	380	5	72
Hand Roll (Cone) 4 oz	120	2	18
Inari (rice filled soybean pocket), 4 pces	420	9	73
Sushi-Nigiri (fish on rice):			
average all types, 1 piece	70	0.5	12
Sushi Plate: Assorted, 6 pieces	420	3	36
Combination (Sushi & Sushi Rolls)			
2 Sushi + 6 small & 3 med. rolls	400	7	72
Sashimi (Sl. Raw Seafood/Beef)			
Ika (Squid), 4 oz	105	2	0
Hamachi (Yellowtail), 4 oz	165	6	0
Maguro (Yellowfin Tuna), 4 oz	120	1	0
Niku (Beef), 5 oz	200	10	0
Saba (Mackerel), 4 oz	160	7	0
Suzuki (Sea Bass), 4 oz	110	0.5	0
Tako (Octopus), 4 oz	95	1	0
Dipping Sauces: Average, 2 Tbsp	30	0	7
Ginger Vinegar Dressing, 2 Tbsp	20	0	5
Edamame (young green soybeans):			
Steamed (in pods), 4 oz	60	3	5
Boiled beans (no pods), 4 oz	160	7	12
Katsu-don Pork with Rice	1100	39	141
Miso Soup with Tofu pieces, 1 cup	85	3	11
Seaweed Salad, 1.5 oz	20	2	0
Sukiyaki (Beef/Tofu/Veg.), 8 oz	400	24	32
Tempura (Batter-fried Shrimp & Veggies)			
3 large shrimp & veggies	320	18	25
1 shrimp only	60	4	3
Teppan Yaki (Steak, Seafood & Veggies)			
10 oz serving	470	30	15
Teriyaki: Beef, 4 oz serving	350	25	4
Chicken, 4 oz serving	260	9	7
Salmon, medium, 6 oz	270	8	3
Sake Wine (16% alcohol), 3 fl.oz	115	0	7
Yakatori, 1 skewer, 2½ oz	140	5	1

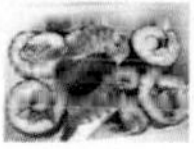

Kosher/Deli Foods

	C	F	Cb
Bagel/Bialy, 1 small, 2 oz	160	2	32
Beiglach (Cheese Knish)	350	17	35
Blintzes: Average, 1 only	120	1	25
With Sour Cream & Preserves	370	10	30
Borscht: (W/o Sour Cream), 1 cup	85	3	14
Diet/Reduced Calorie, 1 cup	30	1	7
Cabbage Roll (meat/rice), 5 oz	170	6	21
Chicken Broth: 1 cup	80	8	0
With vegetables	100	8	5
With noodles	150	9	16
Lowfat, plain, 1 cup	25	1	0
Cholent, 1 medium serving, 1 cup	350	16	48
Chopped Liver: 1 serving, 3 oz	110	6	5
With Egg Salad, ¼ cup	100	7	3
Farfel, dry, ½ cup	90	0.5	21
Hallah (Yeast Bread), 1 slice, 1 oz	85	2	14
Gefilte Fish Balls. Regular, med., 2 oz	55	2	4
With Jelled Broth	80	2	6
Cocktail size, 1 oz	30	1	2
Sweet, medium, 2 oz	65	2	4
With Jelled Broth	95	2	9
Herring: Smoked, 2 oz	120	8	0
In Sour Cream, 2 oz	150	10	0
Kasha, cooked, ½ cup	100	0.5	20
Kipfel (Vanilla/Almdond Cookie), 1 pce	60	2	7
Knaidlach ~ See Matzo Balls			
Knish: Kasha/Potato, 1 only	130	4	22
Cheese, 1 only	350	17	35
Kreplach, beef, 1 piece	40	1	6
Kugel, potato/noodle, 1 serving	300	20	25
Latkes (Potato Pancake), 2 oz	200	11	22
3 Latkes with Sour Cran Apple Sce	750	25	95
Lochshen: Plain, 1 cup	130	2	26
Pudding, 1 cup	380	13	48
Lox (Smoked Salmon), 2 oz	65	2	0
Mandelbrot (Almond Bread),			
1 slice, ¼" thick	45	2	5
Matzo *(See Page 88)*, 1 oz board	110	0.5	21
Matzo Balls: 2 small, or 1 large, 2"	90	3	12
Extra large ball, 3"	180	6	24
Matzo Ball Soup:			
Cup with 2 small or 1 large ball	150	5	27
Bowl with Chicken & Noodles	325	13	34
Jerry's Deli, large bowl	560	17	56
New York Cheesecake, 4 oz	350	24	26
Pierogi, potato/cheese, 1 piece	90	4	11
Reuben S'wich w/ ½ lb Corned Beef	920	60	28
Schmaltz (Rend'd Chicken Fat), 1 Tbsp	90	10	0

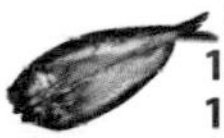

Korean Food

	C	F	Cb
Bibimbab (Veggies & Beef on Rice), 1 cup	565	15	89
Bulgogi (Barbeque Beef), 3.5 oz	325	12	15
Galbi (Short Ribs), 16 oz	975	61	16
Gujeolpan (Pancake with Meat & Vegetables), 1 cup w/ 1 pancake	340	11	39
Japchae (Noodle w/ Veggies & Meat), 1¼ cup	365	19	34
Sides:			
Kimchee (Cabbage Relish), ½ cup	30	0	6
Namool (Assorted Veggies) 1 cup	125	6.5	9
Soups: *Per Serving*			
Muguk (Radish & Chive Soup), 6 oz	105	7	6
Samgyetang (Ginseng Chkn Soup),			
Without Chicken Skin, 1 cup	520	11	60
With Chicken Skin, 1 cup	725	35	60
Yuk Gae Jang (Spicy Beef Soup), 1¼ cup	180	13	5

Lebanese/Middle East

	C	F	Cb
Baba Ghannouj, 2 Tbsp, 1 oz (Eggplant/Sesame Dip)	70	6	2
Baklava, 1 pastry, 1¾ oz (Pastry, Nuts, Syrup)	245	18	18
Cabbage Rolls, 1 roll, 3 oz (Cabbage Leaf, Meat, Rice)	100	3	12
Cous Cous, 1 serving (Semolina, Milk, Fruit, Nuts)	400	21	43
Felafel (Chick Pea Fritter): Fried, 1 medium, 1 oz	60	4	4
Hummus, ¼ cup, 2.2 oz	105	3	5
Fried Kibbi, 1 piece, 3 oz (Wheat, Meat, Pinenuts)	180	8	15
Kafta, 1 skewer, 1½ oz (Ground Lamb Sausage on Skewer)	85	5	2
Kibbeh Naye, 1 cup, 9 oz (Raw Lamb, Bulgur & Spices)	450	18	28
Lebanese Omelet, 1 serving, 4 oz (Egg, Spinach, Pinenuts, Onion)	200	12	13
Pilaf, 1 cup (Rice, Onion, Raisins, Apr., Spice)	400	11	60
Shawourma, 1 serving, 4 oz (Spit-Roast Beef)	280	15	2
Shish Kabob, 1 stick, 2½ oz	130	7	2
Spinach Pie, 1 piece, 3½ oz	290	21	20
Sweet Almond Sanbusak, 1 piece (Pastry, Almonds, Spices)	200	15	11
Tabouli, 1 serving, 4 oz	125	7	13
Tahini Sauce, average, 1 Tbsp	90	8	2

Mexican

	C	F	Cb
Black Bean Soup, 1 bowl	200	3	34
Burritos *(Taco Bell):* Bean	370	10	55
Supreme® Beef	440	18	50
Chili, plain, ¼ cup	90	6	8
Chili con Carne: With Beans, 1 cup	310	17	15
Without Beans, 1 cup	370	28	10
Chimichangas, Beef, 5 oz	400	19	43
Chorizo Sausage, 2 oz	265	23	0
Churros, 1½ oz	150	8	18
Corn Chips, ½ cup, 1 oz	160	10	17
Costillas Ribs, 6 oz	675	52	0
Enchilada, average	330	10	49
Fajitas, Chicken	200	7	20
Guacamole, average, 2 Tbsp, 1 oz	45	4	2
Horchata: *Don Jose,* 1 cup, 8 fl. oz	140	4	25
Cacique, 1 pint bottle, 16 fl. oz	320	7	62
Margarita (with 1½ oz Tequila)	160	0	6
Masa (Pre-mixed for Tamales), 1 oz	80	5	9
Menudo, ½ cup	55	1.5	10
Nachos: *Del Taco,* Regular	395	24	40
Macho Nachos	1145	63	113
Taco Bell: BellGrande®	760	43	80
Supreme®	470	26	42
Nachos: With cheese, peppers, 1 portion (6-8 nachos), 7 oz	600	33	60
W cheese, beans, beef, peppers, 1 portion (6-8 nachos), 9 oz	570	31	56
Nopal Cactus Salad, 1 serving	130	9	11
Papas Fritas (Fried Potatoes) (1), 6 oz	325	18	40
Piloncillo (Brown Sugar): 1 T., 0.46 oz	50	0	13
Cone, small, 3", 3 oz	325	0	81
Quesadilla, Cheese *(Taco Bell)*	490	28	39
Queso Fresco, ¼ cup	80	4.5	8
Refried Beans, ¾ cup, 6 oz	160	3	26
Rice Pudding (Arroz Con Leche), 4 oz	140	3	24
Sopes (Gorditas), 2 oz	120	0	27
Taco *(Taco Bell):* Regular, Crispy	170	10	13
Ranchero Chicken	270	15	21
Taco Supreme®	220	14	14
Double Decker® Taco	340	14	39
Taco Salad with Salsa	840	52	85
Taco Sauce, average, ¼ cup	15	0	3
Taco Shell, regular	50	2	8
Tamales, Beef/Chicken, average 4.5 oz	250	11	27
Taquitos, Beef & Cheese, 4.5 oz	330	15	36
Tostada *(Taco Bell)*	250	10	29
Tortilla, Corn, 6" diameter	70	1	14
Tortilla Chips, 1 oz	150	8	18

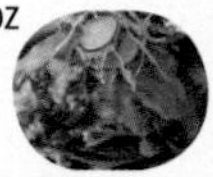

Extra Listings of Mexican Dishes:
• **Fast-Foods Section** *(Taco Bell, Del Taco)*
• **Canned Bean/Chili Products:** *See Page 111*

Mexican (Cont)

	C	F	Cb
Breads: Bolillos, 1 roll, 3½ oz	240	4	42
Telera, 2 oz	150	1.5	19
Mexican Cornbread, 4" square	210	11	19
Cakes, Cookies, Pastries			
Banderilla (Pastry Puff), 1 shell	140	10	8
Bigotes, 7"	570	22	44
Calvos, 2½ oz	320	18	38
Capirotada (Bread Pudding), 10 oz	810	38	107
Cinnamon Cookies, 2	125	8	13
Cocadas, 1 oz	120	6	15
Cortadillo, 1 cookie, 1.9 oz	300	11	48
Concha (All Colors):			
Small (3" diameter), 2½ oz	250	8	38
Medium (4" diameter), 3½ oz	350	11	53
Large (5" diameter), 5½ oz	550	18	84
Cream Puff with Custard, 4¼ oz	255	14	25
Cuerno, 2 oz	200	4.5	34
Cuerno Fine, 2¾ oz	330	17	40
Donut, large, 4", 3½ oz	440	21	58
Elotes, 3½ oz	450	24	51
Empanadas (Average all types):			
Small, 2 oz	230	10	28
Regular, 3 oz	300	14	42
Fiesta Cookie, 2¼ oz	280	8	47
Galletas Mixtas (1), 1 oz	100	2.5	16
Guayaba, 3¼ oz	360	14	53
Jelly Rolls, 3¼ oz	240	4	46
Mantecadites (Almond Shortbread), 4½ oz	670	42	64
Mini Pound Cake, 3 oz	260	12	33
Mini Cupcakes, 1¾ oz	180	8	25
Muffins/Nino Enbuelto, large, 6 oz	465	11	48
Nuez, 3¼ oz	380	17	52
Ojo De Buey, 4 oz	360	15	55
Oreja (Elephant Ear), 3 oz	310	15	38
Pan Dulce (Mexican Sweet Bread), 1 bun	330	10	45
Panquecitos, 2½ oz	260	11	36
Piedras, 4 oz	470	15	76
Polvorones, 3 oz	370	18	48
Puerquitos, 5 oz	600	24	88
Rebanadas, 3½ oz	390	18	51
Roles De Canela (Cinn. Roll), 4½ oz	490	15	81
Roscas, 2¾ oz	360	18	44
Semitas, 3 oz	300	10	46
Sopapillas (flaky pastry puffs), 1 piece	100	7	10
with Honey & Cream	200	14	18
Strawberry Crema Roll (⅙), 2½ oz	240	5	45

Extra Food Listings ~ See CalorieKing.com

Polish

	C	F	Cb
Cabbage Rolls with Sour Cream, 2 sm.	220	10	30
Chicken Casserole w/ Mushrooms, 1 c.	520	27	5
Kielbasa (Sausages, Onions, fried), 2 large	350	28	2
Meatballs in Sour Cream, 3 x 1½" balls	300	16	11
Pierogi, Fruit/Vegetables, 3" ball	80	2	15
Pork Goulash (Pork/Vegetable Stew)	550	21	38
Pot Roast with Vegetables	630	21	28

Soul Foods

	C	F	Cb
Breakfast Sausage, fried, 2 patties	250	17	0
Brunswick Stew, 1 cup, 8.5 oz	320	14	19
Cornbread, homemade, 3 oz	200	7.5	28
Fatback, raw, ¼ oz	60	6.5	0
Ham Hock	90	6.5	2
Hog Maw	45	2.5	0
Hominy, cooked, ¾ cup	110	0.5	25
Hush Puppies, 5 pieces	260	12	35
Kale, cooked, ½ cup	20	0.5	4
Oxtail	70	3.5	0
Pig's Ear, ¼ ear	50	3	0
Pig's Foot, ½ foot	70	4.5	0
Pig's Tail, ⅓ tail	115	10	0
Poke Salad, cooked, ½ cup	16	0.5	3
Pork Brains	40	2.5	0
Pork Chitterlings, simmered, 3 oz	260	25	0
Pork Cracklings, ½ oz	80	6	0
Pork Neck Bones	65	4	0
Pork Skin, 1 cup	70	4.5	0
Pork Tongue, ⅓ tongue	75	5.5	0
Possum	65	3	0
Sousemeat	60	4.5	0
Succotash, ½ cup	80	1	17
Sweet Potato Pie, ⅛ of 9" pie	250	12	34
Tripe, 2 oz	55	2	0
Vienna Sausage, 2 small	90	8	1
1 small	45	4	0.5

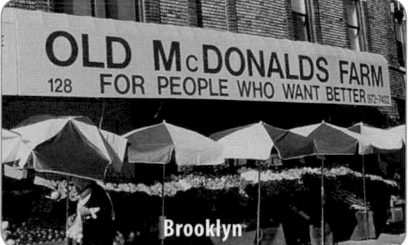

OLD McDONALDS FARM
128 FOR PEOPLE WHO WANT BETTER

Brooklyn

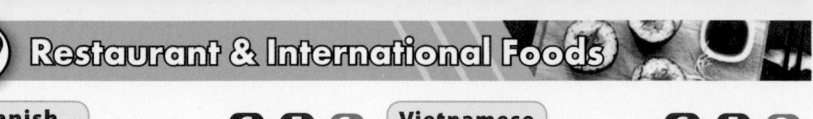

Spanish

	C	F	Cb
Arroz Abanda (Fish with Rice)	340	8	31
Arroz Con Pollo (Rice/Chicken Salad)	500	23	50
Clams Marinara, 8 clams	330	16	22
Cochifrito (Lamb with Lemon/Garlic)	650	25	5
Cochinillo Asado, 2 sl. (Rst Suckling Pig)	300	15	3
Cocido Madrileno			
(Madrid-Style Boiled Dinner)	450	27	18
Flan de Leche (Caramel Custard)	325	9	52
Fritadera de Ternera (Sauteed Veal)	450	27	2
Gazpacho, 1 bowl	60	0	15
Paella a la Valenciana			
(Chicken & Shellfish Rice)	900	42	70
Pollo a la Espanola (Chicken)	475	30	4
Ternera al Jerez (Veal with Sherry)	660	29	6
Zarzuela (Fish & Shellfish Medley)	530	27	40

Thai Foods

	C	F	Cb
Appetizers: Satay Pork, 1 oz	100	4	2
Spring Roll, 1¼ oz	110	6	13
Soups: Tom Yam (Hot & Sour):			
Spicy Shrimp/Seafood, 1 cup	100	4	6
1 bowl	160	7	10
Vegetarian, 1 cup	50	0	11
Curries: Chicken with Ginger, 1 cup	390	34	4
Thick Red Curry withBeef, 1 cup	600	50	7
Thai Chicken Curry, 1 cup	340	23	4
Massaman Curry, 1 cup	680	57	8
Green Curry with Pork, 1 cup	480	44	5
Pad Thai, Large serving, 18 oz	990	38	125
Fish: Steamed with Spicy Thai Sce	450	8	46
Crispy Fried, 5 oz	290	15	9
Spicy Chicken (w/ veggies), stir-fry	450	22	14
Spicy Garlic Tofu w/ veggies, stir-fry	340	18	18
Sticky Thai Rice: Plain 1 cup, 6 oz	170	0.5	36
With Coconut & Sesame Seeds, 1 c.	880	28	120
Stir-fried Rice Noodles, 1 c. 5½ oz	270	9	40
Stir-fried Vegetables, 1 cup	100	3	18
Salads: Green Papaya Salad	160	0	40
Spicy Prawn, 9 shrimp	170	3	15
Thai Chicken, 1 serving	330	9	17
Thai Beef Salad, 1 serving	260	9	15
Thai Noodle, 1 serving	410	13	45
Satay Chicken & Peanut Sauce:			
1 satay stick	390	24	20
Sauces: Peanut Satay, ½ cup, 4 oz	160	10	13

Vietnamese

	C	F	Cb
Banh Cuon (Steam Rice w/ Pork), 1 roll	105	7	8
Bo Nuong (Beef Satay), 2 sticks	265	9	4
Bo Xao Dau Phong			
(Ginger Beef with Onion, Fish Sce)	750	30	10
Ca Chien Gung (Whole Snapper/Ginger)	600	16	6
Canh Chay (Vegetable/Tofu Soup)	80	3	13
Cari (Curry) Chicken, 1 cup	475	29	16
Cari (Curry) Chicken w/ Rice Noodle,			
cup curry & cup cooked noodles	660	29	60
Cari (Curry) Chicken, w/ Steamed Rice,			
cup curry & cup rice	650	29	55
Cuu Xao Lan (Curried Lamb,			
Veggies in Coconut)	900	40	80
Ga Chien (Crisp Chick + Plum Sce)	900	40	105
Ga Nuong (Chicken Satay + Sce)	240	10	4
Ga Xao Rau (Marinated Chicken			
Braised with Vegetables)	800	26	100
Gio Lua (Lean Pork Pie), ⅛ of pie	245	12	0
Goi Cuon (Cold Spring Rolls), each	60	1	7
Rau Cai Xao Chay (Stir Fried Veges)	400	15	65
Thit Bo Vien (Beef Balls), 6 balls	225	14	2
Thit Heo Goi Baup Cai, each			
(Spicy Cabbage Rolls with Pork)	200	7	11
Soup: Per Bowl (1½ Cup)			
Bun Bo Hue (Hot & Spicy Soup			
Without Pork Feet	340	9	35
With Pork Feet	830	45	35
Chicken & Rice Noodle Soup	400	3	55
Pho Bo (Beef Noodle Soup)	410	7	59
Pho Ga (Chicken Noodle Soup)	460	6	58
Pho Tai (Rare Beef & Noodle Soup)	440	7	73
Salad: Per ½ Cup			
Goi Du Du (Green Papaya Salad)	155	3	29
Sauce: Nuoc Cham (Hot Sauce)	5	0	1

Gourmet & Miscellaneous

	C	F	Cb
Ants Eggs/Larvae, 1 Tbsp	20	0	0
Ants, chocolate coated, 3 Tbsp	140	7	2
Bee Maggots, canned, 3 Tbsp	65	2	0
Caviar, black/red, 1 Tbsp	40	3	0
Caterpillars, canned, 2 oz	60	2	0
Frog Legs, fried, 1 pair (large)	125	7	0
Haggis, boiled, 4 oz	350	24	22
Locusts, roasted, 1 oz	35	1	0
Silkworms, raw, 1 oz	60	2	0
Snails in garlic butter, 6 large	200	10	4
Snake, roasted, 4 oz	160	6	0

Updated Nutrition Data ~ www.CalorieKing.com
Persons with Diabetes ~ See Disclaimer (Page 22)

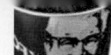

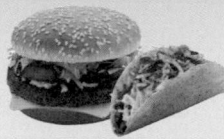

***For More Restaurants &
Full Nutritional Data
~ See CalorieKing.com***

Fast - Foods & *Restaurants*

A&W® (Nov '10)

Burgers:	C	F	Cb
Hamburger	380	19	33
Cheeseburger	420	21	37
Double Cheeseburger	680	38	44
Bacon Cheeseburger	530	30	39
Bacon Double Cheeseburger	760	45	45
Papa Burger	690	39	44
Papa Single Burger	470	25	38
Sandwiches: Crispy Chicken	550	25	52
Grilled Chicken	400	15	31
Chicken Strips: 3 pieces	500	29	32
Hot Dogs: Plain	310	19	23
Coney Chili Dog	340	20	26
Coney Chili Cheese Dog	380	23	28
Corn Dog Nuggets: 5 pieces	180	8	20
8 pieces	280	13	32
Fries/Sides:			
French Fries: Small/Kids, 2½ oz	200	8	28
Regular, 4 oz	310	12	45
Large, 5½ oz	430	17	61
Cheese Fries: 6 oz	390	18	50
Chili Cheese Fries, 7 oz	410	17	52
Cheese Curds, Breaded/Fried, 5 oz	570	40	27
Onion Rings: Reg., Breaded, 4 oz	350	16	45
Large, 5½ oz	480	27	62
Dipping Sauces: BBQ, 1 oz	40	0	10
Honey Mustard, 1 oz	100	6	12
Ranch, 1 oz	160	17	2
Desserts: Per Small Serving			
Polar Swirl: M&M/Oreo, average	700	25	107
Reese's	740	31	97
Sundaes: Choc.;Caramel; Fudge, av.	340	9	55
Strawberry	300	8	47
Soft Serve, Vanilla cone, 5½ oz	260	7	41
Milkshakes: Strawb., Small, 16 fl.oz	670	29	90
Choc.; Vanilla, av., Small, 16 fl.oz	710	30	100
Medium, 20 fl.oz	890	38	123
Floats:			
A&W Root Beer: 20 oz	350	5	77
Large, 32 fl.oz	640	10	136
Diet, 20 oz	170	5	30
Freeze, A&W Root Beer, 16 oz	430	9	79
Sodas:			
Pepsi: Kids, 12 fl.oz, av.	150	0	42
Small, 16 fl.oz	200	0	56
Regular, 20 fl.oz	250	0	70
A&W Root Beer: Regular, 20 fl.oz	270	0	72
Diet, 20 fl.oz	0	0	0
Tea, Lipton Raspberry, Medium, 14 fl.oz	140	0	37

Applebee's® (Nov '10)

Shareable Appetizers: As Served	C	F	Cb
Buffalo Chicken Wings: Classic	710	49	7
Honey BBQ	790	35	59
Hot	720	49	8
Boneless: Classic	1170	69	66
Honey BBQ	1240	55	117
Hot	1170	70	67
Chili Cheese Nachos	1680	107	133
Crunchy Onion Rings	1230	59	161
Dynamite Shrimp	730	54	40
Mozzarella Sticks (9)	940	46	84
Quesadillas: Cheese Grande	1300	87	85
Chicken Grande	1460	90	90
Chicken: Includes Standard Sides			
Chicken Fried Chicken	1250	60	114
Chicken Tenders: Basket	1000	59	81
Platter	1300	77	104
Fiesta Lime Chicken	1230	67	97
Margherita Chicken	750	27	67
Combos: Without Sides or Toppings			
Steak: With Fried Shrimp	630	31	35
With Grilled Shrimp	390	19	2
With Honey BBQ Chicken	530	13	25
With Riblets	950	47	38
Pasta Bowls: As Served			
Chicken Broccoli Alfredo	1200	58	104
Crispy Orange Chicken	1900	73	231
Shrimp Fettuccine Alfredo	1220	62	105
Three-Cheese Chicken Penne	1310	61	120
Realburgers: Without Fries			
Bacon Cheddar Cheeseburger	940	60	48
Cheeseburger	850	52	47
Cowboy Burger	1120	67	74
Fire Pit Bacon Burger	1070	73	50
Hamburger	770	46	47
Quesadilla Burger	1420	104	45
Steakhouse Burger with A1 Sauce	1190	82	63
Ribs & Fajitas: Includes Standard Sides			
Applebees Riblets: Basket	1110	57	89
Platter	1700	88	130
Sizzling Entrees: Includes Sides			
Asian Shrimp	710	15	117
Bourbon Street Steak	700	41	31
Chicken with Spicy Queso Blanco	550	22	37
Steak & Cheese	1070	65	54
Skillet Fajitas: Chicken	1320	53	137
Combo	1410	67	139
Shrimp	1340	65	138
Steak	1360	55	139

Updated Nutrition Data ~ www.CalorieKing.com
Persons with Diabetes ~ See Disclaimer (Page 22)

Applebees® cont... (Nov '10)

Under 500 Calories: Includes Sides	**C**	**F**	**Cb**
Asiago Peppercorn Steak	390	14	26
Asian Crunch Salad with Dressing	490	9	57
Grilled Dijon Chicken & Portobello	450	16	32
Grilled Shrimp & Island Rice	380	4.5	59
Spicy Shrimp Diavolo	500	10	79
Sandwiches: Without Sides			
Bacon, Cheese Chicken Grill	720	33	47
California Turkey Club	1050	63	62
Seafood: As Served			
Double Crunch Shrimp	1280	70	129
Garlic Herb Salmon	750	37	59
Hand-Battered Fish & Chips	1560	105	106
Sliders: Without Fries			
BBQ Pulled Pork	1020	48	89
Cheeseburger	1240	80	81
French Dip	830	49	74
Signature Steaks: Without Sides			
Bourbon Street w/ Mshrms & Onions	600	38	9
Shrimp 'N Parmesan Sirloin	540	28	5
Steak & Toppers: Without Sides			
House Sirloin, 9 oz	310	13	0
New York Strip, 12 oz	590	39	1
Ribeye, 12 oz	590	39	0
Salads: Regular, Without Dressing Unless Indicated			
Apple Walnut Chicken	440	19	17
Grilled Shrimp 'N Spinach	720	53	25
Oriental Grilled Chicken w/ Dressing	1240	77	87
Santa Fe Chicken	900	54	51
Sides: Chili bowl	540	32	24
Loaded Baked Potato	450	35	28
Loaded Mashed Potato	430	29	30
Salads: Caesar, small	90	3.5	10
House, small	230	15	12
Soup: Per Bowl			
French Onion	280	16	19
Tomato Basil Soup	250	14	27
Desserts: As Served			
Maple Butter Blondie	990	52	116
Shooters: Chocolate Moose	450	31	44
Hot Fudge Sundae	340	18	45
Triple Chocolate Meltdown	810	46	91

Arby's® (Nov '10)

Sandwiches:	**C**	**F**	**Cb**
Beef 'n Cheddar Sandwiches:			
Regular	430	19	42
Medium	530	25	42
Large	650	33	44
Roast Beef Sandwiches:			
Regular, 3 oz Beef	350	13	37
Medium, 5 oz Beef	450	19	37
Roastburgers: All American	390	16	40
Bacon Cheddar	430	18	39
Bacon Bleu	450	21	39
Chicken:			
Chicken Bacon & Swiss: Crispy	590	27	54
Roast	470	19	43
Chicken Fillet: Crispy	520	24	51
Roast	400	16	40
Melts:			
Arby's Melt	320	11	38
Ham & Swiss Melt	300	8	37
Market Fresh Sandwiches:			
Corned Beef Reuben	690	32	65
Pecan Grilled Chicken Salad	870	44	88
Roast Ham & Swiss	750	30	85
Roast Turkey Ranch & Bacon	850	37	84
Ultimate BLT	880	46	84
Popcorn Chicken:			
Regular, 4¾ oz	360	16	27
Large, 6½ oz	490	22	38
Toasted Subs:			
Classic Italian	590	30	57
French Dip & Swiss	500	17	59
Philly Beef	570	27	55
Turkey Bacon Club	570	24	56
Regular Combos: Includes Medium Curly Fries & 22 fl.oz Pepsi Without Ice			
Beef 'n Cheddar Sandwich	1245	48	183
Chicken Bacon & Swiss Crispy	1405	56	195
Corned Beef Reuben Sandwich	1505	61	206
Pecan Grilled Chicken Salad S'wich	1645	73	223
Popcorn Chicken	1150	45	160
Roast Turkey & Swiss Sandwich	1525	57	219
Market Fresh Chopped Salads: Without Dressing			
Italian	390	31	10
Turkey Club	250	14	9
Sides & Sidekickers:			
Curly Fries: Small, 4½ oz	410	22	48
Medium, 6 oz	540	29	64
Large, 7 oz	640	34	76
Jalapeno Bites, regular, 5 bites	300	17	32
Loaded Potato Bites, regular, 5 bites	340	20	29
Mozzarella Sticks, regular, 4 sticks	430	23	36
Onion Petals, regular, 3½ oz	330	18	38
Potato Cakes, small, 2 cakes	260	14	16

Continued Next Page ...

Fast - Foods & *Restaurants*

Arby's® cont... (Nov '10)

Kids Menu:	C	F	Cb
Curly Fries, 2¾ oz	240	13	29
Popcorn Chicken, 3½ oz	260	12	20
Jr Roast Beef Sandwich, w/o Mayo	300	9	37
Breakfast: *Per Serving*			
Blueberry Muffin, 3 oz	280	14	33
Biscuits: Plain	250	11	32
Bacon, Egg & Cheese	450	26	34
Ham, Egg & Cheese	420	22	34
Sausage, Egg & Cheese	590	42	35
Croissants: Bacon, Egg & Cheese	390	24	24
Ham & Cheese	270	14	22
Ham, Egg & Cheese	360	20	24
Sausage, Egg & Cheese	530	40	24
Sourdoughs: Bacon, Egg & Cheese	540	27	46
Egg & Cheese	440	19	45
Ham, Egg & Cheese	480	20	46
Sausage Egg & Cheese	530	40	24
Wraps: Bacon, Egg & Cheese	620	33	45
Sausage, Egg & Cheese	740	47	45
Sauces: Cheddar Cheese, side, 1½ oz	45	3	3
Marinara, 1½ oz	35	1.5	4
Tangy Southwest, 1½ oz	230	24	3
Dipping Sauces: Tangy BBQ, 1 oz	45	0	11
Buffalo, 1 oz	10	0.5	2
Honey Dijon Mustard, 1 oz	130	12	5
Desserts:			
Turnovers: Apple with Icing	340	15	48
Cherry Turnover with Icing	340	15	47
Shakes: *17 fl.oz*			
Chocolate; Jamocha, average	620	17	108
Vanilla	540	17	85
Drinks:			
Iced FruiTea: Mandarin Peach, 11 fl.oz	90	0	23
Passion Fruit, 11 fl.oz	100	0	25
Mountain Dew, 22 fl.oz	300	0	84
Pepsi, 22 fl.oz	275	0	77

Arthur Treachers® (Nov '10)

Meals: *With Triple Chips*	C	F	Cb
Boats: Chicken, 9¾ oz	520	33	53
Fish, 10 oz	560	29	57
Shrimp, 9¾ oz	610	29	72
Sides: *Per À la Carte Serving*			
Baked Potato, 8 oz	210	0	48
Batter Dip't Chicken, 2½ oz	260	7	35
Batter Dip't Fish, 3¾ oz	190	6	26
Chips: 1 Regular, 6½ oz	370	20	46
1 Triple, 15 oz	850	45	105
Cole Slaw, 3½ oz	140	9	15
Hushpuppies, 6 pieces, 7 oz	830	30	127
Onion Rings, 1 regular, 4½ oz	260	1.5	56

Atlanta Bread Co® (Nov '10)

Sandwiches:	C	F	Cb
Chicken Salad on Sourdough	440	19	42
Honey Maple Ham on Honey Wheat	410	5	64
Kid's Peanut Butter & Jelly on French	550	15	89
Kid's Grilled Cheese on French	390	15	46
Tuna Salad on French	630	33	57
Turkey on Nine Grain	370	6	50
Veggie on Nine Grain	500	25	52
Signature Sandwiches: *On Focaccia Unless Indicated*			
ABC Special on French Baguette	750	38	57
Bella Chicken	610	38	34
California Avocado	930	50	98
Chicken Waldorf	450	29	26
NY Hot Pastrami on Rye	660	29	59
Turkey Bacon Rustica	960	56	62
Paninis: Chicken Pesto	710	26	80
Chicken Cordon Bleu	670	19	80
Cubano	650	19	80
Italian Vegetarian	570	16	84
Turkey Club	710	24	81
Salads: *Without Dressing*			
Caesar	150	9	7
Balsamic Bleu Salad	330	18	35
Chopstix Chicken Salad	240	10	22
Greek Salad	240	16	15
House Salad	90	2	13
Salsa Fresca Salmon Salad	560	29	40
Soups: *Per 1¼ Cup*			
Broccoli Cheese	250	17	14
Chicken & Sausage Gumbo	190	6	24
Chili, Beef/Frontier, average	290	10	30
Tomato Fennel & Dill	290	23	18
Wisconsin Cheese	290	15	24

For Complete Menu & Data ~ see CalorieKing.com

Au Bon Pain® (Nov '10)

Bagels: *Per Bagel*	C	F	Cb
Asiago Cheese	370	8	57
Cinnamon Crisp	410	7	77
Everything	320	4	60
Jalapeno Double Cheddar	340	10	53
Honey 9 Grain	350	4	69
Cream Cheese Spreads: *Per 2 oz*			
Lite Cream Cheese	120	9	5
Honey Pecan, 2½ oz	200	16	10
Vegetable	170	16	3

Continued Next Page ...

Updated Nutrition Data ~ www.CalorieKing.com
Persons with Diabetes ~ See Disclaimer (Page 22)

Au Bon Pain® cont... (Nov '10)

Breakfast Sandwiches:	C	F	Cb
Egg on a Bagel	430	12	58
With Bacon	490	16	58
With Bacon & Cheese	570	23	59
With Cheese	510	18	59
Smkd. Salmon & Wasabi/Onion Dill Bagel	430	11	64
Café Sandwiches			
Arizona Chicken	710	29	62
Baja Turkey	700	27	71
Caprese	680	32	65
Chicken Pesto	660	24	66
Mozzarella Chicken	680	24	67
Pastrami	590	23	52
Spicy Tuna	470	16	60
Hot Sandwiches and Melts			
Baked Turkey	720	26	79
Eggplant & Mozzarella	670	30	73
Steakhouse on Ciabatta	640	23	73
Wraps: Chicken Caesar Asiago	610	28	61
Mediterranean Wrap	610	29	73
Southwest Tuna	760	41	66
Thai Peanut Chicken	530	15	79
Harvest Rice Bowls:			
Angus Steak Teriyaki	660	18	101
with Brown Rice	620	19	86
Mayan Chicken	550	11	87
with Brown Rice	510	13	72
Breads: Per Piece			
Artisan Honey Baguette, 4¾ oz	340	5	66
Bread Bowl, 9¼ oz	620	3	123
Farm House Rolls, 4½ oz	360	7	63
Focaccia, 4½ oz	360	7	62
Rosemary Garlic Bread Stick, 2 oz	190	5	31
Soups: Per Medium 12 oz Bowl			
Baked Stuffed Potato	350	20	29
Carrot Ginger	140	5	22
Chicken Gumbo	180	8	21
Corn & Green Chili Bisque	260	15	27
Cream of Chicken & Wild Rice	240	14	22
Italian Wedding	170	7	19
Southern Black-Eyed Pea	170	2	29
Tomato Florentine	130	3	18
Vegetarian Chili	220	2	39
Wild Mushroom Bisque	190	9	22
Kid's Menu, Macaroni & Cheese	330	10	24
Salads: Without Dressing			
Apple & Goat Cheese, 10 oz	290	13	39
Caesar Asiago Salad, 6 oz	220	12	18
Chef's Salad, 9 oz	250	15	7

Au Bon Pain® cont... (Nov '10)

Salads (Cont): Without Dressing	C	F	Cb
Garden, 6½ oz	70	2	12
Grilled Chicken Caesar Asiago, 8½ oz	300	13	18
Mandarin Sesame Chicken, 9¾ oz	310	17	29
Mediterranean Chicken, 10¼ oz	290	16	12
Thai Peanut Chicken, 11 oz	240	8	19
Tuna Garden, 10½ oz	240	12	15
Turkey Cobb, 11 oz	330	19	14
Dressing: Caesar, 2 oz	270	28	4
Hazelnut Vinaigrette, 2 oz	270	25	11
Sesame Ginger, 2 oz	230	20	12
Bakery: Per Item			
Brownie, Blondie, 4 oz	460	33	59
Cookies: English Toffee, 1½ oz	250	14	27
Shortbread, 2¼ oz	340	20	37
Croissants: Per Croissant, Filled			
Almond	600	38	55
Apple	280	11	44
Apple Almond	460	23	59
Chocolate	440	22	58
Raspberry Cheese	370	17	46
Sweet Cheese	400	19	49
Desserts: Creme de Fleur	500	25	56
Lemon Pound Cake, 5 oz	520	25	67
Mint Chocolate Pound Cake, 5 oz	530	29	64
Strudel. Apple; Cherry, average	450	25	50
Muffins: Blueberry	490	17	74
Carrot/Cranberry Walnut	550	26	69
Low-Fat Triple Berry	300	3	65
Raisin Bran	480	11	85
Beverages: Caffe Latte, 16 fl oz	260	14	21
Hot Chocolate, 16 fl.oz	460	15	74
Peach Iced Tea, 22 fl.oz	240	0	61
Coffee Blast, 16 fl.oz	440	21	71
Strawberry Smoothie, 16 fl.oz	310	1	66

For Complete Nutritional Data ~ see CalorieKing.com

Auntie Anne's® (Nov '10)

Pretzels: With Butter	C	F	Cb
Almond	390	6	74
Cinnamon Sugar	470	12	84
Garlic	350	5	65
Jalapeno	330	5	63
Original	340	5	65
Original Stix, 6 sticks	340	5	65
Sesame	400	10	67
Sour Cream & Onion	360	5	68

Continued Next Page ...

Fast - Foods & Restaurants

Auntie Anne's® cont...(Nov '10)

Pretzels: *Without Butter*

	C	F	Cb
Almond Pretzel	350	2	74
Cinnamon Sugar	380	1	84
Garlic Pretzel	310	1	65
Jalapeno	300	1	63
Original	310	1	65
Original Stix, 6 sticks	310	1	65
Sesame	360	6	67

Dipping Sauces

Caramel Dip, 1½ oz	130	3	23
Cheese Sce; Hot Salsa Cheese, av., 1 oz	90	7	3
Cream Cheese, 1¼ oz	80	6	1
Heated Marinara Sauce, 2 oz	45	0	7
Sweet Dip, 1½ oz	130	0	32
Sweet Mustard, 1¼ oz	60	2	10

Beverages: *Per Serving*

Auntie Anne's Lemonade, 21 fl.oz	260	0	66
Dutch Ice (20 fl.oz): Blue Raspberry	240	0	62
Kiwi-Banana	220	0	53
Lemonade	300	0	76
Mocha	390	12	73
Pina Colada	300	0	73
Strawberry	230	0	58
Wild Cherry	280	0	69
Dutch Smoothie: *Per 20 fl.oz*			
Blue Raspberry	440	15	72
Kiwi-Banana	420	15	66
Lemonade	470	15	81
Mocha	540	22	79
Pina Colada	470	15	79
Strawberry	430	15	69

Back Yard Burgers® (Nov '10)

Burgers:

	C	F	Cb
American Cheeseburger ⅓ lb	730	44	47
Back Yard Burger ⅓ lb	680	39	47
Black Jack	780	49	48
Bleu Cheeseburger: ⅓ lb	780	47	47
⅔ lb	1270	86	47
Cheddar Cheeseburger: ⅓ lb	790	48	47
⅔ lb	1290	88	47
Jr Burger	530	27	47
Mushroom Swiss	790	49	45
Pepper Jack, ⅓ lb	740	45	47
Swiss Cheeseburger: ⅓ lb	790	48	47
⅔ lb	1290	88	47

Chicken Sandwiches:

Blackened Chicken	540	24	53
Crispy Chicken	590	26	65
Grilled Chicken	350	4.5	47
Hawaiian Chicken	450	11	59

Back Yard Burgers® (Nov '10)

Specialities:

	C	F	Cb
Big Dog	500	33	32
Bak-Pak: Chicken Tender Meal	1110	71	91
Dog	320	18	29
Chicken Tender Meal	1260	79	102
Chili Cheese Big Dog	630	44	34
Garden Veggie Burger	400	8	57

Sides: *Per Serving*

Chili	150	9	8
Seasoned Fries: Regular, 6 oz	640	45	58
Large, 9 oz	960	68	87

Salads: *Without Dressing*

Blackened Chicken	330	15	25
Fried Chicken	410	19	41
Garden Fresh	100	2	20
Grilled Chicken	220	4	23
Side Salad	30	0	6

Dressings: *Per Serving*

Bleu Cheese	220	24	1
Honey Mustard	240	23	7
Ranch	150	15	2

Desserts: *Per Serving*

Cobblers: Apple	360	14	59
Blackberry	290	8	51
Cherry	350	12	59
Peach	330	11	56

Shakes: *Per 12 fl.oz*

Chocolate; Strawberry	630	29	83
Vanilla	620	28	71

For Complete Nutritional Data ~ see CalorieKing.com

Baja Fresh® (Nov '10)

Burritos: *As Served*

	C	F	Cb
Baja Burrito: With Chicken	790	38	65
With Steak	850	46	67
Bare Burrito: With Charbroiled Chkn	640	7	97
Veggie and Cheese	580	10	101
Bean & Cheese Burrito: With Chicken	970	35	96
With Steak	1030	43	97
Vegetarian	840	33	96
Burrito Mexicano: With Chicken	790	13	117
With Steak	860	21	118
Burrito Ultimo: With Chicken	880	36	84
With Steak	950	44	85
Grilled Vegetarian	800	33	94

Fajitas: *As Served, Without Tortilla Chips*

Chicken with Corn Tortillas	860	24	105
Chicken with Flour Tortillas	1140	33	147

Continued Next Page ...

Baja Fresh® cont... (Nov '10)

Nachos:: As Served	**C**	**F**	**Cb**
With Charbroiled Chicken	2020	110	164
With Charbroiled Steak	2120	118	163
With Cheese	1890	108	163
Quesadillas: As Served			
With Charbroiled Chicken	1330	80	84
With Charbroiled Steak	1430	87	84
With Cheese	1200	78	84
Vegetarian	1260	78	96
Tacos: As Served			
Baja Fish Taco, Fried	250	13	27
Grilled Mahi Mahi Taco	230	9	26
Original Baja Style Taco: W/ Chicken	210	5	28
With Charbroiled Shrimp	200	5	28
Salads: As Served, Without Dressing			
Baja Ensalada:			
With Charbroiled Chicken	310	7	18
With Charbroiled Shrimp	230	6	18
With Charbroiled Steak	450	18	18
Tostadas: Charbroiled Fish	1130	55	99
Charbroiled Shrimp	1120	55	99
Charbroiled Steak	1230	63	98
Savory Pork Carnitas	1180	62	100

For Complete Nutritional Data ~ see CalorieKing.com

Baskin Robbins® (Nov '10)

Ice Creams: Per 4 oz Scoop	**C**	**F**	**Cb**
Classic Flavors: Cherries Jubilee	240	12	30
Chocolate	260	14	33
Jamoca Almond Fudge	270	15	31
Mint Chocolate Chip	270	16	28
Old Fashioned Butter Pecan	280	18	24
Oreo Cookies 'n Cream	280	15	32
Pralines 'n Cream	280	14	35
Rainbow Sherbet	160	2	34
Reese's P'nut Butter Cup	300	18	31
Vanilla	260	16	26
Very Berry Strawberry	220	11	28
World Class Chocolate	280	16	31
Premium Churned: Per 2½ oz Scoop			
Light: Aloha Brownie	150	5	26
Cappuccino	140	5	20
Raspberry Chip	140	4	24
Frozen Yogurt, Fat-Free Van., 4 oz	150	0	32
Fruit Blast Bars, all flavors, average	50	0	14
Sorbets: Per 4 oz Scoop			
Lemon; Strawberry	130	0	34
Mango	120	0	32

Baskin Robbins cont... (Nov '10)

Sundaes:	**C**	**F**	**Cb**
Classic Sundaes: Banana Royale	620	28	87
Brownie	920	47	119
Banana Split	1010	34	173
Premium Sundaes:			
Chocolate Chip Cookie Dough	990	43	138
Reese's Peanut Butter Cup	1220	80	109
Soft Serve Sundaes: *Per 10 oz Regular*			
Caramel	580	21	89
Strawberry	450	18	59
Sundae Cups: Oreo	330	15	45
Reese's Peanut Butter Cup	390	24	36
Pralines 'n Cream	330	16	44
Soft Serve:			
'31 Below' Blends: *Per 16 oz Cup*			
Chocolate Oreo	1290	55	187
Fudge Brownie	1390	58	199
Heath	1160	54	151
Jamoca Oreo	860	33	128
Oreo	1000	41	143
Reese's Peanut Butter Cup	1220	67	134
Strawberry Banana	710	23	112
Cups: Vanilla: Kid's, 3 oz cup	140	6	19
Regular, 6 oz cup	280	11	37
Large, 9 oz cup	430	17	58
Fruit Cream:			
Strawberry: Medium, 16 fl.oz	630	19	102
Large, 24 fl.oz	860	25	144
Mango, Medium, 16 fl.oz	635	18	110
Large, 24 fl.oz	870	23	153
Beverages			
Freezes with Orange Sherbet:			
Small	370	4	82
Medium	510	5	112
Cappuccino Blast: *Per Medium, 24 fl.oz*			
Original	480	19	72
Mocha	610	19	104
Fruit Blast: *Per Medium, 24 fl.oz*			
Peach Passion Fruit	370	0.5	94
Strawberry Citrus	330	0	83
Wild Mango	470	1.5	116
Fruit Blast Smoothie: *Per Medium, 24 fl.oz*			
Mango	620	2	148
Peach Passion Banana	540	1	131
Milk Shakes: *Per Medium, 24 fl.oz*			
Choc Chip Cookie Dough	1030	42	137
Vanilla	980	45	125
Chocolate with Vanilla Ice Cream	990	44	131
Strawberry w/ Strawb. Ice Cream	770	31	105
Cones: Cake	25	0	5
Sugar	45	0.5	9
Waffle	160	4	28

For Complete Nutritional Data ~ see CalorieKing.com

Fast - Foods & *Restaurants*

Big Apple Bagels® (Nov '10)

Bagels:

	C	F	Cb
All types, average, 5 oz	340	2	68
½ bagel, 2½ oz	170	1	34

Choice Bagels: Per Bagel

Blueberry Cobbler	390	8	70
Cheddar Nacho	350	6	60
Cinnamon Apple Pie	385	8	68
Cinnamon Bun	400	8	70
Cinnamon Danish	395	8	72
French Toast	370	4	74
Quiche Lorraine	355	8	54
Strawberry White Chocolate	365	4	72
Swiss Melt	370	8	58
White Chocolate Swirl	395	8	70

Cream Cheese: Per 2 Tbsp , 1 oz

Plain	90	9	2
Plain, Lite	60	4.5	3
Other varieties, average	90	8	2
Whipped: Classic Plain	70	7	1
Brown Sugar Cinnamon	70	5	5
Reduced-Fat Spring Veggie	60	5	2

My Favorite Muffin: Per Jumbo, 5¾ oz

Regular: Blueberry	505	24	66
Chocolate Chip	635	33	81
Cinnamon Swirl Cheesecake	640	33	84
Pumpkin Spice	545	24	78
Fat Free: Blueberry	325	0	78
Chocolate Marble	375	0	87
Cinnamon Bun	505	0	126

Sandwiches:

Big Apple Club	795	37	75
Classic Reuben, Overstuffed	960	43	57
Grilled Chicken Bruschetta Pizzaah	345	21	24
Morning Classic	485	11	73
Roast Beef Parmesan Grinder	585	15	76

For Complete Nutritional Data ~ see CalorieKing.com

Biggby Coffee (Nov '10)

Hot Drinks: Per 16 fl.oz, Without Sugar Unless Indicated

Caffe Latte: With 2% Milk	175	7	16
With Non-Fat Milk	115	0	16
With Soy	160	5	19
Cappuccino: With 2% Milk	105	4	10
With Non-Fat Milk	70	0	9.5
With Soy	95	3	11
Chai Latte: With 2% Milk	345	8	53
With Non-Fat Milk	285	0	53
Cocoa Carmella: *With Sugar*			
With 2% Milk	310	9	49
With Whipped Cream	390	15	53
Mocha Mocha: *With Sugar*			
With 2% Milk	275	7.5	46
With Whipped Cream	355	14	50

Biggby Coffee cont... (Nov '10)

Cold Drinks: 16 fl.oz , Without Sugar

	C	F	Cb
Big Chill: Chai with 2% milk	430	6	86
Mocha with Whipped Cream	410	14	65
Original	330	6	69
Creme Freeze: Banana	375	5	84
Berry Fruizen-T w/ Whipped Crm	465	10	90

For Complete Menu & Data ~ see CalorieKing.com

Blimpie® (Nov '10)

Cold Deli Subs: Per 6" Sub on White, Includes Dressing

	C	F	Cb
Blimpie Best, with Provolone	450	17	49
BLT, without Cheese	430	22	43
Club, with Swiss	410	13	49
Cuban, with Swiss	410	11	43
Ham & Swiss Cheese	420	14	49
Roast Beef & Provolone	430	14	46
Tuna without Cheese	470	21	43
Turkey & Provolone	410	13	49
Wraps: Chicken Caesar	560	24	56
Southwestern	530	22	61

Hot Deli Subs: Per 6" Sub on White

Meatball, with Provolone	580	31	50
Pastrami, with Swiss	430	16	42
VegiMax, with Provolone	520	20	56

Salads: Regular, Without Dressing

Buffalo Chicken	220	9	10
Garden	30	0	6
Tuna Salad	270	19	6
Ultimate Club	260	14	10

Dressings & Sauces: Per 1½ oz

Creamy Caesar	210	21	2
Creamy Italian	180	18	4

Soups: Per 8½ oz Serving

Chicken Noodle	130	4	18
Cream of Broccoli with Cheese	250	19	13
Harvest Vegetable	100	1	19
Minestrone	90	3	14
New England Clam Chowder	170	3	28

Desserts:

Brownie	230	10	28
Cookies: Oatmeal Raisin	180	7	27
Sugar	320	16	42

For Complete Nutritional Data ~ see CalorieKing.com

Bob Evans® (Nov '10)

Breakfast	C	F	Cb
Bowls: Border Scramble, 18½ oz	1030	57	75
Sausage, 19½ oz	1025	63	78
Spinach, Bacon & Tomato, 18½ oz	1040	62	81
Country Biscuit	650	45	39
Pot Roast Hash	680	45	30
Hotcakes: Buttermilk (1), w/o topping	335	10	56
Cinnamon (1), without topping	380	12	62
Omelets: Three Cheese	530	40	5
Border Scramble	635	46	14
Egg Lites	420	24	13
Farmer's Market	630	45	14
Western	530	36	8
Crepes: Plain (1)	255	14	27
Blueberry (1)	305	14	40
Dinners: As Served			
Beef: Meatloaf with Gravy	435	22	22
Pot Roast Beef Stew, 20 oz	715	34	67
Pot Roast Stroganoff, 24 oz	815	43	65
Chicken: Chicken & Brocc. Alfredo	870	46	62
Chicken-N-Noodles: Deep-Dish	700	29	66
Slow-Roasted, 13¼ oz	225	4	30
Chicken Parmesan, w/ Sce, 28 oz	1175	58	96
Fried Chicken Strips (1), 1½ oz	135	8	10
Garlic Butter Grilled Chkn Breast	180	6	1
Fish: Fried Haddock, 6½ oz	365	18	27
Garlic Butter Salmon, 8 oz	255	9	1
Potato-Crusted Flounder, 5 oz	175	7	9
Salmon, 7 oz	245	8	0
Wildfire Salmon, 8½ oz	310	9	15
Pork, Cranb. Apple Pork Loin, 11½ oz	390	22	30
Turkey, Slow-Roasted, 4 oz	135	5	3
Seniors: *Without Sides Unless Indicated*			
Chicken Parmesan with Meat Sauce	845	44	57
Country Fried Steak with Gravy	550	37	37
Meatloaf with Gravy	435	22	22
Open-Faced Roast Beef w/ Gravy	475	24	22
Farm Fresh Wraps:			
Chicken Caesar, 11½ oz	605	29	55
Chicken Salad, 10 oz	605	29	66
Turkey Club, 10¼ oz	695	34	58
Fit from the Farm:			
Breakfast: Egg Lites with Tomato	60	0	2
Blueberry-Banana French Toast	325	6	36
Fresh Fruit Plate:			
With Low Fat Cottage Cheese	345	4	69
With Low Fat Strawb. Yogurt	355	2	84
Veggie Omelet	270	2	43

Bob Evans® cont... (Nov '10)

Fit From The Farm (Cont)	C	F	Cb
Dinners: *Includes Menu-Listed Sides, Condiments*			
Chicken, Spinach & Tomato Pasta	525	16	67
Grilled Chicken Breast, 23 oz	480	9	58
Potato Crusted Flounder, 20½ oz	415	8	67
Salads: *With Reduced-Fat Raspberry Dressing*			
Apple-Cranberry Spinach: Regular	390	15	49
Savor Size, 8¼ oz	380	15	47
Sandwiches & Burgers			
Burgers: Bacon Cheeseburger	720	38	35
Cheeseburger	650	31	35
Hamburger	540	22	34
Sandwiches: Fried Chicken Club	635	31	47
Bob-B-Q Pulled Pork	595	24	65
Grilled Chicken Club	510	23	34
Grilled Chicken, plain	370	10	33
Pot Roast	575	28	50
Turkey Bacon Melt	590	28	49
Salads: *Large, Without Dressing Unless Indicated*			
Cobb, 14½ oz	515	31	10
Country Caesar w/ Drssg,16¾ oz	745	53	20
Country Spinach, 10¼ oz	430	25	12
Heritage Chef ,12½ oz	400	25	11
Wildfire Grilled Chicken, 13½ oz	390	13	37
Side Dishes:			
Baked Potato, 10 oz	195	0	50
Bread & Celery Dressing, 6 oz	295	16	31
Coleslaw, 3½ oz	210	14	19
Grilled Mushrooms, 7 oz	85	5	10
Home Fries, 5 oz	165	6	24
Loaded Baked Potato, 11½ oz	395	16	53
Mashed Potatoes, 5½ oz	190	7	16
Gravy/Sauces			
Gravy: Beef, 2 oz	25	1	3
Chicken/Pork Roasted, 2 oz	60	4.5	3
Sauces: Tartar, ¾ oz	115	2	1
Wildfire BBQ, 1 oz	60	0	15
Kid's Menu:			
Mac & Cheese, 6½ oz	320	8	41
Mini Cheeseburger (1)	285	15	22
Plenty-O-Pancakes, 5½ oz	335	12	52
Smiley Face Potatoes, 3 oz	270	16	29
Sundae, Fudge Blast, 4 oz	215	9	31
Dessert:			
Pie: Apple Pie, N.S.A., 6¾ oz slice	500	30	56
Coconut Cream Pie, 7 oz slice	515	29	59

Bojangles® (Nov '10)

Cajun & Southern Style Chicken	C	F	Cb
Breast, average	280	17	12
Leg, average	120	16	11
Thigh, average	310	23	11
Wing, average	160	25	11
Sandwiches			
Cajun Filet: Without Mayonnaise	335	11	41
With Mayonnaise	435	22	41
Grilled Filet: Without Mayonnaise	235	5	25
With Mayonnaise	335	16	25
Snacks: Buffalo Bites	180	5	5
Chicken Supremes, 4 pieces	335	16	26
Biscuit Sandwiches: Plain	245	12	29
Bacon	290	17	26
Bacon, Egg & Cheese	550	42	27
Cajun Filet	455	21	46
Country Ham	270	15	26
Egg	400	30	26
Sausage	350	23	26
Smoked Sausage	380	26	27
Steak	650	49	37
Fixins': Botato Rounds	235	11	31
Cajun Pintos	110	0	18
Dirty Rice	165	6	24
Green Beans	25	0	5
Macaroni & Cheese	200	14	12
Marinated Cole Slaw	135	3	26
Potatoes, without Gravy	80	1	16
Seasoned Fries	345	19	39
Sweet Biscuits: Bo Berry	220	10	29
Cinnamon	320	18	37

For Complete Nutritional Data ~ see CalorieKing.com

Boston Market® (Nov '10)

Sandwiches & Burgers:	C	F	Cb
Boston Chicken Carver	750	29	64
Boston Turkey Carver	700	26	65
Classic Chicken Salad	800	41	65
Half Boston: Chicken Carver	375	15	32
Turkey Carver	350	13	32
Meatloaf Open-Faced	670	38	48
Roasted Turkey Open-Faced	330	6	43

Boston Market® cont... (Nov '10)

Individual Meals: *Without Sides*	C	F	Cb
Beef Brisket, 4 oz	230	13	0
Half Rotisserie Chicken, 12 oz	610	29	1
Pastry Top Chicken Pot Pie, 15 oz	810	48	60
Family Meals: *Without Sides*			
Meatloaf, 7¾ oz	480	36	21
Roasted Turkey, 5 oz	180	3	0
Salads: *Entree Size*			
Caesar Salad: W/o dressing, 6 oz	140	8	7
With 2 oz Caesar Dressing	430	38	9
With 1½ oz Lite Ranch Dressing	210	12	15
Market Chopped Salad:			
Without Dressing	190	9	22
With 2 oz Dressing	480	40	24
Add Extra for:			
5 oz Rotisserie Chicken	180	3	0
3 oz Roasted Turkey	110	2	0
Sides			
Cinnamon-Apples, 5 oz	210	3	47
Creamed Spinach, 6¾ oz	280	23	12
Fresh Steamed Vegetables, 4¾ oz	60	2	8
Fresh Vegetable Stuffing, 4¾ oz	190	8	25
Garlic Dill New Potatoes, 5½ oz	140	3	24
Gravy: Beef, 3 oz	35	1.5	4
Poultry, 4 oz	50	2	7
Green Beans, 3 oz	60	3.5	7
Macaroni & Cheese, 7¾ oz	300	11	35
Mashed Potatoes, 7¾ oz	270	11	36
Potato Salad, 7 oz	390	29	26
Seasonal Fresh Fruit Salad, 5 oz	60	0	15
Sweet Corn, 6¼ oz	170	4	37
Sweet Potato Casserole, 7 oz	460	16	77
Soups			
Chicken Noodle, 14 oz	250	8	23
Chicken Tortilla: With Toppings	410	26	30
Without Toppings	160	8	13
Desserts			
Apple Pie, 5¾ oz	580	30	74
Chocolate Cake, 5 oz	580	34	67
Choc. Chip Fudge Brownie, 3 oz	320	13	49

For Complete Nutritional Data ~ see CalorieKing.com

Boston Pizza® (Nov '10)

Starters: Per Order	C	F	Cb
Cactus Cut Potatoes with Dip, 10 oz	830	70	38
Boston's Pizza Bread, w/o Sauce	500	12	84
Oven Roasted Wings, 9¼ oz	430	30	6
Burgers & Sandwiches:			
Burgers: Prime Rib Original	940	68	47
With Bacon	1000	73	47
Sandwiches: Beef Dip	860	27	108
Boston Brute	810	21	116
Boston Cheesesteak	1140	49	113
Buffalo Chicken	910	33	118
Ciabatta Chicken	750	42	58
Pizzas (Medium): Per Slice			
BBQ chicken	190	6	25
Bacon Double Cheeseburger	250	10	25
Cajun Shrimp	290	16	23
Deluxe	220	7	25
Hawaiian	210	5	28
Meateor	260	11	25
Pepperoni	200	7	24
Szechuan	200	5	27
Tropical Chicken	250	11	26
Tuscan	250	10	29
Pastas: Full Order, Without Garlic Bread			
Boston's Lasagna, 17¼ oz	670	19	90
Chicken & Mushrm Fett., 27½ oz	1200	51	138
Spicy Italian Penne, 29 oz	1420	76	136
Salads: Includes Dressing			
Caesar, full size, 10½ oz	400	37	13
Spinach, full size, 11 oz	430	33	17
Desserts:			
Apple Crisp, 14½ oz	740	19	138
Chocolate Brownie Addiction, 8½ oz	570	18	99

For Complete Nutritional Data ~ see CalorieKing.com

Braum's® (Nov '10)

Frozen Yogurt: Per ½ Cup	C	F	Cb
Chocolate Peanut Butter Cup	180	10	19
Average Fruit Flavors	130	5	19
Ice Cream: Per ½ Cup			
Carb Watch: Chocolate Chip	180	10	17
Other flavors, average	155	11	17
Light: Average all varieties	130	4	19
Premium: Peanut Butter Cup	190	12	18
Other flavors, average	150	6	18

For Complete Nutritional Data ~ see CalorieKing.com

Bruegger's Bagels® (Nov '10)

Bagels	C	F	Cb
Average all flavors, 4¼ oz	320	3	65
Breakfast S'wiches: With Plain Bagel			
Egg & Cheese	470	14	63
With Bacon	480	21	63
With Sausage	560	23	63
Smoked Salmon	460	10	66
Spinach & Cheddar Omelet	500	16	64
Western	760	56	66
Deli Sandwiches: Plain Bagel Unless Indicated			
BLT on Hearty White Bread	720	42	62
Chicken Breast	550	6	81
Garden Veggie	360	2	72
Ham On Honey Wheat Bread	540	16	64
Roast Beef on Hearty White Bread	560	18	59
Turkey	440	8	64
Signature & Classic Sandwiches:			
Herby Turkey/Sesame Bagel	530	14	73
Leonardo da Veggie/Plain White Bread	560	15	76
Roma Roast Beef/Hearty White Bread	770	44	62
Tarragon Chkn Salad/Hrty White Bread	750	37	75
Thai Peanut Chicken/Plain Bagel	580	11	91
Turkey Chipotle Club/Hon. Wheat Bread	800	51	57
Salads: With Dressing			
Caesar	270	17	22
Chicken Caesar	380	20	23
Mandarin Chicken Medley	450	21	37
Sesame Chicken	490	29	30
Cookies: Chocolate Chip	390	17	52
Double Chocolate	390	19	51
Everything	380	18	49
Dessert Bars: Seven Layer	650	43	58
Chocolate Chunk Brownie	310	18	38
Toffee Almond	400	19	53

For Complete Menu & Data ~ see CalorieKing.com

Burgerville® (Nov '10)

Burgers:	C	F	Cb
Cheeseburger	380	20	30
Classic Hamburger	530	30	42
Double Beef Cheeseburger	450	27	30
Half Pound Colossal	750	45	43
Hamburger	320	17	30
Tillamook Cheeseburger	640	39	42
Sandwiches: Crispy Chicken	460	19	54
Deluxe Crispy Chicken	600	30	54
Grilled Chicken, Low-Fat	330	5	45
Nine Grain Turkey Club	540	32	36
French Fries, Regular, 5 oz	360	15	52

For Complete Menu & Data ~ see CalorieKing.com

Burger King® (Nov '10)

Whopper Sandwiches: With Mayo	C	F	Cb
Whopper	670	40	51
Whopper, without Mayo	520	23	51
Double Whopper, with Cheese	1010	66	52
Triple Whopper, with Cheese	1250	84	52
Whopper JR.	340	20	28
New York Whopper Bar:			
Angry Whopper Sandwich	880	55	59
California Whopper Sandwich	850	57	50
Meat Beast Whopper Sandwich	910	60	53
NY Pizza Burger, whole, 6 pieces	2530	144	168
Mshrm & Swiss Stkhouse XT Burger	870	49	54
Original Steakhouse XT Burger	760	46	52
Flame Broiled Burgers:			
BK Stackers: Double	570	37	29
Triple	750	51	30
Quad	930	65	31
Cheeseburger	310	15	28
Double Cheeseburger	460	27	28
Hamburger	260	11	27
XT: A1 Steakhouse	970	61	55
Steakhouse	770	46	53
BK Veggie Burger with Cheese	450	20	44
Chicken & Fish Sandwiches: With Mayo or Sauce			
BK Big Fish	640	31	67
Original Chicken	630	39	46
Premium Chicken	470	18	40
Spicy Chick'N Crisp	460	30	34
TenderCrisp Chicken	800	46	68
TenderGrill Chicken	520	19	49
BK Chicken Fries: Without Buffalo Sauce:			
6 pieces	250	15	16
9 pieces	380	22	24
Kids Crown Shaped Chicken Tenders:			
4 pieces	180	11	13
8 pieces	360	21	25
Macaroni & Cheese	160	5	22
Dipping Sauces: Buffalo	80	8	2
Honey Mustard	90	6	8
Ranch; Zesty Onion, average	145	15	2
Sweet & Sour	45	0	11
French Fries: Small, 4¼ oz	340	17	44
Medium, 5¾ oz	440	22	56
Large, 7 oz	540	27	69
Onion Rings: Small (15)	310	17	36
Medium (20)	400	21	47
Large (24)	490	26	57

Burger King® cont... (Nov '10)

Salads: Without Dressing or Croutons	C	F	Cb
Garden: With TenderCrisp Chicken	410	23	27
With TenderGrill Chicken	230	8	9
Dressings: Ken's Creamy Caesar, 2 oz	210	21	4
Ken's Fat Free Ranch, 2 oz	60	0	15
Breakfast:			
Cheesy Bacon BK Wrapper	380	24	28
Ham Omelet Sandwich	270	12	29
French Toast Sticks: 5 Pieces	380	18	49
Cini-minis with Icing (4)	490	18	74
Biscuits:			
Bacon, Egg & Cheese	420	25	34
Ham, Egg & Cheese	400	22	33
Sausage, Egg & Cheese	550	37	34
Burritos: *Includes Salsa*			
Bacon, Egg & Cheese	300	16	24
Potato, Egg & Cheese	320	17	29
Croissan'wich: Bacon Egg & Chse	340	19	26
Egg & Cheese	300	16	26
Ham Egg & Cheese	330	16	27
Double Croissan'wich:			
With Bacon, Egg & Cheese	420	25	27
With Ham, Bacon, Egg & Cheese	420	24	28
With Ham, Sausage, Egg & Chse	550	35	28
With Sausage, Egg & Cheese	680	49	29
Hash Browns: Small, 2½ oz	400	26	39
Medium	540	35	52
Sourdough Sandwich:			
Ham, Egg & Cheese	420	19	40
Sausage, Egg & Cheese	560	34	41
Desserts/Pies: Dutch Apple Pie	320	14	46
Funnel Cake Sticks with Icing (9)	300	11	49
Hershey's Sundae Pie	300	18	31
BK Fresh Apple Fries, w / Dipping Sce	70	0.5	16
Shakes:			
Chocolate; Strawberry, av., Small, ,16 fl.oz	435	11	78
Medium, 22 fl.oz	650	16	119
Large, 32 fl.oz	960	23	176
Vanilla: Small, 16 fl.oz	370	12	60
Medium, 22 fl.oz	520	16	84
Oreo Sundae Shakes: Per Medium, 22 fl.oz			
Chocolate	920	28	159
Vanilla	790	28	124
Beverages: Mocha Iced Coffee, 16 fl.oz	340	7	63
Frozen Coca-Cola: Small, 16 fl.oz	110	0	31
Medium, 22 fl.oz	140	0	40

For Complete Nutritional Data ~ see CalorieKing.com

Updated Nutrition Data ~ www.CalorieKing.com
Persons with Diabetes ~ See Disclaimer (Page 22)

California Pizza Kitchen
~ See CalorieKing.com

Captain D's Seafood® (Nov '10)

Dinners/Platters: Includes Cole Slaw, French Fries & Hush Puppies

	C	F	Cb
Bite Size Shrimp Dinner	1140	61	120
Catfish Feast	995	57	88
Clam Platter, ½ lb	1450	87	133
Country Style Fish Dinner	1070	59	97
Deluxe Seafood Platter	1610	94	114
Fried Flounder	1530	93	115
Oyster Dinner	1000	58	100
Ultimate Premium Shrimp Platter	1290	65	69
Salads:			
Fried Chicken Salad	205	10	18
Side Salad	20	0	3
Wild Alaskan Salmon Salad	175	1	8
Sides			
Baked Potato, plain	240	0	54
Broccoli, 3.5 oz	40	1	5
Macaroni & Cheese, 4 oz	160	7	17
Dessert, Cheesecake w/ Strawb.	430	26	45

Caribou Coffee® (Nov '10)

Without Whipped Cream Unless Indicated

Classic Hot Beverages: Per Medium

Coffee, with Steamed 2% Milk	90	3.5	9
Coffee Of The Day, with 2% Milk	20	0.5	1
Espresso, 1 medium, 3 shots, 6 fl.oz	0	0	0
Breve	510	45	17
Cappuccino, with 2% Milk	70	3	6
Macchiato, with 2% Milk, 6 fl.oz	20	1	1

Cold Beverages: Per Medium

Iced Americano	5	0	0
Iced Coffee, Cold Pressed	5	0	0
Iced Latte, with 2% Milk	150	6	14
Iced Mocha, Milk Choc., 2% Milk	350	11	51

Coolers: Per Medium With Whipped Cream

Caramel	500	16	88
Coffee	420	17	67
Espresso	370	16	57

Smoothies: Per Medium

Passion Fruit Green Tea	290	0	70
Pom-a-Mango	350	0.5	85
Strawberry Banana, 22 fl.oz	350	0	84

Snowdrift: Per Medium With Milk Chocolate

Cookies & Cream, with 2% Milk	630	18	103
Mint, with 2% Milk	510	13	84

Wild: Per Medium With Whipped Cream

Hot Apple Blast	400	11	76
Mint Cond. Milk Choc., 2% Milk	580	40	67

For Complete Menu & Data ~ see CalorieKing.com

Carl's Jr.® (Nov '10)

Charbroiled Burgers:	C	F	Cb
Big Hamburger	460	17	54
Chili Cheeseburger	780	41	58
Famous Star with Cheese	660	39	53
Kids Hamburger	230	10	24
Super Star with Cheese	920	58	54
The Big Carl	920	59	51
The Six Dollar Burger: Original	890	54	58
Bacon Cheese	950	62	49
Chili Cheese	1000	56	59
Guacamole Bacon	1040	70	53
Low-Carb	570	43	7
Teriyaki	810	43	69
Western Bacon	1020	53	81
Chicken Sandwiches:			
Bacon Swiss Crispy Chicken	750	40	62
Charbroiled: BBQ Chicken	380	7	49
Chicken Club	560	27	44
Santa Fe Chicken	630	35	44
Spicy Chicken Sandwich	420	27	33
Chicken Strips, 5 pieces	610	43	32
Chicken Stars, 6 pieces	320	24	14
Fish: Fish & Chips	730	39	72
Carl's Catch Fish Sandwich	710	37	74
Breakfast: Bacon & Egg Burrito	550	32	37
Breakfast Burger	780	41	64
French Toast Dips, 5 pcs, w/o syrup	460	21	60
Hash Brown Nuggets, 4 oz	350	23	32
Loaded Breakfast Burrito	780	49	51
Sourdough Breakfast Sandwich	470	25	37
Steak & Egg Burrito	650	36	43
Sunrise Croissant Sandwich	590	44	27
Fries: Chili Cheese, 12 oz	980	56	88
CrissCut Fries, 5 oz	450	29	42
Natural Cut: Small, 4¼ oz	320	15	42
Medium, 6 oz	460	22	60
Large, 6½ oz	500	24	65
Onion Rings, 4½ oz	530	28	61
Salads: Without Dressing or Croutons			
Cranb. Apple Walnut Gr. Chicken	300	11	25
Original Grilled Chicken	200	6	13
Dressings: Per 2 oz Pkg			
Blue Cheese	320	34	1
House	220	22	3
Low-Fat Balsamic	35	1.5	5
Shakes: Van.;Choc.;Strawb. av.	710	33	86
Oreo	730	38	81
Malts, average all flavors	780	35	99

Carvel® (Nov '10)

Ice Creams: Per Small, 7½ oz

	C	F	Cb
Cups: Chocolate	410	21	48
Vanilla	450	26	47
No Sugar Added, Vanilla	260	7	51
Dashers: *Per Small 12 oz*			
Mint Chocolate Chip	770	42	95
Peanut Butter Cup	1060	60	95
Strawberry Shortcake	580	29	74
Novelties: Brown Bonnet	390	23	43
Deluxe Flying Saucer with Sprinkles	350	16	49
Flying Saucer, Chocolate	230	10	33
Classic Sundaes: *Small*			
Caramel	700	36	84
Hot Fudge	540	30	60
Strawberry	610	34	67
Beverages			
Blended Drinks: *Per Small, 16 fl.oz*			
Arctic Blender: Cookie Dough	920	40	126
Fried Ice Cream	670	31	85
Peanut Butter	870	33	88
Carvelanche: Butterfinger	730	38	92
M&M; Reese's, average	755	39	87
Smoothies, average all flav.,16 fl.oz	315	0	78
Thick Shake, Strawberry	600	31	70
Thick ShakeFloats: Chocolate	790	34	109
Strawberry	750	39	85
Vanilla	810	39	102

Checkers®

Same Menu & Data as Rally's ~ See Page 231

Cheesecake Factory® (Nov '10)

(Author Estimates)

10" Cheesecake: Per Slice

	C	F	Cb
Adam's P'nut B'cup Fudge Ripple	930	59	93
Banana Cream	860	63	70
Brownie Sundae	970	63	96
Choc Chip Cookie Dough	1910	72	102
Dulce de Leche Caramel	1010	74	83
Kahlua Cocoa Coffee	840	55	80
Key Lime Cheesecake	710	49	64
Original Cheesecake	630	45	53
Vanilla Bean Cheesecake	870	64	69
White Choc. Raspberry Truffle	900	62	80
Appertizer, Avocado Eggrolls, 1 roll	435	27	48
Dinners: *Complete Meal*			
Cajun Jambalaya Pasta	1960	43	290
Chicken Madeira	1430	76	82
Famous Factory Meatloaf	1955	96	162
Fresh Fish Tacos	1130	23	160
Herb Crusted Filet of Salmon	1040	60	68
Lemon-Herb Roasted Chicken	1790	108	94
Salad, BBQ Ranch Chkn, w/o bread	1415	113	65

Charley's Grilled Subs® (Nov '10)

	C	F	Cb

Subs: Regular 7¾" Includes Standard Toppings, Without Sauce or Dressings Unless Indicated

	C	F	Cb
BBQ Cheddar, with Sauce	580	20	69
Bacon 3 Cheese Steak	635	32	54
Buffalo Chicken, with Sauce	530	16	60
Chicken Bacon Club	570	25	53
Chicken Cordon Blue	570	18	54
Chicken Teriyaki with Sauce	520	16	58
Italian Deli	585	25	53
Mushroom Swiss Steak	520	19	57
Philly Cheesesteak	520	19	55
Philly Chicken	515	15	67
Philly Ham & Swiss	515	15	59
Philly Steak Deluxe	525	19	58
Philly Veggie	450	15	62
Sicilian Steak	640	31	53
Turkey Cheddar Melt	470	12	53
Ultimate Club	560	23	54
Salads: *Cheese/Dressings not included*			
Chicken, Teriyaki; Buffalo, average	210	7	13
Fresh Garden Salad	60	2	9
Grilled Steak Salad	210	10	10
Dressings, Italian/Ranch, av., 1 oz	150	15	1
Mayo, 1 Tbsp., ½ oz	100	11	0
Original Lemonade, 16 fl.oz	165	0	40

For Complete Menu & Data ~ see CalorieKing.com

Chevys Fresh Mex® (Nov '10)

	C	F	Cb

	C	F	Cb
Sizzling Fajitas: *As Served*			
Original Famous Chicken	930	32	95
Sizzling Steak	1030	46	94
Mesquite Grilled Tacos: *As Served*			
Chicken	1050	35	125
Fish	1060	39	125
Steak	1110	44	124
Fresh Mex Specialties: *As Served*			
Chili Verde	1030	44	113
Crispy Chicken Flautas	1510	76	156
Red Chile Pork Taquitos	1350	69	136
Signature Enchiladas: *As Served*			
Chicken Mole	950	51	84
Chipotle Chicken	1070	64	87
Shrimp & Crab	1360	97	87
Grande Salads: *With Dressing Unless Indicated*			
Grilled Chicken Caesar	860	69	32
Grilled Fajita	1585	128	70
Santa Fe Chopped, w/o Dressing	670	39	30
Tostada without Dressing	1680	115	105
Soup, Tortilla, 1 bowl	390	17	35
Tamalito (Sweet Corn) (2)	190	7	29
Tortilla (El Machino) (2)	140	4	22

Chick-fil-A® (Nov '10)

Chick-fil-A Sandwiches: W/o Sauce	C	F	Cb
Chargrilled Chicken	300	3.5	38
Chargrilled Chicken Club	410	12	39
Chicken Salad	500	20	52
Cool Wraps: *Without Dressing*			
Chargrilled Chicken	410	12	50
Chicken Caesar	460	15	47
Spicy Chicken	410	12	48
Breakfast: Chicken Biscuit	450	20	48
Bacon, Egg & Cheese Biscuit	520	29	44
Sausage Biscuit	590	41	42
Burritos: Chicken	450	20	43
Sausage	510	29	40
Chick-n-Minis, 1 box, 3 pieces	260	10	30
Chicken, Egg & Cheese Bagel	530	23	50
Cinnamon Cluster	400	15	61
Hash Browns, 2.7 oz	280	19	25
Salads: *Without Dressing & Condiments*			
Chargrilled Chicken & Fruit	230	6	23
Chargrilled Chicken Garden	180	6	11
Chick-n-Strips	470	23	27
Southwest Chargrilled Chicken	240	9	18
Salad Dressings, Sauces & Condiments:			
Garlic & Butter Croutons, ½ oz	60	2	9
Tortilla Strips, ½ oz	80	4	8
Dressings: Blue Cheese, 1 oz	150	16	1
Buttermilk Ranch; Caesar, 1 oz	160	17	1
Light Italian, 1 oz	15	0.5	2
Thousand Island, 1 oz	150	14	5
Sauces: BBQ; Honey Mustard, 1 oz	45	0	11
Buffalo, ¾ oz	10	0	1
Buttermilk Ranch, ¾ oz	110	12	1
Chick-fil-A, 1 oz	140	13	6
Honey Roasted BBQ, ½ oz	60	5	2
Sides: Carrot & Raisin Salad, 6 oz	260	12	39
Chicken Salad Cup, 6 oz	350	24	6
Cole Slaw, 10½ oz	580	50	31
Side Salad w/o Crtons or Dress., 4 oz	70	4.5	5
Waffle Potato Fries: Small, 3 oz	290	16	34
Medium, 4 oz	380	21	45
Large, 4½ oz	430	23	50
Desserts:			
Cheesecake, 3¼ oz	310	23	22
Fudge Nut Brownie, 3oz	370	19	45
Lemon Pie, 1 slice, 4¼ oz	360	13	58
Icedream Cone w/o Toppings	170	4	31
Milkshake, Chocolate, 18¼ oz	750	28	113

Chili's® (Nov '10)

Appetizers: As Served	C	F	Cb
Bottomless Tostada Chips with Salsa	480	39	26
Crispy Onion Str. & Jalap. Stack/Ranch	1020	86	49
Loaded Nachos: Beef (12)	1690	122	60
Chicken (12)	1570	97	64
Skillet Queso with Tostada Chips	920	73	46
Southwestern Eggrolls with Dressing	910	57	72
Triple Dipper: Big Mouth Bites w/ Dress.	740	48	46
Buffalo Boneless Wings, with Dress.	750	60	27
Chicken Crispers without Dress.	600	39	29
Hot Spin. & Artichoke Dip with Chips	570	45	20
Burgers: As Served, On white Bun with Fries			
Big Mouth Bites with Dressing	1810	110	140
Classic Bacon Burger	1520	88	115
Jalapeno Smokehouse with Dressing	2130	139	127
Everything Is Better On The Grill			
Cajun Pasta: As Served			
With Grilled Chicken	1350	70	104
With Shrimp	1310	75	105
Chicken: As Served			
Margarita Grilled Chicken	530	8	67
Monterey Chicken	870	47	53
Fajitas: *Without Tortillas & Condiments*			
Beef	470	25	26
Buffalo Chicken	1040	76	43
Classic Chicken	360	12	23
Trio	530	26	28
+ Condiments only (1)	230	19	7
+ Flour Tortillas only (3)	380	10	62
Quesadillas: As Served			
Bacon Chicken Ranch	1550	94	93
Jalapeno Steak	1520	102	99
Steaks: *Without Sides*			
Classic Sirloin, 8 oz	450	26	19
Flame-Grilled Ribeye, 12 oz	900	68	18
Hand Battered: As Served			
Chicken Crispers w/ Honey Mustard	1750	109	136
Country-Fried Steak	1440	83	123
In House Smoked Ribs: Full Rack Without Sides			
Original	1110	81	33
Memphis Dry Rub	1180	87	34
Shiner Bock BBQ	1230	81	58
Salads: *Large, Includes Dressing Unless Indicated*			
Asian: With Grilled Chicken	930	50	71
With Salmon	1120	69	71
With Steak	1050	63	74
Sweet Endings: Per Slice			
Cheesecake	710	42	68
Chocolate Chip Paradise Pie	1290	68	163
Molten Chocolate Cake	1070	51	143

For Complete Menu & Data ~ see CalorieKing.com

Fast - Foods & *Restaurants*

Chipotle® (Nov '10)

Breads	C	F	Cb
Crispy Taco Shells (3)	180	6	27
Flour Tortillas (Burrito), (1)	290	9	44
Flour Tortillas (Taco), (3)	270	8	39
Meal Components			
Barbacoa, 4 oz	170	7	2
Black Beans, 4 oz	120	1	23
Carnitas, 4 oz	190	8	1
Cheese, 1 oz	100	9	0
Chicken, 4 oz	190	6.5	1
Cilantro-Lime Rice, 3 oz	130	3	23
Lettuce, 1 oz	5	0	0
Pinto Beans, 4 oz	120	1	22
Steak, 4 oz	190	7	2
Condiments			
Salsa: Corn, 4 oz	80	1.5	15
Green Tomatillo, 2 oz	15	0	3
Red Tomatillo, 2 oz	40	1	8
Tomato, 3½ oz	20	0	4
Sour Cream, 2 oz	120	10	2
Vinaigrette, 2 fl.oz	260	25	12
Extras: Chips, serving, 4 oz	570	27	73
Guacamole, 3½ oz	150	13	8

Chuck E. Cheese® (Nov '10)

Appetizers: Includes Condiments	C	F	Cb
Buffalo Wings (12)	900	60	48
Italian Bread Stick (1)	175	9	18
Mozzarella Stick (1)	95	6	6
Pizzas: *Per Medium Slice*			
BBQ Chicken	185	6	24
Cheese	155	5	21
Super Combo	185	8	22
Veggie Combo	160	6	22
Oven Baked Sandwiches:			
Ham & Cheese	685	27	79
Italian Sub	790	39	78
Roasted Chicken Ciabatta	715	28	80
French Fries:			
With Ketchup & Ranch: 4 oz	420	20	55
8 oz	840	40	110
Hot Dog, with Mustard & Relish	310	19	35
Desserts: Apple Dessert Pizza, 1 slice	190	5	33
Chocolate Cake (8"), 1 slice	290	13	41
Cinnamon Stick, w/ Toppings,1 stick	70	2	11

Church's Chicken® (Nov '10)

Chicken: Per Serving	C	F	Cb
Original: Breast, 1 piece	200	11	3
Leg, 1 piece	110	6	3
Thigh, 1 piece	330	23	8
Wing, 1 piece	300	19	7
Spicy: Breast, 1 piece	320	20	12
Leg, 1 piece	180	11	8
Thigh, 1 piece	480	35	20
Wing, 1 piece	430	27	17
Tender Strips: 1 piece	120	6	6
Spicy, 1 piece	135	7	7
Sides: *Per Regular Serving*			
Cajun Rice, 6 oz	130	7	16
Cole Slaw, 6 oz	150	10	15
Corn on the Cob (1)	140	3	24
French Fries, 3½ oz	290	14	38
Honey Butter Biscuits (1), 1¾ oz	190	10	22
Jalapeno Cheese Bombers (4)	240	10	29
Macaroni & Cheese, 6 oz	220	10	24
Mashed Potatoes & Gravy, 6 oz	70	2	12
Okra, 3½ oz	350	22	36
Whole Jalapeno Peppers (2)	10	0	2
Sauces: *Per Packet*			
BBQ; Sweet & Sour	25	0	6
Creamy Jalapeno	80	9	1
Honey Mustard	90	9	3
Purple Pepper	45	0	12
Ranch	105	10	1

Cici's Pizza® (Nov '10)

Buffet: Per ⅒ of 12" Pizza	C	F	Cb
Alfredo	120	3.5	18
Bacon Cheddar	110	4.5	19
Bar-B-Que	150	2.5	25
Beef	150	4	20
Cheese	150	4	19
Ham & Pineapple	150	3.5	21
Pepperoni & Jalapeno	150	4.5	20
Sausage	140	5	20
Spinach Alfredo	120	3.5	19
Zesty Ham & Cheddar	120	4	19
To-Go: *Per ⅒ of 15" Pizza*			
Alfredo	170	6	23
Bar-B-Que	240	6	36
Beef	190	8	24
Pepperoni & Jalapeno	210	7	24
Sausage	220	8	25
Spinach Alfredo	170	6	23
Zesty Ham & Cheddar	160	7	23
Zesty Pepperoni	170	9	23
Zesty Veggie	140	6	24

Updated Nutrition Data ~ www.CalorieKing.com
Persons with Diabetes ~ See Disclaimer (Page 22)

Cinnabon® (Nov '10) C F Cb

	C	F	Cb
Baked Goods: Cinnabon Bites (6)	520	16	78
Caramel Pecanbon (1)	1100	47	156
Cinnabon Stix (5)	410	23	46
CinnaPretzel (1)	750	6	156
Classic Cinnabon (1)	815	32	117
Cup Cakes: 24-Carrot; Cinnacake (1) av.	470	25	55
Average all others (1)	515	25	70
Sweet Roll Icing: Frosting Cup, 1.4 oz	180	11	25

Claim Jumper® (Nov '10) C F Cb

	C	F	Cb
Appetizers: As Served			
Cheese Potatocakes (3)	1105	74	86
Southwest Eggrolls	1165	49	108
Burgers & Sandwiches: Without Sides			
Grilled Cobb Sandwich	1230	77	72
Widow Maker Burger	1490	99	81
Meals: Per Whole Dish, Unless Indicated			
Favorites: Giant Stuffed Baker	1060	50	91
Meatloaf & Mashed Potatoes	1625	95	143
Whiskey Apple Glazed Pork Loin	1475	74	104
Pasta/Pizza:			
Black Tie Chicken, large	3175	199	212
Meatball Calzones	1655	89	134
Spicy Jambalaya w/ Noodles, large	2050	112	182
Rotisserie: Includes Roasted Vegetables Only			
BBQ Baby Back Pork Ribs	1805	126	83
Roasted Tri-Tip & Gravy	895	56	22
Seafood: Oaxacan Style Sea Bass	740	24	81
Tilapia Veracruz	870	34	84
Entree Salads: Per Large Size, Includes Dressing			
Chicken Citrus, Charbroiled	1480	71	139
Salmon Caesar, Broiled	1520	113	56
Soups: Per Bowl, Without Cheese Toast			
Baked Potato Cheddar	445	35	24
New England Clam Chowder	440	33	25
Desserts: Choc. Motherlode Cake	2760	144	340
Lemon Bar Brulee	745	31	105

For Complete Menu & Data ~ see CalorieKing.com

Coldstone Creamery® (Nov '10) C F Cb

	C	F	Cb
Ice Creams			
Amaretto: Like it	330	20	33
Love it	530	31	53
Gotta have it	790	47	80
Sorbet: Average all flavors			
Like it	155	0	38
Love it	250	0	62
Gotta have it	370	0	93

Cosi® (Nov '10)

	C	F	Cb
Flatbread Pizza, Individual:			
Margherita	705	31	96
Pepperoni	805	40	95
Traditional Cheese	685	29	95

Cosi® cont... (Nov '10)

	C	F	Cb
Melts: With Rustic Bread			
Chicken TBM	695	31	49
Pesto Chicken	670	31	52
Steakhouse Gonzola	750	47	49
Tuna Melt	875	40	51
TBM Melt	635	32	49
Sandwiches: With Rustic Bread			
Buffalo Bleu	565	25	47
Fire Roasted Veggie	325	8	44
Italiano	745	42	49
TBM	530	30	46
Soup: Per 10 oz Bowl, w/o Flatbread			
Pollo e Pasta	160	4	14
Tomato Basil Aurora	225	15	18
Salads: Includes Dressing			
Cosi Cobb, 12½ oz	710	55	16
Greek Salad, 14 oz	515	47	19
Grilled Chicken Caesar, 11 oz	620	44	20
Signature Salad, 11¼ oz	610	45	44
Steakhouse, 14 oz	615	49	14

Costco Food Court (Nov '10) C F Cb

	C	F	Cb
Pizza: Per Slice			
Combo, 11oz	680	29	72
Cheese, 10 oz	700	28	70
Pepperoni , 9 oz	620	24	68
Dogs, average, 8 oz	560	32	46
Salad, Chicken Caesar, 20½ oz	670	40	35
Meals: Cheese Burger Fry Combo	860	45	72
Chicken Bake 11½ oz	770	25	78
Ital. Sausage Sandwich, 12½ oz	700	42	46
Beverages: Hot Latte, 9½ fl oz	190	5	24
Hot Mocha, 11¼ fl oz	310	9	45
Mocha Freeze, 16¼ fl .oz	320	7	49
Latte Freeze, 15½ fl.oz	240	7	32
Smoothie, Fruit Smoothie, 16 fl.oz	290	0	72
Desserts: Ice cream Bar, 8 oz	870	65	60
Berry Sundae, 12¼ oz	410	0	87
Yogurt, 12 oz	390	0	82

Cousins Subs® (Nov '10) C F Cb

7½" Subs	C	F	Cb
BLT with Mayo	590	38	47
Cheese Steak	505	19	49
Chicken Cheddar Deluxe w/ Mayo	670	39	51
Club with Mayo	645	35	51
Double Cheese Steak	745	36	49
Italian Special with Dressing	815	51	50
Philly Cheese Steak with Sauce	530	19	55
Roast Beef with Mayo	605	30	50
Seafood with Crab & Mayo	640	38	60

Continued Next Page ...

Fast - Foods & *Restaurants*

Cousins Subs® cont... (Sept '10)

7½" Subs (cont)	C	F	Cb
Three Cheese with Mayo	685	44	50
Tuna with Mayo Blend	645	38	49
Turkey Breast with Mayo	530	28	50
Better Bunch, 5" Mini Subs: *Without Mayo & Cheese*			
Club	190	2	26
Garden Veggie; Hot Veggie, average	140	1	27
Ham; Turkey Breast	175	2	26
French Fries: Small, 2¾ oz	250	13	30
Medium, 4 oz	365	19	43
Large, 5¼ oz	485	25	57
Salads: *Without Dressing*			
Chef Salad	325	14	25
Italian	405	24	24
Tuna Salad	625	46	23

For Complete Nutritional Data ~ see CalorieKing.com

Culver's® (Nov '10)

Butter Burgers:	C	F	Cb
Original: Single; Kids	345	12	35
Double	480	20	36
Triple	615	28	37
Cheddar with Bacon, Single	540	30	31
Cheese: Single; Kids	400	17	36
Double	580	29	37
Culver's Bacon Deluxe: Single	575	35	34
Double	750	47	34
Culver's Deluxe: Single	495	28	35
Double	670	40	34
Mushroom & Swiss, Single	430	20	32
Sourdough Melt, Single	415	20	33
Corn Dog, Kids	260	14	26
Chicken Tenders, 4 pieces	440	20	32
Hot Dog	460	27	46
Kids	435	27	38
Sides			
Crinkle Cut Fries: Kids	275	12	38
Regular	385	17	53
Large	495	22	68
Chili Cheddar Fries, 8¾ oz	605	30	71
Dairyland Cheese Curds, 6½ oz	670	38	54
Mashed Potatoes with Gravy	140	2	26
Sandwiches: Angus Philly Steak	470	21	35
Beef Pot Roast	365	12	33
Crispy Chicken Filet	580	35	50
Flame Roasted Chicken	310	9	36
Grilled Reuben Melt	590	31	41
North Atlantic Cod Filet	665	41	47
Pork Tenderloin (Breaded)	595	26	62
Shaved Prime Rib	505	28	35
Turkey Sourdough BLT	560	32	36

Culver's® cont... (Nov '10)

Dinner Plates: Per Serving	C	F	Cb
Beef Pot Roast	745	36	73
Butterfly Crispy Shrimp, 6 pieces	1320	68	152
Chopped Steak	850	50	63
Fried Chicken: 2 pieces	1790	100	141
4 Pieces	2220	122	159
North Atlantic Cod, Fried, 2 pieces	1865	122	136
Salads: *Without Dressing*			
Chicken Cashew w/ Flame Rstd Chkn	445	24	20
Classic Caesar w/ Flame Roasted Chkn	340	16	14
Garden Fresco	230	10	20
Side Caesar	55	2	5
Side Salad	55	2	6
Desserts:			
Frozen Custard: Chocolate, 1 scoop	295	14	35
Vanilla, 1 scoop	310	18	30
Concrete Mixers: *Medium*			
Chocolate	995	49	122
Turtle	1155	71	114
Classic Sundaes: *Per 2 Scoops*			
Bananas Foster	785	41	93
Turtle	980	60	97
Beverages: Choc. Malt, medium	970	45	122
Chocolate Shake, medium	910	44	114
Root Beer Float, medium	550	18	90

For Complete Nutritional Data ~ see CalorieKing.com

D'Angelo's® (Nov '10)

Sandwiches:	C	F	Cb
Cheeseburger: Pokket	460	23	35
Sub	530	25	49
Wrap	600	31	52
Chicken Stir Fry: Pokket	400	10	39
Sub	470	12	53
Wrap	550	19	57
Classic Vegetable: Pokket	360	13	43
Wrap	520	22	61
Roast Beef: Sub	320	5	46
Wrap	410	12	50
Turkey Breast: Pokket	260	1	31
Sub	330	3	45
Grilled Quesadillas: Number 9	380	19	31
Chicken Stir Fry	360	15	31
Veggie	290	13	33
Salads: *Entree Size With Dressing Unless Indicated*			
Caesar	620	54	28
Chicken Caesar	670	53	21
Chicken Cobb , without Dressing	330	18	14
Greek	320	22	20
Tossed, without Dressing	60	0	13
Turkey, without Dressing	170	1	10

For Complete Menu & Data ~ see CalorieKing.com

Updated Nutrition Data ~ www.CalorieKing.com
Persons with Diabetes ~ See Disclaimer (Page 22)

Dairy Queen® (Nov '10)

Burgers & Sandwiches:	C	F	Cb
GrillBurgers:			
Bacon Cheddar, ¼ lb	650	35	41
½ lb Burger	720	40	42
½ lb Flame Thrower	1060	75	41
Original: Bacon Dbl Cheeseburger	730	41	35
Cheeseburger	400	18	34
Hamburger	350	14	33
Double	540	26	33
Sandwiches: Crispy Chicken	560	28	48
Grilled Chicken	370	16	32
Baskets:			
Chkn Strips: 4 piece with Gravy	1360	63	103
6 piece, with Country Gravy	1640	74	121
Iron Grilled Chicken Quesadilla	1070	50	117
Hot Dogs: All Beef	250	14	21
With Chili & Cheese	430	22	39
Salads: Without Dressing			
Crispy Chicken	460	19	31
Grilled Chicken	280	11	14
Sides			
DQ French Fries, Regular, 4 oz	310	13	43
DQ Onion Rings, Regular, 4 oz	360	16	47
Desserts: Per Medium			
Blizzard Treats: Banana Cream Pie	780	30	115
Butterfinger	740	26	114
Cappuccino Heath	870	38	122
Chocolate Chip	880	50	96
Cookie Dough	1010	40	148
Oreo Cookies	680	25	100
Reese's Peanut Butter Cups	760	31	101
Strawberry CheeseQuake	690	28	92
DQ Blizzard Cakes (10"): *Per 1/10 Cake*			
Oreo	720	31	97
Reese's Peanut Butter Cup	730	34	93
Strawberry CheeseQuake	630	27	84
DQ Dipped Cones: *Per 7¾ oz Cone*			
Butterscotch	490	23	59
Chocolate	470	22	60
DQ Sundaes: Per Medium, 8¼ oz			
Caramel	430	11	75
Hot Fudge	440	14	66
Strawberry	350	10	56
Malts: Per Medium			
Caramel	960	24	163
Chocolate	900	22	154
Strawberry	770	20	128
Moo Latte: Per 16 fl.oz			
Cappuccino	500	18	71
French Vanilla	560	18	88
Mocha	590	23	82

For Complete Nutritional Data ~ see CalorieKing.com

Daphne's® Greek Cafe (Nov '10)

Starters:	C	F	Cb
Hummus & Pita	330	17	37
Fire Feta & Pita	335	19	31
Pita Sandwiches: Without Fries, Rice or Salad			
Crispy Shrimp	430	23	39
Fresh Carved Gyros	665	46	42
Grilled Chicken	480	18	33
Spicy Grilled Chicken	600	29	36
Plates: Without Sides, Pita Bread or Tzatziki			
Grilled Chicken Ka-bobs	325	7	6
Grilled Steak Ka-bobs	220	11	9
Greek Salads: Without Dressing			
Classic	195	6	14
Crispy Shrimp	360	16	20
Falafel	670	40	52
Grilled Chicken	365	11	14
Dressings: Original	105	12	2
Lite Greek	60	6	2
Sides: Falafel, (3 pieces)	280	19	23
French Fries	270	12	37
Grilled Chicken Ka-bob	160	4	3
Pita Bread	230	8	28
Salad & Rice with Orig. Dressing	385	12	50
Spanakopita	220	18	11
Tzatziki	45	4	3

Davanni's® (Nov '10)

Half Hoagies: Includes 6" White Bun, Cheese, Salad, Butter, Dressing, Mayo & Sauce	C	F	Cb
Assorted	390	29	21
BLT	595	48	22
Chicken & Bacon with Honey Mustard	440	22	30
Chicken Parmigiana	365	17	22
Club	385	25	22
Italian Sausage	525	37	28
Pastrami	445	25	22
Pizza	315	18	22
Southwestern Chicken	480	27	25
Three Cheese	385	28	21
Tuna Melt	550	42	24
Turkey	355	22	22
Turkey Bacon Chipotle	465	30	22
Veggie	350	23	25
Calzones: Sausage Green Peppers	790	42	69
Pepperoni Sausage	825	49	66
Pizzas: Per Slice			
5 Meat: Thin Crust	240	12	18
Traditional Crust	300	12	30
Solo, Thin Crust	1010	63	45
The Works: Thin Crust	250	13	18
Traditional Crust	310	14	30
Veggie: Thin Crust	210	9	18
Traditional Crust	265	9	30

Fast - Foods & *Restaurants*

Del Taco® (Nov '10)

Breakfast	C	F	Cb
Breakfast Burrito	280	13	26
Bacon & Egg Quesadilla	430	20	37
Egg & Cheese Burrito	400	18	35
Steak & Egg Burrito	520	25	35
Hash Brown Sticks (5)	210	15	18
Burgers: Cheeseburger	430	22	40
Double Del Cheeseburger	560	35	35
Triple Del Cheeseburger	950	66	40
Burritos:			
Del Beef	470	20	37
Del Classic Chicken	510	33	37
Deluxe Combo	570	25	64
Deluxe Del Beef	510	23	39
Half Pound Red/Green, average	440	10	67
Macho Beef	1010	44	82
Macho Chicken	920	30	111
Macho Combo	990	34	112
Shredded Beef Combo	500	20	55
Spicy Chicken; Veggie Works, av.	615	16	96
Nachos: 4 oz	330	22	28
Del, 7¼ oz	440	23	45
Quesadillas:			
Cheddar; Spicy Jack	480	25	37
Chicken Cheddar; Spicy Jack Chkn	570	30	40
Tacos: Big Fat Chicken	330	14	34
Big Fat Steak	390	18	33
Chicken Del Carbon	150	5	19
Chicken, Soft	220	12	16
Classic	200	12	10
Crispy Fish	300	17	29
Macho	300	17	16
Steak Taco Del Carbon	210	8	18
Salad, Deluxe Taco Salad	850	46	70
Sides: Chips & Salsa, 3 oz	140	8	15
Fries: Small, 5 oz	270	16	31
Macho, 10 oz	550	31	63
Chili Cheese, 10½ oz	570	33	46
Deluxe Chili Cheese, 12 oz	610	36	48
Nachos, Macho, 17 oz	1000	56	94
Shakes: Chocolate, 13½ fl.oz	630	13	117
Strawberry, 13½ fl.oz	600	13	108
Vanilla, 13½ fl.oz	560	13	100

Denny's® (Nov '10)

Breakfast: Without Sides	C	F	Cb
Favorites: T-Bone Steak & Eggs, 16 oz	780	36	4
Country Fried Steak & Eggs, 11 oz	660	42	29
Moons Over My Hammy, 13 oz	780	42	50
Southwest Steak Burrito	910	52	76
Omelettes: Ham & Cheddar, 10 oz	590	44	4
Ultimate, 12 oz	670	54	8
Veggie-Cheese, 13 oz	500	37	10
Scrambles: Heartland, 20 oz	1150	66	97
Meat Lovers, 19 oz	1130	66	80
Slams: All American, 10 oz	820	69	5
French Toast, 15 oz	940	53	68
Grand Slamwich, w/o Hash Browns	1320	90	71
Lumberjack, 15 oz	850	46	60
Sides: Biscuit & Sausage Gravy, 8 oz	580	34	57
English Muffin, with Margarine, (1)	180	3	25
Hash Browns, 5 oz	210	12	26
Oatmeal, with 8 oz milk, 16 oz	270	7	37
Sweets:			
Fabulous French Toast Platter (3)	1010	52	93
Pancakes: *Without Margarine, Syrup or Toppings*			
Buttermilk (3)	510	6	102
Chocolate Chip (3)	720	18	129
Toppings: Maple-flav Syrup, 1½ oz	145	0	36
Sugar-free, 1½ oz	25	0	9
Cherry Topping, 3 oz	85	0	21
Whipped Margarine, 1 Tbsp	50	0	6
Appetizers:			
Mozzarella Cheese Sticks, 8 oz	750	40	195
Smothered Cheese Fries, 10 oz	840	50	74
Burgers & Sandwiches: Without Sides			
Better Burgers:			
Bacon Cheddar, 15 oz	940	52	49
Classic Cheeseburger, 15 oz	870	46	51
Without Cheese, 14 oz	790	40	50
Double Cheeseburger, 23 oz	1480	88	52
Mushroom Swiss, 18 oz	910	49	55
Slamburger, 15 oz	990	54	59
Sandwiches: BLT, w/ Mayo, 7 oz	520	35	35
Club, with Mayo, 11 oz	640	33	55
Grilled Chicken, w/ dressing, 15 oz	880	51	64
Super Bird, without dressing, 12 oz	700	37	53
Melts: *Without Dressing*			
Chicken Ranch, 12 oz	800	30	80
Spicy Buffalo Chicken, 15 oz	870	41	82

Continued Next Page ...

Denny's® cont... (Nov '10)

Dinner Meals
Without Sides, Sauce Or Bread Unless Indicated

	C	F	Cb
Amerian Classics: Chicken Strips, 8 oz	560	24	41
Country Fried Steak w/ Gravy, 13 oz	1000	65	54
Homestyle Meatloaf w/ Gravy, 7 oz	600	46	14
Sizzlin' Skillets: Grilled Chicken	770	34	72
Prime Rib, 19 oz	900	42	77
Steak & Seafood:			
Fit Fare Grilled Tilapia, 17 oz	600	11	66
Grilled Shrimp Skewers, 10 oz	370	10	39
Lemon Pepper Tilapia, 13 oz	640	27	41
T-Bone Steak: 12 oz	740	56	0
With Breaded Shrimp, 13 oz	920	64	20
With Shrimp Skewer, 12 oz	830	60	0
Tilapia Ranchero, 19 oz	470	17	57
Rockstar Menu: All Night Sampler	1120	47	131
Hooburrito, 17 oz	1430	67	164
Salads: *Without Dressing or Bread*			
Chicken Strip Deluxe, 18 oz	590	29	44
Cranberry Pecan Chicken, 9 oz	250	8	11
Grilled Chicken Deluxe, 17 oz	290	10	15
Prime Rib & Bleu, 10 oz	270	16	6
Dressings: *Per 1 oz*			
Bleu Cheese	130	13	1
Caesar	100	10	0
French	75	5	8
Honey Mustard	160	15	5
Ranch	130	14	1
Sides (Dinner)			
Coleslaw, 5 oz	260	22	15
Country-Fried Potatoes, 5 oz	390	28	30
Dinner Rolls, 2 pieces	260	9	38
Garlic Bread, 2 pieces	170	9	21
Ranchero Mashed Potatoes, 4 oz	140	6	50
Soups: *Without Bread*			
Chicken Noodle, 12 oz	165	4	19
Clam Chowder, 12 oz	265	17	24
Vegetable Beef, 12 oz	125	1	18
Desserts			
Cheesecake, 7 oz	640	41	58
French Silk Pie, 7 oz	770	57	59
Hot Fudge Brownie a` la Mode, 9 oz	830	37	122
Oreo Blender Blaster, 14 oz	890	44	113
Oreo Sundae, 9 oz	760	37	103
Beverages			
Flav. Cappuccino; Hot Choc., 8 fl.oz	100	2	28
Milkshakes, Van/Choc, 12 fl.oz	560	26	76
Raspberry Nestea, 16 fl.oz	80	0	21

For Complete Nutritional Data ~ see CalorieKing.com

Dippin' Dots® (Nov '10)

	C	F	Cb
Flavored Ices:			
All flavors, ½ cup, 3 oz	90	0	23
Frozen Yogurt:			
Strawberry Cheesecake, ½ cup	100	0	21
Ice Cream: *Per ½ Cup*			
Banana Split	170	10	16
Chocolate Chip Cookie dough	215	11	26
Peanut Butter Chip	165	10	15
Strawberry	170	10	16
Fat-Free, Fudge, No Sugar Added	90	0	18
Red.-Fat, Vanilla, No Sugar Added	125	6	13

Donato's® Pizza (Nov '10)

	C	F	Cb
Thin Crust Pizza: *¼ Large Pizza*			
Chicken Vegy Medley	495	20	51
Classic Trio	675	37	52
Founder's Favorite	700	38	52
Hawaiian	590	27	56
Thicker Crust Pizza: *¼ Large Pizza*			
Founder's Favorite	860	42	78
Mariachi Beef	795	36	81
Mariachi Chicken	805	35	81
Pepperoni	800	39	76
Serious Cheese	800	38	77
The Works	845	41	81
Vegy	715	29	83
No Dough Pizza - Individual			
Chicken Vegy Medley	495	29	20
Classic Trio	530	37	18
Founder's Favorite	560	38	18
Hawaiian	435	26	22
Mariachi Beef	530	34	23
Mariachi Chicken	495	30	21
Pepperoni	500	35	17
Pepperoni Zinger	585	42	17
Serious Cheese	455	31	17
Serious Meat	655	46	19
The Works	545	37	21
Stromboli: 3 Meat	690	31	67
Cheese	695	31	66
Deluxe	615	25	68
Pepperoni	715	34	67
Vegy	605	24	69
Desserts:			
Apple Timpano, 2 slices	405	9	72
Cinnamon Timpano, 2 slices	525	22	73

For Complete Nutritional Data ~ see CalorieKing.com

Domino's® Pizza (Nov '10)

C   F   Cb

12" Hand-Tossed: *Per Slice, ⅛ Pizza, Includes Cheese*

	C	F	Cb
Beef	205	9	23
Cheese Only	180	6	23
Green Peppers, Onion & Mushroom	180	6	23
Ham	190	6	23
Ham & Pineapple	195	6	24
Pepperoni	205	8	23
Pepperoni & Sausage	235	11	24
Sausage	210	9	24

14" Thin Crust: *Per Slice, ⅛ Pizza, Includes Cheese*

	C	F	Cb
Beef	230	14	18
Cheese Only	190	11	18
Green Pepper Onion & Mushroom	190	11	18
Ham	200	11	18
Ham & Pineapple	210	11	20
Pepperoni	220	14	18
Pepperoni & Sausage	265	17	19
Sausage	235	14	19

12" Deep Dish: *Per Slice, ⅛ Pizza, Includes Cheese*

	C	F	Cb
Beef	245	12	26
Cheese Only	220	10	26
Green Pepper Onion & Mushroom	220	10	26
Ham	230	10	26
Ham & Pineapple	235	10	27
Pepperoni	245	12	26
Pepperoni & Sausage	275	14	27
Sausage	250	12	27

12 "Feast Hand-Tossed: *Per Slice, ⅛ Pizza*

	C	F	Cb
America's Favorite Feast	120	14	10
Bacon Cheeseburger Feast	260	12	25
Barbecue Feast	240	10	30
Deluxe Feast	220	9	26
ExtravaganZZa Feast	280	13	27
Hawaiian Feast	210	7.5	27
MeatZZa Feast	270	13	26
Philly Cheese Steak Feast	220	9	23
Ultimate Pepperoni	250	13	24
Vegi Feast	210	7.5	26

14" Feast Thin Crust: *Per Slice, ⅛ Pizza*

	C	F	Cb
America's Favorite Feast	180	10	19
Bacon Cheeseburger Feast	310	20	21
Barbecue Feast	280	16	27
Deluxe Feast	250	15	21
ExtravaganZZa Feast	320	20	22
Hawaiian Feast	230	13	23
MeatZZa Feast	310	20	21
Philly Cheese Steak Feast	240	14	18
Ultimate Pepperoni	290	19	19
Vegi Feast	220	13	22

Domino's® Pizza cont... (Nov '10)

C   F   Cb

12" Feast Deep Dish: *Per Slice, ⅛ Pizza*

	C	F	Cb
America's Favorite Feast	160	5	24
Bacon Cheeseburger Feast	300	15	28
Barbecue Feast	280	13	30
Hawaiian Feast	250	11	29
Philly Cheese Steak Feast	260	12	25
Ultimate Pepperoni	290	15	27

Oven Baked Sandwiches

	C	F	Cb
Chicken Bacon Ranch	880	46	70
Chicken Parm	760	31	72
Italian	880	45	71
Philly Cheese Steak	690	27	72

BreadBowl Pasta: *Per ½ Bowl*

	C	F	Cb
Chicken Alfredo, 10¾ oz	700	25	93
Chicken Carbonara, 11¾ oz	740	28	94
Italian Sausage Marinara, 12oz	735	27	98
Pasta Primavera, 11 oz	670	24	94

Salads: *Per 2 Servings*

	C	F	Cb
Garden Fresh, 8½ oz	140	7	10
Grilled Chicken Caesar, 9½ oz	180	7	10

Salad Dressings & Condiments: *Per 1½ oz Package*

	C	F	Cb
Blue Cheese	240	25	2
Buttermilk Ranch	230	24	2
Creamy Caesar	210	21	2
Golden Italian	210	22	2
Light Italian	20	1	3

Bread Side Items

	C	F	Cb
Breadsticks: 1 stick, without sauce	105	6	11
8 sticks, without sauce	850	48	88
Cheesy Bread:			
1 stick, without sauce	110	6	11
8 sticks, without sauce	880	48	88
Bread Dipping Sauces: *Per Container*			
Garlic	250	28	0
Marinara	25	0	5
Cinna Stix:			
1 stick, without icing	120	6	14
8 sticks, without icing	960	48	112
Sweet Icing, Dipper Cup	250	2.5	57

Chicken Side Items

	C	F	Cb
Buffalo Chicken Kickers			
without Dipping Sauce (2)	100	4.5	7
Buffalo Wings:			
Barbecue, 2 wings, without sauce	230	14	6
Hot, 2 wings, without sauce	200	14	2
Chicken Dipping Sauces: *Per 1½ oz Container*			
Blue Cheese	240	25	2
Hot	50	4.5	3
Ranch	200	21	2

Updated Nutrition Data ~ www.CalorieKing.com
Persons with Diabetes ~ See Disclaimer (Page 22)

Don Pablos® (Nov '10)

	C	F	Cb
Appetizers: Per Whole Plate, Includes Queso & Garnish, without Guacamole			
Beef Taquitos (6)	625	45	27
Chicken Flautas (6)	565	36	39
Nachos:			
Acapulco Beef, 9 chips	1385	87	69
Cheese, 9 chips	1145	84	39
Quesadillas:			
Mesquite Grilled: Chicken, 4 slices	825	50	62
Steak, 8 slices	1630	100	104
Dips: Per 6 oz Cup, Without Chips			
Queso Blanco	540	45	6
Prairie Fire Bean	355	21	27
Burritos: Entree, Per Burrito, Without Beans			
Chicken	1180	58	105
Spicy Ground Beef & Bean	1285	68	97
Carnitas: Entree, Without Beans			
Pork	985	34	120
Cold Set, Side	160	11	18
Chimichangas: Entree, Without Beans			
Chicken	1100	61	91
Spicy Ground Beef De Oro	1475	80	112
Classic Fajitas: Entree, w/ On., Peppers & Lime, w/o Fajita			
Combo - Steak & Chicken	625	31	47
Grilled Shrimp	425	38	22
Mesquite - Grilled: Chicken	570	27	58
Steak	680	36	36
Add Fixin's: Flour Tortillas (3)	1120	33	180
Corn Tortillas (4)	235	4	48
Guacamole, 1 scoop	70	6	4
Tacos: Crispy Beef (3)	870	41	65
Crispy Chicken (3)	725	31	66
Lunch:			
Combos: Entree, w/o Beverage, Soup or Side Salad			
Don Pablo's	790	36	70
Dos Beef Tacos (Soft)	1085	48	192
Fajitas: Entree, W/ On., Peppers & Lime, w/o Fajita			
Chicken	280	13	29
Steak	335	17	18
Quesadilla & Salad Combo: Entree, w/o Dressing			
Cheese	1045	69	64
Chicken	1045	56	75
Salads:			
Chicken Caesar, with Dressing	1285	76	114
Steak Caesar, with Dressing	1360	82	99
Sides: French Fries, w/o Ketchup, 7 oz	345	10	60
Mexican Rice, 3 oz	120	2	23
Monterey, Jack & Cheddar Chse, 1 oz	110	9	1
Refritos, 5 oz	215	7	27
Sour Cream, 1 scoop	80	8	2

Dunkin Donuts® (Nov '10)

	C	F	Cb
Donuts: Apple N' Spice	240	11	32
Bavarian Kreme	250	12	31
Boston Kreme	280	12	38
Chocolate Frosted	230	10	32
Chocolate Kreme Filled	310	16	37
French Cruller	250	20	18
Jelly Filled	260	11	36
Old Fashioned Cake	280	18	27
Powdered Cake	300	18	30
Strawberry Frosted	230	10	33
Sugar Raised	190	9	22
Vanilla Kreme Filled	320	17	37
Fancies: Apple Fritter	400	15	63
Bow Tie Donut	310	15	39
Chocolate Iced Bismark	350	14	53
Coffee Roll: Original	370	18	49
Chocolate Frosted	380	19	50
Eclair	350	14	53
Fritter: Apple	400	15	63
Glazed	400	15	63
Munchkins: Plain Cake (4)	200	12	20
Glazed, average all varieties (4)	240	12	32
Jelly Filled (5)	300	13	40
Powdered Cake (4)	240	14	24
Sugar Raised (5)	200	13	25
Sticks: Plain Cake	300	20	26
Cinnamon Cake	310	20	30
Glazed: Cake	340	20	38
Chocolate Cake	390	25	40
Jelly	400	20	54
Powdered Cake	320	20	31
Bagels: Plain; Salt	320	2.5	63
Cinnamon Raisin	330	3.5	65
Everything	350	5	65
Multigrain	390	8	65
Onion; Wheat, average	315	3	62
Sesame	360	6	63
Danish: Apple Cheese	330	16	41
Cheese	330	17	39
Strawberry Cheese	320	16	40
Muffins: Chocolate Chip	630	23	98
Blueberry	510	16	87
Reduced Fat	450	10	86
Coffee Cake	660	26	98
Corn	510	17	84
Honey Bran Raisin	500	14	86

Continued Next Page ...

Dunkin Donuts® cont... (Nov '10)

Breakfast	C	F	Cb
Oven Toasted Breakfast Sandwiches:			
Bagels: Egg & Cheese	470	14	66
Bacon Egg & Cheese	510	17	66
Ham Egg & Cheese	510	16	67
Sausage Egg & Cheese	640	29	67
Biscuits: Bacon Egg & Cheese	470	29	36
Sausage Egg & Cheese	610	40	36
Croissant: Bacon Egg & Cheese	510	31	39
Ham Egg & Cheese	510	30	39
Sausage Egg & Cheese	640	43	39
English Muffin:			
Bacon Egg & Cheese	360	16	34
Ham Egg & Cheese	360	15	35
Sausage Egg & Cheese	490	28	35
Sandwiches			
Dunkin' Deli Sandwiches			
Cravings: Chicken Bruschetta	580	26	49
Chipotle Chicken	600	25	50
Pastrami Supreme	750	39	51
Pressed Cuban	680	33	50
Deli Classics: Tuna (Albacore)	660	19	56
Turkey & Cheese	450	13	52
Favorites: Steak & Cheese	470	16	50
Toasted Italian	560	25	52
Turkey & Bacon Club	440	13	51
Salads: With Dressing			
Dunkin' Deli: Caesar	320	29	11
Chicken Caesar	440	33	11
Garden	180	6	21
Soups: Broccoli Cheddar, 1 cup	190	11	14
Chicken Noodle	130	3	19
Beverages			
Cappuccino, without sugar, 10 fl.oz	80	4	7
Coolatta:			
Coffee: with Skim Milk, 16 fl.oz	210	0	51
With Cream, 16 fl.oz	400	23	49
With Milk, 16 fl.oz	240	4	50
Strawberry Fruit, 16 fl.oz	300	0	72
Tropical Orange, 16 fl.oz	220	0	52
Hot Chocolate: Small, 10 fl.oz	210	7	39
White, 1 medium, 14 fl.oz	340	13	56
Iced Coffee: 16 fl.oz	10	0	2
Flavored Coffee: Caramel, 10 fl.oz	10	0	2
Toasted Almond, 10 fl.oz	10	0	1

Eat 'N Park® (Nov '10)

Breakfast	C	F	Cb
Fruit Cup	60	0.5	15
Hash Browns	200	8	28
Home Fries	210	12	24
Oatmeal with Milk	200	4	33
Omelette: Cheese	390	30	2.5
Chicken Fiesta	565	37	10
Ham & Cheese	535	35	4
Veggie	415	30	8
Western	345	21	7
Pancakes, Buttermilk: Plain (1)	75	1	15
Blueberry (1)	85	1	16
Waffles: Belgian (1)	280	12	35
Strawberry (1)	375	18	48
Appetizers:			
Buffalo Chicken Tenders	635	42	27
Fried Cheese Sticks	535	36	26
Grilled Chicken Quesadillas	905	55	51
Onion Rings	245	16	23
Burgers:			
Black Angus: American Grill	610	37	31
BBQ Bacon Cheddar	865	53	53
Mushroom & Onion	710	41	45
Superburger	1085	73	28
Classic: Black Angus	420	21	22
Bacon Cheeseburger	530	31	22
Cheeseburger	465	25	22
Garden Burger	220	4	33
Original, Superburger	565	38	27
Sandwiches:			
BLT	490	15	66
Buffalo Chicken	740	41	59
Chargrilled Chicken	320	6	32
Chicken Portabella Hoagie	845	56	47
Hot Turkey	500	9	71
Reuben on Rye	730	50	31
Santa Fe Turkey & Bacon	880	60	45
Shredded Pot Roast	530	31	28
Turkey Club	835	50	52
Whale of a Cod Fish	880	41	76
Dinners: Baked Lemon Sole, 1 filet	195	10	6
Chargrilled Chicken, 2 pieces	350	9	0
Chicken Fillets (5)	530	26	28
Chicken Parmiiana: Marinara Sauce	960	37	100
With Meat Sauce	985	40	95
Chicken Stir-Fry	390	8	47
Cod Floridian, 2 filets	240	3	8
Ground Sirloin w/ Fried On. Ring	425	26	5
Spaghetti Marinara	695	9	129
Spaghetti with Meat Sauce	830	16	145
T Bone Steak	575	39	1

Continued next page...

Eat 'N Park® cont... (Nov '10)

Salads: Without Dressing	C	F	Cb
Buffalo Chicken Salad	610	35	42
Chicken Fajita	410	12	35
Garden Salad	95	3	15
Grilled Chicken	445	20	30
Grilled Chicken & Strawberry	215	6	13
Grilled Chicken Portobella	310	10	23
Dressings: Per 2 fl.oz			
Bleu Cheese	245	25	3
French Fat Free	75	0	18
Italian Fat Free	20	0	5
House Ranch	215	21	4
Thousand Island	190	19	4
Desserts:			
Grilled Stickies a la Mode	725	39	81
Ice Cream, 2 scoops	230	12	27
Pies: Per Slice			
Apple	525	27	67
Cherry	520	28	63
Peachberry	390	19	51
Strawberry	295	12	45

Edo Japan® (Nov '10)

Meals: Per Bento Box w/o Teriyaki	C	F	Cb
Beef Yakisoba, 20¼ oz	830	30	102
Chicken Yakisoba, 20½ oz	800	25	102
Seafood Grill, 23 oz	860	16	129
Sizzling Shrimp, 22 oz	800	16	122
Sukiyaki Beef, 20¼ oz	900	28	120
Specialties: Without Teriyaki Sauce			
Curry Chicken Bowl, 13¼ oz	500	21	27
Ginger Pork, 14½ oz	650	23	82
Hawaiian Chicken, 15½ oz	590	12	85
Seafood Grill, 17¾ oz	570	4	89
Sukiyaki Beef, 14¾ oz	610	16	80
Teriyaki Chicken, 15 oz	580	12	80

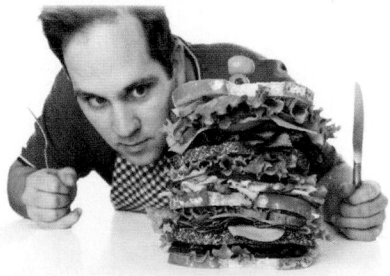

Einstein Bros®/Noahs® (Nov '10)

Bagels:	C	F	Cb
Asiago Cheese	310	5	56
Blueberry	300	1	65
Chocolate Chip	280	2.5	56
Cinnamon Sugar Chicago Style	310	2.5	66
Egg	300	5	54
Everything	270	2	56
Garlic Dip'd	270	2.5	56
Honey Whole Wheat; Plain	260	1	57
Onion Dip'd	270	2.5	56
Poppy Dip'd	280	3	56
Potato	270	4	52
Power Bagel, Fruit & Nut	310	5	61
Sesame Dip'd	280	3	56
Sundried Tomato	260	1.5	54
Gourmet Bagels: Dutch Apple	350	7	66
Green Chile	350	8	58
Spinach Florentine	340	8	57
Six-Cheese	330	6	56
Breakfast Sandwiches			
Egg Way: Original	530	20	62
With Bacon	580	24	59
With Black Forest Ham	570	21	62
Spinach Mushroom & Omelette	540	20	65
Bacon & Spinach Panini	860	51	66
Sausage Ranchero Panini	680	29	64
Vegetable Panini	730	36	68
Wraps: California Chicken	630	28	63
Chipotle Turkey	730	37	70
Bagel Dogs: With Cheddar Cheese			
Original	550	26	56
Original Asiago	560	27	56
Pizza Bagels: Cheese	420	12	63
Pepperoni	470	16	63
Cream Cheese: Per 2 Tablespoons, Whipped			
Reduced Fat: Blueberry	70	5	6
Garlic Herb/Garden Veggie	60	5	3
Honey Almond; Strawberry, av.	70	5	6
Plain; Sun Dried Tomato & Basil	60	5	2
Onion and Chive	70	6	3
Smoked Salmon	60	6	2
Salads: With Dressing			
Bros Bistro	820	68	38
Bros Bistro with Chicken	940	71	39
Chipotle	590	38	53
Chicken Chipotle	710	41	54
Caesar Salad with Chicken	820	66	20
Coffee, Specialty: Per Regular, 12 fl.oz			
Americano Regular 8 fl.oz	1	0	0
Café Latte	140	5	13
Non-Fat	100	1	14
Cappuccino, Whole Milk	150	8	13
Espresso, Regular 2 fl.oz	1	0	0
Mocha, Whole Milk	270	9	38

Fast - Foods & *Restaurants*

El Pollo Loco® (Nov '10)

	C	F	Cb
Burritos:			
BRC	440	12	68
Classic Chicken	550	17	69
Ultimate Grilled	710	23	86
Flame-Grilled Chicken: *Skin On*			
Breast	220	9	0
Leg	90	4	0
Thigh	220	15	0
Wing	90	5	0
Bowls: Chicken Caesar	490	22	44
The Original Pollo	690	10	106
Ultimate Pollo	1050	34	110
Loco Value Menu:			
Chicken Taquito with Avocado Salsa	230	12	20
Chips & Guacamole	250	14	26
Cheese Quesadilla	420	23	35
Loco Salad with Cilantro Dressing	170	14	7
Taco al Carbon	150	5	17
Mexican Favorites:			
Grilled Chicken Nachos	810	40	70
Grilled Chicken Tortilla without Sauce	390	16	37
Soup:			
Chicken Tortilla w/ Tortilla Strips, reg.	210	9	18
Large	450	20	37
Tacos: Crunchy Chicken	190	8	16
Soft Chicken	260	12	18
Salads: Chicken Tostada w/o Dress.	840	42	74
Garden Salad, small, w/o Dress.	70	3.5	8
Dressings: *Per Packet*			
Creamy Cilantro, 3 oz	440	46	3
Light Creamy Cilantro, 2 oz	70	5	6
Light Italian, 2 oz	20	1	2
Ranch, 2 oz	230	24	2
Thousand Island, 2 oz	220	21	6
Condiments: *Per 1½ oz*			
Guacamole	70	6	3
Salsa: Avocado	40	3.5	2
House	10	0	2
Pico de Gallo	15	1	2
Sides			
Corn Cobbette, 5 oz	90	0.5	19
French Fries, 6 oz	330	17	42
Fresh Vegetables w/ Marg., 4 oz	60	3	8
Macaroni & Cheese, 5½ oz	280	17	28
Mashed Potatoes with Gravy, 6 oz	120	1.5	25
Pinto Beans, 6 oz	200	4	29
Refried Beans with Cheese, 6¼ oz	270	7	36
Spanish Rice, 4½ oz	220	2	45
Desserts: Caramel Flan, 5 oz	260	12	34
Churros (2)	300	18	32

For Complete Nutritional Data ~ see CalorieKing.com

Fatburger® (Nov '10)

	C	F	Cb
Burgers: *Without Extras*			
Baby Fat	400	21	37
Fatburger	590	31	46
Kingburger	850	41	69
Turkeyburger	480	21	50
Veggieburger	510	20	60
Sandwiches: *Without Extras*			
Crispy Chicken	560	27	53
Grilled Chicken	430	14	42
Fish	560	31	55
Sides and Fries			
Fries: Fat Fries; Skinny Fries, av.	385	17	53
With Chili, average	485	23	57
With Chili & Cheese, average	595	32	58
Sides: American Cheese, 1 slice	70	5	1
Cheddar Cheese, 1 slice	110	9	1
Chili Cup	200	11	10
with Cheese & Onions	320	20	12
Mayonnaise	90	10	1
Onion Rings	540	29	64
Relish	20	0	5
Shakes: Chocolate	910	45	115
Peanut Butter	950	53	114
Strawberry; Vanilla, average	885	44	112

For Complete Nutritional Data ~ see CalorieKing.com

Fazoli's® Italian Food (Nov '10)

	C	F	Cb
Pasta Bowl: *Per Serving*			
Fettuccine with Alfredo, 20 oz	900	27	126
Fettuccine with Marinara, 20½ oz	660	3	129
Ravioli with Marinara Sce, 12¼ oz	490	15	69
Ravioli with Meat Sauce, 13 oz	570	21	70
Spaghetti w/ Marinara Sce, 20½ oz	660	3	129
Sampler Platter: *Per Serving*			
Classic Sampler Platter, 22¾ oz	880	30	110
Ultimate Sampler Platter, 30 oz	1130	34	153
Oven-Baked Pasta: *Per Serving*			
Chicken Broccoli Penne, 21¼ oz	920	42	77
Chicken Parmigano, 21½ oz	1000	39	108
Baked Spaghetti, 15½ oz	640	22	80
With Meatballs, 18½ oz	890	39	86
Penne with Creamy Basil Chkn, 18¾ oz	970	51	73
Rigatoni Romano, 17¼ oz	880	44	76
Tortellini Robusto, 17½ oz	1020	50	80
Twice-Baked Lasagna, 18½ oz	700	39	47
Pizzas: *Per Slice*			
Cheese, 4 oz	270	11	32
Pepperoni, 4¼ oz	310	14	32

Continued next page...

Fast - Foods & Restaurants

Fazoli's® cont... (Nov '10)

Submarinos	C	F	Cb
Club Italiano, 13 oz	780	36	68
Fazoli's Original, 12¾ oz	880	50	68
Ham 'n' Swiss Supremo, 12 oz	690	31	68
Italian Four Chse & Tomato, 11½ oz	710	37	59
Rstd Red Pepper Chicken, 11¾ oz	780	36	59
Smoked Turkey Basil, 12¾ oz	750	37	68
Salads: *Without Dressing*			
Caesar Side Salad, 4¼ oz	40	2	4
Chicken & Pasta Caesar, 13¼ oz	470	15	38
Cranberry & Walnut Chicken	390	14	27
Crispy Chicken BLT	480	26	31
Grilled Chicken Artichoke	240	4.5	11
Italian Side Salad, 4¼ oz	80	4.5	4
Pasta Side Salad, 6 oz	300	12	38
Salad Dressing: *Per 1.5 oz*			
Caesar	230	25	1
Italian	160	14	7
Fat Free	25	0	6
Honey French	220	18	14
Ranch	220	24	2
Lite Ranch	120	12	2

For Complete Nutritional Data ~ see CalorieKing.com

Firehouse Subs® (Nov '10)

Subs: *Per Medium, Without Mayo or Cheese*

	C	F	Cb
Chicken Salad	760	46	63
Engine Company	390	6	52
Engineer	380	5	55
Ham	410	7	58
Hero	430	7	54
Hook & Ladder	410	7	68
Italian	560	25	55
NY Steamer	410	12	48
Roast Beef	410	6	48
Tuna Salad	610	28	62
Turkey	370	4	54
Veggie	300	5	56

Chili and Salads: *Includes Meat, Cheese and Egg, w/o Dressing*
Chili	370	28	17
Chief's Salad: With Chicken Salad	740	58	16
With Tuna Salad	610	40	16
With Ham	360	18	16
With Turkey	300	15	12
Desserts: Brownie (1)	420	18	63
Chocolate Chip Cookie	290	14	37

Five Guys (Nov '10)

Burgers	C	F	Cb
Bacon Burger	780	50	39
Bacon Cheeseburger	920	62	40
Cheeseburger	840	55	40
Hamburger	700	43	39
Little: Bacon Burger	560	33	39
Bacon Cheeseburger	630	39	40
Cheeseburger	550	32	40
Hamburger	480	26	39
Dogs			
Bacon Dog	625	42	40
Bacon Cheese Dog	695	48	41
Cheese Dog	615	41	41
Hot Dog	545	36	40
Fries: Regular 8½ oz	620	30	78
½ Regular Order	310	15	39

Freshens® (Nov '10)

Frozen Yogurt: Per Serving	C	F	Cb
Soft Serve Yogurt, 1 oz	35	0	7
Smoothies: *100% Juice (21 fl.oz)*			
Blended Fruit: Caribbean Craze	290	0	73
Citrus Mango	490	7	108
Jamaican Jammer	350	0	77
Maui Mango	290	0	74
Orange Sunrise	360	1	82
Peach Sunset	270	0	67
Strawberry: Kiwi	320	0	81
Shooter	250	0	64
Squeeze	310	0	68
Tropical Pineapple	310	4	97
High Protein: Peanut Butter	540	12	84
Chocolate Oreo	610	7	11
Low Calorie: No Sugar Added			
Average all flavors	80	0	50

(Note: Carbs include 1¼ oz Erythritol Sweetener)

Nature's Energy: Acai Energy	320	3	71
Mangosteen	320	0	89
Tart Berry	320	0	82
Yerba Mate	320	0	68
Fro-Yo Blasts:			
Cap'n Crunch & P'nut Butter	510	12	82
Cookie Dough	570	7	112
Oreo Overload	430	3.5	83
Indulgent Shakes: Chocolate	530	4	103
Oreo Cream	610	7	115
Strawberry	490	4	94

Gino's East® ® (Nov '10)

	C	F	Cb
Deep Dish Pizza: *Medium 11" Per ⅙ Slice of Pizza*			
Cheese	410	11	58
Crumbled Sausage	420	21	38
Pepperoni	450	15	57
Spinach	410	11	59
Deep Dish Pizza: *Small 6" ~ Per Whole Pizza*			
Cheese	720	16	116
Crumbled Sausage	800	22	116
Pepperoni	780	20	116

Godfather's™ Pizza (Nov '10)

	C	F	Cb
Golden Pizza: *Per Slice*			
Cheese: Medium, ⅛ pizza	220	8	25
Large,¹⁄₁₀ pizza	250	9	28
Combo: Medium, ⅛ pizza	290	13	27
Large, slice, ¹⁄₁₀ pizza	330	15	30
Original Pizza			
Cheese: Mini, ¼ pizza	150	4	20
Medium, ⅛ pizza	260	7	34
Jumbo, ¹⁄₁₂ pizza	350	10	44
Combo: Mini, ¼ pizza	200	8	21
Medium, ⅛ pizza	350	14	36
Jumbo, ¹⁄₁₂ pizza	480	20	47
Thin Pizza			
Cheese: Medium, ⅛ pizza	170	8	15
Large, ¹⁄₁₀ pizza	210	10	17
Combo: Medium, ⅛ pizza	240	13	17
Large, ¹⁄₁₀ pizza	280	16	20
Sides			
Breadstick (1)	110	2	20
Cheesestick,1 piece, ⅙	130	3.5	18
Potato Wedges, 4 oz	175	8	24

Gold Star Chili® (Nov '10)

	C	F	Cb
Meals			
Bowls: Low Carb Coney, 10½ oz	570	47	7
Veggie Chili, 9 oz	160	2	29
Coney, 5¼ oz	285	14	30
Cheese Coney, 5½ oz	345	18	31
Chili: 8 oz	215	12	8
Tex Mex, 8 oz	210	9	17
Chili Cheese Nachos, 8½ oz	410	25	30
Regular: 2-Way	420	11	58
Bean	490	12	71
Onion	435	11	62
Onion Bean	505	12	75

Gold Star Chili (Cont)® (Nov '10)

	C	F	Cb
Meals (Cont)			
Bowls (Cont): Regular 3-Way	650	30	59
Regular 4-Way	665	30	63
Regular 5-Way	735	30	76
Super 5-Way	1140	51	109
Sandwiches: Chili	210	5	32
Chili Cheese	290	12	30
Salads: *Without Dressing*			
Cafe: 8 oz	160	10	15
With Crispy Chicken	310	15	24
With Grilled Chicken, 10½ oz	250	12	15
Caesar Salad, 6 oz	130	6	12
With Crispy Chicken, 8½ oz	280	11	22
With Grilled Chicken, 8½ oz	210	8	12
South of the Border Chili, 16¾ oz	640	39	55
Sides: Fries, 5 oz	365	19	44
Chili Cheese, 9½ oz	595	36	46
Garlic Bread: Without Cheese, 2 oz	215	13	19
With Cheese, 2½ oz	270	18	19

Golden Corral® (Nov '10)

	C	F	Cb
Breakfast:			
Bacon & Cheese Quiche, 1 sl., 4 oz	280	19	15
Corned Beef Hash, 1 cup	420	30	22
French Toast, 1 slice	240	8	23
Hash Browns, 1 cup	205	14	16
Sausage Links (3)	160	14	1
Sausage Patties (1)	245	21	0.5
Scrambled Eggs, 3½ oz	160	11	2
Split Smoked Sausage (1)	250	23	2
Meals:			
Hot Bar: *Without Sides*			
Awesome Pot Roast, 3 oz	100	4.5	5
Baked Fish with Shrimp & Sauce	160	10	2
Baked Florentine Fish, 3 oz	180	12	2
BBQ: Chicken Leg Quarter, 7¾ oz	490	22	21
Pork, 3 oz	170	8	5
Bone-In Breaded Catfish, 3 oz	210	14	7
Bourbon Street Chicken, 3 oz	170	9	4
Breaded Scallops (10), 2½ oz	140	6	13
Coconut Shrimp (5), 2 oz	200	12	16
Crab Cakes (1), 2 oz	180	15	8
Grilled Lemon Pepper Fish (1), 3 oz	180	11	5
Meatloaf, w/ Topping,1 slice, 4. oz	220	11	12
Sirloin Steak, 4½ oz	230	9	1
Cold Bar: *Per ½ Cup*			
Cajun Potato Salad	230	17	15
Coleslaw	110	9	6
Salads: Seafood	140	10	9
Spinach Applewood Bacon , 1 cup	150	11	7
Tuna	200	14	5

Updated Nutrition Data ~ www.CalorieKing.com
Persons with Diabetes ~ See Disclaimer (Page 22)

(The) Great American Bagel Co® (Nov '10)

	C	F	Cb
Bagels: 4-Grain Honey	390	4	80
Apple Cinnamon Sugar	390	4	78
Asiago Cheese	520	16	72
Banana Nut	410	9	69
Blueberry	370	3.5	75
Cheddar Bacon	600	23	71
Chocolate Chip	420	8	78
Cinnamon Delight	640	18	108
Jalapeno Cheddar	370	7	63
Onion	380	4	74
Plain; Pumpernickel; Salt	360	4	71
Stuffed Pepperoni	570	17	78
Stuffed Spinach	640	20	86
Sun-Dried Tomato Basil	390	4	74
Tomazzo	520	13	77
Veggie	310	3.5	61
Sandwiches: BLT	550	17	72
Chicken Parmigiana	740	22	81
Ham	460	9	71
Roast Beef	465	8.5	71
Cream Cheese Filling: Per 1 oz			
Apple Cinnamon; Blueberry	60	4.5	4
Caramel Apple; Choc. Chip, average	70	4	7.5
Garlic Herb; Plain, average	60	5	1
Salsa; Scallion; Spinach, average	50	4.5	1
Strawberry	55	5	1

Green Burrito (Nov '10)

	C	F	Cb
Burritos: Bean & Cheese	780	36	94
Grilled Chicken	880	46	81
The Green Burrito with Steak	850	32	109
Specialties:			
Super Nachos: Chicken	920	48	93
Ground Beef	1060	61	95
Taco Salad: Chicken	780	44	66
Ground Beef	920	56	69
Steak	810	46	69
Tacos: Fish, with 2 Tortillas	320	15	36
Hard Shell: Chicken; Steak, average	195	9	15
Ground Beef	240	14	15
Soft Shell: Chicken	200	7	17
Ground Beef	250	13	18
Sides: Chips, 2 oz	300	17	35
Chips & Cheese, 5 oz	700	42	62
Guacamole, 1½ oz	60	5	3
Pinto Beans & Cheese, 8½ oz	320	16	43
Rice, 6 oz	290	9	50
Sour Cream, 1½ oz	50	3.5	3

(The) Great Steak & Potato Company® (Nov '10)

	C	F	Cb
Breakfast Sandwiches			
Bacon, Egg & Cheese	600	36	39
Egg and Cheese	500	29	39
Ham and Cheese	430	22	41
Ham, Egg and Cheese	570	32	42
Sausage, Egg and Cheese	700	47	39
Steak, Egg & Cheese	600	34	40
Breakfast Sides:			
Potatoes: Deluxe Home	390	23	44
Fresh Cut Home	380	23	42
Sandwiches: 7"			
Chicken Philly	620	22	62
Great Steak Cheesesteak	740	37	62
Ham Delight	710	33	71
Ham Explosion	710	34	70
Philly Cheesesteak	650	26	62
Super Steak Cheesesteak	750	37	64
Veggie Delight	610	31	66
Sides			
Baked Potato, Plain, 6 oz	160	0	36
Chicken Nuggets, Kids, 2¾ oz	165	9	10
Great Fry: Kids, 6¼ oz	270	13	36
Regular, 10¼ oz	440	20	60
Large, 12½ oz	540	25	72
Potato Skins, 6½ oz	390	26	24
Meat: Per 4 oz Serving, without Sides			
Chicken	140	3	0
Corned Beef, 3 oz	135	8	0
Gyro	210	12	5
Ham	120	4	6
Steak	160	7	0
Turkey	90	1	2
Salads: Without Dressing			
Chef Salad	260	11	15
Garden	60	1	13
Grilled Steak	400	23	18
Sauces: Buffalo 1 oz	10	0	2
Teriyaki , 1 oz	25	0	3
Tzatziki, 1 oz	50	4	2
Breads/Pita			
Bread, 12"White, 7 oz	420	4	82
Bread, 7"Wheat, 4 oz	310	4	56
Pita, 2¾ oz	220	5	38

Fast - Foods & *Restaurants*

Haagen-Dazs® (Nov '10)

Ice Cream: Per ½ Cup	C	F	Cb
Amaretto Almond Crunch	270	17	24
Baileys Irish Cream	260	17	21
Bananas Foster	240	13	27
Banana Split	280	16	31
Butter Pecan	310	23	21
Caramel Cone	320	19	32
Cherry Vanilla	240	15	23
Chocolate	270	18	22
Chocolate Chip Cookie Dough	310	20	29
Chocolate Chocolate Chip	300	20	26
Coffee	270	18	21
Cookies & Cream	270	17	23
Creme Brulee	280	19	23
Dark Chocolate	160	17	21
Dark Chocolate Mint	250	17	19
Dulce de Leche	290	17	28
Mango	250	14	28
Midnight Cookies & Cream	290	17	30
Pineapple Coconut	230	13	25
Pistachio	290	20	22
Frozen Yogurt: *Per ½ Cup*			
Coffee	200	4.5	31
Dulce de Leche	190	2.5	35
Peach	170	2	31
Vanilla Raspberry Swirl	170	2.5	32
Wildberry	180	2	34
Sorbet: *Per ½ Cup*			
Cranberry Blueberry	100	0	25
Raspberry; Strawberry	120	0	31
Zesty Lemon	110	0	28

Ice Cream Bars ~ See Page 109

Hardee's® (Nov '10)

Breakfast	C	F	Cb
Biscuits: Bacon, Egg & Cheese	530	36	36
Biscuit 'N' Gravy	530	34	47
Chicken Fillet	600	34	50
Cinnamon 'N Raisin	300	15	40
Country Ham	440	26	36
Country Steak	630	43	45
Loaded Omelet	610	42	36
Made from Scratch	370	23	35
Monster	770	55	37
Sausage	530	38	36
Sausage and Egg	590	42	36
Smoked Ssge with Egg & Cheese	750	56	38

Hardee's® cont... (Nov '10)

Breakfast Bowls:	C	F	Cb
Loaded Biscuit 'N' Gravy	740	52	49
Low Carb	620	50	6
Breakfast Burrito, Loaded	760	49	39
Breakfast Croissants:			
Sunrise: With Bacon	450	29	28
With Ham	400	23	27
With Sausage	550	38	29
Breakfast Sandwiches:			
Frisco	400	18	27
Texas Toast: Bacon, 4¾ oz	380	21	31
Ham, 6¼ oz	390	18	31
Sausage, 5½ oz	480	30	32
Breakfast Sides:			
Grits, 5 oz	110	5	16
Hash Rounds: Small, 3 oz	250	16	25
Medium, 4¼ oz	390	26	36
Large, 5¾ oz	530	35	49
Burgers:			
Big Shef, 7½ oz	660	46	36
Cheeseburger: Regular, 4½ oz	350	16	36
Double, 7¼ oz	530	32	34
Hamburger, Small, 4½ oz	310	15	32
Thickburger: Original, ⅓ lb	770	48	53
Bacon Cheese, ⅓ lb	850	57	49
Little Thick Cheeseburger, 6 oz	450	23	38
Low-Carb ⅓ lb	420	32	5
Monster, ⅔ lb	1320	95	46
Mushroom 'N' Swiss ⅓ lb	650	36	47
Six Dollar Burger, ½ lb	930	59	57
Chicken Strips: *Without Sauce*			
3 Strips, 3¾ oz	370	26	19
5 Strips, 8½ oz	610	43	32
Sandwiches:			
Big Hot Ham 'N' Cheese	460	20	40
Chicken: Charbroiled BBQ Chicken	400	6	62
Big Chicken Fillet	710	38	62
Charbroiled Chicken Club	630	32	54
Fish, Supreme	630	38	51
Kids Meals: *Incl. Kid's Fries & Small Drink*			
Cheeseburger	560	29	59
Crispy Chicken Strips (2), w/o sauce	450	27	40
Hamburger	520	25	59

Continued next page...

Hardee's® cont... (Nov '10)

Sides:	C	F	Cb
Beer Battered Onion Rings, 4½ oz	410	24	45
Fries:			
Crispy Curls: Small 3 oz	340	17	43
Medium 4¾ oz	410	20	52
Large 5½ oz	480	23	60
Natural Cut: Small, 4¼ oz	320	14	45
Medium, 5¾ oz	430	19	60
Large, 6¼ oz	470	21	65
Dessert, Apple Turnover	290	15	36
Drinks: Hot Chocolate	150	3	18
Malts: Per 16 fl.oz			
Chocolate	780	35	97
Strawberry	775	35	98
Vanilla	710	35	97
Shakes. Per 16 fl.oz			
Chocolate	700	34	85
Strawberry	700	33	86
Vanilla	710	33	87

Harvey's® (Nov '10)

Sandwiches & Burgers	C	F	Cb
Angus Burger	560	26	47
Angus Burger, with Cheese	640	32	49
Angus Patty, 1 patty	320	23	4
Cheeseburger	460	23	39
Hamburger	380	16	37
Grilled Chicken Sandwich	290	5	28
VeggieBurger	290	10	33
Hot Dog, (1)	300	13	32
Breakfast:			
Bacon, 3 Strips	40	3.5	0
Extra Egg (1)	90	6	0
Homefries	300	19	29
Sandwich: Breakfast Club	400	19	36
Breakfast Club Deluxe	530	28	39
Toast, White, 2 slices	180	2	35
Sides:			
Chicken Strips, 3 pieces	320	15	27
French Fries: Regular, 4¼ oz	320	13	49
Large, 5¼ oz	410	16	61
Value, 3 oz	240	10	37
Onion Rings: Regular, 2¾ oz	270	15	33
Large, 5 oz	550	29	65

Harvey's® cont... (Nov '10)

Garnishes:	C	F	Cb
Barbecue Sauce, 1 oz	50	0	12
Canadian Cheddar Cheese, 1 slice	80	6	1
Ketchup, ¼ oz	10	0	2
Light Mayonnaise, ½ oz	45	5	1
Relish, ¾ oz	20	0	5
Dipping Sauce: Per 1½ oz			
Barbecue	90	0	21
Honey Mustard	160	12	13
Plum	80	0	21
Sweet n' Sour	80	0.5	17

Heavenly Ham® (Nov '10)

Meats: Per 3 oz Serving	C	F	Cb
Bone-In Hams: Glazed	190	11	4
Fat Removed	160	3	4
Boneless Hams: Glazed	120	4	4
Fat Removed	90	1	4
Classic Sandwiches: Roast Beef	635	36	50
Swiss Philly	700	46	49
Salads: *Without Dressing*			
Chicken	260	17	14
Taste of Italy	310	20	14
Bread: Croissant	230	12	27
French Batard	210	0.5	46
Multigrain Batard	250	3.5	46
Sliced Wheat Bread	300	5	54
Sauces: BBQ, 1¾ oz	260	26	4
Bistro, ¾ oz	120	13	1
Dill, 1½ oz	170	19	1
Mayonnaise, 1 oz	200	24	0
Ranch, 1½ oz	220	23	2
Spicy Brown Mustard, 1 oz	30	0	0
Sweet Café Spread, 1 oz	100	10	4
That Mustard, 1 oz	150	0	30

Hot Dog on a Stick® (Nov '10)

Menu Items	C	F	Cb
American Cheese on a Stick	270	14	26
Beef Hot Dog on a Bun	460	29	37
Turkey Hot Dog on a Stick	240	11	28
Veggie Dog on a Stick	250	5	35
Pepperjack Cheese on a Stick	260	13	25
French Fries, 4½ oz	390	15	60
Lemonade (16 fl.oz): Original	150	0	38
Sugar Free Lemonade	15	0	3
Cherry	210	0	53

Hungry Howie's Pizza® (Nov '10)

Counts may vary in Florida.

Pizzas: Per Slice	C	F	Cb
Cheese: Small, ⅙ pizza	160	3.5	20
Medium, ⅛ pizza	190	5.5	23
Large, 1/10 pizza	210	5	25
X-Large, ⅛ pizza	395	9	42
Oven Baked Subs: Per ½ Sub			
Deluxe Italian	505	18	61
Ham & Cheese	475	15	61
Steak & Cheese	490	15	64
Turkey Club	555	15	63
Vegetarian	530	21	64
Sides: Chicken Tenders, 2 pieces	140	4.5	11
Howie Wings, 5 wings	180	13	0
Salads: Per Small Size, Without Dressing			
Antipasto	230	15	6
Chef	230	13	8
Garden	40	0.5	7
Greek	250	15	16
Dressings: Per 1 oz			
Creamy Italian	120	12	2
Greek	110	11	2
Ranch	180	19	1
Thousand Island	140	14	4

In-N-Out Burger® (Nov '10)

Burgers:			
Hamburger: With Onion	390	19	39
With Mustard/Ketchup, w/o Spread	310	10	41
Protein Style w/ Lettuce Wrap, no Bun	240	17	11
Cheeseburger: With Onion	480	27	39
With Mustard/Ketchup, w/o Spread	400	18	41
Protein Style w/ Lettuce Wrap, no Bun	330	25	11
Double Double®: With Onion	670	41	39
With Mustard/Ketchup, no Spread	590	32	41
Protein Style w/ Lettuce Wrap, no Bun	520	39	11
French Fries, 4½ oz	400	18	54
Drinks: Milk, 10 fl.oz	180	6	18
Coca-Cola®,16 fl.oz	200	0	54
Lemonade, 16 fl.oz	180	0	40
Root Beer,16 fl.oz	220	0	60
Shakes: Chocolate, 15 fl.oz	690	36	83
Strawberry, 15 fl.oz	690	33	91

IHOP® (Jan '10)

Counts may vary between locations C F Cb

Pancakes: With Toppings Unless Specified			
Buttermilk Without Butter Or Syrup			
Full Stack (5)	750	n/a	100
Short Stack (3)	450	n/a	60
Chocolate Chip (4)	610	n/a	100
Double Blueberry (4)	690	n/a	120
Strawberry Banana (4)	690	n/a	130
Syrup: Regular, 1 Tbsp	50	0	12
Sugar-Free, 1 Tbs	10	0	2
Whipped Butter/Margarine, 1 Tbsp	80	9	0
French Toast & Waffles: W/ Toppings Unless Indicated			
Belgian Banana Pecan Waffle	700	n/a	77
French Toast, 6 pcs, w/o butter/syrup	680	n/a	90
Viva La French Toast Combo	750	n/a	60
International Crepes: With Toppings			
Chicken Florentine (2)	880	n/a	80
Garden Stuffed (2)	800	n/a	90
Nutella (3)	990	n/a	170
Swedish (4)	1080	n/a	90
Omelettes: Full Platter, Without Butter/Syrup			
Big Steak	920	n/a	160
Colorado	1890	n/a	130
Garden	1350	n/a	140
Hearty Ham & Cheese	1630	n/a	130
Spinach & Mushroom	1620	n/a	130
Classic Combos			
Biscuits w/ Gravy & Sausage	1410	n/a	98
Eggs Benedict	980	n/a	100
Smokehouse Combo	1290	n/a	90
Top Sirloin Steak & Eggs	1210	n/a	80
Two x Two x Two, average	670	n/a	55
Signature Favorites: Without Butter/Syrup			
Big Country Fried Steak & Eggs	1620	n/a	160
Breakfast Sampler	1250	n/a	90
Ham Steak & Eggs	1130	n/a	90
Rooty Tooty with toppings, average	950	n/a	80
Split Decision	1120	n/a	90
T-Bone Steak & Eggs	1160	n/a	70
IHOP For Me			
Balsamic-Glazed Chicken	510	20	36
Blueberry Harvest Combo	570	20	76
Simply Chicken Sandwich	440	6	42
Spinach/Mushroom/Tomato Omelette	350	14	24
Tilapia Hollandaise	370	13	15
Turkey Bacon Omelette	470	25	17
Two-Egg Breakfast	380	11	40
Veggie Omelette	360	14	34
Whole Wheat French Toast Combo	470	14	51

Jack in the Box® (Nov '10)

Sandwiches & Burgers	C	F	Cb
Bacon Ultimate Cheeseburger	940	66	45
Hamburger: Original	290	12	32
With Cheese	330	15	32
Deluxe	360	19	33
With Cheese	440	26	34
Jumbo Jack: Original	540	32	45
With Cheese	620	39	45
Junior Bacon Cheeseburger	420	24	32
Sirloin Cheeseburger w/ Bacon	960	64	52
Sourdough Jack	680	46	40
Ultimate Cheeseburger	870	61	44

Chicken & Fish			
Chicken Breast Strips, crispy, (4) w/o sce	560	24	53
Chicken Sandwich	440	23	42
With Bacon	480	26	42
Fish & Chips, small, w/o sce, 8½ oz	670	35	68
Jack's Spicy Chicken Sandwich	570	25	60
With Cheese	650	31	62
Sourdough Grilled Chicken Club	550	29	38

Breakfast			
Biscuit: Bacon, Egg & Cheese	420	24	36
Sausage, Egg & Cheese	570	39	37
Breakfast Jack: Regular	280	11	30
With Bacon	300	13	30
Croissant: Sausage	570	40	32
Supreme	440	26	32
Sandwiches: Extreme Sausage	660	47	32
Sourdough	410	21	34
Ultimate	510	24	41
Hash Brown Sticks (5)	280	19	26
Meaty Burrito, without salsa	600	37	38

Snacks & Sides:			
Bacon Cheddar Potato Wedges, 9¼ oz	710	45	58
Beef Taco, regular, (1)	180	10	17
Egg Rolls, without sauce, (3)	440	22	46
Mozzrella Cheese Sticks (3)	280	16	22
Mozzrella Cheese Sticks (6)	560	33	43
Pita Snack: Crispy Chicken (1)	410	19	43
Grilled Chicken, without salsa, (1)	330	14	31
Stuffed Jalapenos, (3)	220	12	21
Stuffed Jalapenos, (7)	510	29	49
Onion Rings, (8), 4¼ oz	450	28	45
Seasoned Curly Fries, med., 4½ oz	430	25	46

Jack in the Box® cont... (Nov '10)

Bowls:	C	F	Cb
Teriyaki: Chicken, 17½ oz	690	6	133
Steak, 17½ oz	750	11	133

Salads: No Dressing or Condiments			
Chicken Club with Grilled Chicken	350	18	13
Grilled Chicken	240	8	15
Side Salad	20	0	4
Southwest Chicken w/ Gr. Chkn Strips	340	14	29

Sauces & Dressings			
Dipping Sauce: Barbecue, 1 oz	40	0	10
Buttermilk House, 1 oz	130	13	3
Frank's Red Hot Buffalo, 1 oz	10	0	2
Sweet & Sour, 1 oz	45	0	11
Tartar, 1½ oz	210	22	2
Sauce: Mayo-Onion, ½ oz	90	10	1
Soy, ¼ oz	5	0	1
Taco, ¼ oz	0	0	0
Cheese: American, 1 slice	40	3.5	0
Real Swiss, 1 slice	70	6	0

Condiments: Per Package			
Ketchup	20	0	4
Mustard	5	0	0
Sour Cream, 1 oz	60	5	2

Desserts			
NY Style Cheesecake, 3¼ oz	310	17	32
Chocolate Overload Cake, 3¼ oz	300	7	57

Ice Cream Shakes: Per 16 fl.oz With Whipped Topping			
Chocolate Ice Cream	800	38	101
Oreo Cookie Ice Cream	810	43	92
Strawberry Ice Cream	780	38	95
Vanilla Ice Cream	700	38	76

For Complete Nutritional Data ~ see CalorieKing.com

Jack's® (Nov '10)

Sandwiches: Big Bacon Burger	610	41	31
Big Jack Burger	530	33	35
Cheeseburger	380	21	31
Chicken Fillet Sandwich	500	25	43
Double Big Jack Cheese Burger	850	59	35
Double Cheeseburger	540	34	31
Grilled Chicken Sandwich	380	16	32
Hamburger	340	18	31
Chicken, Chicken Fingers, 3 pieces	420	23	28
Fries, Regular	310	13	42
Breakfast, Egg & Cheese Biscuit	360	21	31

For Complete Menu & Data ~ see CalorieKing.com

Jamba Juice® (Nov '10)

Breakfast	C	F	Cb
Ideal Meals: Berry Topper, 16 fl oz	480	9	91
Chunky Strawberry, 16 fl oz	570	17	92
Mango Peach Topper, 16 fl oz	500	9	95
Hot Oatmeal: *With Fruit & Sugar*			
Apple Cinnamon	290	4	60
Blueberry & Blackberry	290	3.5	58
Grab N Go Food:			
California Flat Bread: *With Dressing*			
Four Cheesy, 5¾ oz	420	16	46
MediterraneYum, 6 oz	320	8	49
Smokehouse Chicken, 6 oz	390	10	53
Baked Goods: Per 3¼ oz			
Cheddar Tomato Twist	240	4.5	38
Orange Chocolate Chip Scone	380	15	57
Tart Cherry Scone	360	12	58
All Fruit: Original, 22 fl oz			
Mega Mango	320	1	80
Peach Perfection	300	0.5	75
Pomegranate Paradise	340	0.5	85
Strawberry Whirl	300	0.5	75
Blended With A Purpose: Per 16 fl.oz			
Acai Super-Antioxidant	260	4	53
Coldbuster	240	1.5	56
Protein Berry Workout: With Whey	280	0	52
With Soy Protein	270	1	51
Strawberry Energizer	280	1	67
Classics: Per 16 fl.oz			
Aloha Pineapple	290	1	67
Caribbean Passion	250	1	57
Mango-a-go-go	280	1	65
Strawberry Surf Rider	300	1	72
Creamy Treats: Per 16 fl oz			
Chocolate Moo'd	430	4	86
Orange Dream Machine	350	1.5	75
Peanut Butter Moo'd	470	10	82
Fresh Squeezed Juices: Per 16 fl oz			
Carrot	130	0.5	30
Orange	220	1	52
Jamba Light: Per 16 fl oz			
Berry Fulfilling	150	0.5	32
Mango Mantra	150	0.5	31
Strawberry Nirvana	150	0	31
Shots: Single			
Matcha Energy Shot-Soymilk, 4 fl.oz	70	0	14
Wheatgrass, 1 fl oz	5	0	1

Jersey Mike's Subs® (Nov '10)

Cold Subs: *Per Regular, on Wheat, Without Vinegar, Oil or Mayo*	C	F	Cb
#1 BLT	530	24	55
#2 Jersey Shore Favorite	520	16	59
#3 American Classic	520	16	57
#5 Super Sub	540	17	59
#6 Roast Beef & Provolone	680	23	56
#7 Turkey Breast & Provolone	500	14	56
#8 Club Sub with Mayonnaise	850	50	58
#9 Club Supreme w/ Mayonnaise	900	50	58
#10 Albacore Tuna	870	57	58
#13 Original Italian	640	25	60
#14 Veggie	680	31	57
Hot Subs/Cheese Steaks: Per Regular on Wheat Roll			
#15 Meatball & Cheese	850	50	64
#17 Chicken Philly	590	23	57
Steak Philly	580	22	56
#43 Chipotle Chicken	870	54	60
Chipotle Steak	860	53	58
#18 Chicken Parmesan	610	20	69
#19 BBQ Beef	670	14	75
#20 Pastrami & Swiss	540	16	52
#56 Big Kahuna Steak	630	26	57
#56 Big Kahuna Chicken	640	27	58
Cold Wraps: With Flour Tortilla, w/o Vin./Oil or Mayo			
#1 BLT	590	29	60
#2 Jersey Shore Favorite	580	22	64
#3 American Classic	580	22	63
#5 Super Sub	600	22	65
Salads: Without Dressing			
Chef, 16 oz	240	10	12
Grilled Chicken Caesar, 12½ oz	510	35	11
Tossed, 12 oz	50	0.5	11
Tuna, 18 oz	690	60	15
Dressings: Per 2 Tbsp, 1 oz			
Caesar	150	15	2
Chipotle Mayo	180	20	0
Golden Italian	110	11	3
Ranch	120	12	2
Russian	160	16	4
Condiments: Oil, regular, 1 oz	270	30	0
Mustard, ½ oz	0	0	0
Desserts: Cookie, Choc Chip, 1½ oz	200	11	24
Brownie, Chocolate, 4 oz	440	20	60
Drinks: Mountain Dew, 22 oz	310	0	84
Mug Root Beer, 22 oz	290	0	79
Tropicana Twister Orange, 22 oz	360	0	96

Jimmy John's® (Nov '10)

Subs (8") **C** **F** **Cb**

Figures Based on French Bread w/ Standard Toppings & Mayo, Unless Indicated

	C	F	Cb
#1 Pepe	615	31	50
#2 Big John	535	24	49
#3 Totally Tuna without dressing	650	31	54
#4 Turkey Tom	515	22	50
#5 Vito with Italian Vinaigrette	600	28	52
#6 Vegetarian	580	30	53
JJBLT	635	35	49

Giant Club Sandwiches: Figures Based on French Bread w/ Standard Toppings & Mayo, Unless Indicated

	C	F	Cb
#7 Gourmet Smoked Ham	775	32	69
#8 Billy	800	34	68
#9 Italian Night with Mayo & Vinaig.	950	51	70
#10 Hunter's	805	35	67
#11 Country	770	31	69
#12 Beach Club	730	31	71
#13 Gourmet Veggie Club	775	38	71
#14 Bootlegger	685	25	67
#15 Club Tuna without dressing	845	39	72
#16 Club Lulu	755	33	67
#17 Ultimate Porker	765	39	67

Plain Slims: Figures Based on French Bread without Toppings, Dressing or Mayo

	C	F	Cb
Slim 1 Ham & Cheese	510	10	66
Slim 2 Roast Beef	425	3	64
Slim 3 Tuna Salad	720	31	68
Slim 4 Turkey Breast	400	0.5	65
Slim 5 Salami Capicola & Cheese	600	20	66
Slim 6 Double Provolone	545	16	65
The JJ Gargantuan	990	54	54

Low Carb Options: With Standard Toppings & Mayo, without Bread

	C	F	Cb
Hunter's Club Unwich	470	35	4
The JJ Gargantuan Unwich	740	54	7

Low-Fat Options: W/o Standard Toppings, Dressing or Mayo

	C	F	Cb
#4 Turkey Tom	305	0.5	48
Slim 4 Turkey Breast	400	0.5	65

Sides

	C	F	Cb
Jimmy Chips: BBQ, 1 oz	160	9	17
Jalapeno, 1 oz	150	7	18
Regular, 1 oz	160	8	18
Sea Salt & Vinegar, 1 oz	140	8	16
Skinny, 1 oz	130	5	19
Pickle: Spear	5	0	1
Whole	20	0	4
Cookies, average	420	17	64

Johnny Rockets® (Nov '10)

Original Hamburgers **C** **F** **Cb**

	C	F	Cb
Hamburger #12	900	59	55
Original Burger	820	53	52
Chili Cheese	850	50	53
Patty Melt	690	37	49
Rocket: Single	710	44	45
Double	1020	63	52
Route 66	920	60	55
Smoke House: Single	950	55	68
Double	1360	80	99
St Louis	990	56	53
Streamliner	410	8	57

Sandwiches: Chicken Club

	C	F	Cb
Chicken Club	930	51	58
Grilled Breast of Chicken	560	25	47
Grilled Cheese	540	29	48
Philly Cheese Steak	715	46	48
Tuna Melt	900	62	40
Tuna Salad	800	50	41

Other Favourites

	C	F	Cb
Chicken Tenders without Sauce	610	33	39
Chili Dog	810	55	48
Hot Dog	370	20	34

Extras: Bacon, 2 slices, ½ oz

	C	F	Cb
Bacon, 2 slices, ½ oz	90	7	1
Chili, 3 oz	155	12	5
Grilled Mushrooms, 1 oz	35	3	1
Grilled Peppers & Onions, 1 oz	20	1	3

Starters

	C	F	Cb
Chili Bowl, 13 oz	870	73	24
American Fries, 8 oz	550	22	78
Cheese Fries, 10 oz	780	44	72
Chili Fries, 15 oz	1010	62	85
Onion Rings, 8 oz	790	36	80
Rocket Wings, 9 oz	640	36	26

Desserts: Apple Pie, 10 oz

	C	F	Cb
Apple Pie, 10 oz	800	33	119
A la Mode, scoop, 4 oz	250	16	25
Super Sundae, 13 oz	1110	74	120

Beverages: 20 fl.oz

	C	F	Cb
Root Beer	170	0	49
Coke	170	0	28
Sprite	170	0	45
Lemonade	170	0	49

Shakes: Original, 16 fl.oz

	C	F	Cb
Chocolate	890	44	102
Strawberry	750	44	77
Vanilla	840	44	100

KFC® (Nov '10)

Original Recipe:	C	F	Cb
Breast: 1 piece, 5¾ oz	320	15	4
without skin or breading, 4 oz	150	2.5	0
Drumstick, 1 piece, 1¾ oz	120	7	3
Thigh, 1 piece, 3¼ oz	220	15	5
Whole Wing, 1 piece, 1¾ oz	140	8	4
Spicy Crispy: Breast, 1 piece, 6¼ oz	420	25	12
Drumstick, 1 piece, 2 oz	160	10	5
Thigh, 1 piece, 4 oz	360	27	13
Whole Wing, 1 piece, 1¾ oz	170	12	6
Grilled :			
Breast, 4¼ oz	210	8	0
Drumstick, 1½ oz	80	4	0
Thigh, 2½ oz	160	11	0
Whole Wing, 1¼ oz	80	5	1
Strips & Filets:			
Crispy, 2 Strips, 4 oz	230	7	18
3 Strips, 6 oz	340	11	27
Original Filets, 3½ oz	170	7	4
Popcorn Chicken: Kids, 3 oz	290	19	16
Individual, 4 oz	400	26	22
Large, 5½ oz	550	35	30
Sandwiches: With Sauce			
Crispy Twister, with Crispy Strips	560	23	59
Double Crunch, with Crispy Strip	500	20	51
Double Down: Original	540	32	11
Grilled	480	25	4
Filet Sandwich: Original	480	23	42
Grilled	400	16	33
KFC Snackers:			
Crispy Strip: Regular	290	11	33
Buffalo	250	6	35
Ultimate Cheese	270	8	34
Grilled Fillet Sandwich	400	16	33
Toasted Wraps: With Sauce			
With Crispy Strip	350	17	33
With Grilled Filet	310	15	24
With Tender Roast Filet	310	15	24
Wings: Per Wing Without Dipping Sauce			
Boneless: Fiery Buffalo; Honey BBQ, av.	80	3.5	6
Bone In: Fiery Buffalo; Honey BBQ, av.	80	5	4
Hot Wings: Regular	70	5	3
Fiery Buffalo	80	5	5
Honey BBQ	90	5	7

KFC® cont... (Nov '10)

Dipping Sauces	C	F	Cb
Fiery Buffalo, 1 oz	25	0	6
Creamy Ranch, 1 oz	140	15	1
Honey BBQ, 1 oz	40	0	9
Honey Mustard, 1 oz	120	10	6
Sweet & Sour, 1 oz	45	0	12
KFC Famous Bowls & Pot Pie			
Bowls: Snack Size, 8 oz	320	15	34
Mashed Potato with Gravy, 18½ oz	700	32	77
Chicken Pot Pie, 13 oz	690	40	57
Sides: Per Single Portion			
BBQ Baked Beans, 4½ oz	200	1.5	39
Biscuit, 2 oz	180	8	23
Cole Slaw, 4½ oz	180	11	19
Corn on the Cob (3"), 2½ oz	70	0.5	16
Cornbread Muffin, 2 oz	210	9	28
Macaroni & Cheese, 4¾ oz	180	9	20
Mashed Potatoes with Gravy, 5 oz	120	4	19
Potato Wedges, 3½ oz	260	13	33
Salads: Without Dressing or Croutons			
Crispy Chicken BLT	320	12	24
Crispy Chicken Caesar	300	11	22
House Side Salad	15	0	2
Grilled Chicken BLT	230	8	7
Grilled Chicken Caesar	210	7	5
Dressings:			
Original Ranch Fat Free, 1½ oz	35	0	8
Creamy Parmesan Caesar, 2 oz	260	26	4
Light Italian, 1 oz	10	0.5	2
Croutons, Parm. Garlic, Pouch (1)	70	3	8
Desserts:			
Lil' Buckets Parfait Cups:			
Chocolate Cream, 4 oz	280	14	37
Lemon Creme, 4½ oz	390	14	60

Kilwin's® ~ *see CalorieKing.com*

Koo◆Koo◆Roo® ~ *see CalorieKing.com*

Kohr Bros® ~ *see CalorieKing.com*

Kolache® ~ *see CalorieKing.com*

Updated Nutrition Data ~ www.CalorieKing.com
Persons with Diabetes ~ See Disclaimer (Page 22)

Krispy Kreme® (Nov '10)

Doughnuts	C	F	Cb
Apple Fritter	380	20	47
Caramel Kreme Crunch	380	19	49
Chocolate Glazed Cruller	290	15	37
Chocolate Iced Cake	280	14	36
Chocolate Iced Custard Filled	300	17	35
Chocolate Iced Glazed	250	12	33
Chocolate Iced Kreme Filled	350	20	39
Chocolate Iced with Sprinkles	270	12	38
Cinnamon Apple Filled	290	16	32
Cinnamon Bun	260	16	28
Cinnamon Twist	240	15	23
Dulce de Leche	300	18	31
Glazed: Chocolate Cake	300	15	42
Cinnamon	210	12	24
Cruller	240	14	26
Kreme Filled	340	20	39
Lemon Filled	290	16	35
Maple Iced	240	12	32
Original	200	12	22
Raspberry Filled	300	16	36
Sour Cream	300	13	43
Powdered: Cake	290	14	37
Strawberry Filled	290	16	33
Sugar	200	12	21
Traditional Cake	230	13	25
Doughnut Holes: Orig. Glazed (4)	200	11	25
Glazed Cake, Regular/Choc. (4)	210	10	29

Chiller Beverages: *Without Whipped Cream Topping*
Fruity Chillers:

	C	F	Cb
Average all flavors, 12 fl.oz	175	0	43
20 fl.oz	295	0	71

Kremey Chillers: *Includes Whipped Cream Topping*

	C	F	Cb
Orange & Kreme: 12 fl.oz	630	28	92
20 fl.oz	970	40	150
Lemon Sherbert: 12 fl.oz	630	28	95
20 fl.oz	980	40	155
Choc./Mocha: Average, 12 fl.oz	670	29	104
average 20 fl.oz	1050	41	171
Lotta Latte: 12 fl.oz	670	28	49
20 fl.oz	1050	40	79

For Complete Menu & Data ~ see CalorieKing.com

Krystal® (Nov '10)

Burgers:	C	F	Cb
Big Angus	550	35	46
Double, with Bacon & Cheese	850	59	48
Krystal: Original, Single	130	6	20
Double	290	13	33
Bacon Cheese	200	11	20
Cheese	160	8	20
Double Cheese	350	17	34
Chik	300	16	27
Pups: Chili Cheese	230	14	16
Corn	240	14	22
Plain	150	8	15
French Fries			
Medium, 4¼ oz	310	13	46
Chili Cheese, 8¼ oz	570	29	62
Sides			
Large Chili, 12 oz	300	11	33
Chik'n Bites, Small, 3 oz	200	7	20
Salad, Crispy Chicken, 11 oz	370	21	20
Breakfast Items			
Biscuits: Bacon, Egg & Cheese	440	24	34
Chik	400	18	43
Gravy	350	18	41
Plain	260	13	32
Sausage	420	28	32
Kryspers	150	7	19
Sandwich, Krystal Sunriser	200	11	16
Scramblers: Original, with Bacon	330	16	27
With Sausage	420	26	27
4-Carb Scramblers: With Bacon	450	31	2
With Sausage	620	52	3
Desserts:			
Apple Turnover, fried	220	8	34
Lemon Icebox Pie	320	9	56
Drinks: Per 16 fl.oz with ¼ ice			
Coca-Cola Classic	120	0	32
Diet Coke	0	0	0
Sprite	110	0	31

For Complete Menu & Data ~ see CalorieKing.com

**For Menu Updates,
Check Author's Website
www.CalorieKing.com**

Fast - Foods & Restaurants

La Rosa's Pizzeria® (Nov '10)

Pizzas:

	C	F	Cb
Focaccia Style: *Per Slice, ⅛ of Medium Pizza*			
Florentine	240	13	24
Roma	300	18	23
Hand Tossed: *Per Slice, ⅛ of Medium Pizza*			
Cheese	230	8	29
Double Pepperoni	300	14	29
Big 4 Meat	325	15	29
Big 4 Pick 4	280	11	30
Big 4 Veggie	240	7	30
Pan Crust: *Per Slice, ⅛ of Medium Pizza*			
Cheese	300	16	30
Double Pepperoni	370	22	30
Big 4 Meat	325	15	29
Big 4 Pick 4	275	11	30
Big 4 Veggie	235	7	30
Traditional Crust: *Per Slice, ⅛ of Medium Pizza*			
Cheese	200	10	19
Double Pepperoni	280	16	20
Big 4 Meat	285	16	20
Big 4 Pick 4	240	12	20
Big 4 Veggie	200	8	21
Calzones: *Per Calzone, No Dipping Sauce*			
3 Meat & 3 Cheese	1080	55	102
3 Veggie & 3 Cheese	860	34	105
Cheese & Pepperoni	960	45	101
Cheese	840	34	101
Philly Cheesesteak	870	39	90
Sausage Pelucci	1040	52	92
Pasta Dinner: *Without Bread, Soup or Salad*			
Cheese Ravioli	660	26	80
Lasagna with Meat Sauce	735	38	61
Spaghetti: With Meatballs	870	28	119
With Alfredo Sauce	975	50	104
With Meat Sauce	700	18	104
With Traditional Sauce	640	12	113
Ziti Chicken Alfredo	980	42	102
Ziti Sausage Pelucci	765	20	115
Appetizers: *Without Dipping Sauce*			
Boneless Wings: BBQ (1), 1½ oz	75	3	8
Hot (1), 1½ oz	80	5	6
Chicken Tenders, 8½ oz	540	31	30
Four Taste Sampler, 23½ oz	1570	99	82
French Fry Basket with Provolone	860	56	73
Mozzarella Cheese Sticks, 6½ oz	635	43	36
Onion Twists, Regular, 7¼ oz	460	27	48

For Complete Nutritional Data ~ see CalorieKing.com

La Salsa Fresh Mexican Grill® (Nov '10)

	C	F	Cb
Appetizers: Salsa & Chips, 14½ oz	700	32	87
With Guacamole, 14½ oz	970	55	103
Nachos:			
Black Beans: With Carnitas	1570	83	141
With Chicken	1600	83	148
With Steak	1580	84	142
Pinto Beans: With Carnitas	1560	83	139
With Chicken	1590	83	146
With Steak	1565	84	139
Burritos:			
Black Beans: With Cheese	1100	48	132
With Carnitas	1205	51	132
With Chicken	1240	52	139
With California Steak	815	35	89
Pinto Beans: With Cheese	1070	48	115
With Chicken	1200	52	122
With Steak	1175	54	115
Baja Fish Burrito	875	53	58
Overstuffed Grilled Burrito:			
With Carnitas	1200	59	108
With Chicken	1260	59	110
With Steak	1290	66	109
Grande, Black Beans:			
With Carnitas	810	34	91
With Chicken	810	33	93
With Steak	820	35	91
Tacos: Baja Fish	395	22	29
Baja Shrimp	320	19	30
Guadalajara Carnitas	320	15	30
Quesadillas: *With Chips unless indicated*			
Classic: Carnitas	1160	68	82
Chicken	1155	67	83
Steak	1165	69	82
Grande, Pinto Beans:			
With Carnitas	1335	71	114
With Chicken	1330	71	116
With Steak	1330	72	115
Favorites: *Without Chips*			
Stuffed Fajita Quesadilla:			
With Carnitas	855	51	53
With Chicken	865	52	56
With Shrimp	800	49	54
With Steak	885	55	53
Fire Roasted Bowl:			
Black Beans: With Chicken	730	32	74
With Steak	735	34	73
Without Meat	630	29	71
Pinto Beans: With Chicken	730	32	73
With Steak	720	34	70
Without Meat	620	29	69

Little Caesars® (Nov '10)

14" Pizza: Per Slice, ⅛ Pizza

	C	F	Cb
Original Crust: 3 Meat Treat	350	18	30
Hula Hawaiian: With Ham	270	9	33
With Canadian Bacon	280	9	34
Ultimate Supreme	310	14	31
Vegetarian	270	10	32
Deep Dish:			
Just Cheese	320	13	38
Pepperoni	360	16	38
Hot-N-Ready: Just Cheese	240	9	30
Pepperoni	280	11	30
Baby Pan! Pan!: *Per Pan*			
Cheese & Pepperoni	360	18	33
Caesar Wings: Barbecue, 1 wing	70	4	3
Mild/Hot, 1 wing	60	4.5	1
Oven, Roasted, 1 wing	50	3.5	0
Caesar Dips: *Per 1½ oz Container*			
Buffalo	140	14	4
Buffalo Ranch	230	24	3
Buttery Garlic	380	42	0
Cheezy	210	21	3
Chipotle	220	24	2
Ranch	250	26	3
Bread: *Per Piece*			
Crazy Bread, 1 stick	100	3	15
Italian Cheese Bread	130	7	13
Pepperoni Cheese Bread	150	8	13
Sauce, Crazy, 4 oz	45	0	10

Lone Star Steakhouse® (Nov '10)

Appetizers: Per Serving

	C	F	Cb
Chicken Tenders, 12 oz	1095	66	91
Lone Star Wings, 11 oz	955	62	15
Texas Rose, 15½ oz	1260	83	108
Meals: *Served Without Sides, Toppings & Sauce*			
Mesquite Grilled Steaks:			
Cajun Ribeye, 16 oz	1250	101	0
Chopped Steak, 10 oz	900	71	0
Delmonico, 11 oz	860	69	0
Five Star Filet, 9 oz	740	60	0
NY Strip, 14 oz	1035	80	0
San Antonio Sirloin, 12 oz	770	55	0
T-Bone, 20 oz	1540	124	0
Texas Ribeye, 14 oz	1090	88	0

Lone Star® cont... (Nov '10)

	C	F	Cb
Meals (Cont): *Served Without Sides, Toppings & Sauce*			
Mesquite-Grilled Specialties:			
Baby Back Ribs, 12 oz	970	80	0
Grilled Chicken, 6 oz	185	2.5	0
Grilled Pork Chops, 16 oz	1430	100	0
Shrimp Dinner, 3½ oz	105	2	1
Sweeet Bourbon Salmon, 6 oz	240	11	0
Slow Roasted, Prime Rib, 16 oz	1250	10	0
Salads: *Per Serving , Without Dressing*			
El Paso Salad	385	23	21
Grilled Chicken Caesar	455	10	31
Lettuce Wedge	505	48	12
Dressings: *Per Serving*			
Bleu Cheese	250	26	4
Honey Mustard	265	27	8
Ranch	210	22	2
Texas Ranch	215	22	3
Thousand Island	200	18	9
Wish Bone	310	32	4
Sides: *Per Serving*			
Baked Potato	665	18	114
Sauteed Mushrooms	115	8	6
Sauteed Onions	95	7	8
Steamed Mixed Vegetables	70	1	14
Texas Rice	80	2	12
Desserts: *Per Serving*			
Big Brownie Blast	1390	69	178
Homemade Cobbler, average all	240	8	43
Homemade Ice Cream	255	19	19

Long John Silver's® (Nov '10)

	C	F	Cb
Sandwiches: *Includes Toppings And Condiments*			
Chicken, 6½ oz	440	30	47
Fish, 6¼ oz	470	23	49
Ultimate Fish, 7 oz	530	27	50
Seafood			
Battered Fish, 1 piece, 3¼ oz	260	16	17
Battered Shrimp, 3 pieces, 1½ oz	130	9	8
Breaded Clam Strips, 3 oz	320	19	29
Buttered Lobster Bites, snack box, 3¼ oz	230	9	24
Grilled Pacific Salmon, 2 filets, 4½ oz	150	5	2
Grilled Tilapia, 1 filet, 4 oz	110	2.5	1

Continued next page...

213

Long John's cont...® (Nov '10)

Seafood (Cont)	C	F	Cb
Lobster Stuffed Crab Cake, 2¼ oz	170	9	16
Popcorn Shrimp, 1 snack box, 3 oz	270	16	23
Shrimp Scampi, 8 pieces	200	13	3
Chicken, Chicken Plank, 1 piece	140	8	9
Freshside Grille: Per Plate, Without Sides			
Grilled Pacific Salmon, 2 filets	150	5	2
Grilled Tilapia, 1 filet	110	2.5	1
Freshside Grille Side Dishes: Per Serving			
Rice, 2½ oz	80	0.5	18
Vegetable Medley, 2 oz	25	1	4
Sauces & Condiments:			
Dipping Sauces: Per 1 fl.oz			
Cocktail	25	0	6
Tartar	100	9	4
Louisiana Hot Sauce, 1 tspn	0	0	0
Ketchup, 1 packet, ¼ oz	10	0	2
Malt Vinegar, ½ oz	0	0	0
Sides			
Breadstick, 2 oz	170	3.5	29
Broccoli Chse Soup, 1 bowl, 7½ oz	220	18	8
Cole Slaw, 4 oz	200	15	15
Corn Cobbette w. Butter Oil, 3½ oz	150	10	14
Crumblies, 1 oz	170	12	14
Fries: Platter Portion, 3 oz	230	10	34
Combo Portion, 4 oz	310	14	45
Hushpuppy, 1 pup, 1 oz	60	2.5	9
Rice, 5 oz	180	1	37

For Complete Menu & Data ~ see CalorieKing.com

Macaroni Grill (Nov '10)

Appetizers: Inc. Sauce & Garnish	C	F	Cb
Calamari Fritti	650	43	42
Crab-Stuffed Mushrooms	310	24	4
Romano's Sampler, 3 Choices	800	52	50
Tomato Bruschetta	560	17	77
Meals: As Served, Includes Sides			
Grilled Specialties:			
Calabrese Strip	1130	65	47
Grilled Pork Chops	1380	77	96
Grilled Salmon	750	35	55
Honey Balsamic Chicken: Lunch	540	13	54
Dinner	640	15	54

Macaroni Grill (Nov '10)

Meals (Cont): As Served, Includes Sides			
Classico Italian:	C	F	Cb
Lunch: Chicken Marsala	620	34	46
Chicken Scaloppine	740	45	46
Eggplant Parmigiana	800	47	65
Parmesan-Crusted Sole	1190	71	101
Spaghetti Bolognese	570	19	72
Dinner: Chicken Marsala	650	33	49
Chicken Scaloppine	910	59	59
Parmesan-Crusted Sole	1710	105	131
Rosemary Spiedini:			
Grilled Chicken Spiedini	360	10	17
Italian Sausage Spiedini	720	40	43
Jumbo Shrimp Spiedini	230	5	15
Handcrafted Pasta: *As Served*			
Capellini Pomodoro	390	14	55
Carmela's Chicken Rigatoni	1080	58	100
Lobster Ravioli	520	30	32
Pasta Milano	750	24	93
Penne Rustica	980	38	94
Pollo Caprese	550	20	45
Seafood Linguine	650	22	75
Shrimp Portofino, lunch	560	34	37
Neapolitan Pizzas: *Per Whole Pizza*			
Italian Sausage	970	39	95
Margherita	720	20	95
Quattro Formaggio	950	34	111
Salads: As Served, Includes Dressing			
Caesar	260	20	14
Chicken Caesar	650	42	29
Parmesan-Crusted Chicken	960	63	49
Scallops & Spinach	360	18	16
Salad Dressings: Per 1 fl.oz			
Caesar	150	16	2
Mediterranean Vinaigrette	130	14	3
Parmesan Peppercorn Ranch	120	12	2
Desserts: Per Serving			
Italian Sorbetto with Biscotti	220	2	48
Tiramisu	1120	80	88

For Complete Nutritional Data ~ see CalorieKing.com

McDonald's® (Nov '10)

Burgers/Sandwiches	C	F	Cb
Hamburger	250	9	31
Cheeseburger	300	12	33
Double Cheeseburger	440	23	34
Big Mac	540	29	45
Big N' Tasty	460	24	37
Big N' Tasty with Cheese	510	28	38
Quarter Pounder	410	19	37
With Cheese	510	26	40
Double with Cheese	740	42	40
Angus: Bacon & Cheese	790	39	63
Deluxe	750	39	61
Mushroom & Swiss	770	40	59
Filet-O-Fish	380	18	38
McChicken	360	16	40
McRib	500	26	44
Southern Style Crispy Chicken Sndwch	400	17	39

Premium Chicken Classic Sandwiches:			
Crispy Chicken	530	20	59
Crispy Chicken Club	630	28	60
Crispy Chicken Ranch BLT	580	23	62
Grilled Chicken	420	10	51
Grilled Chicken Club	530	17	52
Grilled Chicken Ranch BLT	470	12	54

Snack Wraps:			
Chipotle BBQ: With Crispy Chicken	330	15	35
With Grilled Chicken	260	9	28
Honey Mustard: With Crispy Chicken	330	16	34
With Grilled Chicken	260	9	27
Ranch: With Crispy Chicken	340	17	33
With Grilled Chicken	270	10	26

French Fries:			
Small, 2½ oz	230	11	29
Medium, 4 oz	380	19	48
Large, 5½ oz	500	25	63
Ketchup, 1 package	15	0	3

Chicken McNuggets®			
Chicken McNuggets: 4 pieces	190	12	11
6 pieces	280	17	16
10 pieces	460	29	27

Chicken Selects® Breast Strips			
Strips: 3 pieces	400	24	23
5 pieces	660	40	39
Sauces: Barbecue, 1 oz	50	0	12
Creamy Ranch, 1¼ oz	170	18	2
Spicy Buffalo, 1¼ oz	60	6	1
Sweet 'N Sour, 1 oz	50	0	12
Tangy Honey Mustard, 1¼ oz	60	2	10

McDonald's® cont... (Nov '10)

Breakfast Menu	C	F	Cb
Biscuit: Regular	260	12	33
Large	320	16	39
Bacon Egg & Cheese: Regular	420	23	37
Large	480	27	43
Sausage with Egg: Regular	510	33	36
Large	570	37	42
Southern Style Chicken, Regular	410	20	41
Big Breakfast, Regular Biscuit	740	48	51
English Muffin	160	3	27
Grape/Strawberry Jam	35	0	9
Hash Brown (1), 2 oz	150	9	15
Hotcakes: Plain (3)	350	9	60
With Margarine (2 pats), no Syrup	430	18	60
With Margarine (2 pats) & Syrup (1)	610	18	105
McGriddles: Bacon, Egg & Cheese	420	18	48
Sausage	420	22	44
Sausage, Egg & Cheese	560	32	48
McMuffin: Egg	300	12	30
Sausage	370	22	29
Sausage with Egg	450	27	30
McSkillet: Burrito with Sausage	610	36	44
Burrito with Steak	570	30	44
Sausage Burrito, 4 oz	300	16	26
Sausage Patty, 1½ oz	170	15	1
Scrambled Eggs (2), 3¼ oz	170	11	1

Happy Meals:			
With 4 Chicken McNuggets:			
+ Small Fries + Apple Juice	510	23	63
+ Small Fries + 1% Low Fat Milk	520	25	52
+ Apple Dipper/ Dip + 1% Choc Milk	390	15	46
With Hamburger:			
+ Small Fries + Apple Juice	580	20	84
+ Small Fries + Sprite (12 oz)	590	20	88
+ Apple Dippers/Dip + Low-Fat Milk	460	12	66
With Cheeseburger:			
+ Small Fries & Apple Juice	630	24	85
+ Small Fries + 1% Low-Fat Milk	640	26	74
+ Apple Dippers/Dip & 1% Choc Milk	520	13	80

Mighty Kids Meals:			
With 6 Chicken McNuggets:			
+ Small Fries + Apple Juice	610	28	68
+ Apple Dippers/Dip + 1% Choc Milk	550	21	65
With Double Cheeseburger:			
+ Small Fries + Apple Juice	770	34	86
+ Apple Dippers/Dip + Low-Fat Milk	640	26	69

Continued Next Page ...

McDonald's® cont... (Nov '10)

	C	F	Cb
Premium Salads: *Without Dressing*			
Bacon Ranch Salad: W/o Chicken	140	7	10
With Crispy Chicken	370	20	20
With Grilled Chicken	260	9	12
Caesar Salad: Without Chicken	90	4	9
With Crispy Chicken	330	17	20
With Grilled Chicken	220	6	12
Southwest Salad: W/ Crispy Chicken	430	20	38
With Grilled Chicken	320	9	30
Fruit & Walnut, Snack Size, 1 pkg	210	8	31
Side Salad, 3 oz	20	0	4
Butter Garlic Croutons, ½ oz	60	1.5	10
Salad Dressings: *Per Package*			
Newman's Own: Creamy Caesar, 2 fl.oz	190	18	4
Creamy Southwest, 1½ fl.oz	100	6	11
Ranch, 2 fl.oz	170	15	9
Low-Fat: Balsamic Vinaig., 1½ fl.oz	40	3	4
Family Recipe Italian, 1½ fl.oz	60	2.5	8
Desserts/Cookies			
Apple Dippers: 1 package, 2½ oz	35	0	8
With Low-Fat Caramel Dip	100	0.5	23
Baked Hot Apple Pie, 2¾ oz	250	13	32
Cinnamon Melts, 4 oz	460	19	66
Cookies: Chocolate Chip Cookie, (1)	160	8	21
McDonaldland® Cookies, 2 oz	260	8	43
Oatmeal Raisin (1), 1 oz	150	6	22
Sugar Cookie (1), 1 oz	160	7	21
Fruit 'n Yogurt Parfait: Reg., 5¼ oz	160	2	31
Without Granola, 5 oz	130	2	25
Ice Cream: Kiddie Cone, 1 oz	45	1	8
Vanilla Reduced-Fat Cone, 3¼ oz	150	3.5	24
McFlurry™: M&M® Candies, 12 fl.oz	620	20	96
Oreo® Cookies, 12 fl.oz cup	550	17	88
Sundaes: Hot Caramel Sundae, 6½ oz	340	8	60
Hot Fudge Sundae, 6¼ oz	330	10	54
Strawberry Sundae, 6¼ oz	280	6	49
Peanuts (for Sundaes), ¼ oz	45	3.5	2
Triple Thick Shakes: *Average all Flavors:*			
12 fl.oz cup	425	10	74
16 fl.oz cup	565	14	98
21 fl.oz cup	750	18	130
32 fl.oz cup	1125	27	197
Fruit Juice: Apple, 6.8 fl.oz box	100	0	23
Orange: Small, 12 fl.oz	140	0	33
Medium, 16 fl.oz	180	0	42
Large, 21 fl.oz	250	0	57

McDonald's® cont... (Nov '10)

	C	F	Cb
Sodas:			
Coca-Cola or Sprite: *Without Ice*			
Child, 12 fl.oz cup	110	0	29
Small, 16 fl.oz cup	150	0	40
Medium, 21 fl.oz cup	210	0	58
Large, 32 fl.oz cup	310	0	86
Diet Coke	0	0	0
Hi-C Orange Lavaburst: *Without Ice*			
Child, 12 fl.oz cup	120	0	32
Small, 16 fl.oz cup	160	0	44
Medium, 21 fl.oz cup	240	0	64
Large, 32 fl.oz cup	350	0	94
Powerade Mountain Blast: *Without Ice*			
Child, 12 fl.oz cup	70	0	20
Small, 16 fl.oz cup	100	0	27
Medium, 21 fl.oz	150	0	39
Large, 32 fl.oz	220	0	58
Milk: 1% Low-Fat, 8 fl.oz	100	2.5	12
1% Chocolate, 8 fl.oz carton	170	3	26
Iced Tea, no added sugar	0	0	0
Coffee Drinks, Black, 16 fl.oz	0	0	0
Coffee Cream 1 package, ½ fl.oz	20	2	0
Sugar Packet (1), 0.15 oz	15	0	4
Iced Coffee:			
Regular or flavors (average):			
Small, 8 fl.oz	130	5	21
Medium, 11½ fl.oz	190	8	29
Large, 17 fl.oz	270	11	45
With Sugar-Free Vanilla Syrup:			
Small, 8 fl.oz	60	5	8
Medium, 11½ fl.oz	90	8	11
Large, 17 fl.oz	120	11	16
McCafe Coffees:			
Cappuccino			
Whole Milk: Small, 12 fl oz	120	7	9
Medium, 16 fl oz	140	8	11
Large, 20 fl oz	180	10	13
Nonfat Milk: Small, 12 fl oz	60	0	9
Medium, 16 fl oz	80	0	12
Latte			
Whole Milk: Small, 12 fl oz	150	8	11
Medium, 16 fl oz	180	10	13
Nonfat Milk: Small, 12 fl oz	90	0	13
Medium, 16 fl oz	110	0	15
Mocha			
Whole Milk: Small, 12 fl oz	280	11	40
Medium, 16 fl oz	330	12	48
Nonfat Milk: Small, 12 fl oz	240	5	41
Medium, 16 fl oz	280	6	50

For Complete Menu & Data ~ see CalorieKing.com

Manhattan Bagel® (Nov '10)

Bagel (East Coast): Per Bagel	C	F	Cb
Blueberry, 3¾ oz	270	1	60
Chocolate Chip, 3¾ oz	290	2.5	58
Cinnamon Raisin, 4 oz	330	1	70
Egg; Jalapeño Cheddar, 4 oz	320	2	67
Pumpernickel, 3½ oz	250	1.5	55
Salt; Spinach, average, 4¼ oz	320	1	68
Sun-Dried Tomato, 4 oz	310	1	66
Cream Cheese: Plain, 1¾ oz	180	16	4
Reduced-Fat, 1¾ oz	150	12	5

For Complete Nutritional Data ~ see CalorieKing.com

Marie Callender's® (Nov '10)

Tasters: Per Complete Dish as Served	C	F	Cb
Crispy Chicken Tenders	1000	68	57
Crispy Green Beans	810	52	75
Loaded Potato Skins	710	42	51
Burgers and Sandwiches: *Without Fries*			
Original Burger	870	59	39
Albacore Tuna Melt	1050	72	55
Roasted Turkey Croissant Club	1070	76	50
Smoked Ham Stack	880	61	51
Main Meals: *Per Complete Meal as Served*			
Americana Classics:			
Artichoke & Mushroom Chicken	1030	76	38
Callender's Fish & Chips	1280	92	85
From The Grill: Grilled Lemon Chkn	730	44	41
Grilled Atlantic Salmon, Cajun Style	840	60	29
St. Louis BBQ Ribs	1260	82	58
Pasta Perfecto: *Includes Garlic Bread*			
Chicken & Broccoli Fettuccini	1480	87	119
Double Shrimp Pasta	1490	95	97
Pies, Chicken Pot Pie, w/out Sides	1140	79	68
Home-Style Soups & Chili:			
Chili, without Cornbread, 1 cup	280	8	34
Hearty Vegetable, 1 bowl	90	0	18
French Onion, with Garlic Bread, 1 crock	710	43	52
Crisp Salads: *Includes Dressing*			
Chicken Ginger-Sesame	1070	47	130
Gorgonzola, Pecan & Field Greens	940	54	80
Traditional Caesar	490	35	28
Sides: Cornbread, 1 piece, 2 oz	170	6	26
French Fries, 4 oz	380	20	45
Honey Butter, 1 oz	170	16	8
Desserts: *Per Slice Unless Indicated*			
Pies: Apple	570	31	70
Banana Cream, with Meringue	510	24	66
Chocolate Cream, with Meringue	570	26	77
Pumpkin, with Whipped Cream	530	23	70
Razzleberry	660	39	71

Breakfast & Other Menu Items ~ see CalorieKing.com

Max & Erma's® (Nov '10)

Appetizers:	C	F	Cb
Black Bean Roll-Ups w/out dressing	575	10	95
Entrees: As Served			
Caribbean Chicken (lunch)	535	20	59
Salads: *Without Breadstick*			
Hula Bowl with 3 oz dressing	585	10	78
Baby Greens Salad, with dressing	120	11	6
Sides:			
Fruit Salad, 4½ oz	55	0	17
Garlic Breadstick (1)	150	6	20
Fruit Smoothie	125	0.5	29

Mazzio's® (Nov '10)

Appetizers: Per Serving	C	F	Cb
Cheese Dippers, w/o sauce, ⅓ order	405	18	47
Nachos: Beef w/ Jalapenos, ½ order	485	34	20
Cheese with Jalapenos, ½ order	425	30	19
Rstd. BBQ Tossed Chkn Wings, ⅕ order	190	12	7
Calzones: *Per ⅒ Whole, Without Sauce*			
Ham Bacon & Cheddar	245	7.5	32
Pepperoni	260	10	33
Pastas: *Without Garlic Toast*			
Fettuccine Alfredo	1060	56	107
Spaghetti with Marinara Sauce	640	8	120
Lasagna: with Alfredo Sauce	1265	94	55
with Meat Sauce	950	52	64
Sandwiches: *Without Chips or Pickle*			
Wheatberry:			
Chicken, Bacon & Swiss	1020	70	48
Ham & Cheddar	745	47	47
Mazzio's Sub	770	49	45
Hoagie: Chicken, Bacon & Swiss	1360	72	120
Ham & Cheddar	1090	50	119
Mazzio's Sub	1110	52	117
Turkey & Swiss	1060	40	118
Pizzas: *Per ⅛ Medium Pizza*			
Cheese: Original Crust	235	9	30
Thin Crust	180	9	18
Chicken Club: Original Crust	260	9	31
Thin Crust	205	9	19
Mazzio's Works: Original Crust	305	14	31
Thin Crust	255	15	20
Meatbuster: Original Crust	285	13	30
Thin Crust	235	13	19
Pepperoni: Original Crust	255	11	30
Thin Crust	200	11	18
Sausage: Original Crust	275	12	30
Thin Crust	225	12	19
Sides: Breadsticks, w/o sce, ¼ order	150	3	26
Garlic Toast, w/o sce, 1 pce, 1½ oz	160	10	15

For Complete Nutritional Data ~ see CalorieKing.com

Mimi's Cafe® (Nov '10)

Breakfast	C	F	Cb
Hot Off The Griddle: *Without Sides*			
Belgian Waffle	395	17	50
French Toast	305	13	40
Gourmet: *Without Sides*			
Brie Cheese Lorraine Crepes	550	41	21
Eggs Florentine Benedict	690	50	36
Sandwiches and Burritos: *Without Sides*			
Chipotle Burrito	965	44	84
Ciabatta Breakfast Sandwich	945	53	77
Three Egg Omelettes: *Without Sides*			
Capresse	475	38	8
Mardi Gras	620	45	5
Lunch:			
Burgers: *Without Sides*			
French Quarter	1480	105	68
Turkey Pesto Ciabatta	1250	73	83
Dinner:			
Just Enough Dinner: *As Served, Without Soup or Salad*			
Artichoke Asiago Chicken Spaghettini	1265	76	81
BBQ Pork Chop	850	40	86
Santa Fe Shrimp & Chicken Fettuccine	925	55	70

Miami Subs® (Nov '10)

Burgers	C	F	Cb
Deluxe Burger	785	59	31
Deluxe Cheeseburger	860	65	32
Deluxe Bacon Cheeseburger	920	70	32
Platters: Chicken Breast	745	41	57
Gyros	1420	93	81
10 Wings with Fries & Blue Cheese	1020	67	50
Salads: Caesar with Dressing	460	34	26
Chicken Caesar with Dressing	610	39	28
Chicken Club	490	25	23
Garden	310	18	21
Greek	285	15	24
Cheesesteaks (6"): Original	410	11	45
Classic	420	11	44
Chicken Philly Classic	550	27	47
Works	530	23	51
Pitas: Gyros	660	39	47
Chicken	390	13	34
Subs (6"): Ham & Cheese	450	18	49
Italian Deli	515	25	49
Meatball	490	22	49
Tuna	470	18	44
Turkey	485	19	51
Sides: Mozzarella Sticks	755	57	34
Onion Rings	870	68	56
Spicy Fries: Regular	530	39	39
Large	1040	72	85

Mr. Goodcents® (Nov '10)

	C	F	Cb
Cold Sub: Per ½ Sub on Wheat Bread			
Centsable	480	20	58
Italian Sub	640	37	55
Mr. Goodcents Original	510	25	56
Oven Roasted Chicken Breast	350	6	55
Penny Club	350	6	57
Pepperoni & Cheese	740	46	55
Roast Beef	350	6	55
Tuna Salad	490	21	63
Veggie Sub	290	4	58
Hot Sub: Per ½ Sub on Wheat Bread w/ Cheese			
Chicken Bacon Ranch w/ Cheddar	630	29	57
Meatball with Mozzarella	670	33	65
Philly Jack 'n Cheese	490	16	60
Pasta:			
Alfredo Sauce on Mostaccioli	1290	80	106
Chicken Alfredo on Mostaccioli	1370	70	112
Chicken Parmesan on Mostaccioli	660	10	100
Red Sauce on Mostaccioli	520	4	100

Mr. Hero® (Nov '10)

7" Hot Subs & Burgers	C	F	Cb
Burgers: Cheeseburger	775	55	47
Romanburger	860	62	48
Meatball Sub	725	47	47
Steak Subs: Tuscan	625	31	42
Hot Buttered Cheesesteak	670	42	45
Zesty Bacon & Swiss	615	32	42
7" Deli Subs: Original Italian	640	39	47
Tuna & Cheese	725	54	44
Turkey	470	20	46
Ultimate Italian	675	40	46
4½" Taste Buddies: Per Sandwich			
Bacon Cheeseburger	430	30	33
Grilled Italiano	440	32	32
Tuna 'n Cheese	485	38	31
Zesty Chicken	495	25	48
Pasta, Spag./Rigatoni with Meatballs			
In Marinara Sauce & Breadstick	1115	36	153
Salads: Without Dressing Unless Indicated			
Grilled Chicken	165	2.5	13
Tuna Delight with Mayonnaise	495	48	10
Sides:			
Breadsticks, w/ Marinara Sauce (2)	445	17	64
Cheese Sauce, 1½ oz	55	4	4
Jalapeno Poppers. 4½ oz	430	28	37
Mozzarella Sticks, w/ Marinara Sce	565	43	12
Onion Petals, w/ Tangy Sce, 5¾ oz	695	46	64
Fries, Potato Waffer, 5¾ oz	430	30	38
Desserts: Oreo Cookie Cheesecake	260	17	24
Strawberry Swirl Cheesecake	280	19	22

Mrs Fields Cookies® (Nov '10)

	C	F	Cb
Brownies: *Per 2.6 oz Brownie*			
Butterscotch Blondie	350	14	52
Double Fudge	360	20	45
Pecan Fudge	360	20	46
Special Walnut Fudge & Blondie	330	16	43
Toffee Fudge	360	19	47
Walnut Fudge	360	20	45
Cake, Chocolate Chip, 1 piece, 3 oz	350	17	45
Cookies:			
Bite Size Nibblers: Cinn, Sugar (3)	170	8	22
Debra's Special (3)	170	7	23
Peanut Butter (3)	180	10	20
Semi-Sweet Chocolate (3)	170	8	24
Triple Chocolate (3)	170	9	23
White Chunk Macadamia (3)	180	9	23
Butter (1)	200	8	29
Cut Out (1)	400	19	56
Debra's Special (1)	200	9	28
Peanut Butter (1)	210	12	24
Semi-Sweet Chocolate (1)	210	10	29
with Walnuts(1)	220	11	29
Triple Chocolate (1)	210	11	28
White Chunk Macadamia (1)	230	12	27
Muffins: Blueberry (1), ¾ oz	70	3	10
Chocolate Chip (1), ¾ oz	80	4	11
Mandarin Orange (1), ¾ oz	80	3	9
Raspberry (1), ¾ oz	70	3	10

For Complete Nutritional Data ~ see CalorieKing.com

Nathan's Famous® (Nov '10)

	C	F	Cb
Burgers:			
Burger with Cheese, 10¼ oz	705	43	45
Double Burger w/ Cheese, 15½ oz	1180	84	45
Bacon Cheeseburger, 10¾ oz	785	50	45
Super Cheeseburger, 13½ oz	985	72	47
Nathan's Famous Hot Dogs:			
Original, 3½ oz	295	18	24
Cheese Dog, 5 oz	390	25	30
Chili Dog, 5 oz	400	23	33
Corn Dog with Stick, 3¼ oz	380	21	39
Chicken:			
Chicken Tenders (3), 6¼ oz	525	39	24
Chicken Tender Platter, 17½ oz	1245	90	80
Grilled Chicken Breast Platter, 15 oz	840	56	58

Nathan's®cont... (Nov '10)

	C	F	Cb
Sides:			
Fries: French: Regular, 6½ oz	465	34	35
Large, 9 oz	635	46	49
Super, 14 oz	999	73	75
Cheese: Regular, 8 oz	565	42	41
Large, 11 oz	735	54	55
Super, 18 oz	1200	89	163
Mozzarella Sticks (3), w/ Sauce, 5½ oz	390	28	20
Onion Rings, regular, 5½ oz	545	45	36
Wraps:			
Grilled Chicken Caesar	700	34	60
Krispy Southwest Chipotle	750	39	62

New York Fries

~ See CalorieKing.com

Ninety Nine (Nov '10)

	C	F	Cb
Appetizers: *Serves 4*			
Boneless Wings & Skins Sampler (4)	1660	111	70
Calypso Coconut Shrimp (4)	600	32	60
Outrageous Potato Skins (4)	1140	86	43
Steak & Chse Spring Rolls (4), w/ Sce	900	55	62
Sandwiches: *Without Sides*			
Chicken Parmigiana	880	36	92
Triple-Decker Turkey Club	950	37	107
Steakburger: Bacon & Cheese	940	57	46
Mushroom & Cheese	950	58	49
Steakburger	810	47	45
with Cheese	890	53	46
Sweet & Smokey	1060	61	67
Meals: *Without Sides*			
Cape Cod Seafood Trio	650	40	20
Captain's Combo Platter	1410	96	73
Fish & Chips	1160	76	60
Grilled Chicken Fajitas	1350	54	101
Smothered Sirloin Tips	820	40	9
Salads: Boneless Buffalo Wing	1030	57	74
Pecan Crusted Chicken	880	44	80
Wild Bleu Chicken & Spinach	1190	79	52
Sides:			
Double Bleu Iceberg Wedge	450	41	9
Garl. Red-Skin Mashed Pot., 2 scoops	260	12	34
Honey Butter Biscuit w/ Honey Butter	230	12	27
Perfect: Rice Pilaf, 2 scoops	260	6	46
French Fries, Kids, 8 oz, raw wt.	510	34	4
Desserts: Apple Fortune	860	38	1
Little Midnight Fudge Hero	430	23	
Strawberry Mimosa Cake	680	33	

Fast - Foods & *Restaurants*

Noodles & Company® (Nov '10)

Meals: Per Regular Order
Small Order: Halve the figures of regular

	C	F	Cb
American: Buttered Noodles	620	16	84
Mushroom Stroganoff	780	31	100
Spaghetti	670	18	101
Spaghetti with Meatballs	900	35	104
Wisconsin Mac & Cheese	900	31	119
Asian: Bangkok Curry	490	13	85
Chinese Chop Salad	310	15	40
Indonesian Peanut Saute	950	23	165
Japanese Pan Noodles	690	9	133
Pad Thai	700	20	117
Mediterranean: Pasta Fresca	780	22	111
Penne Rosa	810	26	119
Pesto Cavatappi	910	30	124
The Mediterranean Salad	310	13	39
Whole Grain Tuscan Linguine	770	26	108
Proteins: Braised Beef	190	10	0
Meatballs	230	17	3
Organic Tofu	180	11	4
Parmesan Crusted Chicken Breast	190	8	17
Sauteed Beef	210	12	1
Seasoned Chicken Breast	130	2.5	0
Salads: Caesar	320	28	11
Cucumber Tomato, side	80	0	18
Tossed Green, side	60	6	3
Sides: Potstickers, 3 Pieces	200	4.5	31
Ciabatta Roll (1)	160	1.5	31
Soups: Chicken Noodle, regular	300	4	44
Thai Curry, regular	480	19	70
Tomato Basil Bisque, regular	420	23	45

Nothing But Noodles® (Nov '10)

Noodle Bowls

	C	F	Cb
American: Beef Stroganoff	510	31	33
Buttery Noodles	650	44	46
Santa Fe Pasta	705	54	40
Southwest Chipotle	715	58	41
Spicy Cajun Pasta	660	50	44
Asian: Pad Thai Noodles	600	10	118
Sesame Lo Mein	410	11	64
Spicy Japanese Noodles	420	8	74
Thai Peanut	570	20	89
Italian: Basil Pesto	575	42	36
Cappelini Primavera	500	28	56
Fettuccini Alfredo	725	56	36
Margherita Pasta	475	31	36
Marinara Pasta	485	11	77
Three-Cheese Macaroni	445	21	45

Complete Menu & Data ~ see CalorieKing.com

O'Charley's® (Nov '10)

Appetizers: As Served

	C	F	Cb
Barbacoa Quesadillas	1170	73	64
Chicken Tenders, w/ Chipotle BBQ Sce	1040	37	119
Over-Loaded Potato Skins	1260	98	43
Southwestern Twisted Chips	1280	89	111
Spicy Jack Cheese Wedges (7)	880	60	55
Three-Cheese Shrimp Dip	870	49	86
Top Shelf Combo	1880	130	105
Brunch: With Sides & Rustic Bread			
Omelettes: Ham & Cheese	1210	76	76
Prime Time Prime Rib, 10 oz	1420	91	78
Spinach & Mushroom	1110	67	80
Meals: Without Sides Unless Indicated			
Chicken: Boneless Buffalo Tenders (5)	880	66	27
Teriyaki Sesame, with Rice Pilaf	1030	25	151
Pasta: Chicken Parmesan	1500	77	138
Outrgs. Chkn & Spinach Lasagna	1210	73	72
Prime Rib	1530	101	90
Seafood:			
Catfish Platter with Tartar Sauce	1430	121	46
Gr. Salmon with Rice Pilaf, 6 oz	560	27	32
Gr. Shrimp with Rice Pilaf & Sce	290	7	32
Steak & Ribs: Per Serving, Without Sides			
Baby Back Ribs: ½ Rack	740	48	38
1 full rack	1480	96	76
Filet Mignon, 9 oz	450	28	0
Grilled Top Sirloin, 7 oz	430	28	1
Louisiana Sirloin with Cajun Butter	680	40	3
Sides: French Fries, adult size	390	24	40
Potato: Baked, plain	240	5	50
Loaded	480	29	54
Smashed	370	12	47
Salads: Without Dressing Unless Indicated			
Apple Crunch Salad	920	56	79
Black & Bleu Caesar with Dressing	1050	79	22
California Chicken	700	37	48
Tortilla Chicken	610	27	41
Soup: Per Cup			
Chicken Harvest	160	8	12
Chicken Tortilla	150	9	12
Creamy Wild Mushroom	150	14	7
Desserts: Cinnamon Sugar Donuts	1130	54	139
Ooey Gooey Caramel Pie, 1 slice	730	28	106
Ultimate Choc. Choc. Cake, 1 sl.	1080	59	151

For Complete Menu & Data ~ see CalorieKing.com

Old Country Buffet

~ See CalorieKing.com

Olive Garden® (Nov '10)

Appetizers	C	F	Cb
Bruschetta	610	13	100
Muscles di Napoli	180	8	13
Sicilian Scampi	500	22	43
Stuffed Mushrooms	410	28	19
Entrees:			
Lunch: Eggplant Parmigiana	620	26	70
Fettuccine Alfredo	800	48	69
Five Cheese Ziti al Forno	770	32	89
Lasagna Classico	580	32	35
Dinner: Chicken Parmigiana	1090	49	79
Fettucini Alfredo	1220	75	99
Manicotti Formaggio	940	46	81
Garden Fare Selections (Lower Fat)			
Lunch: Capellini Pomodora, 13 oz	480	11	78
Linguine alla Marinara, 10½ oz	310	4	55
Shrimp Primavera, 19 oz	510	9	79
Venetian Apricot Chicken	200	3	32
Dinner: Capellini Pomodora, 21 oz	840	17	141
Linguine alla Marinara, 17 oz	430	6	76
Shrimp Primavera, 26 oz	730	12	110
Venetian Apricot Chicken	380	4	32
Desserts: Black Tie Mousse Cake	760	48	73
Chocolate Gelato	620	25	89
Tiramisu	510	32	48

(The) Old Spaghetti Factory® (Nov '10)

Appetizers: Per Serving	C	F	Cb
Shrimp, Spinach & Artichoke Dip	150	10	10
Sicilian Garlic Cheese Bread	330	19	28
Toasted: Beef Ravioli, 4 oz	200	4.5	30
Cheese Ravioli, 4 oz	210	6	30
Entrees, Lunch/Dinner:			
Classics:			
Spaghetti: With Clam Sauce, 15 oz	660	14	104
With Marina Sauce, 15 oz	560	5	108
With Meat Sauce, 15 oz	610	9	105
With Sicilian Meatballs, 21 oz	960	31	114
Factory Favorites:			
Chicken Parmigiana, 19 oz	830	32	80
Spinach & Cheese Ravioli, 11 oz	480	16	63
Spinach Tortellini w/ Alfredo Sauce	930	56	86
Signature Selection: Chicken Penne	910	32	105
Crab Ravioli, 11 oz	810	46	73
Lasagna Vegetariano 20¾ oz	830	48	68
Meatloaf, Italian Style, 18½ oz	1180	68	83

On the Border® (Nov '10)

Appetizers: As Served	C	F	Cb
Border Sampler	2010	135	105
Fajita Quesadillas: Chicken	1240	85	59
Steak	1230	90	59
Burritos & Chimichangas:			
Includes Rice, Without Beans & Sauce			
Burrito, Classic Shredded Beef	1010	39	105
Chimichangas: Chicken	1300	76	107
Ground Beef	1400	88	107
Dinner: *Includes Rice, Without Beans*			
Enchiladas: Gr. Pepper Jack Chkn	1110	50	104
Ranchiladas	1490	83	106
Suiza	1010	44	111
Fresh Grill: *Served As Listed*			
Carne Asada	930	35	103
Chicken Salsa Fresca	520	9	60
Jalapeno-BBQ Salmon	590	21	45
Queso Chicken	1130	50	115
Tomatillo Chicken	850	24	108
Salads: *Without Dressing*			
House, Side	200	12	20
Sizzling Fajita Chicken	710	46	25
Sides: *Per Serving*			
Mexican Rice	290	5	54
Pico de Gallo	10	1	1
Sour Cream	60	5	2
Sauce: *Per Serving*			
Chipotle Honey	230	4	48
Habanero Fire	120	9	9
Tequila Lime Chile	170	14	6
Dressings: *Per Serving*			
Ranch Dressing	230	23	2
Smoked Jalapeno Vinaigrette	230	23	8

For Complete Nutritional Data ~ see CalorieKing.com

Orange Julius® (Nov '10)

Fruit Drinks: Per 16 fl.oz	C	F	Cb
Bananarilla	320	7	65
Blackberry	280	7	55
Mango	150	0.5	38
Orange	130	0.5	33
Raspberry	200	1	51
Strawberry Banana	300	7	60
Premium Fruit Smoothies: *Per 20 fl.oz*			
Blackberry Storm	680	15	128
Orange Swirl	540	12	103
Raspberry Creme	650	15	118
Tropi-Colada	530	10	99
Fat Free: Mango Passion	370	0	86
Strawberry Xtreme	390	0	89
Nutrition Boosts: Fiber Plus, 0.2 oz	5	0	4
Heart Health, 0.15 oz	15	0	3
Joint Care, 0.2 oz	20	0	5

221

Fast - Foods & *Restaurants*

Outback Steakhouse® (Nov '10)

Aussie-Tizers:	C	F	Cb
Per Whole Dish, With Sauce/Dressing			
Alice Springs Chkn Quesadilla, Sm	1115	70	69
Regular	2140	133	128
Aussie Cheese Fries: Small	1210	87	77
Regular	2135	151	139
Bloomin' Onion	1565	84	185
Gold Coast Coconut Shrimp	565	22	68
Kookaburra Wings, Hot	2145	185	28
Seared Ahi Tunah: Small	355	23	12
Regular	480	29	17

Burgers & Sandwiches

	C	F	Cb
Bacon Cheese Burger	1130	80	44
With Fries	1485	99	88
Grilled Chicken & Swiss Sandwich	695	33	50
With Fries	1050	52	93
Roasted Filet Sandwich	765	20	88
With Fries	1115	39	131
The Bloomin Burger	1175	72	76
With Fries	1525	91	119
The Outbacker Burger	760	45	43
With Fries	1115	64	86

Steaks: *Meat Only ~ Add Extra for Sides*

	C	F	Cb
New York Strip, 14 oz	715	37	0.5
Outback Special: 6 oz Sirloin	330	19	0.5
9 oz Sirloin	445	23	0.5
12 oz Sirloin	560	27	0.5
Prime Rib, 8 oz	535	45	2
16 oz	1060	90	2
Ribeye, 14 oz	1195	99	0.5
Teriyaki Marinated Sirloin, 9 oz	420	12	17
The Melbourne, P/house, 20 oz	1010	58	1
Victoria's Filet: 6 oz	520	42	0.5

Outback Favorites: *With Set Sides As Per Menu*

	C	F	Cb
Alice Springs Chicken	1650	113	73
Baby Back Ribs, full rack	2365	179	67
Grilled Chicken on the Barbie	585	26	32
New Zealand Rack of Lamb	1815	149	48
No Rules Parmesan Pasta	910	53	89
With Chicken	1355	77	91
With Chicken & Scallops	1365	77	94
With Chicken & Shrimp	1365	78	92
With Scallops	1320	76	97
With Shrimp	1275	77	92
Sweet Glazed Rstd Pork Tenderloin	850	43	73

Outback Steakhouse® (Nov '10)

Fish & Seafood:	C	F	Cb
Without Sides Unless Indicated			
Atlantic Salmon	360	21	1.5
Lobster Tails without Butter	230	2	6
Shrimp en Fuego Fettuccini	1185	55	95
Tilapia with Lump Crab Meat	505	29	8

Perfect Combinations: *Without Sides Unless Indicated*

	C	F	Cb
Filet & Shrimp Scampi	615	38	18
Outback Special:			
Grilled Shrimp, with 6 oz Sirloin	550	35	7
With 9 oz Sirloin	610	33	9
With 12 oz Sirloin	725	36	9
Ribs & Alice Spring Chicken	1270	98	7
With Aussie Fries	1625	118	50

Salads: *Without Dressing Unless Indicated*

	C	F	Cb
Chicken Caesar	1045	74	27
Queensland Salad: Without Dressing	840	59	23
With Ranch Dressing	1050	79	30
Classic Roasted Filet Wedge	565	30	27

Soups: *Per Bowl*

	C	F	Cb
Baked Potato	775	48	73
Cream of Broccoli	410	30	24
Onion	435	32	28

Add On Mates:

	C	F	Cb
Grilled Scallops with Butter	320	23	9
Lobster Tail with Butter	325	24	5
Lobster & Mushroom Topping	395	36	8
Sauteed Mushrooms	135	3	18

Sides: Aussie Fries

	C	F	Cb
Aussie Fries	355	19	43
Baked Potato: Plain	330	4.5	65
With Bacon	380	9	65
With Butter	520	26	65
With Cheese	355	7	65
Loaded	530	25	66
With Sour Cream & Chives	390	10	66
Blue Cheese Pecan Salad	525	36	35
Fresh Seasonal Veggies w. Butter	145	11	11
Garlic Mashed Potatoes	370	25	32
Potato Boats	165	2	32
Sweet Potato	595	21	99
Without butter	420	4	92

Desserts: *Per Single Serving*

	C	F	Cb
Classic Cheesecake without Sauce	185	9	26
Chocolate Thunder from Down Under	480	38	34
Nutter Butter Peanut Butter Pie	880	56	89

For Complete Menu & Data ~ see CalorieKing.com

Updated Nutrition Data ~ www.CalorieKing.com
Persons with Diabetes ~ See Disclaimer (Page 22)

Panda Express® (Nov '10)

Appetizers	C	F	Cb
Chicken Egg Roll, (1), 3 oz	200	12	16
Chicken Potsticker (3)	220	11	23
Veggie Spring Roll (2)	160	7	22
Meals			
BBQ Pork, 4½ oz	360	19	13
Beef & Broccoli, 5½ oz	150	6	12
Beijing Beef, 5½ oz	850	50	67
Black Pepper Chicken, 6oz	250	14	12
Eggplant & Tofu, 6 oz	310	24	19
Kung Pao Chicken, 6 oz	300	19	13
Mongolian Beef, 7 oz	230	11	17
Orange Chicken, 5½ oz	400	20	42
Sweet & Sour Pork, 5½ oz	400	23	36
***Rice & Noodles**: Per Serving*			
Chow Mein, 8¼ oz	400	12	61
Fried Rice, 10 oz	570	18	85
Steamed Rice, 8¾ oz	420	0	93

Panera Bread® (Nov '10)

	C	F	Cb
Bagels: Blueberry	330	1.5	67
Plain	290	1.5	59
Spreads: Plain Cream Cheese, 2 oz	180	18	2
Reduced Fat, average, 2 oz	130	12	2
Sandwiches: Per Full Sandwich			
Cafe:			
Sierra Trky on Focc w/ Asiago Chse	970	54	80
Smoked Ham & Swiss on Rye	700	28	65
Smoked Turkey Breast on Country	560	17	68
Tuna Salad on Honey Wheat	750	47	64
Signature:			
Asiago Roast Beef, on Asiago Cheese	690	27	64
Bacon Turkey Bravo on Tom. Basil	830	29	88
Italian Combo, on Ciabatta	1040	45	94
Salads: Full Size, With Dressing			
Asian Sesame Chicken, 11¼ oz	400	20	29
Caesar, 9¾ oz	390	27	25
Classic Cafe, 9¾ oz	170	11	18
Greek, 13½ oz	380	34	14
Soups: Per 12 oz Unless Indicated			
Broccoli Cheddar	290	16	24
Cream of Chicken & Wild Rice	320	17	33
French Onion, with Croutons, 13¼ oz	240	12	24
Low-Fat: Chicken Noodle	110	4	10
Garden Vegetable with Pesto	160	3.5	28
Muffins: Choc. Chip Muffie, 2¾ oz	280	12	40
Pumpkin Muffie, 2¾ oz	290	11	45
Wild Blueberry, 4½ oz	440	17	66

Papa Gino's® (Nov '10)

Appetizers: Small, 2 Servings	C	F	Cb
BBQ Chicken Tenders, 8½ oz	520	18	55
Buffalo Chicken Tenders, 8½ oz	450	19	36
Cheese Breadsticks, 13¼ oz	970	39	116
Cinnamon Sticks, 7¼ oz	620	19	100
French Fries, 12¼ oz	540	23	80
Mozzarella Sticks, 11 oz	950	59	69
Pastas: Entree Size			
Papa Platter, Penne; Spaghetti, 19½ oz	990	32	135
Ravioli, 13½ oz	590	24	71
Spaghetti & Meatballs, 19½ oz	890	29	123
Spagh. Chkn Parmigiana, 23½ oz	1070	39	129
Pizzas: Per Slice			
Large Thin Crust: BBQ Chicken	270	7	38
Buffalo Chicken	240	7	31
Cheese	220	6	31
Chicken and Roasted Garlic	290	10	34
Chicken Pepper	270	9	32
Meat Combo	320	15	32
Papa Roni	320	15	32
Pepperoni	270	11	31
Super Veggie	240	7	35
The Works	300	12	33
Single Sliced Pizza			
Thick Crust: Cheese, 7 oz	450	13	62
Pepperoni, 7 oz	480	15	64
Subs: Per Small Sub			
BLT	720	35	71
Italian	910	48	69
Meatball	740	32	76
Meatball Parmesan	840	41	76
Steak	630	25	65
Steak & Cheese	720	32	68
Super Steak	760	32	76
Tuna	740	39	67
Turkey Club	630	23	70
Salads: Without Dressing or Bread Stick			
Buffalo Chicken Tender	330	15	29
Caesar	190	10	19
with Chicken	320	11	14
Chicken Bacon Cheddar	530	33	22
Chicken Tender	320	14	29
Garden	180	8	25
Side: Caesar	70	4	6
Garden	70	3	10
Dressings: Bleu Cheese, 1 oz	150	15	2
Caesar, 3 oz	400	44	2
Ranch, 3 oz	280	30	4
Honey Dijon Fat-Free, 1½ oz	60	0	13

Papa John's® (Nov '10)

Original Crust (14"): Per ⅛ Pizza	C	F	Cb
BBQ Chicken & Bacon, 5¼ oz	350	12	44
Spicy Italian, 5¼ oz	380	18	38
Spinach Alfredo, 4 oz	290	11	36
The Meats, 3¾ oz	370	17	38
The Works, 5½ oz	330	14	39
Thin Crust (14"): *Per ⅛ Pizza*			
BBQ Chicken & Bacon, 4 oz	290	13	29
Spicy Italian, 4 oz	320	20	22
Spinach Alfredo, 2¾ oz	230	13	20
The Meats, 3¾ oz	310	19	22
The Works, 4¼ oz	270	15	23
Wings: Without Sauce			
BBQ, 2 wings, 2½ oz	190	12	6
Buffalo, 2 wings, 2½ oz	170	13	3
Dipping Sauces: *Per 1 oz Container*			
Barbeque	45	0	11
Blue Cheese	160	16	1
Buffalo	15	0.5	2
Ranch	100	10	1
Sides: *Without Dipping Sauce*			
Breadsticks (2)	290	4.5	54
Cheesesticks (4), 4¾ oz	370	16	41
ChickenStrips (2), 2½ oz	130	4.5	10
Cinnamon Sweetsticks (4), 6¾ oz	580	16	98

Papa Murphy's® (Nov '10)

Original Crust: Per 1/12 Family Size Pizza	C	F	Cb
BBQ Chicken	340	13	37
Cheese	270	11	30
Cowboy	350	18	32
Gourmet: Chicken Garlic	320	14	30
Classic Italian	350	18	31
Vegetarian	300	14	31
Hawaiian	290	11	33
Murphy's Combo	360	18	33
Pepperoni	320	15	31
Rancher	330	16	31
Specialty of the House, average	320	15	32
Veggie Combo	300	13	33
Stuffed Pizza: *Per 1/16 Family Size Pizza*			
5 Meat	370	16	39
Big Murphy	370	16	40
Chicago Style	370	16	40
Chicken and Bacon	370	15	39

Papa Murphy's® cont... (Nov '10)

Thin Crust deLITEs: Per 1/10 Large Pizza	C	F	Cb
Cheese	140	7	13
Hawaiian	160	7	15
Pepperoni	170	9	13
Veggie	160	9	13
Salads: *Without Dressing or Croutons*			
Club	280	16	12
Garden	200	12	16
Italian	280	20	14

Pei Wei Asian Diner (Nov '10)

First Tastes: Per Whole Dish, Without Sauce	C	F	Cb
Crab Wontons	340	20	26
Crispy Potstickers	300	16	24
Edamame	320	14	18
Minced Chicken with Lettuce Wraps	620	22	72
Vegetable Spring Rolls	210	7	35
Noodles & Rice Bowls: *Per Whole Meal, 2 Servings*			
Dan Dan Noodle, Chicken	780	20	106
Fried Rice: Beef	1040	32	136
Chicken	1000	24	132
Lo Mein Noodles: Beef	1080	40	136
Chicken	1120	40	134
Pad Thai Noodles: Beef	1580	52	218
Chicken	1440	40	210
Teriyaki Bowl: *Includes White Rice*			
Beef	1100	26	162
Chicken	1120	26	160
Shrimp	1060	24	160
Japanese Chili Ramen: Beef	980	32	128
Chicken	1000	32	126
Vegetable Tofu	1080	40	138
Signature Dishes: *Per Whole Meal, 2 Servings, W/o Rice*			
Honey Seared: Chicken	840	24	102
Shrimp	860	30	102
Sweet & Sour: Chicken	720	20	96
Shrimp	740	26	94
Soup: *Per Serving*			
Hot & Sour: Per Cup	190	8	12
Per Bowl	250	10	16
Thai Wanton: Per Cup	150	8	6
Per Bowl	140	8	7
Salads: *Per Whole Meal, Serves 2, Without Dressing*			
Asian Chopped Chicken	340	8	24
Spicy Chicken	1010	38	120
Dressings: *Per 2 oz Serving*			
Lime Vinaigrette	220	20	8
Sesame Ginger	220	21	6
Sauces: Lettuce Wrap	50	3	3
Sweet Chile	140	0	17

Updated Nutrition Data ~ www.CalorieKing.com
Persons with Diabetes ~ See Disclaimer (Page 22)

Pepe's Mexican® (Nov '10)

Burritos:	C	F	Cb
Beef & Bean	510	24	52
Beef & Bean Suizo	640	34	55
Chicken & Bean	480	21	51
Chicken & Bean Suizo	610	31	54
Pork & Bean	470	19	51
Pork & Bean Suizo	600	29	54
Flautas: Beef, plain	160	9	10
Beef with Cheese & Sauce	190	12	11
Chicken, plain	190	10	16
Chicken with Cheese & Sauce	230	13	17
Tacos: Beef Crisp	210	11	16
Beef Soft Corn	250	10	28
Beef Soft Flour	250	11	24
Chicken Crisp	190	9	15
Chicken Soft Corn	230	8	27
Chicken Soft Flour	230	9	23
Pork Crisp	170	6	16
Pork Soft Corn	220	6	27
Pork Soft Flour	220	7	24
Tostadas:			
Beef & Bean	380	23	26
Beef & Bean Suiza	440	29	26
Chicken & Bean	360	21	21
Chicken & Bean Suiza	410	26	25
Pork & Bean	350	20	26
Pork & Bean Suiza	410	25	26
Taco Salads: Beef: With 4 oz salsa	550	26	52
Without Taco Shell	330	19	20
Chicken: With 4 oz salsa	520	23	51
Without Taco Shell	300	16	19
Pork: With 4 oz salsa	500	20	52
Without Taco Shell	290	13	19

Peter Piper Pizza (Nov '10)

Appetizers:			
Breadsticks (2), 2½ oz	250	10	36
Chicken Strip (2), 4¾ oz	300	9	26
Wing (2), 1¾ oz	110	8	0

Pizza: Per Slice
Original Crust: *Per ⅛ of 14" Pizza*

	C	F	Cb
Cheese	300	9	37
Ham & Pineapple	280	7	38
Pepperoni	300	10	36
Pepperoni & Sausage	310	11	37
Sausage	310	10	38

Peter Piper Pizza cont... (Nov '10)

Pizza: Per Slice

Hand-Tossed Crust: *Per ⅛ of 14" Pizza*	C	F	Cb
Cheese	290	9	38
Ham & Pineapple	280	7	39
Pepperoni	290	10	37
Pepperoni & Sausage	310	11	38
Sausage	310	19	39
Pan Crust: *Per ⅛ of 14" Pizza*			
Cheese	290	9	38
Ham & Pineapple	310	7	46
Pepperoni	330	10	44
Pepperoni & Sausage	340	11	45
Sausage	340	11	46
Thin Crust: *Per ⅛ of 14" Pizza*			
Cheese	150	5	14
Ham & Pineapple	130	4	15
Pepperoni	150	6	13
Pepperoni & Sausage	150	7	14
Sausage	150	7	14
Signture Pizzas			
Original Crust: *Per ⅛ of 16" Pizza*			
5 Meat Supreme	320	13	33
California Veggie	240	6	33
Chicago Classic	270	9	33
New York 3 Cheese w. Pepperoni	340	14	32
Smokehouse	340	13	33
The Werx	290	10	33
Hand-Tossed Crust: *Per ⅛ of 16" Pizza*			
5 Meat Supreme	320	13	34
California Veggie	240	6	34
Chicago Classic	270	9	34
New York 3 Cheese w. Pepperoni	340	14	34
Smokehouse	340	13	34
The Werx	280	10	34
Pan: *Per ⅛ of 16" Pizza*			
5 Meat Supreme	340	13	39
California Veggie	260	6	39
Chicago Classic	290	9	39
New York 3 Cheese w. Pepperoni	360	15	39
Smokehouse	360	14	39
The Werx	310	10	39
Thin Crust: *Per ⅛ of 16" Pizza*			
5 Meat Supreme	190	9	14
California Veggie	130	4	14
Chicago Classic	150	6	14
New York 3 Cheese w. Pepperoni	200	10	14
Smokehouse	200	10	14
The Werx	160	7	14
Salads: Without Dressing or Croutons			
Chicken Caesar, 8 oz	200	8	10
Family, 4 oz	20	0	
Italian Chef, 13 oz	290	16	
Side, 5 oz	20	0	

P.F. Chang's® (Nov '10)

Starters: Small Plate, Per Serving	C	F	Cb
Crab Wontons, w/o Plum Sauce (2)	165	10	13
Egg Roll (1)	175	8	22
Lettuce Wraps: Chicken (1)	160	7	17
Vegetarian (1)	140	7	11
Pork Dumplings: Without Potsticker Sauce			
Pan-Fried (1)	70	4	6
Steamed (1)	60	2	6
Shrimp Dumplings: Without Sauce			
Pan-Fried (1)	60	2	6
Steamed (1)	45	0	6
Spare Ribs: Northern Style (1)	345	19	11
Changs BBQ, without Slaw, (1)	345	24	7
Spring Rolls, without Sauce, (2)	155	8	17
Meals: Per Whole Dish without Rice			
Beef: A La Sichuan, 18 oz	910	36	75
Mongolian, 18 oz	1010	45	60
Orange Peel, 15 oz	850	39	63
Chicken: w/ Black Bean Sce, 27 oz	900	48	42
Chang's Spicy, 18 oz	970	39	69
Kung Pao Chicken, 15 oz	1150	69	42
Orange Peel Chicken, 15 oz	1000	45	60
Sesame Chicken, 24 oz	1030	42	75
Sweet & Sour Chicken, 15 oz	1110	57	114
Duck, VIP , 12 oz	1300	58	110
Seafood: Cantonese Scallops, 14 oz	490	28	34
Cantonese Shrimp, 14 oz	430	20	20
Lemon Pepper Shrimp, 18 oz	470	20	38
Shrimp w/ Candied Walnuts, 21 oz	1130	72	75
Vegetarian Plates:			
Buddha's Feast, steamed, 12 oz	110	0	22
Coconut Curry Vegetables, 26 oz	1020	72	52
Ma Po Tofu, 30 oz	1050	69	51
Lunch Bowls: Per Whole Dish w/ White Rice, w/o Soup			
Moo Goo Gai Pan, 28 oz	780	22	94
Sesame Chicken, 28 oz	1070	30	152
Shrimp with Lobster Sauce, 24 oz	680	20	90
Sides: Small, Per Whole Dish			
Garlic Snap Peas, 4½ oz	95	3	11
Green Tea Soba Noodles, 6 oz	425	18	56
Shanghai Cucumbers, 6 oz	60	3	5
Sichuan Asparagus, 7½ oz	150	9	15
Spinach Stir-Fried w/ Garlic, 7½ oz	80	4.5	8
Soups: Hot & Sour, 1 cup, 7 oz	80	3	9
1 bowl, 34 oz	390	15	44
Egg Drop : 1 cup, 7 oz	60	3	8
1 bowl, 34 oz	290	15	39
Desserts: Banana Spring Rolls (4)	940	40	136
Great Wall of Chocolate Cake (4)	1530	72	244
Mini Tiramisu (1)	100	11	10

Piccadilly Cafeteria® (Nov '10)

Meals: Without Sides	C	F	Cb
Beef: Angus Chopped Steak, 5¼ oz	435	31	0
10 oz	885	65	5
Liver with Onion Sauce	365	20	22
Meatballs & Spaghetti	815	40	80
Chicken: & Dumplings, 8 oz	285	10	7
Breast, Blackened, 1 order	295	14	3
Florentine, 8 oz	465	9	44
Lemon Pepper, half	1545	105	22
Parmigiana, 1 order	1240	36	135
Sesame Glaze, 9 oz	715	34	57
Tetrazzini, 1 order	375	21	18
Pork Chops: Smothered, 8 oz	730	34	46
Blackened with Fettuccine	660	30	35
Southwest, with Mexican Rice	955	31	113
Seafood: Blcknd Shrimp Fettuccine	825	40	73
Cajun Baked Tilapia	330	20	4
Crawfish Etoufee	555	14	84
Tilapia w/ Shrimp Cream Sauce	280	6	10
Mediterranean Tilapia	240	8	8
New Orleans Sauteed Shrimp	835	40	78
Salads: Without Dressing			
Ambrosia, 6½ oz	285	14	43
Italian Rotini, 3½ oz	285	19	26
Piccadilly Fruit Salad, 5¾ oz	70	0	18
Potato, 4 oz	170	7	24
Spinach	95	5	7
Savory Sides:			
Baked Macaroni & Cheese, 5¼ oz	310	17	26
Breaded Okra, 3¼ oz	240	13	26
Broccoli & Rice, 5 oz	385	17	42
Candied Sweet Potatoes, 4½ oz	305	0	77
Carrot Souffle, 5 oz	390	17	58
Cauliflower with Cheese Sauce	175	10	5
Mashed Potatoes, 5 oz	115	4	19
Turnip Greens, 1 order	60	2	11
Soups: Per Cup:			
Seafood Gumbo	225	6	32
Shrimp & Corn	200	10	19
Tomato-Macaroni	110	1	22
Bread:			
Corn Sticks (1)	155	9	16
Garlic Bread, 1 slice	205	10	25
Desserts:			
Buttermilk Chess Pie, 1 slice	635	30	87
Coconut Cream Pie, 1 slice	550	33	59
Peach Cobbler, 8 oz	545	22	82
Red Velvet Cake, 1 slice	835	54	83

Pita Pit ~ *see CalorieKing.com*

Pizza Hut® (Nov '10)

Fit'n Delicious (12"): Per Slice, 1/8 Pizza

	C	F	Cb
Chkn, Mushroom & Jalapeno, 3¼ oz	170	4.5	22
Chicken, Onion & Green Pepper, 3¼ oz	180	4.5	23
Green Pepper, Onion & Tomato, 3 oz	150	4	24
Ham, Onion & Mushroom, 3 oz	160	4.5	23
Ham, Pineapple & Tomato, 3 oz	160	4.5	24
Tomato, Mushroom & Jalapeno, 3 oz	150	4	23

Hand-Tossed Style (12"): Per Slice, 1/8 Pizza

Cheese Only, 3¼ oz	220	8	26
Dan's Original, 3½ oz	260	12	26
Hawaiian Luau, 3½ oz	240	10	27
Ham & Pineapple, 3¼ oz	200	7	27
Italian Sausage & Onion, 3½ oz	240	11	27
Meat Lover's, 3¾ oz	300	16	25
Pepperoni, 3 oz	230	10	25
Pepperoni & Mushroom, 3¼ oz	210	8	26
Spicy Sicilian, 3½ oz	250	11	26
Supreme, 3¾ oz	260	12	26
Triple Meat Italiano, 3½ oz	260	12	25
Veggie Lover's, 3¾ oz	200	7	27

P'Zone: Per ½ P'Zone

Classic, 8 oz	630	23	77
Meaty, 8½ oz	710	31	76
Pepperoni, 7¾ oz	630	24	76

Pan (12"): Per Slice, 1/8 Pizza

Cheese Only, 3¼ oz	240	11	27
Dan's Original, 4 oz	280	14	27
Ham & Pineapple, 3½ oz	230	9	28
Hawaiian Luau, 3½ oz	260	12	28
Italian Sausage & Onion, 3¾ oz	270	13	28
Meat Lover's, 4 oz	330	18	27
Pepperoni & Mushroom, 3½ oz	240	10	27
Spicy Sicilian, 3¾ oz	270	13	27
Supreme, 4 oz	290	14	27
Triple Meat Italiano, 3½ oz	290	15	27
Veggie Lover's, 3¾ oz	230	9	28

Personal Pan (6"): Per Pizza

Cheese Only, 7¼ oz	590	24	69
Ham & Pineapple, 7½ oz	550	20	71
Meat Lover's, 9¼ oz	830	46	68
Supreme, 9 oz	720	36	69
Veggie Lover's, 8¼ oz	550	20	70

Pizza Mia (12"): Per Slice, 1/8 Pizza

Cheese; Pepperoni, average, 2½ oz	200	7.5	24

Stuffed Crust (14"): Per Slice, 1/8 pizza

Cheese Only, 4½ oz	350	14	39
Ham & Pineapple, 5 oz	340	13	41
Meat Lover's, 5¾ oz	480	26	39
Supreme, 5¾ oz	420	21	40
Veggie Lover's, 5½ oz	330	13	40

Pizza Hut® cont... (Nov '10)

Thin 'n Crispy (12"): Per 1/8 Slice

	C	F	Cb
Cheese Only, 2¼ oz	190	8	22
Ham & Pineapple, 2½ oz	180	6	23
Meat Lover's, 3 oz	280	16	22
Supreme, 3 oz	240	12	23
Veggie Lover's, 3 oz	180	6	23

Appetizers: Breadsticks (1), 1½ oz | 150 | 7 | 19 |
| Cheese Breadsticks (1), 2 oz | 180 | 7 | 20 |

Wings: Per 2 Pieces without Dipping Sauce

Baked: Hot, 1½ oz	100	6	1
Mild, 1½ oz	110	7	1
Bone Out: Buffalo, 2½ oz	190	9	18
Honey BBQ, 3 oz	220	8	27
Crispy Bone In: Buffalo, 2½ oz	230	15	16
Honey BBQ, 3 oz	260	14	24
Traditional: All American, 1½ oz	80	5	0
Garlic Parmesan, 2 oz	180	16	1

Dipping Sauces: Marinara, 3 oz | 60 | 0 | 12 |
| Blue Chse; Ranch, av., 1½ oz | 225 | 24 | 2 |

Pastas, Tuscani: Per ½ Pan

Bacon Mac N Cheese, 12½ oz	520	22	54
Chicken Alfredo, 11½ oz	630	33	56
Lasagna, 11¼ oz	600	33	43
Meaty Marinara, 11 oz	520	24	50

Desserts: Cinnamon Sticks, 2 | 170 | 6 | 26 |
Hershey's Choc. Dunkers, 2	200	9	26
With Chocolate Sauce, 1½ oz	320	12	50
Dipping Cup, White Icing, 2 oz	170	0	44

Pizza Ranch® (Nov '10)

Pizzas, 12": Per 1/8 Slice

	C	F	Cb
Thin Crust: Beef; BBQ Chicken	130	6	12
Bacon Cheeseburger	140	7	12
California Chicken	165	9	13
Canadian Bacon	120	5	12
Chicken Broccoli Alfredo	135	7	13
Prairie (Veggie)	130	6	
Roundup	150		
Stampede	160		
Texan	160		

Original Crust ~ Add 40 Cals and 9g Carb
Skillet Crust ~ Add 10 Cals & and 2 g Co
Broasted Chicken: Breast, 1 pie
   Leg, 1 piece
   Thigh, 1 piece
   Wing, 1 piece
Sides, Potato Wedge
For Complete Menu

Fast - Foods & *Restaurants*

Planet Smoothie® (Nov '10)

Cool Blended Smoothies:
Per 22 fl.oz Unless Indicated

	C	F	Cb
PB & J	500	16	87
Shag-a-delic	290	0	74
The Last Mango	340	1	85
Twig & Berries	280	0	74
Vinnie del Rocco	370	0	92

Energy Smoothies: Per 22 fl.oz Unless Indicated

	C	F	Cb
Berry Bada-Bing	350	0.5	92
Chocolate Elvis	440	17	72
Frozen Goat	220	0	56
Grape Ape	210	0	54
Pink Promise, 16 fl.oz	210	0	45
Road Runner	300	0	75
Spazz	270	0	69

Protein Smoothies: Per 22 fl.oz Unless Indicated

	C	F	Cb
Workout Blast: Big Bang	260	0	67
Chocolate Chimp	190	1.5	45
Mr Mongo: Chocolate	270	1.5	66
Strawberry	330	0	86

Pollo Tropical® (Nov '10)

Entrees: ¼ *Chicken*

	C	F	Cb
Dark Meat: With skin, 4 oz	270	17	0
Without skin, 3 oz	180	9	0
White Meat: With skin, 6 oz	350	17	0
Without skin, 5 oz	230	7	0

Tropichops:

	C	F	Cb
Chicken, White Rice/Black Beans:			
Regular, 17 oz	530	10	90
Large, 30 oz	1090	27	142
Chicken, Yellow Rice/Vegetables:			
Regular, 10 oz	330	5	51
Large, 23 oz	840	22	93
Pork, White Rice/Black Beans:			
Regular, 18 oz	680	22	92
Large, 31 oz	1260	49	145
?ork, Yellow Rice/Vegetables:			
?gular, 13 oz	490	18	54
?e, 24 oz	1000	44	97
?n: Regular, 19 oz	580	12	110
?oz	950	21	178
?ides, Toppings, Tortillas			
?verage	1145	38	153
?obb Chicken	950	41	57
?es	290	14	32
	500	24	69
	310	8	63
	360	18	29
	400	21	30

Popeye's® (Nov '10)

Chicken: Mild & Spicy with Skin

	C	F	Cb
Breast, average	355	21	8
Leg, average	105	6	3
Thigh, average	290	22	7
Wing, average	145	10	5
Big Deals: Delta Mini (1), 3½ oz	300	13	30
Chicken Biscuit, 3½ oz	350	20	30
Loaded Chicken Wrap, 6 oz	400	17	44
Sides: Biscuit, 2 oz	240	13	26
Cajun Rice, regular, 4 oz	170	6	22
Coleslaw, regular, 5 oz	260	23	14
Corn on the Cob (1), 7¾ oz	190	2	37
French Fries, 3 oz	310	17	35
Mashed Potatoes, regular, 4 oz	100	3	17
With Gravy, 5 oz	120	4	18
Red Beans & Rice, regular, 6 oz	320	19	31
Dessert, Cinn. Apple Turnover, 3 oz	250	12	34

Port of Subs® (Nov '10)

Figures Based on West Coast Outlets

Light Submarine: Per 5" Sub (Five Grams of Fat or Less)
Without Cheese, Oil or Mayonnaise

	C	F	Cb
#2 Ham Turkey	330	5	46
#5 Smoked Ham & Turkey	320	5	46
#6 Vegetarian, no Cheese	240	2	44
#7 Roast Beef	315	4	43
#8 Turkey	315	4	47
#9 Peppered Pastrami	295	4	44
#10 Roasted Chicken Breast	305	3	44
#14 Smoked Ham	300	4	44
#18 Roast Beef & Turkey	315	4	45

Cold Submarine S'wiches: Per 5" Sub With Standard
Toppings, Oil & Vinegar, Without Mayo/Mustard

	C	F	Cb
#1 Ham, Salami, Capicolla & Pepperoni with Provolone	530	26	45
#2 Ham & Turkey with Provolone	435	15	46
#3 Salami & Turkey with Provolone	465	20	46
#4 Ham & Salami with Provolone	470	21	45
#5 Smkd Ham & Turkey with Cheddar	430	15	47
#6 Vegetarian with Avocado & Olives	600	33	49
#7 Roast Beef with Provolone	420	14	43
#8 Turkey with Provolone	420	14	47
#9 Peppered Pastrami with Swiss	440	17	44
#10 Rstd Chicken Brst w./Provolone	410	13	45
#11 Ham with American	380	20	45
#12 Salami with Provolone	480	25	45
#13 Peppered Pastrami Turkey Swiss	510	26	44
#14 Smoked Ham with Swiss	445	17	45
#15 Salami & Pepperoni w/ Provolone	510	27	45
#16 BLT Sandwich	520	30	43
#17 Tuna without Cheese	420	18	45
#18 Rst Beef & Turkey w. Provolone	420	14	45

Updated Nutrition Data ~ www.CalorieKing.com
Persons with Diabetes ~ See Disclaimer (Page 22)

Port of Subs® cont... (Nov '10)

Figures Based on West Coast Outlets

Grillers: 5" Serving	C	F	Cb
BBQ Pork Griller	780	18	104
Grilled Chicken	520	13	58
Hot Pastrami	540	15	58
Italian	555	21	58
NY Steak & Cheese	615	18	57
Sandwiches:			
Turkey, Bacon & Avocado: 5 inch	495	20	46
8 inch	805	35	73
12 inch	1500	95	104

Fresh Salads: *With Oil & Vinegar Unless Indicated*

	C	F	Cb
Caesar Salad with Dressing: 6 oz	335	30	7
With Grilled Chicken, 13 oz	540	34	15
Chefs Salad, 11 oz	390	25	13
Garden Salad, 8 oz	95	5	10
Grilled Chicken, 13 oz	300	10	16
Tuna Salad, 11 oz	310	23	12
Sides: Macaroni Salad	330	22	28
Potato Salad	230	12	28
Dessert:			
Brownie, 5 oz	300	10	48
Chocolate Chunk Cookie, 4½ oz	560	29	72

Pret A Manger® (Nov '10)

Baguettes:	C	F	Cb
Chicken Mozzarella	500	16	68
French Brie & Basil	500	20	58
Smoked Salmon & Cream Cheese	520	20	64
Slims,			
Roasted Beef, Arugula & Parmesan	290	8	28
Sandwiches:			
Avocado & Parmesan	570	27	59
Balsamic Chicken & Avocado	520	25	58
Chicken & Bacon	480	20	58
Classic Turkey Club	520	21	59
Smoked Ham & Egg	450	16	48
Slims: Avocado & Parmesan	285	14	30
Balsamic Chicken & Avocado	260	11	32
Chicken & Bacon	240	13	29
Classic Turkey Club	260	11	30
Wraps:			
Jalapeno Chicken, Hot	400	21	46
Spicy Falafel Hot	540	24	61
Swedish Meatball Ragu, Hot	700	37	49
Soup: Per Medium 12 oz Serving			
Angus Steak Chili with Beans	345	11	35
Moroccan Lentil	435	20	54
Souper Reuben	300	17	23
Veggie Split	330	5.5	29

Pret A Manger® cont... (Nov '10)

Salads: Per Pack, w/o Dressing	C	F	Cb
Cobb & Greens	430	24	30
Grilled Chicken & Avocado	430	28	41
Grilled Chicken Caesar	400	16	24
Red, White & Greens	300	17	14
Bakery: Banana Cake	420	24	48
Carrot Cake	460	29	47
Chocolate Brownie	390	20	51
Chocolate Cake	470	19	71
Raspberry Bar	390	18	55
Smoothies: Mango, 8 oz	130	0	33
Raspberry, 8 oz	120	0	28

For Complete Menu ~ See CalorieKing.com

Pretzelmaker® (Nov '10)

Pretzels:	C	F	Cb
Bites			
Salted, Small, 3½ oz	250	1	52
Whirl & Salt, 4 oz	270	3.5	52
Pretzel Dogs: Mini (6)	300	19	23
Whirl & Salt (1)	480	29	38
Pretzels: Caramel Crunch	300	4	58
Cinnamon Sugar	330	4	65
Garlic	310	4	60
Italian Parmesan	310	3.5	60
Ranch	320	4.5	60
Salted	310	4	59
Unsalted	280	1	59
Sauces: Per 1½ oz Container			
Caramel	140	0	35
Cheddar Cheese Icing	80	5	4
Cream Cheese	200	20	2
Ketchup	20	0	4
Mustard	5	0	1
Nacho Cheese	80	5	4
Pizza	20	0.5	6
Beverages: Per 20 fl.oz			
Blended Drinks:			
Cool Cappuccino	640	21	
Mango Madness	520	1	
Mocha Mania	620		
Power Pomegranate	490		
Rockin' Raspberry	65		
Strawberry Banana	6		
Lemonade: Original, 44 fl oz			

Fast - Foods & *Restaurants*

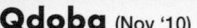

Qdoba (Nov '10)

	C	F	Cb
Burritos: *With 13" Flour Tortilla*			
Grilled Chicken	520	18	55
Ground Beef	570	25	55
Pulled Pork	490	13	64
Signature Burritos: *With 13" Flour Tortilla*			
Ancho Chile BBQ	420	11	70
Grilled Vegetables	390	12	59
Quesadillas: *With 13" Soft Flour Tortilla*			
Grilled Chicken	960	54	56
Shredded Beef	960	52	60
3-Cheese Nachos: *With Meat & Tortilla Chips Only*			
Grilled Chicken	750	36	76
Ground Beef	800	43	76
Pulled Pork	720	31	85
Tacos: *With Crispy Shell*			
Grilled Chicken (1)	120	6.5	8
Ground Beef (1)	140	9	9
Pulled Pork (1)	110	4.5	11
Shredded Beef (1)	120	5.5	10
Taco Salads: *With Crunchy Tortilla Bowl*			
Grilled Chicken	595	2	44
Ground Beef	645	39	44
Breakfast Items: *With 10" Flour Tortilla*			
Breakfast Burrito: *With Spicy Chorizo, Egg & Potato*			
With 3-Cheese Queso Sauce	460	21	44
With Fajita Ranchero Sauce	400	15	43
Condiments: *3-Cheese Queso, 2 oz*	100	8	3
Ancho Chile BBQ, 2 oz	90	2.5	16
Black Beans, 6 oz	210	1.5	35
Cheese, 1½ oz	170	14	0
Cilantro Lime Rice, 6 oz	330	8	60
Fajita Vegetables, 2 oz	30	1.5	4
Grilled Vegetables, 3½ oz	60	3.5	5
Guacamole, 3 oz	130	11	7
Mango Salsa, 4 oz	60	0	14
Pico de Gallo, 2 oz	10	0	1
Pinto Beans, 6 oz	190	1.5	34
Sour Cream, 2 oz	60	4	3

Quizno's Subs® (Nov '10)

~~d~~ on Quizno's Standard Portion Sizes. Figures may not
for Baltimore, Boise, Cleveland, Denver, Des Moines,
Springfield.
~~~~ular: With Cheese & Dressing Unless Indicated
Value Subs:

~~iss~~	770	44	63
~~, ~~ Cheddar	780	43	64
	1220	94	60
~~ar~~	770	44	63

Quizno's Subs® cont... (Nov '10)

*Based on Quizno's Standard Portion Sizes. Figures may not
apply for Baltimore, Boise, Cleveland, Denver, Des Moines,
Raleigh, Springfield.*

Subs (Cont): *Regular, w/Cheese & Dressing Unless Indicated*

Signature:	C	F	Cb
Baja Chicken	780	36	64
Bourbon Grille Steak	830	35	76
Chicken Carbonara	840	42	60
Double Cheese Cheesesteak	1030	63	65
Honey Mustard Chicken	830	41	66
Mesquite Chicken	790	39	61
Prime Rib and Peppercorn	930	53	66
Steakhouse Beef Dip	860	45	65
Torpedos: Beef Bacon & Cheddar	790	32	85
Italian	895	47	82
Pesto Turkey	675	24	85
Turkey Club	815	38	84
Bullets:			
Beef, Bacon & Cheddar	385	18	38
Italian	445	25	36
Pesto Turkey	330	13	38
Tuna Melt	525	37	35
Turkey Club	405	21	38
Sammies: *With Cheese & Dressing Unless Indicated*			
Alpine Chicken	380	19	28
Bistro Steak Melt	395	24	30
Cantina Chicken, without Cheese	265	6	35
Italiano	410	25	28
Roadhouse Steak, without Cheese	250	4	38
Sonoma Turkey	380	23	29
Veggie	330	19	29
Kids Sammies:			
Cheesy	230	10	25
Ham & Cheese	200	6	25
Turkey & Cheese	200	6	26
Soups: *Per Bowl*			
Broccoli Cheese	305	18	26
Chicken Noodle	155	3.5	25
Chili, with 2 Crackers	275	7	34
Tomato Basil	205	9	19
Regular Salads: *With Flatbread & Dressing*			
Chicken Caesar	920	67	39
Classic Cobb	800	56	40
Honey Mustard Chicken	920	65	48
Raspberry Chipotle	710	30	70

Updated Nutrition Data ~ www.CalorieKing.com
Persons with Diabetes ~ See Disclaimer (Page 22)

Rally's/Checkers® (Nov '10)

Burgers/Sandwiches	C	F	Cb
Bacon Double Cheeseburger	650	42	32
Big Buford	670	40	41
Cheese Double Cheese	510	31	31
Chili Cheeseburger	320	15	30
Crispy Fish Sandwich	430	19	51
Rallyburger	390	22	32
Wings: Classic Honey BBQ, 5 pieces	390	17	18
Extra Hot, 5 pieces	355	21	2
Parmesan Garlic, 5 pieces	480	35	1
Fries:			
Chili Cheese Fries, 7¾ oz	550	34	48
French: Medium, 4 oz	350	21	36
Large, 4½ oz	400	24	42

Ranch 1® (Nov '10)

Sandwiches: Chicken & Cheese	C	F	Cb
Sandwiches: Chicken & Cheese	390	12	39
Chicken Philly, 9¼ oz	410	13	40
Crispy Chicken, 11½ oz	710	39	60
Crispy Spicy Chicken, 11½ oz	545	17	68
Grilled Spicy Chicken, 10¼ oz	365	7	46
Ranch 1 Classic, 9½ oz	685	47	37
Bowls: Chicken Teriyaki, 19¼ oz	505	7	78
Fajitas, Chicken, 10 oz	540	24	53
Chicken, Rice, 11 oz	275	6	28
Popcorn Chicken: Small, 5½ oz	325	12	30
Large, 7½ oz	420	15	38
Kids Meal, 2 oz	110	4	10
Salads: Complete			
Grilled Chicken Caesar, 13¼ oz	430	30	14
Mandarin Chicken, 19¼ oz	815	43	78
Southwest Chicken, 17½ oz	745	50	44
Fries: Medium, 5¾ oz	380	21	43
Large, 8 oz	530	29	58
Kids Meal, 4 oz	280	15	31
Cheese: Regular, 9 oz	495	27	54
Large, 14 oz	755	42	80

Red Hot & Blue® (Nov '10)

BBQ Platters: Without Sides	C	F	Cb
Five Meat Treat	1165	85	15
Memphis Half Chicken	1510	103	11
Pulled Chicken	365	24	6
Smoked Sausage	950	67	36
BBQ Sandwiches: Regular, Without Sides			
Beef Brisket	415	17	36
Carolina Chopped Pork	460	23	34
Smoked Sausage	470	23	37
Ribs, Half Slab: Dry	1350	100	32
Sweet	1315	95	40

Red Hot & Blue cont... (Nov '10)

Salads: Without Dressing	C	F	Cb
Grilled Chicken Caesar	755	45	45
RH & B Chopped Salad	935	55	54
Smokehouse Salad	770	44	44
Southern Fried Chicken	690	30	58
Soup, Corn Chowder, 1 bowl	320	17	22
Sides: BBQ Beans	215	4	37
Mashed Potatoes with Gravy	335	15	47
Potato Salad	510	32	46

Red Lobster® (Nov '10)

Lunch	C	F	Cb
Starters:			
Chilled Jumbo Shrimp Cocktail	120	0.5	9
Crispy Calamari & Vegetables	1520	97	115
Lobster, Crab & Seafood Mushrooms	380	21	20
Pan Seared Crab Cakes	280	14	13
Classics: *Per Lunch Portion*			
Cajun Chicken Linguini Alfredo	630	27	45
Crab Linguini Alfredo	560	25	47
Crunchy Popcorn Shrimp	280	14	26
LightHouse Menu, Grilled/Broiled: *½ Portion Serving*			
Main Lobster Meat, 1½ oz	45	0.5	0
Rainbow Trout	220	10	6
Salmon	270	9	6
Tilapia	210	3	9
Signature Combinations:			
Admiral's Feast	1500	87	110
Seaside Shrimp Trio	1030	57	68
Ultimate Feast	620	30	29
Dinner			
Starters: Clam Strips	370	22	31
Lobster, Artichoke & Seafood Dip	1200	74	101
Mango-Jalapeno Shrimp Skewers	560	22	58
Parrot Isle Coconut Shrimp	590	33	54
Lobster & Crab Entrees:			
Lobster & Shrimp Pasta	1020	50	86
North Pacific King Crab Legs	390	3.5	2
Rockzilla	130	1.5	0
Snow Crab Legs Meat, 3½ oz	160	1	0
Sides: Fries	330	17	40
Home-Style Mashed Potatoes	180	9	22
Garden Salad	90	3	13
Garden Salad with Shrimp	105	3	13
Dipping Sauces: Per 1½ oz			
Cocktail Sauce	40	0	9
Sweet & Spicy Glaze	100	0	24
Tartar Sauce	190	19	6
100% Pure Melted Butter	350	38	2

For Complete Nutritional Data ~ see CalorieKing.com

Red Robin® (Nov '10)

Appetizers: As Served	C	F	Cb
Chili Chili Con Queso	1375	88	109
Creamy Artichoke & Spinach Dip	1115	60	101
Guacamole, Salsa & Chips	815	47	88
Just-in-Quesadilla	1070	55	69
Nachos: Chili	1955	132	130
With Chicken	2085	134	132
RR's Buzzard Wings	1075	84	4
Towering Onion Rings	1775	112	171

Entrees: With Sides, Dressings & Sauce			
Arctic Cod Fish & Chips	1120	67	83
Clucks & Fries: Regular Style	1450	92	100
Buffalo Style	1695	121	100
Ensenada Chicken Platter	755	41	26
Grilled Chicken alla Caprese	645	34	35
Jumbo Shrimp & Slaw Plater	1255	56	148
Red's Rice Bowl	830	10	137
Shrimp & Cod Duo	1435	84	133
Steak Sliders (3)	1125	58	91

Sandwiches & Burgers: With Standard Components

Gourmet Burgers:			
A.1. Peppercorn	1025	59	70
Bacon Cheeseburger	1030	69	51
Bleu Ribbon	999	57	70
Burnin' Love	935	60	55
Cheeseburger	930	60	53
Guacamole Bacon	1045	64	54
Natural	570	24	51
Pub	955	55	57
Royal	1195	83	52
Sauteed 'Shroom	960	56	58
The Banzai	1035	62	68
Whiskey River BBQ	965	53	68
Other Favorite Burgers: Garden	560	23	73
Grilled Turkey	640	37	50
Lettuce-Wrap Your Burger	420	27	8

Sandwiches:			
Chicken: Blackened	695	34	52
Bruschetta	680	31	55
California	835	44	52
Crispy	910	54	70
Teriyaki	905	48	64

Other Favorite Sandwiches:			
Crispy Cod	605	29	61
Grilled Salmon	855	50	53

Wraps:			
Caesar's Chicken	850	43	69
Whiskey River BBQ Chicken	1110	62	84

Rita's ~ see CalorieKing.com

Rocky Rococo® (Nov '10)

Pastas: Per Serving	C	F	Cb
Can't Decide, 14 oz	465	9	77
Fettuccine with Alfredo Sauce:			
Regular, 14 oz	460	14	66
Light, 7 oz	230	7	33
Spaghetti with Meatballs:			
Regular, 15 oz	630	16	89
Light, 7½ oz	315	8	45
Spaghetti with Tomato Sauce:			
Regular, 14 oz	470	4	87
Light, 7 oz	235	2	44

Pizzas: Per Slice, ⅛ Pizza			
Cheese	380	9	54
Garden	390	10	56
Pepperoni	425	13	54
Sausage	495	19	54
Sausage Mushroom	500	19	55

Sides:			
Breadsticks: With Marinara Sce (6)	420	7	72
With Jalapeno Cheese Sauce (6)	530	18	72
Wheat Muffin (1)	200	4	38

Roly Poly® (Nov '10)

Wraps: Per 6" White Wrap Unless Indicated

Ham & Smoked Pork:	C	F	Cb
Italian Classic	335	12	32
Key West Cuban Mix	330	9	44
Peachtree Melt	310	11	27
Pork Melt	310	11	26
Porky's Nightmare	320	12	28
Chicken: Basil Cashew Chicken	300	10	30
Catalina Chicken Salad	315	11	28
Chicken Caesar	310	11	30
Chicken Cordon Bleu	310	11	26
Chicken Fajita	315	9	28
Chicken Popper	285	8	29
Cobb Salad	255	12	27
Delhi Chicken	325	12	33
Hickory Chicken	350	10	25
Oriental Chicken	270	4	29
Santa Fe Chicken	305	11	28
Tuna: Popeye's Tuna On Wheat	305	4	31
Classic Tuna Melt	340	17	26
Texas Tuna Melt	310	12	30
Thai Hot Tuna	340	11	30
Tuna Luau	325	14	34

Round Table® Pizza (Nov '10)

Appetizers	C	F	Cb
Buffalo Wings, 6 pieces	420	30	6
Garlic Bread, 6 pieces	420	21	54
with Cheese, 6 pieces	600	36	54
Garlic Parmesan Twists, 3 pieces	510	15	78
Honey BBQ Wings, 6 pieces	480	27	12
Pizzas (Large 14"): Per Slice, ½ Pizza			
Original Crust: Cheese	230	9	25
Chicken & Garlic Gourmet	250	11	25
Chicken Smokehouse	270	12	26
Gourmet Veggie	240	10	27
Guinevere's Garden Delight	220	8	26
Hawaiian	220	8	27
Italian Garlic Supreme	270	14	25
King Arthur Supreme	270	13	26
Maui Zaui, with Polynesian Sce	260	10	29
Montague's All Meat Marvel	290	15	25
Pepperoni	240	11	24
Smokehouse Combo	290	14	26
Pan Crust: Cheese	300	11	38
Chicken & Garlic Gourmet	340	13	39
Chicken Smokehouse	360	14	40
Gourmet Veggie	320	12	41
Guinevere's Garden Delight	300	10	39
Hawaiian	300	10	40
Italian Garlic Supreme	360	16	39
King Arthur Supreme	340	14	39
Maui Zaui w/ Polynesian Sauce	340	12	43
Montague's All Meat Marvel	360	15	38
Pepperoni	320	13	38
Skinny Crust: Cheese	190	9	18
Chicken & Garlic Gourmet	220	11	18
Chicken Smokehouse	240	12	19
Gourmet Veggie	200	10	20
Guinevere's Garden Delight	180	8	19
Hawaiian	190	8	20
Italian Garlic Supreme	240	14	18
King Arthur Supreme	240	13	19
Maui Zaui with Polynesian Sauce	220	10	22
Montague's All Meat Marvel	260	15	18
Pepperoni	210	11	18
Sandwiches:			
Chicken Club	800	43	59
Ham Club	740	40	60
RT Pizza	410	18	78
Turkey Club	720	38	59
Turkey Sante-Fe	730	40	57

For Complete Nutritional Data ~ see CalorieKing.com

Rubio's Mexican Grill® (Nov '10)

Burritos: Without Chips	C	F	Cb
Baja: Grill Chicken	630	28	55
Steak	720	38	56
Bean & Cheese	760	37	78
Carnitas Rajas	790	33	77
Fish	750	41	75
Grilled Mesquite Shrimp	730	34	75
Grilled Veggie	680	27	75
Mahi Mahi	650	34	59
Big Burrito Especial: Chicken	820	31	102
Steak	900	38	102
Health Mex: Chicken	520	14	69
Mahi Mahi	560	20	67
Nachos: Grande	1270	78	117
Grande Chicken	1340	78	114
Grande Steak	1430	87	114
Quesadillas: Cheese	1120	70	87
Chicken	1200	70	89
Tacos:			
Regular: Fish, Especial	320	18	31
Grilled Chicken	250	12	23
Grilled Mesquite Shrimp	220	10	23
Grilled Steak	220	10	22
World Famous Fish	270	13	30
Grilled Gourmet: Chicken	320	17	24
Garlic Herb Shrimp	340	19	23
Portobello & Poblano	290	17	26
Steak	350	21	24
Health Mex: Chicken	130	1	22
Mahi Mahi	170	4	21
Street: Carnitas	100	4.5	9
Chicken	90	2.5	9
Steak	120	6	9
Salads: Includes Dressing/Sauce			
Chicken Chipotle Ranch	480	32	23
Chicken Chopped	500	25	37
Chicken Grilled Grande Bowl	630	27	62
Chicken Surfside Citrus	500	30	34
Wrapsalads: Includes Dressing/Sauce			
Chicken Chipotle Ranch	770	45	62
Chicken Chopped	780	38	72
Chicken Surside Citrus	800	43	73
Salsas: Per 1 oz			
Picante	20	1	2
All Other Varieties	5	0	1
Desserts:			
Brownie, 3 oz	430	22	57
Churro, 1½ oz	170	8	22

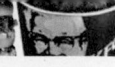
Ruby Tuesday® (Nov '10)

	C	F	Cb
Appetizers: *Per ¼ Order without Sides or Sauce*			
Asian Dumplings	115	5	12
Cheddar Fries	335	20	28
Fried Mozzarella	145	6	13
Jumbo Lump Crab Cake	70	4	4
Southwestern Spring Rolls	175	10	15
Thai Phoon Shrimp	190	13	12
Burgers: *Without Sides*			
Handcrafted: Alpine Swiss	1050	62	79
Boston Blue	1200	71	87
Ruby's Classic	930	55	65
Smokehouse	1220	73	88
Prime: Triple Prime	1110	82	49
Triple Prime Bacon Cheddar	1330	101	49
Triple Prime Cheddar	1270	96	49
Premium Sandwiches: *Without Sides*			
Avocado Turkey Burger	885	54	54
Buffalo Chicken Burger	790	41	63
Chicken BLT	800	40	63
Fresh Grilled Chicken	870	41	51
Turkey Burger	700	39	50
Premium Seafood: *Without Sides*			
Asian Glazed Salmon	370	26	15
Crab Cake Dinner	270	17	13
Creole Catch	195	8	2
Herb Crusted Tilapia	400	24	11
New Orleans Seafood	315	18	4
Salmon Florentine	415	31	7
Ribs & Platters: *Without Sides*			
Asian Sesame Glazed, Half	540	32	19
Chicken Tender Dinner	380	17	11
Classic BBQ, Half	485	24	26
Memphis Dry Rub, Half	460	29	6
Fit & Trim Choices: *Served With Broccoli and White Cheddar Mashed Potatoes*			
BBQ Grilled Chicken	590	4	11
Creole Catch	445	23	36
Creole Shrimp Salad	450	17	44
Vegetarian Pasta Marinara	490	10	81
Petite Salads: Creole Shrimp	250	8	25
Grilled Chicken	360	11	25
Grilled Salmon	385	8	25
Steaks & Chicken: *Without Sides*			
Chef's Cut 12 oz Sirloin	740	50	1
Chicken Bella	400	15	10
Chicken Florentine	390	14	8
Cowboy Sirloin	570	29	23
Peppercorn Mushroom Sirloin	460	22	12
Petite Sirloin	300	16	1
Rib Eye	820	63	1
Top Sirloin	390	22	1

Ruby Tuesday® cont... (Nov '10)

	C	F	Cb
Pasta Classics: *Without Sides*			
Chicken & Broccoli	1565	96	94
Chicken & Mushroom Alfredo	1220	59	89
Parmesan Chicken	1420	77	111
Parmesan Shrimp	1050	57	89
Shrimp Carbonara	1370	96	81
Vegetarian Pasta Marinara	490	10	81
Perfect Lunch Combinations:			
Minis: Buffalo Chicken	620	23	69
Ruby	635	35	50
Salmon Cake	700	33	67
Turkey	550	28	54
Vegetarian	680	27	95
Soups: Broccoli & Cheese Soup	380	32	14
Clam Chowder	320	20	18
Tortilla Soup	285	13	31
Garden Fresh Salads: *Without Dressing*			
Carolina Chicken	705	24	30
Creole Shrimp	445	17	44
Garden	395	17	49
Grilled Chicken	700	22	34
Grilled Salmon	745	17	44
Dressings *(Per 1 oz):* Blue Cheese	180	19	1
Balsamic Vinaigrette	35	3	4
Honey Mustard	90	8	5
Italian	60	6	2
Ranch	100	11	1
Signature Parmesan	150	16	1
Thousand Island	70	7	3
Signature Sides: French Fries	395	18	55
Baked Potato: Plain	280	2	56
Loaded Baked Potato	590	29	58
Blue Cheese Coleslaw	330	32	11
Brown-Rice Pilaf	230	9	30
Creamy Mashed Cauliflower	135	8	13
Garlic Cheese Biscuit	90	4	10
Onion Rings	350	21	35
Sauteed Baby Portob, Mshsrms	100	4	10
White Cheddar Mashed Potatoes	170	10	21
Desserts: Blondie for One	625	27	88
Double Chocolate Cake	895	40	124
Italian Cream Cake	990	56	110
New York Cheesecake	735	60	84
Cookies: Chocolate Chip	180	9	24
White Choc. Macadamia Nut	200	12	23
Drinks: Ruby's Root Beer Float	400	14	68
Lemonade: Pomegranate	235	0	59
Other Fruit Flavors	190	0	48

For Complete Menu ~ see CalorieKing.com

Runza® (Nov '10)

Burgers	C	F	Cb
Legendary: ¼ lb Cheeseburger Runza	430	21	32
½ lb Double Cheeseburger Runza	640	32	37
¼ lb Bacon Cheeseburger	510	29	36
¼ lb Legend Supreme	770	37	62
¼ lb Swiss Mushroom	450	25	36
Junior: Cheeseburger	330	17	28
Cheeseburger Runza	310	14	30
Swiss Mushroom	380	21	26
Sandwiches			
BBQ Chicken, grilled	390	9	46
Buffalo Chicken grilled	440	13	36
Cheese Runza	560	21	66
Deluxe Chicken, crispy	480	19	51
Original Runza	500	17	65
Polish Dog	420	26	30
Smothered Chicken, grilled	380	10	41
Swiss Mushroom Runza	590	25	68
French Fries: Small, 3 oz	280	15	31
Medium, 4½ oz	410	23	46
Large, 7 oz	630	35	70
French Onion Dip, 2 oz	90	6	4
Frings, 6½ oz	540	28	64
Onion Rings: Medium, 4 oz	370	20	41
Large, 6½ oz	590	32	66
Salads: *Without Dressing*			
Tossed, with Crispy Chicken	440	27	29
Tossed, with Grilled Chicken	280	13	13
Dressings: Caesar	410	45	3
Fat-Free Hidden Valley Ranch	60	0	15
Soups: *Per Bowl*			
Boston Clam Chowder	320	23	33
Broccoli Cheese	360	27	35
Cauliflower Cheese	330	26	32
Chicken Noodle	170	5	21
Homemade Chili	310	10	26
Potato with Bacon	310	20	40
Vegetable Cheese	330	22	28
Wisconsin Cheese	430	35	36
Kids Meals: *Includes Small Fries, Without Drink*			
Mini Corn Dogs (5)	550	32	56
Chicken Strips (2)	460	25	42
Jr Hamburger	500	24	55
Kids Runza Sandwich	530	24	64
Desserts & Drinks			
Chocolate Chip Cookie (1)	310	16	34
Shakes: Cappuccino, reg., 12 floz	470	18	65
Vanilla, regular, 12 fl.oz	470	16	69
Pepsi Runza Slushie, med., 18 fl.oz	220	0	60

Ryan's® Grill, Buffet & Bakery (Nov '10)

Entrees: *Without Sides*	C	F	Cb
BBQ Ribs, 1 rib, 3½ oz	180	12	7
BBQ Chicken, 1 spoon, 2¾ oz	150	6	9
Carved Turkey Breast, 1 slice, 2 oz	90	3.5	0
Chicken Fried Steak, 1 piece, 2¼ oz	210	13	15
1 piece, with gravy, 2½ oz	220	13	16
Chicken Pot Pie, 1 spoon, 4½ oz	290	18	24
Fried Breaded Catfish, 1 filet, 6¼ oz	340	16	12
Fried Fish. 1 piece, 1½ oz	90	5	4
Fried Shrimp, 11 shrimp, 2 oz	150	8	16
Fried Tilapia, 1 piece, 1 oz	70	2.5	4
Grilled Chicken Breast, plain, 4 oz	180	4	0
Grilled Pork Chop: Plain (1), 3 oz	170	9	0
BBQ; Teriyaki, average, 1 chop	190	10	4
Grilled Teriyaki Chicken Thighs, 1 oz	60	2.5	4
Macaroni & Cheese, 1 spoon 3½ oz	120	2.5	19
Meat Lasagne, 1 piece, 6 oz	250	11	22
Meatloaf, 1 slice, 2 oz	100	6	6
Mexican Casserole, 1 spoon, 4½ oz	190	9	21
Pizza: Cheese, 1 slice, 3 oz	200	8	21
Pepperoni, 1 slice, 3 oz	250	13	21
Rotisserie Chicken. Breast, (1), 4¾ oz	280	13	0.5
1 Leg, 2¾ oz	120	9	0.5
1 Thigh, 4¼ oz	250	16	1
Sirloin Steak, 3 oz	180	9	0
Spaghetti, 1 spoon, 3 oz	130	2.5	23
Spag. Sce with Meat, 1 spoon, 2 oz	140	8	10
Taco Meat, 1¼ oz	70	4	3
White Turkey w/ 1 spoon gravy, 4¼ oz	90	2	4
Sides:			
Baked Potato, plain, 6½ oz	180	0	31
Baked Beans, 4 oz	90	1	20
Breaded Fried Okra, 3 oz	220	12	28
Brussel Sprouts, 2¾ oz	40	2	6
Corn Cobbet (1) 2¾ oz	90	3	4
Garlic Mashed Potatoes, 3 oz	90	4	11
Glazed Baby Carrots with Sauce, 2 oz	60	3	7
Gr. Vegetables with Broccoli, 1¾ oz	40	3	2
Pinto Beans, 3¼ oz	70	1	14
Rice Pilaf, 1½ oz	60	1	12
Steamed Cabbage with Bacon, 1¾ oz	60	5	2
Yellow Squash with Onions, 1¾ oz	40	3.5	2
Desserts: Cheesecake, plain,1 slice	370	19	45
Ice Cream Cone (flat bottom)	15	0	3
Key Lime Pie, 1 slice, 2¾ oz	280	12	39
Lem. Creme Cake, sug. free,1 slice	170	15	9
Cookies: Oatmeal Raisin (1)	120	5	16
Sugar Cookie (1)	120	5	17

7-Eleven® (Nov '10)

	C	F	Cb
Breakfast			
Big Eats: *Per Sandwich*			
Sausage, Egg & Cheese Biscuit	500	30	41
Egg, Ham & Cheese Croissant	360	25	25
Sausage, Egg & Cheese Muffin	360	23	25
Roller Grill Items: *Per Item*			
Hot Dogs: Big Bite, ¼ lb	360	34	2
Biggest Big Bite, ⅓ lb	480	45	3
Bratwurst Sausage (1)	370	34	4
Breakfast Bite Sausage (1)	250	21	2
Buffalo Chicken Bite (1)	170	14	11
Cheese & Jalapeno Taquito (1)			
Cheeseburger Bite (1)	440	38	2
Sauces: Casa Buena Chedd. Chse, 2 oz	110	9	5
Casa Buena Premium Chili, 1 oz	15	0.5	2
Big Eats Sandwiches: *Per Sandwich*			
Smkd Tky w/ Jack Chse/Wheat Bread	460	22	42
With Southwest Mayo	540	26	49
Ham & Havati Chse on Onion Roll	420	15	43
Egg Salad On White Bread	520	29	42
Tuna Salad On Wheat Bread	450	19	48
Turkey & Cheddar On Wheat Sub	280	6	37
Turkey & Swiss On Pita Bread	460	14	64
Bakery Stix™ Treats: *Per Stick (3½ oz)*			
Grilled Cheese; Ham & Cheese	280	12	32
Salads: Tuna Macaroni, 8 oz	270	8	29
Reser's Coleslaw, 3½ oz	130	7	17
Reser's Macaroni Salad, 3½ oz	220	15	20
Reser's Potato Salad, 3½ oz	200	10	19
Bakery:			
Brownie, Iced, 3¼ oz	380	15	58
Donuts: Chocolate Iced (1)	400	19	52
Chocolate Iced Yeast Raised (1)	330	16	41
Long John, Chocolate, 3½ oz	390	20	49
Beverages			
Fr. Vanilla Iced Cappuccino	140	3	26
Hershey's S'Mores Cocoa, 8 fl oz	200	7	36
Fountain Drinks *(Assumes ⅓ Ice)*			
Coca-Cola/Pepsi/Dr.Pepper/7Up:			
Gulp, 20 oz	195	0	51
Big Gulp, 32 oz	310	0	82
Super Gulp, 44 oz	430	0	112
Double Gulp, 64 oz	625	0	163
Diet Coke/Diet Pepsi, 16 oz	1	0	0
Slurpees: Average All Flavors,			
12 oz size	95	0	24
22 oz size	175	0	44
28 oz size	220	0	56
40 oz size	315	0	80
Hawaiian Punch; Dr Pepper, avg.,			
12 oz size	180	0	48
22 oz size	330	0	88
28 oz size	420	0	112
40 oz size	600	0	160

Saladworks® (Nov '10)

	C	F	Cb
Salads: *Without Dressing*			
Autumn Harvest	310	12	43
Bently	245	10	11
Buffalo Bleu	250	7	24
Chicken Caesar	285	4	19
Cobb	270	16	13
Fire Roasted Cabo Jack	370	18	31
Garden Deluxe	240	2	92
Greek	185	10	19
Mandarin Chicken	230	7	37
Nuevo Nicoise	230	5	73
Sophie's Salad	310	14	35
Tivoli	430	20	74
Dressings: *Per 1 oz Ladle*			
Bistro Balsamic	250	27	8
Bistro Balsamic Lite	40	0	10
French; Lemon; 1000 Island, average	260	24	10
Honey'd Mustard	80	0.5	18
House Healthy: Ranch	160	16	4
Royal Caesar; Italian, average	180	15	9
Lite Ranch	95	7	5
Oriental Sesame	170	8	22
Royal Caesar	290	31	2

Extra Menu Items ~ See CalorieKing.com

Sandella's Flatbread Cafe (Nov '10)

	C	F	Cb
Wraps			
Buffalo Chicken	455	17	53
Chicken Fajita	445	13	54
Pacific Chicken	420	11	56
Pesto Turkey	480	18	58
Sweet & Spicy Chicken	355	4	55
Paninis: Chicken Delicato	535	22	51
Spinach, Ham & Swiss	510	19	53
Turkey & Mozzarella	495	19	54
Tuscan Chicken	580	25	56
Quesadillas: California	410	16	53
Chicken Fajita	385	8	52
Mediterranean	470	24	55
Grilled Flatbread: Aloha	570	20	70
Brazilian Chicken	460	15	51
Pesto Chicken	665	33	57
Spinach & Bacon	680	41	52
Vegetarian	685	19	61
Chopped Salads: Aloha	295	11	36
Greek	305	9	18
Rice Bowls: Black Bean & Rice	705	7	133
Chicken Fajita	630	9	102

For Complete Menu & Data ~ see CalorieKing.com

Sbarro's® (Nov '10)

Entrees	C	F	Cb
Baked Ziti with Sauce	700	41	43
Chicken Parmigiana	520	22	16
Meat Lasagna	650	37	36
Spaghetti with Sauce	820	28	120
Pizza: *Per Slice (Thin Crust)*			
Cheese	460	13	60
Pepperoni	730	37	61
Sausage	670	31	60
Supreme	630	27	63
Stuffed Pizza: *Per Slice*			
Spinach & Broccoli	790	34	89
Pepperoni	960	42	89

Schlotzsky's® (Nov '10)

	C	F	Cb
Oven-Toasted Sandwiches: *Per Medium Sandwich*			
Angus: Beef & Provolone	760	29	81
Corned Beef Reuben	910	40	80
Corned Beef	580	13	78
Pastrami Reuben	910	39	80
Pastrami & Swiss	905	36	83
BLT	560	21	74
Chicken & Pesto	570	14	73
Chicken Breast	515	6	78
Chipotle Chicken	550	14	68
Dijon Chicken	575	11	79
Homestyle Tuna	565	16	73
Santa Fe Chicken	620	15	76
Smoked Turkey Breast	520	9	77
Smoked Turkey Reuben	895	38	84
Turkey & Guacamole	565	13	82
Turkey Bacon Club	785	32	77
Original Style: The Original	770	34	78
Cheese	790	38	76
Ham & Cheese	735	27	80
Turkey	830	35	80
Panini: Classic Swiss & Tomato	625	26	63
Grilled Chicken Romano	570	16	62
Italiano	735	32	67
Mozzarella & Portobello	485	15	63
Smoked Ham Crostini	645	23	67
Smoked Turkey & Guacamole	600	21	69
Wraps: Asian Chicken	535	12	80
Feta & Portobello	620	39	55
Grilled Chicken & Guacamole	690	36	60
Homestyle Tuna	455	17	55
Parmesan Chicken Caesar	555	21	61

Schlotzsky's® cont... (Nov '10)

8" Pizzas: *Per Pizza*	C	F	Cb
BBQ Chicken & Jalapeno	715	16	99
Baby Spinach Salad	455	7	80
Bacon, Tomato & Portobello	620	23	75
Combination Special	640	25	76
Double Cheese	595	21	74
Fresh Tomato & Pesto	555	19	73
Grilled Chicken & Pesto	685	22	75
Mediterranean	560	20	74
Pepperoni & Double Cheese	685	30	74
Smoked Turkey & Jalapeno	655	21	78
Thai Chicken	725	23	85
Vegetarian Special	540	17	74
Salads: *Without Dressing/Croutons Unless Indicated*			
Baby Spinach & Feta	115	7	6
Caesar Salad with Croutons	105	5	10
Chicken	290	15	12
Garden	50	1	12
Greek	135	8	13
Grilled Chicken Caesar with Croutons	220	8	12
Ham & Turkey Chef	255	13	14
Pasta	70	3	12
Potato	240	13	29
Turkey Chef	310	18	14
Kid's Meals: *Without Cookie or Drink*			
Cheese Pizza	480	13	73
Cheese Sandwich	395	15	48
Ham & Cheese Sandwich	425	16	49
Pepperoni Pizza	525	17	73
Turkey Sandwich	300	5	49
Desserts			
Brownie	415	22	54
Carrot Cake	715	42	80
New York Style Cheesecake	350	23	30
Cookies: Chocolate Chip	160	8	22
Fudge Chocolate Chip	160	8	22
Oatmeal Raisin	150	6	22
Sugar	160	7	22
White Chocolate Macadamia	170	9	21

Second Cup® ~ see CalorieKing.com

Shakey's® (Nov '10)

Pizzas (12"): Per ⅒ Pizza	C	F	Cb
Cheese: Pan Crust	185	6	26
Thin Crust	150	6	18
Firehouse: Pan Crust	255	12	27
Thin Crust	220	12	19
Garden Veggie: Pan Crust	185	6	27
Thin Crust	150	5	19
Margherita: Pan Crust	175	5	26
Thin Crust	135	4.5	18
Rustic Garlic Chicken: Pan Crust	190	5.5	26
Thin Crust	155	5.5	18
Shakey's Special: Pan Crust	210	6.5	31
Thin Crust	195	10	18
Texas BBQ Chicken: Pan Crust	205	5	29
Thin Crust	170	5	21
Ultimate Meat: Pan Crust	280	14	26
Thin Crust	245	13	18
Additional Toppings: Beef	35	3	0
Cheese	15	1	0
Chicken	15	0.5	0
Ham	10	0.5	0
Pepperoni	25	2.5	0
Sausage	45	4	0
Sharables: Per Serving			
Chicken Strips (5)	620	31	48
Mojo Potatoes (5)	215	11	25
Mojo Supreme, serves 4-6	1950	120	160
Shakey's Spicy Wings (6)	495	29	27
Shakey's Famous Chicken: Per Piece			
Fried Chicken: Breast	475	26	16
Leg	170	19	6
Thigh	350	24	10
Wing	130	9	3.5

Sheetz® (Nov '10)

	C	F	Cb
Breakfast: Plain Bagel, Without Cheese Condiments or Dressing Unless Indicated			
Shmagelz: Bacon & Egg	530	27	53
Egg & American Cheese	440	19	50
Egg, Ham & Provolone	525	21	55
Shmiscuitz: Bacon & Egg	540	35	39
Egg & American Cheese	450	27	36
Egg, Ham & Swiss Cheese	550	30	41
Egg, Sausage & American Cheese	625	44	36
Shmuffins: Bacon & Egg	410	25	29
Egg & American Cheese	320	17	26
Egg & Ham	310	11	30
Egg, Sausage & Cheddar Cheese	495	34	26
Egg & Steak	395	16	27

Sheetz® cont... (Nov '10)

Cold Subz: Per 6" White Sub, Without Cheese, Toppings or Condiments Unless Indicated	C	F	Cb
American Cheese	350	11	45
BLT	455	19	50
Chicken Salad with Tomatoes	500	23	55
Italian	365	10	47
Rst Beef w/ Lettuce, Tom., Olives., On.	310	5	50
Tuna Salad w. Lettuce, Tom., Pickles	465	18	57
Turkey & Provolone	395	12	48
Hot Subz: Per 6" White Sub, Without Cheese, Toppings or Condiments Unless Indicated			
Chicken & American Cheese	470	15	45
Meatball with Marinara Sauce	380	13	49
Pepperoni	440	20	45
Steak & Swiss Cheese	535	19	47
Ciabataz: Without Cheese, Toppings or Condiments Unless Indicated			
Chicken Salad	480	25	51
Deli with Provolone Cheese	475	23	45
Ham & Swiss Cheese	410	15	46
Tuna Salad w/ Lettuce, Tom., Pickles	455	20	54
Turkey w/ Provolone, Lettuce & Tom.	395	14	47
Hot Dogz: Without Cheese, Toppings Or Condiments Unless Indicated			
Hot Dogz with Chili & Onions	310	19	27
Nachoz:			
Nachoz Bueno with Nacho Cheese	515	23	65
Nachoz Grande with Nacho Cheese	515	23	65
Saladz: Without Dressing			
Chef with Shredded Cheese	250	12	13
Crispy Chicken w/ Shredded Chse	370	16	31
Garden with Shredded Cheese	130	8	8
Grilled Chicken	145	4	7
Steak	210	8	8
Taco with Shredded Cheese	355	10	38
Sidez:			
Chili, Mac & Cheese	130	6	14
Cole Slaw	200	9	28
Fryz: Bag, 3¼ oz	160	6	23
Cup, 5 oz	260	10	36
Cheese, 14½ oz	670	32	81
Smokehouse, 15¼ oz	985	53	103
Coffeez™: Per 16 fl.oz			
Capo'ccino: Creme Burlee	280	8	50
Fat-Free French Vanilla	140	0	34
Hot Chocolate, medium	250	4	52

Updated Nutrition Data ~ www.CalorieKing.com
Persons with Diabetes ~ See Disclaimer (Page 22)

Shoney's® (Nov '10)

Breakfast

	C	F	Cb
Off The Grill: *Per Plate*			
Bacon, Egg & Cheddar Croissant	790	57	30
Sirloin Steak & Eggs	580	36	3
Platters: Pancakes, with Bacon	665	11	110
with Sausage Patties	775	21	110
Skillets: Big Biscuit	980	56	93
Fiesta	1030	76	42
Sunrise Special	1470	62	191

Lunch/Dinner:

	C	F	Cb
Starters: Angus Steak Chili	620	37	50
Chicken Enchilada Soup	445	22	50
Chicken Strips	1270	84	87
Onion Rings, Jumbo	980	69	102
Burgers: *Without Sides*			
All American	1160	93	40
BBQ Bacon Cheeseburger	1470	117	45
Classic	1360	111	40
Mushroom Swiss	1195	89	42
Chicken: *Without Sides*			
Sandwiches: Blackened Chicken	720	36	40
Grilled Chicken Sandwich	720	36	40
Croissant, Chicken Salad	645	33	39
Classic Sandwiches: *Without Sides*			
Philly Cheese Steak	1140	74	61
Reuben	835	45	44
Slim Jim	695	36	57
Turkey Club	1250	83	60
Croissant, BLT	580	48	26

Entrees: *With Standard Sides Unless Indicated*

	C	F	Cb
Chicken: Blackened w/ BBQ Sauce	585	18	39
With Honey Mustard	785	44	33
Chicken Strips	1320	88	91
Grilled with BBQ Sauce	450	20	14
With Honey Mustard	650	46	22
Fish: Fish & Chips Basket	1310	74	102
Fish Sandwich, without sides	1190	63	105
Grilled Salmon	515	34	27
Pan-Blackened Catfish Fry	915	60	66
Southern Catfish Fry	1465	78	137
Pasta: Baked Spaghetti	1460	54	145
Lasagna: Half Portion	730	44	58
Full Portion	1140	65	93
Skillets:			
Artichoke & Crabmeat Casserole	1410	80	134
Lemon Chicken w/ Mshrm & Rice	1220	67	91
Slow-Cooked Pot Roast	835	45	57

Shoney's® cont... (Nov '10)

Entrees (Cont): *With Standard Sides*

	C	F	Cb
Steak: Half-O-Pound	1325	103	62
Porterhouse Steak, 16 oz	2170	136	97
Ribeye, 10 oz	1485	90	97
Smothered Liver & Onions	775	46	48
Steakhouse Sirloin, 8 oz	1380	83	97
T-Bone, 12 oz	1725	110	100
Salads: *Entrée* Fried Chicken	1095	70	93
Grilled Chicken	1060	56	70
Salmon	870	60	49
Kid's Menu: Cheeseburger	790	56	41
Fish Wrap	490	32	25
Grilled Cheese	450	32	24
Mac & Cheese	965	54	83
Sides: Baked Potato, plain	225	0	51
Biscuit (1)	190	9	23
Fries: Chili Cheese Fries	680	42	61
French	520	30	56
Homefries	120	6	15
Fruit Bowl	60	0	15
Garlic Grecian Bread, 1 slice	330	24	23
Loaded Potato Mix	115	13	8
Mashed Potatoes	240	11	31
Onion Rings	490	35	51
Wild Rice	150	4	25
Desserts: Apple Crisp	810	38	81
Hot Fudge Cake	710	30	101
Key Lime Cheesecake	830	58	74
Pies: Peanut Butter, 1 slice	570	35	57
Strawberry, 1 slice	350	13	53
Sundaes: Banana Split	545	21	93
Hot Fudge	535	25	68
Peach	370	17	46
Strawberry	375	17	47

Sizzler® (Nov '10)

Burgers & Sandwiches:

	C	F	Cb
Burgers: Mega Bacon Chseburger	1010	61	48
Sizzler Burger: 1/3 lb	620	30	47
1/2 lb	760	40	47
Sandwiches: Grilled Chicken Club	665	31	48
Malibu Chicken	645	32	57

Hot Entrees: *Without Sides, Dipping Sauces & Condiments Unless Indicated*

	C	F	Cb
Chicken: Hibachi Chkn Breast (1)	200	7	7
With Hibachi Sauce, 1 oz	245	7	17
Lemon-Herb Chicken Breast	215	11	1
With Lemon Herb Sauce, 1 oz	260	15	2

Continued Next Page ...

Sizzler® cont... (Nov '10)

Hot Entrees: Without Sides, Dipping Sauces & Condiments Unless Indicated

	C	F	Cb
Seafood: Gr. Salmon w/ Rice Pilaf	545	26	42
Fish 'n Chips	1035	49	111
Fisherman's Platter	820	34	82
Gr. Shrimp Fettuccine Alfredo	985	55	64
Shrimp: Grilled Skewers (2)	545	26	42
Shrimp Fry (12)	435	12	48
Shrimp, Shrimp, Shrimp	970	41	92
Steaks: Bacon Wrapped Sirloin	555	35	5
Classic, 8 oz	320	14	2
Classic Trio	700	32	32
Porterhouse, 18 oz	1365	107	1
Rib Eye, 12 oz	950	62	1
Ultimate Sizzlin' Trio	1420	87	92

Prepared Salads: Per 4oz Serving w/out Dressing

Ambrosia	125	4	22
Caesar	50	4	2
Carrot Raisin	110	6	12
Creamy Cole Slaw	70	4	6
Greek	45	4	2
Macaroni	225	12	27
Potato	325	27	18
Seafood	160	11	11

Salad Dressings: Per 2 Tbsp, 1 oz

Honey Mustard	110	8	9
Italian, Low Fat	40	3	3
Ranch	115	12	1
Signature Blue Cheese	105	11	1
Thousand Island	95	9	5

Salad Bar Items: Bacon Bits, 2 oz	110	6	6
Cottage Cheese, 2 oz	50	2	2
Garbanzo Beans, 2 oz	50	0	8
Kidney Beans, 2 oz	50	0	8
Peas, 2 oz	30	0	6
Turkey Ham, 2 oz	75	6	2

Sides: W/out Condiments/Toppings

Baked Potato	265	4	51
Brocoli, 5 oz	50	0	7
Cheese Toast, 1 slice	235	19	13
French Fries, 5 oz	285	13	42
Fresh Baked Roll	165	1	33
Rice Pilaf, 5 oz	225	4	39

Soups: Per 6 oz Bowl

Chicken Noodle	100	2	14
Clam Chowder	325	18	35
French Onion	55	2	6
Minestrone	70	1	14
Split Pea	115	1	19

Dessert Bar: Chocolate Syrup, 1 oz	90	0	21
Choc/Vanilla Soft Serve, 4 oz	135	4	24

For Complete Menu & Data ~ see CalorieKing.com

Skyline Chili® (Nov '10)

Burritos:

	C	F	Cb
All Chili Burrito	560	30	37
All Chili Deluxe Burrito	650	35	45

Meals: Per Regular Serving

Black Bean & Rice, 3-Way	800	40	74
Black Bean & Rice, 4-Way	810	40	77
Black Bean & Rice, 5-Way	880	40	89
Black Bean & Rice, Spaghetti	490	12	79
Bowls: Chili	270	16	6
Chili Bean	270	12	17
Chili Cheese	440	30	6
Coney	870	69	9
Loaded Chili	580	40	18
Vegetarian Black Beans & Rice	320	9	46
Chili Spaghetti: Regular	450	18	43
With Beans	520	17	61
With Beans & Onions	530	17	64
Coneys: Regular with Cheese	340	22	17
Without Cheese	220	12	17
Steamed Potatoes: Plain	310	0	72
Cheddar	740	41	72
Chili	440	8	74

Salads: Without Dressing

Buffalo/Classic Chicken, average	150	7	7
Garden	80	5	6
Greek Chicken	170	8	9
Greek	60	4	5
Southwestern Chicken w/ Tortilla Chips	760	44	65

Wraps: Without Dressing

Buffalo/Classic Chicken, average	520	21	55
Greek Chicken	510	21	54
Southwest Chicken	670	30	65
Sides: Cheese	230	19	1
Chili	130	8	3
Crackers, 1 bowl	100	3	20
French Fries	630	33	79

For Complete Nutritional Data ~ see CalorieKing.com

Smoothie King® (Nov '10)

Fruit Smoothies: Per 20 fl.oz Cup
Figures Include Turbinado. Without Turbinado, deduct 100 calories and 23 carbs.

	C	F	Cb
Build Up, High Protein Smoothies:			
Almond Mocha	365	9	42
Banana	320	9	32
Chocolate	365	9	42
Get Energy: Acai Adventure	435	5	92
Go Goji	435	0	104
Green Tea Tango	280	3	52

Continued on Next Page....

Smoothie King® cont...(Nov '10)

Fruit Smoothies: Per 20 fl.oz Cup
Figures Include Turbinado. Without Turbinado,
deduct 100 calories and 23 carbs.

	C	F	Cb
Snack Right: Banana Berry Treat	365	0	86
Berry Punch	360	0	91
Fruit Fusion	355	1	76
Grape Expectations	400	0	95
Stay Healthy: Cranberry Cooler	495	0	120
Cranberry Supreme	555	1	130
Mangosteen Madness	385	0	94
Orange KA-BAM	465	0	117
Trim Down: Blackberry Dream	365	1	88
MangoFest	285	0	72
Muscle Punch	365	1	84
Passion Passport	395	0	96
Peach Slice	315	0	72
Raspberry Collider	340	0	86
Raspberry Sunrise	390	0	95
Slim-N-Trim: Chocolate	295	2	57
Orange Vanilla	215	1	46
Strawberry	375	1	84
Strawberry Kiwi Breeze	375	0	90
Youth Fountain	255	0	61
The Shredder: Chocolate	310	3	36
Strawberry	355	1	56
Youth Fountain	255	0	61

32 fl.oz Cup: Multiply 20 fl.oz figures by 1.5
40 fl.oz Cup: Multiply 20 fl.oz figures by 2

Kids Kup Smoothies

	C	F	Cb
Berry Interesting	275	0	69
Choc-A-Laka	245	3	44
Gimme-Grape	265	0	64
Smarti Tarti	200	0	49

Snappy Tomato (Nov '10)

Pizza: Per Slice, ⅛ of Pizza	C	F	Cb
Buffalo Grilled Chicken	250	8	32
Cheese Pizza	220	7	30
Hawaiian Pizza	370	18	33
Meat Topper	430	23	31
Pepperoni Pizza	340	17	31
Ranch Pizza	370	21	31
Snapperoni Pizza	390	22	31
Supreme Pizza	340	17	32
Veggie Pizza	240	8	33
Oven Baked Hoagie Sandwiches: *W/o Toppings, Sauce/Dressing*			
Grilled Chicken	490	11	71
Steak & Cheese	670	28	73
Snappetizers: *Without Sauce*			
Snappy Wings (2), 3 oz	150	5	12

Sonic Drive-In® (Nov '10)

Burgers	C	F	Cb
Sonic: With Mayonnaise	655	37	55
With Mustard	550	26	54
Bacon Cheeseburger	785	48	57
Cheeseburger: With Mayonnaise	720	42	56
Super Sonic with Mayonnaise	985	64	58
Green Chili Cheeseburger	630	31	56
Jalapeno	555	26	55
Jr.	315	15	30
Jr. Deluxe	350	20	28
Thousand Island Burger	610	32	56
Coneys/Toaster Sandwiches/Wraps			
Coneys: Extra-Long Chili Cheese (1)	660	39	55
Corn Dog (1)	215	11	23
Toaster Sandwiches: Chicken Club	740	46	55
Bacon Cheeseburger	670	39	52
Wraps: Crispy Chicken	485	23	49
Grilled Chicken	390	14	39
Fritos Chili Cheese	670	39	66
Chicken: Chicken Strip Dinner (4)	930	43	100
Jumbo Popcorn Chicken:			
Small, without Sauce, 4 oz	380	22	27
Large, without Sauce, 6 oz	560	32	41
Salads: *Without Dressing*			
Crispy Chicken	340	19	24
Grilled Chicken	250	10	12
Dressings: Honey Mustard, 2 oz	180	16	10
Italian Fat-Free, 2 oz	40	0	10
Light Ranch, 2 oz	110	5	14
Original Ranch, 2 oz	190	20	2
Sides: *Per Medium Serving*			
French Fries: Plain 4 oz	330	13	48
With Cheese 5 oz	420	21	51
With Chili & Cheese, 7 oz	490	27	54
Mozzarella Sticks, w/o sauce, 5 oz	440	22	40
Onion Rings, 5½ oz	440	21	55
Tater Tots: Plain, 2½ oz	200	13	20
With Cheese, 3½ oz	300	21	22
With Chili & Cheese, 5½ oz	370	27	26
Breakfast			
Burritos: Bacon, Egg & Cheese	450	27	38
Sausage, Egg & Cheese	480	31	38
SuperSonic	570	36	48
French Toast Sticks: with Syrup (4)	580	31	70
without Syrup (4)	500	31	49
Sandwiches			
CroiSonic: Bacon	510	36	29
Sausage	600	46	29
Toaster: Bacon, Egg & Cheese	530	32	40
Sausage, Egg & Cheese	620	42	40

Continued Next Page ...

Sonic Drive-In® cont... (Nov '10)

Desserts: *Per Regular*

	C	F	Cb
Banana Split	510	18	80
Vanilla Cone	250	13	31

Floats/Blended: *Regular*

	C	F	Cb
Diet Coke; Diet Dr Pepper	260	14	29
Coca-Cola	330	14	49

Fruit Smoothies: Strawb., reg.

	C	F	Cb
Strawb., reg.	500	0	124
Strawberry-Banana, regular	460	0	113

Shakes: Banana, regular

	C	F	Cb
Banana, regular	500	26	60
Chocolate, regular	560	26	74
Pineapple; Strawberry, reg. av.	525	26	67

Single Topping Sundaes: *Regular*

	C	F	Cb
Chocolate	490	22	67
Hot Fudge	520	27	63
Pineapple	450	22	58
Sonic Blast, average, regular	730	38	87

Drinks: Barq's Root Beer, 20 fl.oz

	C	F	Cb
Barq's Root Beer, 20 fl.oz	190	0	52
Cranberry Juice: Regular	170	0	46
Large, 20 fl.oz	210	0	56

For Complete Nutritional Data ~ see CalorieKing.com

Souplantation® (Nov '10)

Soups: *Per Cup*

	C	F	Cb

Regular Soup:

	C	F	Cb
Chesapeake Corn Chowder	290	17	30
Classical Minestrone	120	2	20
Cream of Mushroom	290	24	15
New Mexican Corn with Chicken	200	10	19
Vegetarian Harvest	200	10	23

Breads: Sourdough

	C	F	Cb
Sourdough	150	0.5	27
Buttermilk Cornbread, 1 piece	140	2	27

Focaccia, Garlic Asiago

	C	F	Cb
Garlic Asiago	160	8	19

Hot Tossed Pastas: *Per Cup*

	C	F	Cb
Creamy Bruschetta	360	16	43
Garden Vegetable with Meatballs	310	10	44
Vegetarian Marinara with Basil	260	4	44

Prepared Salads: *Per ½ Cup*

	C	F	Cb
BBQ Potato	170	9	21
Carrot Raisin	90	3	17
Dijon Potato with Garlic Dill Vinegar	150	12	9
Greek Couscous w/ Feta & Pinenuts	210	10	25
Thai Noodle with Peanut Sauce	190	10	18

Dressing & Croutons: *Per 2 Tbsp*

	C	F	Cb
Balsamic Vinaigrette	180	19	1
Blue Cheese Dressing	130	13	3
Honey Mustard Dressing	150	13	8
Fat Free	25	0	7
Italian Dressing, Fat-Free	45	0	10
Ranch Dressing	150	15	4
Fat Free	50	0	2
Thousand Island Dressing	90	9	3
Croutons, Garlic Parmesan, 5 pieces	80	5	6

Souplantation® cont... (Nov '10)

Muffins:

	C	F	Cb
Chocolate Brownie	180	8	26
Fruit Medley Bran	130	0.5	29
Blueberry/Lemon	140	4	24

Desserts: *Per ½ Cup*

	C	F	Cb
Apple Cobbler	360	10	67
Apple Medley	70	0	18
Banana Royale	80	0	20
Rice Pudding	110	2	20
Vanilla Pudding	150	4	27
Chocolate Chip Cookie, small	75	3	10
Chocolate Lava Cake, ½ cup	330	8	62
Chocolate Syrup, 2 Tbsp	110	3	20
Granola Topping, 2 Tbsp	110	4	16

For Complete Nutritional Data ~ see CalorieKing.com

Southern Tsunami® (Nov '10)

Sushi: *Per Pack*

	C	F	Cb
Blue Crab Roll, 9 oz	455	14	63
Classic Miso Roll, 11 oz	465	9	64
California Roll w/ Brown Rice, 9½ oz	305	7	53
Cream Cheese Roll, 10 oz	530	20	64
Crunchy Shrimp Roll, 10¼ oz	520	20	69
Dragon Roll: (Seawater Eel), 10 oz	470	14	72
Eel Roll (Freshwater Eel), 10 oz	505	16	69
Eel Roll (Sea Eel), 10 oz	450	11	71
M&M Roll: Shrimp & Avocado, 7½ oz	335	5	62
Tuna & Cucumber, 8 oz	320	1	60
Marina Plate, 7¾ oz	380	7	57
Meteor Special, 9¼ oz	395	3	73
Nigiri: Fish Roe, 1 piece,1½ oz	60	0	10
Fresh Salmon, 1 piece, 1¼ oz	70	1	9
Fresh Water Eel, 1 piece, 1½ oz	100	4	11
Octopus, 1 piece, 1 oz	60	1	9
Sea Eel, 1 piece, 1½ oz	85	3	11
Shrimp, 1 piece, 1 oz	45	0	9
Smoked Salmon, 1 piece, 2 oz	95	1	16
Tilapia, 1 piece, 1 oz	50	1	9
Tuna, 1 piece, 1 oz	50	0	7
Yellowtail, 1 piece, 1¼ oz	55	1	9
Ocean Crab Roll, 10 oz	415	8	66
Orange Roll, 10½ oz	405	6	71
Rainbow Roll, 12½ oz	500	8	70
Spicy Roll: Baby Shrimp, 9¾ oz	420	8	68
Salmon, 10 oz	485	14	64
Tuna, 10 oz	460	9	64
Tempura Roll, 11 oz	540	11	87
Tsunami Roll, 9 oz	470	12	74
Vegetable Combo: 12 pieces, 9½ oz	355	6	68

Updated Nutrition Data ~ www.CalorieKing.com
Persons with Diabetes ~ See Disclaimer (Page 22)

Spaghetti Warehouse® (Nov '10)

Appetizers: Per Serving	C	F	Cb
Bruschetta	550	37	48
Garlic Cheese Bread	1330	90	81
Mozz. Fritta w/ Tomaato Sce & Ranch	930	60	66
Stuffed Mushrooms	310	19	14
Toasted Ravioli w/ Tomato Sauce	980	46	106
Meals: Without Soup, Salad or Bread			
Baked Penne	780	37	81
Chicken Alfredo	760	25	76
Chicken Florentine	990	47	91
Chicken Tettrazini	690	19	85
Fettuccini Alfredo	600	24	76
Four Cheese Manicotti	810	41	70
Seafood Mediterranean	680	26	84
Shrimp Alfredo	700	25	78
Spaghetti: With Beer Chili	450	8	75
With Italian Sausage	670	18	82
With Marinara Sauce	400	4	76
With Meatballs	770	27	91
With Meat Sauce	500	8	83
Feasts: Fettuccini	1430	80	120
Lasagna	1650	96	109
Spaghetti	1270	62	122
Ultimate Italian	1500	76	120

Starbucks® (Nov '10)

Brewed Coffee	C	F	Cb
Figures based on 16 fl.oz Grande Without Whipped Cream			
Latte Misto (Au Lait): W/ Whole Milk	130	7	9
With Nonfat Milk	70	0	10
With Soy Milk	100	3	12
Espresso Hot			
Caffe Americano	15	0	3
Caffe Latte: With Whole Milk	220	11	18
With Nonfat Milk	130	0	19
With Soy Milk	170	4.5	23
Caffe Mocha: WithWhole Milk	290	12	40
With Nonfat Milk	220	2.5	42
With Soy Milk	250	6	45
Cappuccino: With Whole Milk	140	7	11
With Nonfat Milk	80	0	12
With Soy Milk	110	3	15
Caramel Macchiato: W/ Whole Milk	270	10	34
With Nonfat Milk	190	1	35
Cinn. Dolce Latte: With Whole Milk	290	10	39
With Nonfat Milk	210	0	41
Espresso: 1 doppio, 2 fl.oz	10	0	2
1 solo, 1 fl.oz	5	0	1
Con Panna, 1 fl.oz	30	2.5	2

Starbucks® (Nov '10)

Espresso Iced	C	F	Cb
Figures Based on 16 fl.oz Grande Without Whipped Cream			
Caffe Americano	15	0	3
Caffe Latte: With Whole Milk	150	7	12
With Nonfat Milk	90	0	13
With Soy Milk	120	3	17
Caffe Mocha: With Whole Milk	220	8	35
With Nonfat Milk	170	2.5	36
With Soy Milk	200	4.5	38
White Choc. Mocha: W/ Whole Milk	430	15	60
With Nonfat Milk	350	6	61
With Soy Milk	390	9	65
Frappuccino Blended Coffee:			
Figures For 16 fl.oz Frappuccino's			
Based On Whole Milk, Without Whipped Cream, Unless Indicated			
Caffe Vanilla	300	3	66
Caramel	260	3	55
Cinnamon Dolce; Coffee	240	3	51
Coffee	240	3	50
Double Chocolaty Chip	290	8	53
Espresso	190	2.5	38
Java Chip	320	7	65
Mocha	260	3.5	54
White Chocolate Mocha	300	4.5	59
Frappuccino Blended Creme: With Whipped Cream			
Cinnamon Dolce	350	16	49
Strawberries & Creme	450	17	70
White Chocolate	610	19	92
Tazo Green Tea	440	16	70
Vanilla Bean	390	16	58
Frappuccino Light Blend: With Skimmed Milk			
Caffe Vanilla	170	0	42
Caramel; Cinnamon Dolce	130	0	32
Java Chip	200	3.5	42
Mocha	140	1	34
Tazo Iced Tea Drinks:			
Black/Green/Passion, Shaken	80	0	21
Black/Green/Passion, Lemonade	130	0	33
Vivanno Smoothies:			
Chocolate with 2% Milk	270	4.5	48
Orange Mango with 2% Milk	260	1.5	52
Strawberry with 2% Milk	280	2	54
Kid's Drinks & Others: Per 12 fl.oz unless indicated			
Apple Juice	190	0	48
Apple Juice, Steamed, 8 fl.oz	110	0	28
Hot Chocolate, 2% Milk w/ Whip	290	13	39
White Hot Choc., 2% Milk w/ Whip	380	15	48

Continued Next Page ...

Starbucks® cont... (Nov '10)

Drink Extras:	C	F	Cb
Caramel Drizzle, 1 teaspoon	15	0.5	3
Flavored Syrup: 1 Tbsp	35	0	9
Sugar-Free, 1 Tbsp	0	0	0
Mocha Sauce, 1 Tbsp	25	0.5	6
Sweetened Whipped Cream:			
Grande/Venti, Cold, 1 oz	110	11	3
Grande/Venti, Hot, 1 oz	70	7	2
Breakfast Specialities:			
Bacon, Gouda on Artisan Roll	380	20	31
Egg White, Spinach, Feta Wrap	280	10	33
Egg White/Turkey Bacon S'wich	340	10	47
Ham, Cheddar on Artisan Roll	370	16	32
Oatmeal, 1¼ oz	140	2.5	25
with brown sugar, ½ oz	190	2.5	38
Sandwiches, Panini & Wraps:			
Chicken & Vegetable Wrap	290	9	36
Egg Salad	490	22	54
Tarragon Chicken Salad	480	11	62
Tuna Melt Panini	390	12	49
Turkey & Swiss with Mayo	390	13	36
8-Grain Roll, Plain	350	8	67
Bagels: Asiago	310	4.5	54
Multigrain	320	4	62
Plain	300	1	64
Bars & Brownies: Blueberry Oat Bar	370	14	47
Double Chocolate Brownie	410	24	46
Marshmallow Dream Bar	210	4	43
Rich Toffee Pecan Bar	380	22	42
Cakes: Per Slice			
Pound: Iced Lemon, 4½ oz	490	23	68
Marble, 3¾ oz	350	13	53
Raspberry Swirl, 4½ oz	430	16	67
Starbucks Classic Coffee Cake, 4 oz	440	19	63
Reduced Fat Cakes:			
Banana Chocolate Chip	390	7	79
Cinnamon Swirl	340	9	62
Very Berry	350	10	58
Cookies: Chocolate Chunk	360	17	50
Outrageous Oatmeal	370	14	56
Croissants: Butter	310	18	32
Chocolate	300	17	34
Doughnuts: Chocolate	420	21	57
Old-Fashioned Glazed	420	21	57
Muffins: Apple Bran	350	9	64
Blueberry Streusel	360	11	59
Zucchini Walnut	490	28	52
Scones: Blueberry	460	22	61
Maple Oat Pecan	440	18	59
Petite Vanilla Bean	140	5	21

Starbucks® cont... (Nov '10)

Sweet Rolls & Danish	C	F	Cb
Apple Fritter	420	20	59
Cheese Danish	420	25	39
Double Iced Cinnamon Roll	490	20	70
Morning Bun	350	16	45
Parfaits: Dark Cherry Yogurt, 8 oz	310	4	61
Greek Yogurt & Honey, 6 oz	290	12	43
Strawb. & Blueb. Yogurt, 8 oz	300	3.5	60

Ice Cream ~ See Page 106
For Bottled Drinks ~ See Page 37
Coffee Mix (VIA) ~ See Page 35

Steak Escape® (Nov '10)

Sandwiches & Burgers	C	F	Cb
7" Sandwiches: Cajun Chicken	410	5	58
Classic Italian	470	11	60
Vegetarian	310	1	65
Turkey Club	380	2	62
Wild West BBQ	455	6	60
12" Sandwiches: Cajun Chicken	630	10	80
Classic Italian Sub	760	22	85
Vegetarian	440	2	93
Turkey Club	580	3	88
Wild West BBQ	730	12	84
Kids Sandwiches: Chicken	205	7	29
Ham or Turkey	185	1	31
Steak	210	3	29
Grilled Salads: Side Salad	40	0.5	8
With Chicken or Steak, average	180	6	11
With Ham or Turkey	130	2	8
Fresh Cut Fries:			
Kids Meal Fries, 3 oz	250	13	34
12 oz cup	500	26	67
16 oz cup	650	34	87
Loaded French Fries:			
Bacon & Cheddar, 10¾ oz	905	44	88
Ranch & Bacon, 10¾ oz	1045	71	84
Kids Chicken Tenders (2)	240	11	21
Portions: Chicken, 8 oz	240	8	0
Ham; Turkey, 6 oz	150	1	6
Steak, 8 oz	260	10	0
Smashed Potatoes: Plain, 13¾ oz	245	0	53
With Chicken, 20 oz	385	4	56
With Ham or Turkey, 20 oz	340	2	59
With Steak, 20 oz	395	5	56
With Turkey, 20 oz	340	2	59

For Complete Nutritional Data ~ see CalorieKing.com

Updated Nutrition Data ~ www.CalorieKing.com
Persons with Diabetes ~ See Disclaimer (Page 22)

Steak 'n Shake® (Nov '10)

	C	F	Cb
The Original Steakburgers:			
Single	280	11	30
Double 'n Cheese	440	25	31
Triple	510	30	30
Bacon 'n Cheese Double	480	28	31
Cheesy Cheddar	480	27	32
Guacamole	770	55	47
Spicy Chipotle	710	49	42
Chili: 3-Way, 1 bowl	830	36	94
5-Way, 1 bowl	1170	63	99
Deluxe, 1 bowl	1220	74	81
Sandwiches: Grilled Chicken	470	23	51
Spicy Chicken	560	29	51
Turkey Club	420	16	45
Salads: Without Dressing:			
Apple Walnut Grilled Chicken	410	17	45
Fried Chicken	470	26	34
Grilled Chicken	270	10	30
French Fries: Regular	440	21	60
Large	640	30	87
Cheese: Regular	610	34	67
Large	1170	67	117
Soups: Per 6 fl.oz Cup, without Crackers or Toppings			
Chicken Gumbo	70	1.5	11
Vegetable	60	1.5	12
Breakfast: Bacon Strips (4)	110	9	2
Bacon Bagel	390	12	51
Biscuit & Sausage Gravy	560	29	60
Classic Stack O' Cakes w/ Bacon	810	21	137
Cheddar Scrambler	530	37	17
Hash Browns (6)	310	21	27
Sausage Patties (2)	450	41	2
Sourdough: Sausage Melt	900	69	34
Steakburger Melt	680	47	32
Apple Pie à la mode	640	33	80
Sundaes: Chocolate Chip Cookie	840	43	107
Hot Fudge	540	29	64
Strawberry	390	22	47
Walnut Brownie Fudge	820	42	106
Coke Float	520	22	74
Shakes: Per Regular			
Banana; Mocha	700	23	111
Butterfinger	910	31	146
Chocolate; Vanilla, average	700	23	112
Cookies 'n Cream	1010	34	163

Subway® (Nov '10)

	C	F	Cb
6" Sandwiches (6g Fat or Less)			

Figures based on 9-grain wheat bread and toppings: lettuce, tomato, onion, green peppers and cucumbers. **Cheese, oil or mayo not included.**

	C	F	Cb
Black Forest Ham	290	4.5	48
Oven Roasted Chicken Breast	320	4.5	49
Roast Beef	310	4.5	46
Subway Club	320	5	48
Sweet Onion Chicken Teriyaki	380	4.5	60
Turkey Breast	280	3.5	47
Turkey Breast & Black Forest Ham	300	4	48
Veggie Delite	230	2.5	45

6" Toasted Sandwiches: *Figures based on 9-grain wheat bread, lettuce, tomato, onion, green peppers, cucumbers and cheese.* **Oil or mayo not included.**

	C	F	Cb
Big Philly Cheesesteak	520	18	54
BLT	360	13	45
Chicken & Bacon Ranch	570	28	49
Italian B.M.T.	450	20	48
Meatball Marinara	580	23	71
Spicy Italian	520	28	48
Subway Melt	380	11	49
The Feast	540	22	51
Tuna	530	30	46

Flatbread Sandwiches (8g Fat or Less): *Figures based on flatbread, lettuce, tomatoes, onions, green peppers and cucumbers. Cheese, oil or mayo not included.*

	C	F	Cb
Black Forest Ham	320	7	47
Oven Roasted Chicken Breast	350	8	48
Roast Beef	340	8	46
Subway Club	350	8	47
Sweet Onion Teriyaki	410	7	60
Turkey Breast	310	6	47
Turkey Breast & Black Forest Ham	330	7	48
Veggie Delite	260	5	45

Low-Fat Footlong Sandwiches: *Figures based on 9-grain wheat bread, lettuce, tomato, onion, green peppers and cucumbers.* **Cheese, oil or mayo not included.**

	C	F	Cb
Black Forest Ham	570	9	95
Oven Roasted Chicken Breast	640	9	98
Roast Beef	630	9	92
Subway Club	640	10	96
Sweet Onion Chicken Teriyaki	760	9	121
Turkey Breast & Black Forest Ham	590	8	96
Veggie Delight	460	4.5	91

Continued Next Page ...

Subway® cont... (Nov '10)

Kid's Meals Sandwiches: **C** **F** **Cb**

Kids Pak Figures based on 9-grain wheat bread, lettuce, tomatoes, onions, green peppers.

	C	F	Cb
Black Forest Ham	180	2.5	31
Roast Beef	200	3	30
Turkey Breast	190	2.5	31

6" Breakfast Omelet Sandwiches: Figures based on regular egg and 9-grain bread

	C	F	Cb
Double Bacon, Egg & Cheese	520	25	47
Egg & Cheese	420	18	46
Steak, Egg & Cheese	490	20	48
Western Egg & Cheese	450	19	47

Salads (6g Fat or Less)

Includes lettuce, tomato, onions, green peppers, olives, cucumber. No Dressing or Croutons.

	C	F	Cb
Black Forest Ham	110	3	12
Oven Roasted Chicken Strips	130	2.5	10
Roast Beef	140	3.5	10
Subway Club	140	3.5	12
Sweet Onion Chicken Teriyaki	200	3	25
Turkey Breast	110	2	12
Turkey Breast & Ham	120	3	12
Veggie Delite	50	1	10

Sandwich Components: For 6" Sub or Salad

Cheese: *Per ½ oz*

	C	F	Cb
Cheddar	60	5	0
Processed American, Swiss	40	3.5	1
Pepperjack; Provolone	50	4	0
Shredded Monterey Cheddar	50	4.5	1

Meats: Chicken Strips, 2½ oz

	C	F	Cb
Chicken Strips, 2½ oz	80	1.5	0
Ham, 2 oz	60	2	2
Roast Beef, 2½ oz	80	2.5	1
Seafood Sensation, 2½ oz	190	16	7
Subway Club, 3 oz	90	2.5	2
Tuna, 2½ oz	260	24	0

Sauces & Dressings:

	C	F	Cb
Chipotle Southwest, 1½ Tbsp	100	10	1
Honey Mustard, Fat-Free, 1½ Tbsp	30	0	7
Mayonnaise: 1 Tbsp, ½ oz	110	12	0
Light, 1 Tbsp, ½ oz	50	5	0.5
Mustard, Yellow or Deli Brown. 2 tsp	5	0	0.5
Olive Oil Blend, 1 tsp	45	5	0
Ranch Dressing, 1¼ Tbsp	110	11	1
Sweet Onion, Fat-Free, 1¼ Tbsp	40	0	9

Subway® cont... (Nov '10)

Soups: Per Bowl   **C** **F** **Cb**

	C	F	Cb
Chicken & Dumpling	170	5	23
Chicken Tortilla	110	1.5	11
Chili Con Carne	340	11	35
Chipotle Chicken Corn Chowder	140	3	22
Cream of Potato with Bacon	240	13	26
Fire-Roasted Tomato Orzo	130	1	24
Golden Broccoli & Cheese	180	11	16
Minestrone	90	1	17
New England Style Clam Chowder	150	5	20
Roasted Chicken Noodle	80	2	12
Rosemary Chicken & Dumpling	90	1.5	14
Spanish Style Chicken with Rice	110	2.5	16
Tomato Garden Vegetable w. Rotini	90	0.5	20
Vegetable Beef	100	2	17
Wild Rice with Chicken	230	11	26

Cookies & Desserts

	C	F	Cb
Apple Slices, 1 package, 2½ oz	35	0	9
Chocolate Chip Cookie, 1½ oz	210	10	30
Dannon Light & Fit Yogurt, 6 oz	80	0	16
Oatmeal Raisin Cookie, 1½ oz	200	8	30

Sweet Tomatoes®

~ Same Menu & Data as Souplantation (See Page 242) ~

Swiss Chalet® (Nov '10)

Starters:

	C	F	Cb
Garlic Loaf	650	35	74
Chalet Chicken Wings (8), with sauce	550	34	23
Cheese Perogies (7)	420	10	69
Caesar Salad with Dressing	420	37	16

Burgers/Sandwiches/Wraps: Without Sides

	C	F	Cb
Bacon Cheese Burger,without garnish	890	54	46
Hamburger without garnish	710	39	44
Veggie Burger without garinsh	330	12	52
Chicken on a Kaiser, dark meat	510	14	42
Chicken Quesad. w/o sour crm/salsa	620	23	72

Rotisserie Chicken: *Meat Only*

	C	F	Cb
Double Leg with Skin	630	38	4
Half Chicken, with Skin	610	31	5
Quarter Chicken: Leg, without Skin	220	10	0
Leg meat with Skin	310	19	2
Breast meat without Skin	180	3.5	0
Breast meat with Skin	300	11	3
Chicken Pot Pie, 1 pie	550	34	63
Chicken Stir-Fry: With Rice	750	30	89
Without Rice	430	26	26

From the Grill: Without Sides

	C	F	Cb
BBQ Ribs: Half Rack	650	42	6
Full Rack	1300	85	11

Updated Nutrition Data ~ www.CalorieKing.com
Persons with Diabetes ~ See Disclaimer (Page 22)

Swiss Chalet® cont... (Nov '10)

Entree Salads:	C	F	Cb
Bacon Ranch	530	37	22
Chalet Chopped	440	27	29
Spinach Chicken Salad, w/o tortilla	170	2	14
Dressing/Sauce:			
Caesar Dressing, ½ oz	90	14	0
Chalet Dressing, 1 Tbsp, ½ oz	80	11	1
Chalet Dipping Sauce, 3½ oz	25	1	2
Greek Dressing, ½ oz	70	7	0
Sides: Oven-Baked Potato, 10 oz	220	0	48
Gravy, 4 oz	45	1.5	7
Mashed Potatoes, 5 oz	150	4	27
Sauteed Mushrooms, 6 oz	220	16	11
Seasoned Rice, 6 oz	240	3.5	48
Desserts/Pies: Apple Pie	440	19	65
Caramel Pecan Cheesecake	660	41	68
Chocolate Lava Cake	430	23	53
Coconut Cream Pie	540	33	57
Cranb. Rasp. Frozen Yogurt	110	2	22
Lemon Meringue Pie	400	11	73
Old Fashioned Carrot Cake	610	39	63
Pecan Pie	590	29	79

Taco Bell® (Nov '10)

Burritos	C	F	Cb
Regular:			
½ lb Combo	450	18	52
½ lb Nacho Crunch	520	25	54
7-Layer	510	18	68
Cheesy Bean & Rice	480	21	60
Fresco Style: Bean	340	8	56
Supreme: Chicken	340	8	50
Steak	330	8	49
Grilled Stuft:			
Beef	700	30	79
Chicken	650	24	77
Steak	640	24	76
Supreme: Beef	420	15	52
Chicken	390	12	51
Steak	380	12	51
Chalupas			
Baja: Beef	410	26	31
Chicken	390	23	29
Steak	380	23	29
Nacho Cheese: Beef	370	22	31
Chicken	340	18	0
Steak	330	19	30

Taco Bell® cont... (Nov '10)

Gorditas:	C	F	Cb
Baja: Beef	340	18	30
Chicken	320	15	29
Steak	310	15	28
Nacho Cheese: Beef	290	14	31
Chicken	270	10	30
Steak	260	11	29
Supreme: Beef	300	13	31
Chicken	270	10	29
Steak	270	11	29
Nachos: Regular	330	21	31
BellGrande	770	42	78
Supreme	440	24	42
Tacos: Crunchy Supreme	200	12	15
Double Decker	330	13	38
Supreme	360	15	41
Soft Taco: Beef	210	9	21
Grilled Steak	250	14	20
Ranchero Chicken	270	11	21
Supreme, Beef	240	11	24
Fresco Style: Crunchy	150	7	13
Soft: Beef	180	7	22
Grilled Steak	160	4.5	21
Ranchero Chicken	170	4	22
Specialities:			
Crunchwrap, Supreme	540	21	71
Enchiritos: Beef	370	17	35
Chicken	350	14	34
Steak	340	14	33
MexiMelt	280	14	23
Pizza, Mexican, 7½ oz	540	30	47
Quesadillas: Chicken	520	28	41
Steak	510	28	40
Taco Salads: Chicken Ranch	910	54	71
Chipotle Steak	900	57	70
Fiesta: With Shell	770	41	75
Without Shell	460	24	41
Express with chips	660	34	67
Tortada, Bacon Ranch	570	24	57
Volcano: Burrito	800	42	81
Nachos	1000	62	89
Taco	240	17	14

Continued next page...

Taco Bell® cont... (Nov '10)

Sides	C	F	Cb
Cheesy Fiesta Potatoes, 4¾ oz	270	16	28
Guacamole, 1½ oz	70	6	4
Mexican Rice, 3 oz	130	3.5	21
Pintos 'n Cheese	180	6	19
Salsa, 1½ oz	10	0	2
Sour Cream, Reduced Fat, 1½ oz	60	4	4

Why Pay More!™

	C	F	Cb
Burritos: Bean	370	10	55
Beefy 5 Layer	550	22	69
Caramel Apple Empanada	310	15	39
Cheese Roll-Up	200	10	19
Cinnamon Twists	170	7	26
Crunchy Taco,	170	10	12

Note: Nutritional data for New York residents may vary slightly. Please check Taco Bell website

Taco Cabana® (Nov '10)

Burritos:	C	F	Cb
Bean & Cheese	730	35	77
Black Bean	450	8	82
Stewed Chicken	660	25	73

Flameante Chicken: Per Serving

	C	F	Cb
¼ Chicken Dark Dinner	950	41	82
¼ Chicken White Dinner	800	23	87
½ Chicken Dinner	1250	54	88
Sizzling Fajitas: Chicken Dark	730	21	97
Chicken White	740	20	98
Steak	760	24	98

Tacos:

	C	F	Cb
Crispy: Beef	180	10	11
Chicken	160	7	13
Soft: Bean & Cheese	300	14	32
Beef	230	9	22
Black Bean	200	4	34
Carne Guisada	190	6	21
Chicken	210	7	23

Sides: Per Serving

	C	F	Cb
Black Beans	80	0	14
Borracho Beans	140	3	20
Guacamole, 3 oz	110	9	7
Queso, 3 oz	200	15	5
Refried Beans	250	13	24
Rice	120	0.5	25
Salsa, all types, 1 oz	10	0	1
Ranch Dressing, 1 oz	35	4	1
Sour Cream, 3 oz	160	14	3
Tortillas: 6" Flour	120	3	19
6" Table Corn	70	1	15

Taco Del Mar® (Nov '10)

Mondito Refried Burritos:

C	F	Cb

Per Burrito. Includes Tortilla, Rice, Beans, Meat & Salsa Unless Indicated

	C	F	Cb
Beef, 11 oz	555	19	71
21¾ oz	1070	36	134
Cheese, without meat, 9¾ oz	460	13	69
Chicken, 11 oz	545	17	70
21¾ oz	1030	32	131
Fish, with Cabbage & White Sauce	505	21	61
Pork, 11 oz	545	18	71

Enchiladas: Per Enchilada, Include Tortilla, Meat, Cheese, Rice, Beans, Sauce, Lettuce & Salsa Unless Indicated

	C	F	Cb
Beef, 23½ oz	1030	37	115
Cheese, without meat, 19¾ oz	820	27	112
Chicken, 23½ oz	990	33	113
Pork, 23½ oz	990	35	114

Nachos & Chips: Includes Chips, Cheese, Beans Salsa, Sour Cream & Guacamole

	C	F	Cb
Nachos, refried, 1 tray, 16¾ oz	1190	65	110
Chips & Salsa only, 1 tray 7 oz	590	27	78

Quesadillas: Per Quesadilla. Includes Tortilla, Meat Cheese & Salsa Unless Indicated

	C	F	Cb
Beef, 12½ oz	800	37	66
Cheese, without meat, 10 oz	710	35	63
Chicken, 12½ oz	770	33	64
Pork, 12½ oz	770	35	65

Tacos: Per Taco. Includes Shell, Meat, Cheese, Lettuce & Salsa Unless Indicated

	C	F	Cb
Hard: Beef; Chicken average, 4¾ oz	265	14	17
Fish, 4½ oz	270	15	23
Pork, 4¾ oz	260	14	17
Soft: Beef; Chicken average, 5¾ oz	270	10	28
Fish, 5¾ oz	270	11	34
Pork, 5¾ oz	260	10	28

Taco Salads, Refried: Includes Shell, Beans, Lettuce, Meat, Cheese, Salsa, Sour Cream & Guacamole Unless Indicted

	C	F	Cb
Beef, 21 oz	930	49	75
Chicken, 21 oz	900	45	73
Pork, 21 oz	900	46	74

Sides: Black Beans, 4¼ oz

	C	F	Cb
Black Beans, 4¼ oz	140	2	24
Refried, 4¼ oz	160	3.5	24
Pinto, 4¼ oz	90	0	20
Rice & Pinto, 11 oz	320	3	66
Rice & Black Bean, 11 oz	370	5	69
Rice & Refried Beans, 11oz	390	7	69

Sauce: Enchilada, 3 oz

	C	F	Cb
Enchilada, 3 oz	35	0	7
Guacamole, ¾ oz	40	3.5	2

Desserts: Per 1

	C	F	Cb
Brownie, Oreo, 3¼ oz	400	17	59
Cookies: White Choc. Macadamia	270	16	30
Average all flavors, 2½ oz	240	12	21

Taco John's® (Nov '10)

Burritos:	C	F	Cb
Bean Burrito	360	9	56
Beef Grilled Burrito	600	32	52
Beefy Burrito	440	20	45
Chicken & Potato Burrito	470	19	56
Chicken Grilled Burrito	590	29	50
Combination Burrito	400	14	50
Crunchy Chicken & Potato Burrito	600	28	65
Meat & Potato Burrito	500	23	58
Super Burrito	450	18	54
Tacos: Soft Shell Taco	220	11	21
Taco Bravo	340	13	40
Taco Burger	270	12	28
10 Grams of Fat or Less!			
Crispy	180	10	13
Chili, without Cheese	160	6	17
Soft Shell without Cheese	190	8	20
Specialties: Taco Salad w/o dressing	520	33	37
Chicken Taco Salad w/o dressing	480	27	35
Crunchy Ckn Taco Salad w/o dressing	660	40	47
Super Nachos: Small	450	27	38
Regular	810	48	74
Super Potato Oles: Small	620	39	53
Regular	1030	65	87
Quesadilla Melt: Cheesy	440	23	43
Fajita Beef	540	28	49
Fajita Chicken	510	23	47
Crunchy Chicken without sauce	450	27	24
Snacks: Chips & Queso	430	25	43
Cini-Sopapilla Bites	210	5	37
Sides: Potato Oles: Small	430	26	45
Medium	600	36	62
Large	770	46	80
Kid's Meal portion	290	18	31
Refried Beans: With cheese	320	6	47
Without cheese	260	1.5	47
Mexican Rice	250	6	45
Condiments: Nacho Cheese, 3 oz	120	9	5
Salsa, 2 oz	20	0	4
Sour Cream, 2 oz	120	12	2
House Dressing, 1½ oz	70	7	2
Ranch Dressing, 1½ oz	140	16	3
Desserts: Apple Grande	270	12	39
Choco Taco	390	20	48
Churro	190	7	15

Taco Mayo® (Nov '10)

Burritos:	C	F	Cb
Bean	495	16	71
Beef	490	23	41
Super Beef	540	23	57
Super Chicken	405	16	39
Melts: Tamale	615	34	50
Tostada	525	32	35
Quesadillas: Chicken	675	37	46
Fajita Chicken	700	39	47
Fajita Steak	725	40	47
Tacos: Crispy Taco, Beef	160	9	10
Soft Taco: Beef	230	11	17
Chicken	185	6	16
Salads: Acapulco, Chicken	680	50	35
Steak	705	51	35
SalsaLita Steak	305	8	33
Taco Steak	445	25	30
Sides: Mexicali Rice	160	1	36
Refried Beans	295	9	43
Potato Locos, Small	380	24	36

Taco Time® (Nov '10)

Burritos:	C	F	Cb
Beef, Bean & Cheese	490	17	55
Chicken B.L.T.	690	39	43
Big Juan: Chicken	580	16	70
Ground Beef	630	23	73
Casita: Chicken	490	17	42
Ground Beef	540	24	46
Crisp Burrito: Chicken	380	17	33
Ground Beef	430	21	36
Pinto Bean	360	14	47
Soft Burrito: Beef	430	16	43
Pinto Bean	370	10	54
Veggie	520	17	73
Tacos:			
Soft Tacos: *Per 7 oz Unless Indicated*			
Chicken	360	9	40
Ground Beef	420	16	43
Junior, 5¼ oz	310	13	28
Super Soft Wheat Taco: Beef	590	23	63
Chicken	530	16	60
Other Favorites: Cheddar Melt	250	12	25
Nachos Grande	930	43	96
Tostada: Bean	230	13	21
Chicken	320	13	22
Ground Beef	380	20	25

Continued next page...

Fast - Foods & *Restaurants*

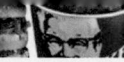

Taco Time® cont... (Nov '10)

Sides	C	F	Cb
Cheddar Fries, med. 7 oz	500	35	39
Mexi Fries®, medium, 6 oz	390	26	38
Mexi-Rice, 3½ oz	80	0.5	17
Stuffed Fries, medium, 7 oz	460	28	42
Refritos with Chips, 6 oz	230	7	29
Salads: Regular: Chkn Taco, 9½ oz	310	13	22
Ground Beef Taco, 9 oz	370	20	24
Tostada Delight: Chicken, 9 oz	450	19	35
Ground Beef, 9 oz	490	26	36
Salsas, Sauces & Dressings			
Chipotle Ranch Dressing, 1 oz	170	18	1
Guacamole, 1 oz	50	4.5	2
Salsa Fresca, 1 oz	10	0	2
Desserts: Churro: Plain	210	16	17
With Cinnamon & Sugar	250	16	27
Crustos	290	6	58
Empanada, average	240	7	41

Target Food Court (Nov '10)

Entrees:	C	F	Cb
Beef Hot Dog	380	23	27
Bratwurst	400	24	27
Chicken Tenders	220	8	18
Italian Sausage	440	29	27
Jalapeno & Cheddar Sausage	410	26	26
Kids: Chicken Nuggets	180	12	9
Hot Dog	330	19	28
Macaroni & Cheese	310	12	39
Mini Beef Hot Dogs	320	15	34
Sandwiches: Ham & Cheddar	460	14	48
Pita Melts, average	240	10	23
Turkey & Provolone	440	12	51
Turkey Club	570	27	44
Salads: California	600	32	44
Chicken Caesar	560	36	19
Soups: Broccoli & Cheese	190	11	16
Chicken Noodle	130	1	18
Snacks: French Fries	230	9	33
Nachos with Cheese & Jalapenos	530	25	67
Popcorn	300	16	32
Yogurt Parfait	300	8	50
Treats: Blueberry Muffin	410	18	56
Brownie	340	15	45
Chocolate Chip Cookie	510	26	68
Cinnamon Roll	480	20	65
Pretzels: Bavarian with Butter	490	6	93
Cheddar	540	15	87
Smoothies: Mango	220	0	54
Strawberry	250	0	62

For Complete Nutritional Data ~ see CalorieKing.com

TCBY® (Nov '10)

Soft Serve Frozen Yogurt: Per 4 oz	C	F	Cb
Average all flavors	110	2	23
Golden Vanilla	120	2	23
Peanut Butter Cup	130	2	26
No Sugar Added, Fat Free:			
Average all flavors	80	0	22
Sorbet: *Per 4 oz (½ Cup)*			
Average all flavors	100	0	25
Hand-Scooped Frozen Yogurt			
Butter Pecan: Kid's, 2½ oz	150	7	17
Small, 4 oz	240	11	27
Regular, 8 oz	480	22	54
Large, 11¾ oz	705	32	80
Chocolate Chocolate: Kid's, 2½ oz	120	3	60
Small, 4 oz	190	5	30
Regular, 8 oz	385	10	60
Large, 11¾ oz	565	14	89
Peaches/Strawberries & Cream:			
Kid's, 2½ oz	110	2.5	18
Small, 4 oz	175	4	29
Regular, 8 oz	350	8	58
Large, 11¾ oz	515	12	85
P'nut Butter Delight: Kid's 2½ oz	170	8	21
Small, 4 oz	270	13	34
Regular, 8 oz	540	26	68
Large, 11¾ oz	800	38	99
Vanilla Bean: Kid's, 2½ oz	110	3	18
Small, 4 oz	175	5	29
Regular, 8 oz	350	10	58
Large, 11¾ oz	515	14	85
No Sugar Added Hand-Scooped			
Choc. Choc. Swirl: Kid's, 2½ oz	80	0	20
Small, 4 oz	130	0	32
Regular, 8 oz	260	0	64
Large, 11¾ oz	375	0	94
Vanilla Fudge Brownie: Kid's, 2½ oz	100	2	21
Small, 4 oz	160	3	34
Regular, 8oz	320	6	68
Large, 11¾ oz	470	9	99

Teriyaki Stix® (Nov '10)

Bowls:	C	F	Cb
Chicken	705	8	111
With Vegetables	735	8	118
Curry	705	15	110
Orange Chicken	770	16	113
Veggie	590	0.5	134
Sandwiches: *Without Cheese or Dressing*			
Ham	185	2	30
Roast Beef	260	3	43
Stacked Club	725	17	96
Turkey	270	2.5	44
Smoothies: Jungle Mist	270	0	73
Raspberry Razzle	215	0	57
Watermelon Wave	270	0	71

The Taco Maker® (Nov '10)

Burritos	C	F	Cb
Regular: Bean	405	16	52
Beef	365	12	44
Chicken	505	20	44
Crispy: Bean	395	26	31
Beef	245	5	41
Soft Shell: Beef	365	13	45
Chicken	435	18	46
Max: ½ lb Beef	420	18	51
Nachos: Regular, Cheese	300	23	7
Deluxe: Beef	440	32	13
Chicken	510	36	13
Guacamole	505	40	16
Tacos: Regular: Beef	90	5	3
Chicken	140	9	2
Plates:			
Burrito Grande: Beef	430	17	53
Chicken	500	21	53
Fajita Dinner			
Chicken; Carnitas, average	800	38	72
Fiesta Dinner: Beef	550	23	54
Chicken	765	36	54
Quesadilla Dinner, Cheese	1100	62	95
Taco Salads: *Without Dressing*			
Beef	740	42	49
Chicken	550	23	45
Fries: Regular	150	6	21
Baked Potatoes: Papa Taco: Bean	270	4	54
Beef	445	19	54
Chicken	520	24	54
Potato, Bacon & Cheese	525	27	52
Turkey	505	23	56

ThunderCloud Subs® (Nov '10)

Subs: Small, with Standard Toppings	C	F	Cb
Classic: BLT	405	17	40
Roast Beef	290	6	40
Smoked Chicken	295	4	40
Turkey	280	4	41
Hot Subs: Meatball	650	32	56
Hot Pastrami	430	13	41
Signature Subs: Club	480	19	43
California Club	510	23	45
N.Y. Italian	570	30	42
Office Favorite	850	46	81
Texas Tuna	700	45	44
Veggie Delite, with Hummus	360	10	53

Tim Hortons® (Nov '10)

Breakfast:	C	F	Cb
Sandwiches: *Regular, With Standard Ingredients*			
Bagel BELT	450	14	58
Bacon, Egg & Cheese	420	23	34
Egg & Cheese	370	19	34
Sausage, Egg & Cheese	540	35	35
Hashbrowns, 1¾ oz	100	5	12
Lunch:			
Sandwiches: *Regular, With Standard Ingredients*			
BLT	450	18	53
Chicken Salad	380	9	55
Egg Salad	390	13	52
Ham & Swiss	440	12	56
Toasted Chicken Club	460	7	70
Turkey Bacon Club	440	8	63
Soups: Per 10 oz Bowl			
Chicken Noodle	110	2.5	19
Chili	300	16	18
Cream of Broccoli	160	9	16
Hearty Potato Bacon	250	13	23
Hearty Vegetable	70	0	14
Minestrone	130	1.5	25
Split Pea with Ham	150	2.5	27
Turkey & Wild Rice	120	1.5	24
Vegetable Beef Barley	130	1.5	21

Continued next page...

Tim Hortons® Cont... (Nov '10)

Bagels:	C	F	Cb
Plain	260	1.5	52
Blueberry; Cinnamon Raisin	270	1	55
Everything	280	2	53
Onion	260	1.5	53

Timbits: *Low-Fat*

	C	F	Cb
Cake, Glazed: Chocolate	70	2.5	10
Sour Cream	90	4.5	12
Old Fashion, Plain	70	5	5
Filled, all varieties	60	2	10
Yeast: Apple Fritter	50	1.5	9
Honey Dip	60	2	9

Baked Goods: *Per Serving*

Cookies:

	C	F	Cb
Caramel Chocolate Pecan	230	11	32
Chocolate Chunk	230	9	35
Oatmeal Raisin Spice	220	8	35
Peanut Butter	280	16	27
Triple Chocolate	250	13	31

Donuts:

	C	F	Cb
Cake: Chocolate Glazed	260	10	39
Old Fashioned Plain	260	19	20
Sour Cream Plain	270	17	27
Filled: Blueberry	230	8	36
Boston Cream	250	9	37
Canadian Maple	260	9	41
Strawberry	230	8	36
Honey Cruller	320	19	37
Yeast, Apple Fritter	300	11	49

Desserts:

	C	F	Cb
Low Fat Yogurt: Creamy Vanilla	160	2.5	32
Strawberry	150	2.5	28

Beverages:

	C	F	Cb
Cafe Mocha, 10 fl.oz	160	7	25
Cappuccino: French Vanilla, 10 fl.oz	240	7	39
Iced Original:			
With Small Milk, 10 fl.oz	180	1.5	39
With Small Cream, 10 fl.oz	300	15	41
Coffee w/med. sugar/cream, 10 fl.oz	75	3.5	9
Hot Chocolate, 10 fl.oz	240	6	45

T.J. Cinnamons® (Nov '10)

Bakery	C	F	Cb
Cinnamon Roll, 5¼ oz	505	10	73
Cinnamon Twist (1), 2½ oz	260	14	33
Pecan Sticky Bun: (1), 6½ oz	690	22	91
4-Pack	2750	90	363
Sticky Bun Smear w/ Pecans, 1¼ oz	180	12	18
T.J. Cream Cheese Icing, 1 oz	115	5	18

Beverages: *Per 12 fl.oz Serving*

	C	F	Cb
Mocha Chill: W/o Whipped Cream	265	4	46
With Whipped Cream	305	7	47

Togo's Eatery® (Nov '10)

Sandwiches: *Regular 6" Roll*

	C	F	Cb
Chef's Creations: BBQ Ranch Chkn	750	27	88
Chipotle Roast Beef with Provolone	990	49	66
Pacific Cobb	710	36	68
Pastrami Reuben with Swiss	990	55	67

Cold: *Includes Standard Sides & Mayo Unless Indicated*

	C	F	Cb
Albacore Tuna	660	28	73
Black Forest Ham & Cheese	670	31	67
Chicken Salad with Almonds	650	29	74
Roast Beef & Avocado	720	29	70
The Italian with Canola Oil	860	43	71
Turkey & Avocado	640	26	74
Turkey Bacon Club	680	32	68
Hot: BBQ Beef	670	19	85
Chicken	630	20	72
Hot Pastrami	750	33	69
Meatball	690	27	78
Sicilian Chicken	710	28	73
Vegetarian: Avocado & Cheese	740	40	73
Avocado & Cucumber	560	25	75
Egg Salad & Cheese	750	39	70

Salad Wraps: *Includes Whole Wheat Wrap, Standard Toppings & Dressing*

	C	F	Cb
Asian Chicken with Asian Dressing	670	32	74
BBQ Chicken Ranch w/ Buttmlk Ranch	630	26	77
Cobb with Blue Cheese	680	36	63
Farmer's Market with Balsamic Vin.	440	14	72
Santa Fe Chicken with Spicy Pepitas	800	44	75

Salads: *Per Full Salad, without Dressing*

	C	F	Cb
Asian Chicken	200	9	17
BBQ Chicken Ranch	230	3.5	31
Chicken Caesar	210	6	17
Cobb	330	20	12
Taco, including shell	600	39	36

Tropical Smoothie Cafe® (Nov '10)

Breakfast:	C	F	Cb
Wraps: Early Bird	615	24	68
Western	635	28	57

Lunch:			
Bistro Sandwiches: *Without Cheese & Sauce*			
Cranberry Walnut Chicken Salad	735	40	71
Hummus Veggie	670	26	84
The Italian	460	16	38
Turkey Bacon Ranch	430	13	37
Turkey Guacamole	595	14	75
Ultimate Club	525	19	43
Wasabi Roast Beef	375	11	33
Toasted Wraps: Buffalo Chicken	625	26	60
Jamaican Jerk Chicken	625	17	79
King Caesar	605	29	56
Sesame Chicken	805	23	113
Totally Turkey	615	25	55

Gourmet Salads: *Includes Standard Dressing*			
Cranberry Walnut Chicken	475	38	20
Sesame Chicken	580	19	73
Thai Chicken	500	11	74
TSC Signature	350	13	37

Low Fat Smoothies: *With Turbinado*			
Blimey Limey	470	0	117
Blue Lagoon	330	1	80
Hawaiian Breeze	380	0	92
Island Fever	420	0.5	103
Rockin Raspberry	425	0.5	103
Strawberry Beach	450	0	109
Sunrise Sunset	410	0.5	100

Supercharged: *With Turbinado*			
Health Nut	530	7	92
Lean Machine	470	0.5	115
Muscle Blaster	485	3	91
Peanut Paradise	690	18	99
Stress Defender	465	0	112

Simply Indulgent Smoothies: *With Turbinado*			
Beach Bum	565	5	125
Chocolate Chiller	555	7	117
Peanut Butter Cup	720	21	123
Tropi-Colada	510	5.5	115

With Splenda, deduct 200 calories & 50g carbs

Tubby's® (Nov '10)

Subs: Per Regular Sandwich	C	F	Cb
Burger Subs: Big Tub	670	56	55
Burger Special	900	59	59
Cheeseburger	910	60	59
Pizza Burger	930	60	62
Taco Burger	825	47	67
Deli Subs: Club Sub	700	41	53
Ham & Cheese	570	30	54
Tubby's Famous	665	39	55
Turkey & Cheese	625	32	51
Turkey Club Sub	850	39	83
Specialty Subs: BLT	635	42	50
Cold Veggie	460	14	66
Italian Sausage	730	45	56
Tuna	415	18	47
Veggie Stir Fry	650	27	89
Chicken Subs:			
Chicken & Broccoli	550	23	56
Chicken & Cheddar	545	23	54
Chicken Club Sub	705	41	53
Chicken Fajita Sub	445	12	57
Grilled Chicken	345	5	52
Steak Subs:			
Mushroom Steak	835	26	52
Pepper Steak	710	46	52
Pizza Steak	985	57	85
Steak & Cheese	825	56	51
Steak Special	745	46	58

Uno Chicago Grill® (Nov '10)

Appetizers: Per Single Serve	C	F	Cb
Crispy Cheese Dippers, 3¾ oz	280	16	27
Pizza Skins, ⅕ pizza, 5 oz	410	28	29
Shrimp & Crab Fondue, 3¼ oz	220	16	13
Burgers: *Without Sides*			
BBQ w/ Bacon & Cheddar (2)	1400	92	64
Sliders (2)	1200	80	52
Uno Burger (2)	1080	72	48
Entrees: *Without Side or Breadstick*			
Baked Stuffed Chicken (2)	360	18	6
Chicken Milanese (2)	860	58	42
Chicken Thumb Platter (2)	480	18	34
Fisherman's Platter (2)	1540	110	148
Smoke, Sizzle & Splash: *Without Sides or Breadstick*			
Baked Haddock (2)	580	34	12
Lemon Basil Salmon	480	34	0
The Chop House Classic	520	18	0
Flatbread Pizza: *Per ⅓ pizza*			
Mediterranean	280	15	29
Pepperoni, Gluten-Free Crust	340	15	41
Spicy Chicken	350	16	34

Fast - Foods & *Restaurants*

Villa Fresh Italian® (Nov '10)

Pizza (18"): Per Slice (⅙ Pizza)

	C	F	Cb
Neapolitan: Cheese	525	19	60
Sausage and Cheese	675	32	61
Pepperoni and Cheese	635	29	60
Stuffed: Meat	880	42	83
Spinach and Mushroom	790	35	87
Sicilian, Deluxe	945	39	105
Stromboli:			
Sausage and Cheese	880	44	83
Pepperoni and Cheese	745	33	83
Pasta & Italian Specialties:			
Baked Ziti	680	35	63
Meat Lasagna	1235	81	86
Spinach and Cheese Lasagna	1065	60	88
Spaghetti	2710	122	349
Chicken Francais	225	11	4
Chicken Cacciatore	780	68	11
Italian Sausage and Peppers	645	64	3
Sauteed Fresh Vegetables	465	43	19

Vocelli Pizza® (Nov '10)

Pizze: Per Slice (⅛ Pizza)

	C	F	Cb
Grande: Cheese	260	6	38
Pepperoni	410	20	38
Gourmet: Deluxe	390	16	40
Meat Magnifico	490	25	38
Philly Steak	360	13	38
Panini: Per Sandwich			
Chicken	900	38	81
Italian	910	42	77
Vegetarian	750	31	83
Insalata: Per Plate			
Antipasta	630	50	16
Chicken Caesar	220	4.5	4
Mediterranean	270	18	20
Tuscany Chicken	350	16	15
Antipasti: Croutons, 1 package	30	1	5
Bruschetta, 1 slice	150	8	14
Buffalo Wings (10)	560	39	3
BBQ Wings (10)	610	33	26
Pepperoni Sticks, 2½ slices	470	26	36
Dressings: Per 1½ oz Packet			
Blue Cheese	230	25	2
Italian	200	21	4
Ranch	260	28	2

Wahoo's Fish Taco® (Nov '10)

Bowls: W/ White Rice & Blk Beans

	C	F	Cb
Blackened Chicken	860	15	127
Charbroiled Chicken	855	15	126
Charbroiled Fish	930	22	126
Teriyaki Fish	930	22	127
Classic Burrito, A la Carte:			
Carne Asada	480	19	53
Carnitas	605	25	54
Charbroiled/Blackened: Fish, av.	545	23	53
Chicken, average	495	18	52
Mushroom	405	16	55
Shrimp	400	16	53
Veggie w/ White Rice & Black Beans	635	19	98
Tacos, A la Carte:			
Blackened Chicken	185	5	22
Carne Asada	180	5	22
Carnitas	235	8	23
Veggie w/ White Rice & Black Beans	215	4	36
Sides: Brown Rice	350	7	64
White Beans	285	3	54
Salads: Chips Not Included			
Blackened Chicken	415	22	14
Carne Asada	400	23	16
Charbroiled Fish	485	29	14

For Complete Nutritional Data ~ see CalorieKing.com

WAWA® (Nov '10)

Breakfast	C	F	Cb
Bagels: Plain	290	1	60
With Butter	490	23	60
Cinnamon Raisin	290	1	63
With Cream Cheese	410	13	65
Everything	310	6	56
Bowls: Per Bowl, without Syrup			
Creamed Chipped Beef On Rye	330	10	50
Pancake: Without Syrup	330	10	56
With Bacon	370	12	57
With Sausage	490	24	57
With Turkey Sausage	420	16	57
Scrambled Egg: With Bacon	370	25	9
With Sausage	490	36	10
Ciabatta Melts: On Shorti Rolls without Extras			
Scrambled Eggs: With Bacon	530	20	58
With Beef Cheesesteak	640	21	60
With Ham & Swiss	670	27	62
Italian Style	640	26	60
Sizzlis: Without Hashbrowns			
Bagels: Bacon, Egg & Cheese	360	14	42
Pork Roll, Egg & Cheese	400	16	43

WAWA® Cont... (Nov '10)

Lunch:	**C**	**F**	**Cb**
Bagel Sandwiches: *With Plain Bagel, w/o Toppings*			
BLT	390	8	62
Chicken Salad	630	29	66
Ham	380	4	62
Cold Hoagies: *On Shorti Roll without Toppings*			
Egg Salad	540	32	46
Tuna Salad	580	36	48
Turkey	320	5	46
Soups: *Per Medium Serving*			
Cream of Broccoli	220	13	19
Maryland Crab	120	1	20
Minestrone	140	3.5	23
Sides: *Per Medium Serving*			
Chili	250	8	32
Macaroni & Cheese	460	21	50
Mashed Potatoes	530	33	52
Meatballs in a Cup	360	25	20
Shephard's Pie	490	28	43
Stuffing	400	23	42
Dinner:			
Breaded Chicken Strips:			
3 piece	240	13	16
5 piece	400	22	27
Hot Dogs: *Without Toppings, Mustard or Sauce*			
Regular	230	15	21
Big Bacon Cheese Dog	640	40	41
Kielbasa	310	17	21
Hot Hoagies: *On Shorti Roll without Toppings*			
Beef Cheesesteak	360	7	42
Chicken Cheesesteak	340	6	42
Homestyle Roast Beef	420	12	46
Meatballs	560	28	60
Sides, *Per Medium Serving*			
Creamy Tortellini with Bacon	420	25	33
Soups: *Per Medium Serving*			
Italian Wedding	130	4.5	16
Loaded Potato	410	26	28
Toasted Flatbreads: Pepp. Pizza	750	42	59
Salsa Chicken	560	19	58
Turkey Quesadilla with Sour Cream	520	18	61
Bakery			
Croissant, Plain	280	14	35
Muffins: Banana Walnut	670	34	83
Blueberry	610	30	78
Chocolate Chip	680	34	86
Corn	640	29	87
Beverages: Per 24 oz			
Hot Cappuccinos: Original	370	13	63
English Toffee	340	9	63
Smoothie, Strawberry Banana	450	3.5	104

Wendy's® (Nov '10)

Burgers & Sandwiches	**C**	**F**	**Cb**
Burgers: ¼ lb Single	470	21	43
½ lb Double, with Cheese	750	42	44
¾ lb Triple with Cheese	1030	63	44
Baconator, Double	980	63	46
Double Stack	360	18	27
Jr. Bacon Cheeseburger	350	19	28
Jr. Cheeseburger Deluxe	300	14	29
Sandwiches: Chicken Club	630	31	55
Crispy Chicken	350	15	38
Homestyle Chicken	470	18	52
Spicy Chicken	460	16	54
Ultimate Chicken Grill	370	7	42
French Fries: Kid's, 2½ oz	210	10	28
Small, 4 oz	330	15	45
Medium, 5 oz	410	19	56
Large, 6½ oz	540	25	73
Chicken Nuggets, 5 pieces	230	14	13
Boneless Chicken Wings:			
Honey BBQ	570	18	69
Spicy Chipotle	500	20	48
Sweet & Spicy Asian	540	18	62
Sauces: Barbecue Nugget	45	0	11
Heartland Ranch Dipping	120	12	3
Garden Sensations Salads: *With Dressing*			
Apple Pecan Chicken	350	12	29
Baja	550	33	36
BLT Cobb	460	26	12
Spicy Chicken Caesar	450	25	25
Sides:			
Hot Stuffed Baked Potatoes:			
Bacon & Cheese	440	12	70
Broccoli & Cheese	330	2	69
Sour Cream & Chives	320	4	63
Chili Large, 16 oz	330	10	32
Mandarin Orange Cup, 5 oz	90	0	21
Frosty: Choc/Van., small, average	310	8	52
Frosti-cino, small	380	11	63
Frosty Shakes: Choc. Fudge, large	540	13	94
Strawb/Vanilla, large, average	510	13	89
Twisted Frosty: Chocolate/Vanilla	480	16	77
M&M's, Chocolate/Vanilla, average	555	19	87
Oreo, Chocolate/Vanilla	440	14	72

For Complete Nutritional Data ~ see CalorieKing.com

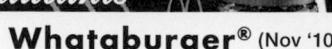

Wienerschnitzel® (Nov '10)

Hot Dogs:	C	F	Cb
Original: *On Standard Bun*			
BBQ Bacon	380	21	33
Chili	290	13	31
Chili Cheese	340	17	31
Deluxe	270	12	30
Pastrami	390	22	29
Plain	270	13	27
Stadium	280	13	30
Big Original: *On Pretzel Bun*			
Kraut	500	24	65
Pastrami	650	35	66
Stadium	510	24	67
Angus All Beef: *On Pretzel Bun*			
Chicago	600	27	69
Chili Cheese	620	37	59
Corn Dogs: Regular	250	17	15
Mini (6)	320	22	22
Sandwiches: Chicken Deluxe	430	21	37
Italian Sausage	350	17	31
Pastrami	580	34	36
Polish Sausage	490	29	39
Sides: Chili Cheese Fries	540	38	39
Fries: Regular	300	22	25
Large	430	31	35
Jalapeno Poppers (3)	210	11	21
Breakfast:			
Biscuits: Egg, Bacon, Cheese	440	25	36
Egg, Sausage, Cheese	540	34	40
Burritos: Egg, Bacon, Cheese	490	25	39
Egg, Sausage, Cheese	590	34	43
French Toast Sticks	490	29	49
Syrup, 1 oz	120	0	31
Desserts:			
Cones: Plain, 6 oz.	300	11	49
Chocolate Dipped, 6 oz.	490	29	57
Floats: Mountain Dew; Root Beer, av.	440	12	84
Tropicana Strawberry Lemonade	450	12	82
Freezees: Butterfinger	620	24	100
Oreo; M&M	630	25	99
Reese's Peanut Butter Cup	630	26	97
Sundaes: Caramel, Hot Fudge avg.	400	15	65
Chocolate	390	14	64
Pineapple; Strawberry	370	14	59
Shakes, average all flavors	650	23	110
Drinks: *16 fl.oz, without ice*			
Lipton Raspberry Iced Tea	180	0	45
Mountain Dew	230	0	61
Mug Root Beer	210	0	57
Pepsi	200	0	55

Whataburger® (Nov '10)

Burgers/Sandwiches	C	F	Cb
Justaburger	290	15	26
Whataburger: Burger	620	30	58
With Bacon & Cheese	780	43	59
Double Meat	870	49	58
Triple Meat	1120	68	58
Jr.	300	15	28
Sandwich: Grilled Chicken	470	19	49
Whatacatch	450	24	44
Whatachick'n	550	27	57
French Fries: Small, 3 oz	320	18	36
Medium, 4½ oz	480	27	55
Large, 6 oz	640	36	73
Onion Rings: Medium, 4¼ oz	400	25	37
Large, 6½ oz	600	38	56
Chicken Strips (2 pieces)	300	16	22
Salads: *Without Dressing*			
Chicken Strips Salad	350	16	33
With Shredded Cheddar Cheese	520	29	34
Garden Salad	50	0	11
With Shredded Cheddar Cheese	220	13	12
Grilled Chicken Salad	220	7	18
With Shredded Cheddar Cheese	390	20	19
Dressing: *Per 2 oz*			
Buttermilk Ranch	310	33	3
Honey Mustard	250	21	15
Thousand Island	150	13	10
Malts:			
Chocolate; Strawb.: Small, 15¾ oz	670	15	123
Medium, average, 25¼ oz	1045	25	188
Vanilla: Small, 15¾ oz	600	17	98
Medium, 25¼ oz	940	27	155
Shakes:			
Chocolate; Strawb.: Small, 15¾ oz	630	16	111
Medium, average, 25¼ oz	995	26	171
Vanilla: Small, 15¾ oz	560	17	87
Medium, 25¼ oz	890	28	139
Breakfast: Cinnamon Roll	390	9	71
Hash Brown Sticks (4)	200	12	20
Texas Toast, 1 slice	150	7	20
Biscuits: Plain	300	17	32
With Bacon	350	20	32
With Gravy	560	33	54
With Sausage	540	37	32
Honey Butter Chicken	560	34	50
Biscuit Sandwiches:			
With Egg & Cheese	450	28	33
With Bacon, Egg & Cheese	500	32	33
With Sausage, Egg & Cheese	690	49	33

Updated Nutrition Data ~ www.CalorieKing.com
Persons with Diabetes ~ See Disclaimer (Page 22)

Whataburger® cont... (Nov '10)

Breakfast (Cont)	C	F	Cb
Breakfast On A Bun: With Bacon	360	21	25
With Sausage	550	38	25
Breakfast Platter (Biscuit/Eggs/Hash Brown):			
With Bacon	730	45	93
With Sausage	920	63	93
Pancakes: Plain (3)	540	7	104
With Bacon	580	11	104
With Sausage	780	28	104
Taquito: With Bacon & Egg	380	21	27
With Bacon, Egg & Cheese	420	24	27
With Potato & Egg	430	23	57
With Potato, Egg & Cheese	470	27	57
With Sausage & Egg	410	24	27
With Sausage, Egg & Cheese	450	28	27
Dessert: Hot Apple Pie, 3 oz	250	12	31

White Castle® (Nov '10)

Sandwiches & Burgers	C	F	Cb
Cheeseburger	170	9	15
Double	300	17	20
Whitecastle Hamburger	140	6	13
Double	240	12	21
Sandwiches:			
Chicken Ring with Cheese	380	30	16
Chicken Breast with Cheese	390	28	20
Chicken Supreme	420	31	20
Fish with Cheese	340	24	18
Surf & Turf with Cheese	540	38	27
Sides			
Chicken Rings: 6 rings, 5 oz	530	47	12
9 rings, 7½ oz	790	71	18
Clam Strips, regular, 4½ oz	210	17	5
Fish Nibblers, regular, 5 oz	320	16	28
French Fries, 5½ oz	370	25	33
Mozzarella Cheese Sticks, 3 sticks	440	33	22
Onion Chips, 6 oz	670	50	46
Onion Rings Homestyle, 5 oz	480	33	40
Sauces & Condiments: Per Packet			
Ketchup, ¼ oz	10	0	2
Mayonnaise, ¼ oz	60	7	0
Ranch Dressing, 1 oz	150	17	1
Sauces: BBQ,¼ oz	10	0	3
Cheese, 1½ oz	130	10	6
Seafood, 1 oz	30	0	7
White Castle Zesty Zing, 1 oz	120	11	4

Winchell's® (Nov '10)

Baked Products	C	F	Cb
Donuts: *Per Donut*			
Buttermilk Bars: Choc Iced; Glazed	420	19	61
Jelly Filled:			
Apple with Cinnamon Crumb	450	18	65
Raspberry with Glaze	480	15	78
Strawberry with Sugar	460	15	74
Old Fashioned: Glazed; Maple Iced	410	18	60
Raised Round: Choc. Iced; Glazed	220	9	31
Sugared	230	9	34

WingStreet (Nov '10)

Chicken	C	F	Cb
Crispy Bone In Wings: *Per 2 Pieces*			
All American, 2 oz	200	14	8
Buffalo, Mild/Med./Hot, 2¾ oz	230	15	16
Cajun, 2¾ oz	240	14	19
Garlic Parmesan, 2½ oz	300	25	9
Bone Out Wings: *Per 2 Pieces*			
All American, 2 oz	150	8	11
Buffalo, Mild/Medium, 2½ oz	190	9	18
Cajun, 2¾ oz	200	8	21
Garlic Parmesan, 2½ oz	260	19	11
Traditional Wings: *Per 2 Pieces*			
All American, 1¼ oz	80	5	0
Buffalo, Medium/Hot, 2 oz	110	6	8
Cajun, 2¼ oz	120	5	11
Garlic Parmesan, 2 oz	180	16	1
Sides: Apple Pies, 2 pies, 3 oz	330	17	40
Fried Cheese Sticks (4), 4¼ oz	380	24	29
Wedge Fries, half order, 4¼ oz	320	18	35

Woody's Bar-B-Q (Nov '10)

Entrees	C	F	Cb
½ Chicken	840	56	0
Baby Back Ribs, ½ Rack, 14 ribs	520	40	2
Beef Prime Rib, 3 oz	230	19	1
Chicken Breast: 1 piece	250	14	4
Spicy Breaded, 1 piece	200	8	14
Chicken Tenders, 2 pieces	190	7	18
Chicken Wings, 2 pieces	210	13	4
Homestyle Meat Loaf, 4 oz	340	26	10
Hot Dog	330	28	8
Pulled Pork, ½ cup	250	19	4
Sausage, 5 pieces	260	16	20
Shrimp, 6 shrimp	180	1	33
Spare Ribs, ½ slab, 4 oz	270	21	0

For Complete Nutritional Data ~ see CalorieKing.com

257

Fast - Foods & *Restaurants*

Yoshinoya® (Nov '10)

Bowls: *Without sauce unless indicated*	C	F	Cb
Beef Bowl: Regular	685	27	81
Large	970	38	116
Beef Bowl w/ Vegetables, regular	605	20	84
Beef & Chicken Combo, large	995	30	131
Chicken Bowl: Regular	610	12	94
Large	910	17	140
Chicken Bowl w/ Teriyaki Sce, reg.	740	12	125
Shrimp Bowl: Grilled	505	3	96
with Seafood Sauce	635	3	126
Vegetable Bowl, regular	390	2.5	86
Kids: Beef	350	11	49
Chicken	360	7	53
Soups: Chicken Vegetable	70	1.5	7
Clam Chowder	210	7	34
Miso Soup	60	1.5	8
Salads: Chicken	360	14	14
Garden	50	0	9
Macaroni	350	21	37
Dessert, Cheese Cake	330	19	35

Z Pizza® (Nov '10)

Pizzas: *Small 10", Per ⅙ Slice*	C	F	Cb
Berkeley Soy Cheese Veggie	180	8	19
California	150	6	19
Casablanca	190	9	18
Greek	150	6	17
Italian; Mexican; Napoli	180	8	18
Provence	160	7	20
Santa Fe	180	7	20
Thai	170	6	19
Tuscan	160	7	18
ZBQ	170	5	21
Sandwiches: Hot Meatball Sub	670	34	45
Pollo Latino Sandwich	350	11	38
Supersub	460	23	34
Turkey Breast Sandwich	400	14	35
Z-Tuna Sandwich	670	32	68
Calzones: Meat Calzone	770	37	77
Veggie Calzone	750	27	102
Salads: *Small w/o Dressing*			
Arugula	260	20	14
Caesar Side	200	17	8
California	100	6	10
Pear and Gorgonzola	530	44	25
ZBQ	220	11	17

Zaxby's (Nov '10)

Zappetizers	C	F	Cb
Onion Rings, without Sauce	625	41	55
Spicy Fried Mushroom without Sauce	430	28	37
Tater Chips, 5½ oz	795	53	75
Meal Dealz: *Without Sauce or Drink*			
Big Zax Snak	765	34	78
Buffalo Wings	740	39	53
Nibbler with Zac Sauce	1295	66	126
Most Popular: *As Served*			
Chicken Finger Plate: Regular	1055	50	91
Large	1590	73	147
Wings & Things, Regular	1140	57	80
Sandwich Baskets: *Includes Fries*			
Cajun Club	1185	57	107
Zaxby's Club	1215	68	102
Wings & Fingerz: *Without Sauce*			
Buffalo Chicken Fingerz: 5 pieces	425	20	8
10 pieces	845	40	18
Buffalo Wings: 5 pieces	370	23	0
10 pieces	735	46	1
Boneless Wings, 5 pieces	390	20	29
Chicken Fingerz, 5 pieces	420	20	8
10 pieces	840	40	17
Zax Kidz:			
Kiddie Cheese, no drink	435	20	55
Kiddie Finger, no drink	390	17	34
Zalads: *With Texas Toast, w/o Dressing Unless Indicated*			
Blue : With Blackened Chicken	590	27	36
With Buffalo Chicken & Sauce	755	39	45
Caesar Zalad:			
With Fr. Chicken, w/o Texas Toast	665	34	31
With Gr. Chicken, w/o Texas Toast	515	23	24
House Zalad: With Fried Chicken	760	40	42
With Grilled Chicken	610	29	35
Zensation, without Texas Toast	840	39	76
Salad Dressings: *Per 1¼ oz Packet*			
Blue Cheese	180	19	2
Honey French	150	12	9
Honey Mustard	150	3	6
Lite Vinaigrette	50	2	7
Mediterranean	140	14	4
Ranch	160	16	2
Thousand Island	230	24	3
Sides: Celery Basket, 2½ oz	5	0	2
Cole Slaw, 2¾ oz	115	8	10
Crinkle Fries, 8 oz	590	25	84
Texas Toast, 3 wedges, 1½ oz	145	6	20

Zero Subs® ~ *see CalorieKing.com*

Notes on Cholesterol

- **Cholesterol** is a white waxy substance produced mainly by our liver. It is also found in animal food products. Plant foods have no cholesterol.

- **Cholesterol is essential to life.** It is a structural part of every body cell wall and is the building block for vitamin D, sex hormones, and bile acids which help in the digestion of dietary fats.

- **The body makes sufficient cholesterol** for its needs and does not rely on cholesterol in the diet. Dietary fats have a major influence on blood cholesterol levels - more so than dietary cholesterol.

- A high blood cholesterol level increases the risk of atherosclerosis - the thickening of arteries that can reduce or block blood flow to the heart, brain, eyes, kidneys, sex organs and other body parts.

  This in turn increases the risk of heart attack, stroke, blindness, kidney failure, impotence and other blood circulatory problems.

  Other risk factors which increase the risk of atherosclerosis include high blood pressure, smoking, obesity and uncontrolled diabetes.

BLOOD CHOLESTEROL

CHECK YOUR RISK!

Total Cholesterol Level (mg/dl)		Risk of Heart Attack
240 and above	~	High Risk
200 - 239	~	Borderline/High
Below 200	~	Desirable

- ❤ **Know your cholesterol level, particularly if there is a family history of heart disease or stroke. If level is high, see your doctor.**

- ❤ **All adults should have their cholesterol, HDL and triglycerides tested at least every 5 years.**

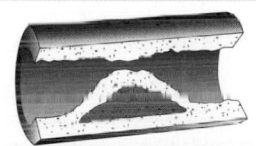

▲ **Atherosclerosis can clog arteries and impede blood flow to the heart or other body organs.**

▼ **A thrombus (blood clot) can form on unstable, festering atherosclerotic plaque and rapidly block blood flow. A heart attack or stroke can result.**

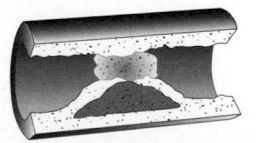

HEART ATTACK WARNING SIGNALS

Many victims die before reaching the hospital by ignoring warning signals and delaying medical help.

Symptoms vary and commonly include:

- **Chest pain,** vice-like squeezing or burning sensation in center of the chest or between the shoulder blades, or in the mid-back. Pain may even feel like severe indigestion.

- **Pain** may be felt in the arms, shoulders, neck or jaw.

- **Shortness of breath** often occurs with or before chest discomfort.

- **Other signs,** with or without pain, include a cold sweat, nausea or light-headedness.

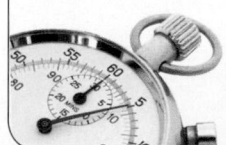

If you experience any of the above symptoms call IMMEDIATELY for medical help. Every minute counts.

Call 9-1-1 *or your emergency number*

Fats & Cholesterol Guide

The amount and type of dietary fat has the greatest influence on blood cholesterol levels.

Fats in food are a mixture of 3 basic types: saturated, monounsaturated, and polyunsaturated. Animal fats are mainly saturated while plant oils and fish oils are mainly mono- and polyunsaturated.

Saturated fats have subgroups known as long-chain, medium-chain, and short-chain fats. Most of the long chain fats raise blood cholesterol, and increase the risk of blood clots and thrombosis leading to artery blockage.

Long-chain saturated fats are found mainly in full-cream milk, cheese, butter, cream, fatty meats and sausages, and processed foods.

Monounsaturated fats tend to more selectively lower 'bad' LDL cholesterol and maintain the protective 'good' HDL cholesterol in the bloodstream – but only if they replace saturated fats in the diet.

Foods rich in monounsaturates include canola and olive oils, canola margarine, peanuts, and avocados.

Polyunsaturated fats consist of two main classes. **Omega-6** polyunsaturates tend to lower blood cholesterol. Rich sources include safflower, sunflower and corn oils.

Omega-3 polyunsaturated fats can lower blood cholesterol; significantly lower blood triglycerides; and reduce the rise of thrombosis, heart arrythmmia, and artery spasm.

Best practical omega-3 sources include canola oil and margarine, soybean oil and fish.

A balanced intake of the two omega classes is important for optimal health. For most Americans, slightly increasing omega-3 intake would help attain a more ideal balance.

Trans fats from hydrogenated vegetable oils and shortenings should also be avoided. They are common in commercial baked and fried food products such as cakes, muffins, pastries, doughnuts, fried snacks and french fries.

Note: All fats are high in calories and need to be limited for weight control.

DIETARY FATS COMPARISON

■ Saturated Fat   ▨ Monounsaturated Fat
Polyunsaturated Fats:
▨ Linoleic (Omega-6) ■ Alpha-Linolenic (Omega-3)

OILS — PERCENTAGE CONTENT

	Saturated	Monounsaturated	Linoleic (Omega-6)	Alpha-Linolenic (Omega-3)
CANOLA OIL	7	63	20	10
LINSEED/FLAX OIL	9	19	17	55
SAFFLOWER OIL	9	14	77	
GRAPESEED OIL	10	22	68	
SUNFLOWER OIL	11	23	66	
CORN OIL	14	32	52	2
OLIVE OIL	14	76		10
SOYBEAN OIL	15	23	54	8
PEANUT OIL	19	45	34	2
COTTONSEED OIL	26	16	58	
PALM OIL	51	39		10

SPREADS & FATS
Saturated Fat includes 'Trans Fats'   ☐ WATER CONTENT

LIGHT MARGARINE	14	14	21	51	
CANOLA MARGARINE	18	45	12	6	19
POLYUNSATURATED MARG	24	20	36	20	
BUTTER	57		18	2	24
LARD	41	47		12	
BEEF FAT	44	37	4	15	

GOOD SOURCES OF OMEGA-3 FATS

Plant Sources	Omega-3 Fats (Grams)
Canola Oil, 1 Tbsp, ½ fl.oz	1.5g
Flaxseed Oil, 1 Tbsp	8g
Soybean Oil, 1 Tbsp	1.2g
Canola Margarine, 1 Tbsp, ½ oz	1g
Soybeans, cooked, ½ cup, 4 oz	0.5g
Walnuts, ½ oz	0.5g

FISH - *Per 4 oz Serving*

High Content: Salmon (Chinook), Tuna,	3g
Trout (Lake), Sardines, Herring, Mackerel	3g
Medium Content:	
Salmon, (Pink/Red/Coho), 4 oz	2g

Fair Content: Per 4 oz Serving

Bass, Catfish, Cod, Grouper, Hake, Halibut, Kingfish, Perch, Pollock, Shark, Trout (Rainbow), Tuna, Crab, Oysters, Blue Mussels, Shrimp, Squid   } 0.5-1g

How Much Is Needed?

As little as 1-2 grams daily of omega-3 fats may benefit general health. High doses of fish-oil supplements should only be taken as directed by your doctor.

Cholesterol in Food

Dietary Cholesterol

Cholesterol in food varies in its effect on blood cholesterol level (BCL) from person to person. Much depends on the amount and type of fat and fiber eaten at the same meal.

Any elevating effect of dietary cholesterol on BCL is more likely to occur when the diet is high in saturated fat. Little elevation, if any, generally occurs when dietary fats are balanced in favor of monounsaturated and polyunsaturated fats (including omega-3 fats).

For example, while fish does contain cholesterol, the omega-3 fats can prevent any increase in BCL. Conversely, a meal containing no cholesterol but rich in saturated fat may result in a significant increase in BCL.

Consequently, the need to be overly-concerned about dietary cholesterol is being de-emphasized in favor of the approach of limiting total fat, saturated fat, and trans fat in particular – and substituting unsaturated fats.

The liver usually cuts back its own cholesterol production in response to cholesterol in the diet. Many people can consume normal amounts of high-cholesterol foods without concern.

However, it is difficult to identify just who is at risk - the so-called 'hyper-responders'. Because over 50% of Americans have a BCL above ideal levels, the **American Heart Association** advises all Americans to be prudent and limit their cholesterol intake to less than 300mg daily, as well as to adopt a heart-healthy diet.

This limitation still allows the inclusion of most foods that are regularly eaten – even the overly-maligned egg.

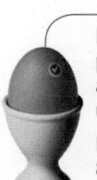

Eggs contain a modest 5 grams of fat per large egg, barely 2 grams of which are saturated, the rest being mono-unsaturated and polyunsaturated.

By comparison, a cup of whole milk has 8g fat of which almost 5g is saturated.

CHOLESTEROL COUNTER

Cholesterol is found only in foods of animal origin. Plant foods contain no cholesterol.
AHA recommends limiting dietary cholesterol to less than 300mg/day.

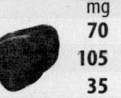

	Chol mg
Meat - Average all types:	
Lean Meat, cooked, 4 oz	70
Fatty Meat, cooked, 4 oz	105
Fat, thick strip, 2 oz	35

Note: While lean meat and fat have similar amounts of cholesterol, choose lean meat to limit fat intake.

	Chol mg
Chicken/Turkey, average, 4 oz	90
Organ Meats: Liver, fried, 4 oz	500
Brains, beef, pan fried, 3 oz	1700
Sausages: Frankfurter, 1.5 oz	25
Salami, 2 slices, 2 oz	40
Bacon: 3 slices, cooked, 1 oz	20
Fish: Fish fillets, average, ckd, 4 oz	70
Tuna/Salmon, canned, 3 oz	30
Scallops, 9 medium, 3 oz	30
Shrimp, 12 large, raw, 3 oz	130
Oysters, raw, 6 medium, 3 oz	45
Lobster, Crab, raw, 3 oz	80
Eggs (Chicken), 1 large	210
1 medium	180
Egg White, *Egg Beaters*	0
Milk/Yogurt: Whole, 1 cup, 8 fl.oz	35
1% Milk, 1 cup	10
Skim/Non-fat, 1 cup	5
Soy Milk, Tofu, Tempeh	0
Cheese: Natural/Hard/Cream, 1 oz	30
Cottage, lowfat, 4 oz	5
Ricotta, part skim, 4 oz	25
Fats: Butter, 2 Tbsp, 1 oz	60
Margarine, Oils (vegetable)	0
Mayonnaise, 1 Tbsp	10
Cream: Heavy, whipping, 2 T, 1 oz	40
Half & Half/Sour, 2 Tbsp, 1 oz	10
Ice Cream: Regular, ½ cup, 4 fl.oz	30
Fruit, Vegetables, Avocados	0
Nuts, Seeds, Grains	0
Coffee, Tea, Soda, Beer, Wine	0

For Comprehensive Food Listings ~ see CalorieKing.com

Blood Cholesterol ~ Diet Hints

1. Maintain a healthy weight.
If overweight, lose weight with a low-fat meal plan and daily exercise.

2. Reduce saturated fat intake by:
(a) eating less dairy fat. Choose low-fat or fat-reduced varieties of milk, yogurt, soy drinks, cheese, and ice cream.

(b) replacing saturated fats with fats and oils rich in monounsaturated and polyunsaturated fats. Choose vegetable oils such as canola, olive, sunflower and soybean. Avoid solid frying fats.

Take Control and *Benecol* (spreads) contain plant stanol esters which can lower total and LDL cholesterol.

(c) eating less fat from meat and poultry. Choose lean cuts of meat and skinless chicken. Go easy on lunch meats, salami and fatty sausages. Enjoy fish.

(d) eating less saturated and trans fats from baked and fried fast-foods. Avoid deep-fried foods. Avoid donuts, cakes, pastries and cookies unless made with healthier fats and oils.

3. Increase your soluble fiber intake.
Foods rich in soluble fiber include beans, lentils, chick peas, hummus, nuts, seeds, psyllium-seed husks and psyllium-fiber supplements. Oat bran, rice bran and barley are also good sources, as are fruit, veggies and avocados. (*See Fiber Guide - Page 264-269*).

4. Eat more soy bean products such as:
soy drinks, tofu, tempeh (cultured soy beans), soy flour and soy vegetarian foods. Soy protein in place of animal protein can significantly decrease high blood cholesterol levels as well as 'bad' LDL cholesterol and blood triglycerides while 'good' HDL cholesterol is maintained. For best results, eat at least 25g of soy protein per day (from 3-4 servings).

5. Eat more fruit, vegetables, and whole grains in place of high-fat foods. Aim for 2 fruits and 5 servings of vegetables per day. They also contain valuable antioxidants. The fat of avocados (and most nuts) is mainly unsaturated and can lower blood cholesterol levels.

6. Limit cholesterol to 300mg per day.
(Extra Notes ~ See Previous Page)

7. Avoid brewed unfiltered coffee (espresso; plunger-style). Several cups per day may raise blood cholesterol. Filtered coffee is fine.

8. Spread your food intake over the day.
Have 5-6 small meals per day rather than just 2-3 large meals. Nibbling, versus gorging, favors lower blood cholesterol.

ALCOHOL - WINE

Alcohol is a mixed bag. Moderate amounts of 1-2 drinks daily appear to reduce the risk of heart attack and ischemic stroke in older persons.

However, larger amounts increase the risk of high blood pressure, obesity, heart failure and hemorrhagic stroke, and can aggravate hypertriglyceridemia: as well as many other health hazards. (*See Alcohol Guide – Page 23*)

The speculative benefits of moderate alcohol intake have been overstated in the media. The overriding harmful effects of excess alcohol do not allow its recommendation for any aspects of health promotion.

Fruit, Vegetables & Tea Also Protect:
Red wine and red grapes (more so than white) contain antioxidants which may help protect cholesterol in the blood from becoming oxidized.

Many fruits, vegetables, grains, nuts and tea also contain protective antioxidants.

Fats in the diet affect more than blood cholesterol levels. They can also strongly influence blood clot formation and thrombosis, as well as blood flow and ultimate oxygen delivery to body parts and organs.

While advanced atherosclerosis can impede blood flow to the heart and other organs, it is thrombosis (complete blockage by blood clots) or arterial spasm which commonly results in a heart attack or stroke.

Plant and fish oils rich in omega-3 fats lessen the risk of blood clots, thrombus formation, and artery spasm by reducing platelet stickiness and adhesion to artery walls. This reduces the risk of atherosclerotic plaque becoming unstable and reactive.

Omega-3 fats also improve blood flow by reducing blood viscosity and increasing the flexibility of red blood cells (RBC) that need to flex and twist on themselves in order to squeeze through tiny narrow capillaries often half their diameter.

A diet high in saturated fats has the opposite effect by stiffening RBC membranes and increasing blood viscosity, thereby hindering blood flow. The stiffening of the RBC membrane also reduces its ability to release vital oxygen to body cells and take up carbon dioxide.

Stiff red blood cells may also form aggregates that resemble coin stacks. In narrow blood vessels, this further impedes blood flow and impairs oxygen release through the much-lessened surface area of red blood cell membranes exposed to blood. (Smoking, lack of exercise, and stress can have similar adverse effects on thrombosis, red blood cell flexibility, and blood flow.)

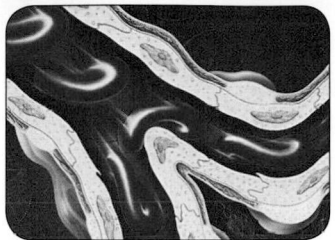

▲ **Picture of Healthy Blood Flow**

Flexible red blood cells twist and slide through tiny capillaries - often half the diameter of red blood cells.

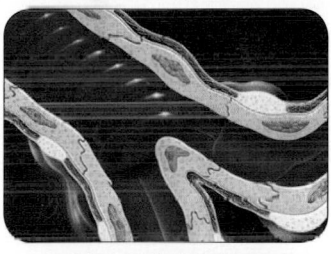

▲ **A Not-So-Healthy Picture!**

Red blood cells have lost their flexibility and ability to twist and slip through capillaries. They are stacked up, thereby impeding blood flow.

A diet high in saturated fats can contribute to this picture - as can smoking, lack of exercise, and stress.

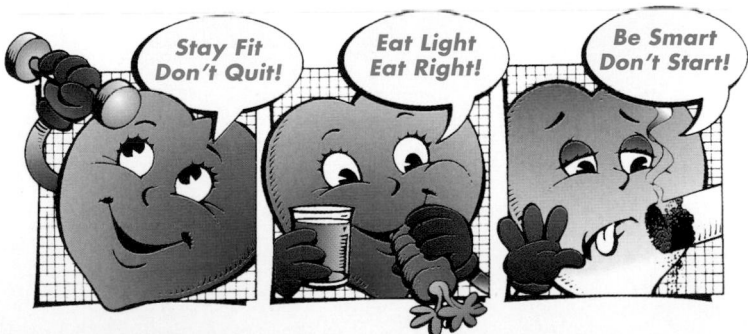

Fiber Guide

Introduction

Fiber is the general term for those parts of **plant** food that we cannot digest (although bacteria in the large bowel partly digests fiber through fermentation). It is not found in foods of animal origin (meats, dairy products).

Fiber promotes intestinal health, bowel regularity, can benefit diabetes and blood cholesterol levels, and may help prevent colon cancer. High-fiber foods also assist weight control.

Most Americans don't eat enough fiber - less than 20 grams/day - instead of a healthier **25 to 35 grams/day.**

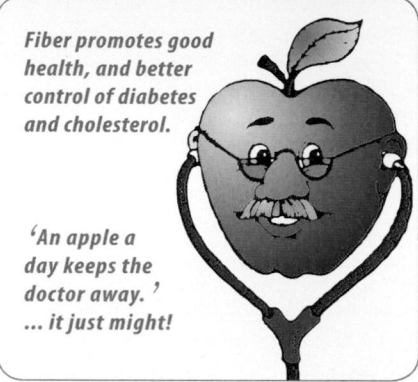

Fiber promotes good health, and better control of diabetes and cholesterol.

'An apple a day keeps the doctor away.' ... it just might!

Types of Fiber

Plant foods contain a mixture of different fibers in varying proportions. Insoluble and soluble fiber categories are based on their solubility in water. All types of fiber are beneficial to the body.

◆ **Insoluble fibers** (cellulose, hemi-celluloses, lignin) make up the structural parts of plant cell walls.

Best food sources are wheat bran, corn bran, rice bran, wholegrain cereals and breads, beans and peas, nuts, seeds, and the skins of fruits and vegetables.

These fibers absorb many times their own weight in water. They create a soft bulk and hasten the passage of waste products through the intestines.

They promote bowel regularity, and aid in the prevention and treatment of uncomplicated forms of **constipation, diverticulosis and hemorrhoids.**

The risk of colon cancer may also be reduced by fiber's diluting effect on potentially harmful substances.

◆ **Soluble fibers** (pectin, gums, mucilages) are found mainly within plant cells, soy milk (whole bean) and products.

Types of Fiber (Cont)

Best Sources of Soluble Fiber: Fruits and vegetables, oat bran, barley, beans and peas, prunes, psyllium and flax seed.

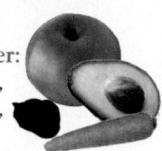

These fibers form a gel which slows both stomach emptying and the absorption of sugars from the intestines. **This helps to control blood sugar levels.**

Weight control is also aided by the slower emptying of the stomach and the feeling of **fullness provided by soluble fiber.**

Some soluble fibers can lower **blood cholesterol** by binding bile acids and excreting them. More body cholesterol must then be broken down to supply bile acids for emulsification of dietary fats. **Rice bran, while not high in soluble fiber, can also lower blood cholesterol.**

◆ **Resistant starch** is that part of starchy foods (approx. 10%) which is tightly bound by fiber and resists normal digestion. Friendly bacteria in the large bowel ferment and change the resistant starch into short-chain fatty acids, which are important to bowel health and may protect against colon cancer.

Starchy foods include bread, cereals, rice, pasta, potatoes and legumes.

Fiber & Weight Control

Fiber can assist weight control in several ways. Fiber-rich foods such as fresh fruit and vegetables, potatoes and wholegrain bread contain few calories for their large volume (due to their low-fat, high water content).

Their bulk fills the stomach and satisfies the appetite much sooner than fiber-depleted foods. The extra chewing time also contributes to satiety, and gives the stomach time to register a feeling of fullness. Excessive calories are less likely to be consumed.

Fiber-depleted foods and drinks are more concentrated in calories; e.g. fats, sugar, candy, soft drinks, fruit juices, alcohol. They require little or no chewing. Large amounts with excessive calories can be consumed before the appetite is satisfied.

Example: Whereas one fresh apple might satisfy the appetite, an apple juice drink with the equivalent sugars and calories of 2-3 apples only minimally satisfies the appetite. (See illustration below.)

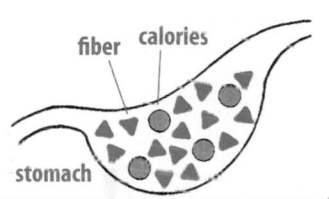

High-fiber foods fill the stomach. Fewer calories are consumed.

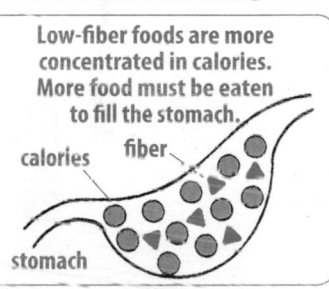

Low-fiber foods are more concentrated in calories. More food must be eaten to fill the stomach.

EFFECTS OF REMOVING FIBER FROM FOOD

2-3 pieces of fresh fruit produces 1 glass of fruit juice. The removal of fiber concentrates the sugar and calories.

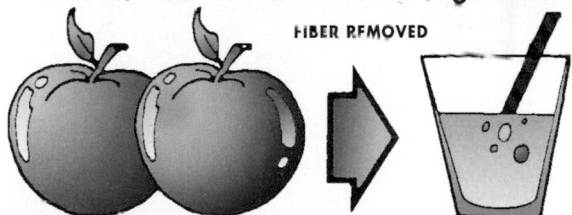

FIBER REMOVED

Fresh Fruit		Fruit Juice
High Fiber	←	Negligible Fiber
Low Calorie Density	←	High Calorie Density
Long Eating Time	←	No Eating Time (Drink)
Satisfies Hunger	←	Does Not Satisfy Hunger
Sugar Slowly Absorbed	←	Sugar More Quickly Absorbed
Less Insulin Required	←	More Insulin Required

Fiber Guide - Constipation

Constipation

Constipation can reasonably be defined as a failure to have a bowel movement at least every second day – and just as importantly, without straining or pain.

Typically, constipated stools are too hard, too narrow and too small.

The **main cause** is simply a lack of dietary fiber. Other contributing factors include insufficient fluids, too little exercise, emotional stress, gastrointestinal disease, lack of proper dentition to chew high-fiber foods, and some medications (e.g. some antacids, antidepressants, pain medications).

Note: Check with your doctor to rule out any underlying medical problem – especially if you have a change in bowel habits in middle-age or later years.

DESIRABLE FIBER INTAKE

Adults: 25-35gm per day
Children (under 18): Age + 5gm
Example: 6-year old (6 + 5)=11gm

SAMPLE FOOD QUANTITIES
For 35 Grams of Fiber/Day

	Fiber
Breakfast Cereal (higher-fiber)	5g
plus 4 slices wholegrain Bread	6g
plus 3 servings fresh Fruit	9g
plus 1 medium Potato (w. skin)	
or 1 cup Brown Rice	4g
or ½ cup wholegrain Pasta	
plus 3-4 servings Veggies/Salad	6g
plus 1 cup Bean Soup	
or ¼ cup Baked/Soy Beans	
or ½ cup Corn/Peas/Lentils	5g
or 1¼ oz Almonds (natural)	
or 3 medium Figs	

HINTS TO INCREASE FIBER AND AVOID CONSTIPATION

① **Breakfast is an important** contributor to daily fiber intake. Eat high-fiber breakfast cereals (bran-based cereals, oatmeal etc.). Add 1-2 tablespoons of unprocessed bran.
Dried fruits, chopped nuts, soy grits, and seeds are also excellent additions to cereals.

Note: A gradual increase in fiber will prevent bloating, gas or pain. People intolerant to bran may benefit from psyllium-based fiber supplements and cereals.

② **Drink adequate water daily.** Fiber works by absorbing many times its own weight in water.

③ **Eat wholegrain breads,** or fiber-enriched breads. They have over double the fiber of regular white bread.

④ **Enjoy fruit as fresh fruit** with skin rather than as fruit juice. Enjoy wholegrain pasta, barley, brown rice, nuts and seeds.

⑤ **Eat more vegetables,** salads and legumes – especially cooked beans, lentils, potatoes with skins, avocado, broccoli, brussels sprouts, cabbage, carrots, celery, and peas.

⑥ **Add bran** (barley/rice/wheat) or soy grits to soups, casseroles, yogurt, desserts, cookies, cakes. Also use whole-meal flour or soy flour in place of white flour. Use nuts, seeds, and ground linseed.

⑦ **Snack** on fresh or dried fruits, carrot or celery sticks, popcorn, nuts or seeds, wholegrain crackers, high-fiber bars (low-fat). Limit amounts if overweight.

⑧ **Exercise regularly** to strengthen abdominal muscles and stimulate the gut. Keep up water intake, especially in warm weather.

⑨ **Avoid** indiscriminate and regular use of harsh laxatives. They can overstimulate the intestinal muscles and may make normal bowel activity impossible. It may take several weeks to restore normal bowel function.

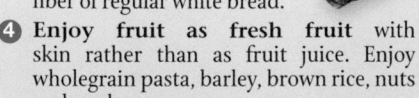

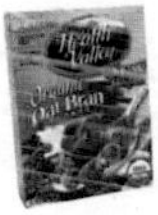

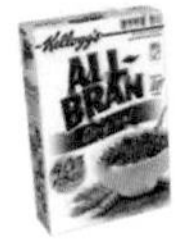

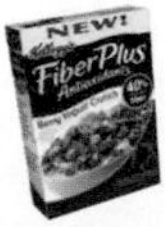

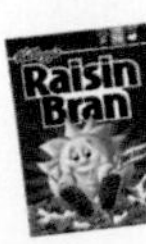

Fiber ~ Fiber (grams)

Breakfast Cereals **Fiber**

General Mills:
Basic 4, 1 cup, 2 oz	3
Cheerios (Honey Nut; Multigrain), 1 c., 1 oz	2
Multi-Bran Chex, 1 cup, 2 oz	7
Oatmeal Crisp Almond, 1 cup, 2 oz	4
Raisin Nut Bran, 1¼ cup, 2 oz	6
Total, average all types, ¾ cup, 1 oz	3
Wheat Chex, 1 cup, 2 oz	6
Wheaties ¾ cup, 1 oz	3

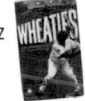

Health Valley:
Amaranth Flakes, ¾ cup, 1 oz	3
Crunches & Flakes, ¾ cup, 1.9 oz	4
Fiber 7 Flakes, ¾ cup, 1 oz	7
Golden Flax, ¾ cup, 1.9 oz	6
Granola (Low-Fat), ⅔ cup, 2 oz	6
Healthy Fiber Flakes, ¾ cup, 1.1 oz	4
Oat Bran Flakes, all types, ¾ cup, 1 oz	2
Oat Bran O's, ¾ cup, 1 oz	3
Real Oat Bran, ½ cup, 1.7 oz	5

Kellogg's:
All-Bran, ½ cup, 1.1 oz	10
All-Bran w. Extra Fiber, ½ cup, 1 oz	13
All-Bran Bran Buds, ⅓ cup, 1.1 oz	13
Corn Flakes, Fruit Loops, Smacks 1 cup, 1 oz	1
Cocoa/Rice Krispies Treats, 1¼ cup, 1 oz	0
Complete: Wheat Flakes, ¾ c., 1 oz	5
Oat Bran Flakes, ¾ cup, 1.1 oz	4
Corn Pops, 1 cup, 1.1 oz	0
Cracklin' Oat Bran, ¾ cup, 1.7oz	6

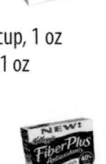

FiberPlus Antioxidants:
Berry Yogurt Crunch, 1 c., 1.9 oz	10
Cinnamon Oat Crunch ¾ c., 1.1 oz	9
Frosted Mini Wheats, 24 bisc., 2 oz	5
Granola w. Raisins, ⅔ cup, 2.1 oz	3
Raisin Bran, 1 cup, 2.1 oz	7
Smart Start, Strong Heart, Cinnamon Raisin, 1 cup, 1.8 oz	4
Special K, 1 cup, 1.1 oz	0.5

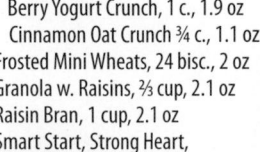

Breakfast Cereals (Cont) **Fiber**

Kashi:
GoLEAN Cereal, 1 cup, 1.8 oz	10
GoLEAN Crunch!, 1 cup, 1.9 oz	8
GoLEAN Bars, avg. (1)	6
Good Friends Original, 1 cup, 1.9 oz	12
Cinna-Raisin Crunch, 1 cup, 1.8 oz	8
Heart to Heart, ¾ cup, 1.2 oz	5
7 Whole Grain Pilaf, ½ cup, cooked, 5 oz	7
7 Whole Grain Puffs, 1 cup, 0.7 oz	1

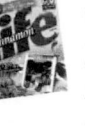

Quaker:
Cap'n Crunch, ¾ cup, 1 oz	1
100% Natural Granola, avg., ½ cup, 1.8 oz	3
Crunchy Corn Bran, 1 cup, 1 oz	5
Life Cereal, ¾ cup, 1.1 oz	2
Oat Bran, ½ cup, 1.4 oz	6
Oatmeal, average, 1 packet	3

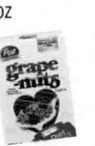

Post:
100% Bran, ⅓ cup, 1 oz	9
Alpha Bits, 1 cup, 1 oz	2
Blueberry Morning, 1 cup, 1.9 oz	5
Cocoa/Fruity Pebbles, 1 cup, 1 oz	0
Cranberry Almond Crunch, 1 cup, 1.8 oz	3
Fruit & Bran, 1 cup, 1.9 oz	6
Grape-Nuts, ½ cup, 2 oz	7
Great Grains, ⅔ cup, 1.9 oz	5
Honey Bunches of Oats, ¾ cup, 1.1 oz	2
Shredded Wheat & Bran, ½ cup, 2 oz	8

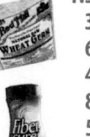

Brans & Supplements, Metamucil
Oat Bran: 1 Tbsp (level)	1
⅓ cup, (5⅓ Tbsp), 1 oz	5
Rice Bran, raw. ¼ cup, 1 oz	6

Wheat Bran (unprocessed):
Raw, 1 Tbsp	1.5
2 Tbsp (level), ¼ oz	3
¼ cup, (4 Tbsp), ½ oz	6
Wheat Germ: Raw, ¼ cup, 1 oz	4
Psyllium Seed Husks, 2 Tbsp	8
Fibersure, 1 heaping tsp	5
Metamucil: Orange, 1 rnd Tbsp, 11g	3
Fiber Wafers (2)	6

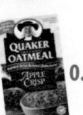

Hot Cereals, Oatmeal
Bulgur (cracked Wheat), ckd, 1 cup	8
Corn/Hominy Grits, dry, 3 Tbsp, 1 oz	0.5
Cream of Wheat, cooked, ¾ cup	1
Oatmeal (uncooked ⅓ cup), ckd, ⅔ cup	3

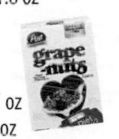

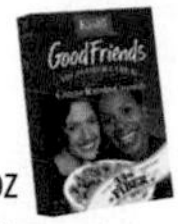

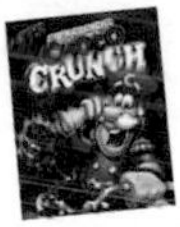

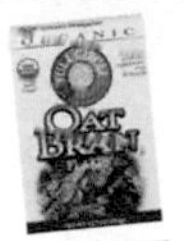

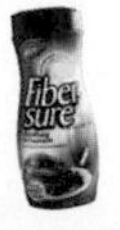

Fiber Counter

Breads & Crackers | Fiber

Bread: White, 1 slice, 1 oz — 0.6
Whole-wheat, 1 slice, 1 oz — 1.5
Wholegrain, 1 slice, 1 oz — 2
Rye, Pumpernickel, 1 oz — 1.5
Bagel/Roll/Bun, 1 medium, 2 oz — 1.5
Pita, whole wheat, 6½" pocket — 4.5
Crackers: Graham, average, 2 — 0.4
Saltine, 4 crackers — 0.4
Crispbreads (Rye), average, 2 — 4
Matzo 1 board, 1 oz — 1
Rice Cakes, average, 1 cake — 0.3
Tortilla: Regular, 6" — 0.5
Whole-wheat, 6" — 1.3

Barley, Pasta, Rice & Flours

Barley, pearled, raw, ¼ cup, 1.7 oz — 8
Rice: White, cooked, 1 cup — 0.6
Brown, cooked, 1 cup — 3.5
Rice-A-Roni, average, 1 cup, prepared — 1.5
Spaghetti/Noodles: Cooked, 1 cup — 2
Whole-Wheat, cooked, 1 cup — 4
Flour: Wheat, All-purpose, 1 cup, 4½ oz — 3.5
Whole-Wheat, 1 cup, 4½ oz — 15
Cornmeal, stone ground, 1 cup, 4½ oz — 13
Carob Flour, 1 cup, 3½ oz — 41
Rye Flour, 1 cup, 3½ oz — 15
Soy Flour: Defatted, 1 cup, 3½ oz — 17
Full-fat, raw, 1 cup, 3 oz — 8
Soy Meal, defatted, 1 cup, 4½ oz — 14

Frozen Entrees & Dinners

Average All Brands: Per Serving
Beans/Chili base, average — 6-10
Potato/Pasta base, average — 4-6
Vegetable base, average — 3
Meat/Chicken base, average — 2-3
Pizzas, ¼ large, average — 3
Vegetarian Soy Burgers, 1 pattie — 4

Soups

Chicken Noodle, 1 cup — 0.5
Tomato Soup, average, 1 cup — 0.5
Vegetable Soup, average, 1 cup — 3
Health Valley: Per 1 Cup Serving
Black Bean; Minestrone — 8
Tomato — 1
5-Bean Vegetable; Lentil & Carrots — 10
Mushroom Barley; Vegetable — 4
Split Pea — 8

Fast Foods & Restaurants | Fiber

Hamburgers: Small, average — 1.5
Large/Whopper, average — 2.5
Hot Dog, Regular — 1.5
French Fries: Small serving, 2½ oz — 2.5
Regular/Medium, 3½ oz — 3.5
Chicken Nuggets, 6 pack — 0.5
Chicken Sandwich, average — 2
Taco, average — 4
Sundaes, Shakes, Soft Drinks — 0
Arby's: Baked Potato w. Broc. & Cheese — 8
Roast Beef Sandwich, regular — 2
Denny's: Grilled Chicken Salad, no bread — 4
Classic Burger, no fries — 4
Club Sandwich, no fries — 2
Grilled Chicken Sandwich, no fries — 4
Domino's ("12"): Classic/Thin, 1 slice — 1
Deep Dish, 1 slice — 3
Feast Pizza, Classic/Thin, 1 slice — 2
McDonald's: Big Mac — 3
Hamburger; Quarter Pounder — 3
Egg McMuffin — 1
Grilled Chicken Caesar Salad — 3
Pizza Hut: Per 1 Slice, Medium
Pan Pizza: Cheese, Pepperoni — 1
Supreme — 2
Thin 'n Crispy, Supreme — 2
Hand-Tossed, average all varieties — 2
Subway: Sandwich, white roll, avg. — 4
w. Honey Wheat Roll, average — 3.2
Salads, average — 4

Cakes, Cookies, Snack Bars

Apple/Fruit Pie, 1 serving, 4 oz — 2
Cake: w. plain flour, 1 serving, 3.4 oz — 1.5
w. whole-wheat flour, 1 serving — 3
Carrot Cake, 4 oz — 4
Cookies, oatmeal, (3 small/1 large) — 1
Donuts, Medium, 1.7 oz — 0.7
Fruit Cake, 1 serving, 1½ oz — 2
Fig Bars, 1 cookie, ½ oz — 0.7
Muffins, Oat Bran (2 small, 1 large), 4 oz — 5
Granola Bars, average, 1 bar — 2
Atkins Advantage Bars, average — 7
Clif Bars, 2.5 oz — 5
Curves, Chocolate Peanut Bar, 25g — 5
Fi-Bar Chewy & Nutty 1 bar — 1
FiberPlus, all bars, 36g — 9
Health Valley: Fruit/Granola Bars — 3
Cereal Bars — 3
Luna Bars, avg., 1.7 oz — 3
Special K, Protein Meal Bar, 1.6 oz — 5

Fiber Counter

Chocolate, Chips, Popcorn | Fiber
Cheese Balls/Curls/Twists	1
Chocolate, Hard Candy, 1 oz	0
Chocolate with nuts/fruit, 2 oz bar	1.5
Mars Bar, 1.8 oz	1
Potato Chips, corn chips, 1 oz	1
Popcorn, 3 cups	3
Pretzels, Twists (6)	1

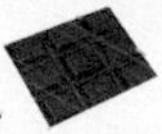

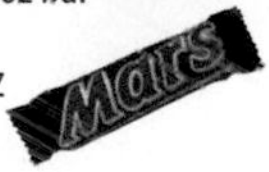

Nuts, Seeds
Almonds: Natural, 25 nuts, 1 oz	3.5
Blanched (skins removed), 1 oz	3
Cashews, Filberts, Pecans, 1 oz	1.7
Peanuts, Mixed Nuts, Coconut, 1 oz	2.5
Peanut Butter, 2 Tbsp, 1 oz	2
Pistachio Nuts, dried, shelled, 1 oz	3
Walnuts, Black/English, dried, 1 oz	2
Seeds: Amaranth, 2½ Tbsp, 1 oz	3.5
Flax Seeds, 3 Tbsp, 1 oz	7
Psyllium Seed Husks, 5 Tbsp, 1 oz	20
Quinoa Seeds, 3 Tbsp, 1 oz	1.7
Sesame Seeds, whole, 1 oz	3.4
Sesame Butter/Tahini, 2 Tbsp, 1.1 oz	1.4
Sunflower kernels, ¼ cup, 1 oz	3.8
Teff Seeds, 1 oz	3.8

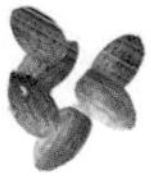

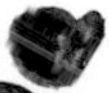

Fruit – Fresh
Apples: 1 medium, 5½ oz (whole)	
with skin + core	3.7
with skin, no core	3.2
without skin, no core	1.7
Apricots, 2 medium, 4 oz	1.5
Avocado, average, ½ medium	6.7
Banana, 1 medium, 6 oz (w. skin)	
Blueberries, raw, ½ cup, 2½ oz	1.7
Cherries, sweet, raw, 8 fruits, 1.6 oz	1
Grapefruit, average, ½ fruit, 10 oz	1.4
Grapes, 1 medium bunch, seedless, 7 oz	2
Kiwifruit, 1 medium, 2.7 oz	2.3
Mango, 1 medium, 11 oz (whole)	1.6
Melons, Cantaloupe, 4 oz (edible)	1
Nectarine, 1 medium, 4 oz	1.9
Olives, average all types, 7 jumbo, 2 oz	1.5
Oranges, 1 medium (7-8 oz w. skin)	
5½ oz (peeled)	3.8
Passionfruit, 2 medium, 2½ oz	5
Peaches, 1 large, 6 oz	2
Pears, raw, 1 medium, 6 oz	4.5
Pineapple, 1 slice, 3 oz	1.2
Plums, 2 medium, 6 oz	1.8
Strawberries, 6 medium/3 large, 2 oz	1
Watermelon, 4 oz (edible)	0.5

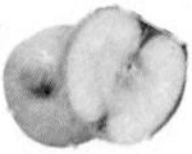

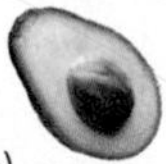

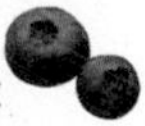

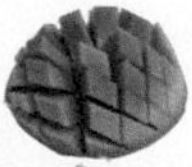

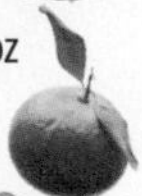

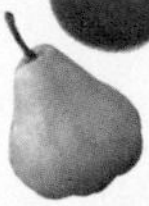

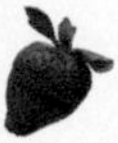

Fruit – Dried, Juice | Fiber
Dried Fruit: Apricots, 8 halves, 1 oz	2.2
Dates (3 med)/ Raisins (2 Tbsp), 1 oz	1.5
Figs, 3 medium, 1½ oz	5
Prunes, 4 medium, 1 oz	2
Fruit Juice: Orange/Apple etc, 1 glass	<0.5
Prune Juice, 5 oz	1.4
Carrot Juice, 8 oz	1.8

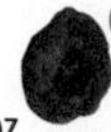

Vegetables
Asparagus, 4 medium spears	1.3
Bean Sprouts, ½ cup, 2 oz	1
Beans: Snap/Green, ½ cup, 2 oz	2
Baked Beans in Tom Sce, ½ c, 4½ oz	5
Dried Beans, ckd, average, ½ cup	7
Beets, ckd, slices, ½ cup, 3 oz	1.7
Broccoli, cooked, ½ cup, 3 oz	2.4
Brussels Sprouts, ckd, ½ cup, 3 oz	3.5
Cabbage: White, ckd, ½ cup, 2½ oz	1
Red, ckd, ½ cup, 2½ oz	2
Carrots, 1 medium (7½"), ½ cup, 3 oz	2.5
Cauliflower, cooked, 3 flowerets, 2 oz	1.5
Celery, raw, diced, 1 cup, 3½ oz	1.6
Chick Peas (Garbanzos), ckd, ½ c., 3 oz	6.5
Corn: Kernels, cooked, ½ cup, 2½ oz	2.5
Corn on the Cob, 1 ear, 5 oz	4
Cucumber/Lettuce/Mushrooms, 2 oz	0.5
Eggplant, raw, sliced, ½ cup, 1½ oz	2
Lentils, cooked, ½ cup, 3½ oz	8
Mixed Vegetables, frozen, cooked, ½ cup	3
Onions, Raw, 1 medium, 4 oz	1.5
Spring Onions, chop., ¼ cup, 1 oz	0.7
Peas: Green, Raw, 2½ oz	3.7
Cowpeas (Black-eyed), ckd, ½ cup	10
Split Peas, ckd, ½ cup, 3½ oz	8
Peppers, sweet, raw, 1 large, 6 oz	3
Potatoes: 1 medium, with skin, 5 oz	4
without skin	2.5
½ cup mashed, 3½ oz	1.5
French Fries, small, 2.6 oz	3
Spinach, cooked, ½ cup, 3 oz	2.2
Squash: Summer, cooked, ½ cup, 3 oz	2.5
Winter, cooked, ½ cup, 3½ oz	2.4
Tomatoes, 1 medium, 4½ oz	1.5
Tomato Sauce, 1 cup	0.3
Soybean Products: Miso, ½ c., 5 oz	7
Tempeh, cooked, 1 piece, 3 oz	
Tofu, ½ cup, 4.4 oz	

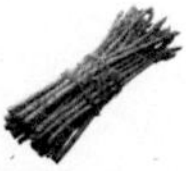

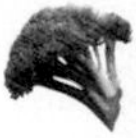

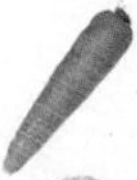

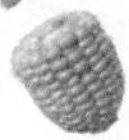

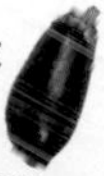

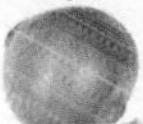

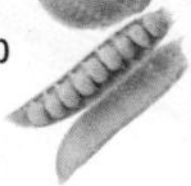

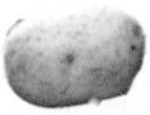

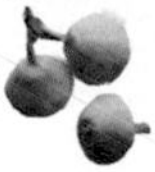

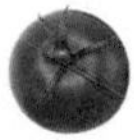

Salads: Side Salad, average
Bean Salad, ½ cup	
Coleslaw, ½ cup	
Potato Salad, ½ cup	

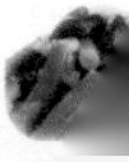

Protein Guide

General Notes

- **Protein has many important body functions.** It builds and repairs muscle, and is the basis of our body's organs, hormones, enzymes, and antibodies to fight infection.

- **Protein is also an emergency fuel** in the absence of sufficient carbohydrate and fats. For this reason, weight loss should be gradual so as to preserve protein levels in muscle, the heart and other body organs.

- **It is easy to obtain sufficient protein, even if vegetarian. Plant proteins are not inferior to animal proteins.** In fact, eating more soy and other plant proteins, and less animal protein, may help to build stronger bones and prevent osteoporosis, and may help to control blood cholesterol levels.

- **When changing to a vegetarian diet,** include soybeans, and other beans, soy milk drinks (calcium-enriched), lentils, tofu, tempeh, nuts and wholegrain breads and cereals. Milk, yogurt, cheese and eggs can enhance nutrient intake.

Protein & Muscle

- Although muscles are built of protein, protein is not a special fuel for working muscle cells – carbohydrates and fats are.

- In fact, a diet high in protein (and fat) and low in carbohydrate can significantly reduce the performance of endurance sports athletes. **Carbohydrates** are the best fuel for muscles exercised for long periods.

- Any **extra protein** required by athletes and body-builders can easily be obtained from the extra food eaten to satisfy hunger and energy needs.

- ₋emember, **excessive protein** intake ⌐ not build bigger muscles. Any excess is ₋rted and stored as fat. Excess protein ⌐ strain the kidneys, which excrete the ⌐ducts of protein metabolism.

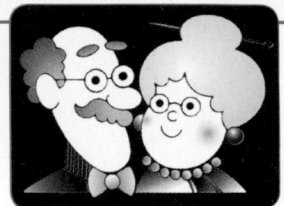

Elderly people (and dieters) must eat sufficient food to ensure adequate protein intake.

Inadequate protein leads to a drop in immune response with greater susceptibility to illness and infections. Muscle strength and muscle mass also drop.

Protein needs are easily met with sensible eating. Athletes who eat enough food for their energy needs can obtain sufficient protein.

RECOMMENDED DAILY PROTEIN INTAKE ~ HEALTHY RANGE ~
(Lower figure is RDA)

		PROTEIN
Children:	1-3 yrs	13g-26g
	4-8 yrs	19g-38g
	9-13 yrs	34g-64g
Males:	14-18 yrs	52g-120g
	19+	56g-120g
Females:	14+	46g-110g
Pregnancy:		71g-120g
Breastfeeding:		71g-120g

Note: On lower-calorie diets, aim for higher amounts of protein within the Healthy Range.

Pro ~ Protein (grams)

Meat   **Pro**

Steak: Average all cuts, lean (no fat)
Small (4 oz raw/3 oz ckd)	23
Medium (6 oz raw/4¼ oz ckd)	34
Large (10 oz raw/7¼ oz ckd)	57
Roast Beef, lean, 2 slices, 3 oz	24
Ground Beef patty, lean, ckd, 3 oz	21
Lamb chop, broiled, 3 oz	22
Liver, cooked, 3 oz	23
Veal cutlet, 1 medium	23
Pork, cooked, lean, 3 oz	24
Bacon, 3 medium slices	6
Ham, roasted, 2 pieces, 3 oz	18
Ham, luncheon, 2 slices, 1½ oz	7
Pastrami (Oscar Mayer), 3 sl., 1¾ oz	10
Sausages: Bologna, 2 sl., 2 oz	7
Braunschweiger, 2 sl., 2 oz	8
Pork link, thick, 2 oz	6
Frankfurter, 1⅓ oz	5
Salami, hard, 3 slices, 1 oz	7
Vegetarian (Boca Burger), 1 pattie	13

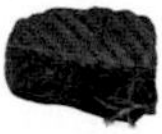

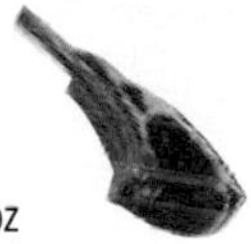

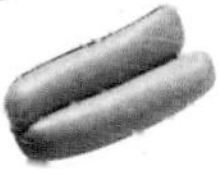

Chicken/Turkey (Without Skin)
Chicken, ckd; Breast, Roasted, 4 oz	36
Leg/Thigh,Roasted, 2 oz	14
½ Whole Chicken	60
Drumstick, Rstd, 1 med., 3 oz	13
Turkey, cooked: Light meat, 3 oz	28
Dark meat, lean, 3 oz	24

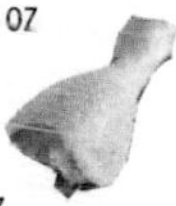

Fish
Fresh Fish: *Per 4 oz, cooked*
Cod, Flounder/Sole, Pollock	28
Catfish, Haddock, Halibut, M/Mahi	28
Ocean Perch, Swordf., Orange Roughy	28
Canned Fish: Tuna, Light, 3 oz	25
White, 3 oz	23
Salmon, pink, 3 oz	17
Salmon, red, 3 oz	17
Sardines, 3 whole (3"), 1¼ oz	9
Anchovies, 1 can, 1½ oz	13
Shellfish: Crabmeat, 3 oz	17.5
Clams, raw, 4 large/9 sml, 3 oz	11
Crayfish, cooked, 3 oz	20
Lobster, cooked, 3 oz	17
Oysters, raw, 6 medium, 3 oz	7
Scallops, 2 lge/5 small, 1 oz	5
Shrimp, raw, 6 large, 1½ oz	8.5
Fish Products: Fish Sticks, 4 sticks	10
Fish Portions, in batter, 4 oz	13
Gefilte Fish, 1 medium ball, 2 oz	8

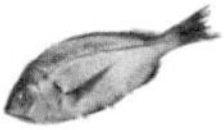

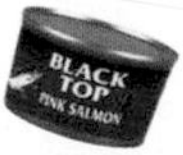

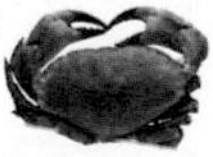

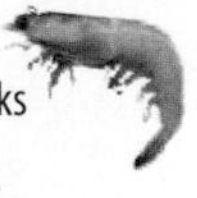

Eggs   **Pro**
1 Large Egg, whole	6
Egg Yolk	3
Egg White	3
Omelet: Plain, 2 eggs	13
Ham & cheese	17
Egg Substitutes (liquid):	
Egg Beaters, ¼ cup, 2 oz	4.5
Better 'n Eggs/Scramblers, ¼ cup, 2 oz	6

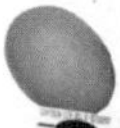

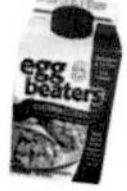

Milk, Yogurt, Ice Cream
Milk: Whole: 2%, 1 cup	8
Low-Fat (1%); Fat-Free, 1 cup	8.5
Chocolate Milk, 1 cup	8
Thick Shake, Chocolate, 10 oz	9
Vanilla, 10 oz	11
Soymilk (fortified), average, 1 cup	7
Soy Dream Enriched, shelf-stable, 1 cup	7
Yogurt: Plain, 6 oz	10
Fruit flavors: 6 oz	8
8 oz	11
Ice Cream: Rich, ½ cup	2
Regular, Vanilla, ½ cup	2.5
Sherbet, ½ cup	1
Custard, baked, ½ cup	7

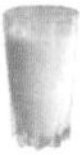

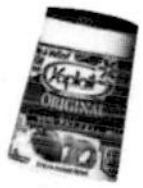

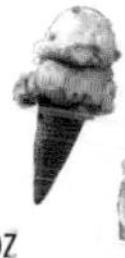

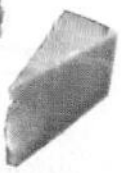

Cheese
Hard Cheeses, average, 1 oz	7
Cottage Cheese, ½ cup	13
Cream Cheese, avg., 1 oz	2
Ricotta, part skim, ½ cup	14

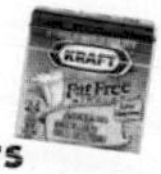

Bread, Bagels, Biscuits
Bread (w. enriched flour): 1 slice, 1 oz	2
4 thin slices, 4 oz	8
4 thick slices, 6 oz	1.2
Bagel, plain 2 oz	6
Biscuits, 1 oz	2
Pita Bread, 1 pita, 1½ oz	4
Pumpernickel, 1 slice, 1 oz	3

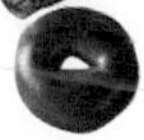

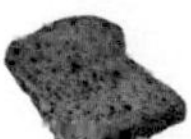

Infant/Baby Foods   **Pro**
Infant Formula Milk:
Enfamil/Gerber/Similac
Regular/Low Iron , 5 fl.oz	2.2
With Iron, 5 fl.oz	2.2
Isomil/Nursoy/ProSobee	3

Baby Cereals:
Average all brands
Dry, 4 Tbsp, ½ oz	1
Jars (w. fruit), 4½ oz	1

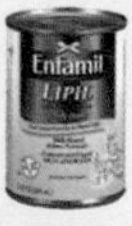

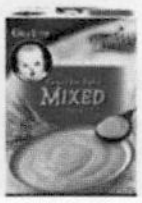

Protein Counter

Breakfast Cereals — Pro

Hot Cereals, cooked:

Bulgur, cooked, 1 cup, 5 oz	9
Oatmeal: Reg., non-fortified, 1 cup	6
Instant, fortified, avg., 1 pkt	4
Quaker, all flavors, ½ cup	5
Corn/Hominy Grits: 1 cup	3
Quaker: Reg., 3 Tbsp, 1 oz	2
Instant White, 1 packet	2
Cream of Wheat, 1 cup	4

Brands ~ Ready-To-Eat

Arrowhead: Average all varieties, 1 oz	3
General Mills: Basic 4, 1 cup, 2 oz	4
Cheerios, Original, 1 cup, 1 oz	3
Cocoa Puffs, 1 cup, 1 oz	1
Kix, 1⅓ cups, 1 oz	2
Multi-Bran Chex, 1 cup, 2 oz	4
Country Corn Flakes, 1 cup, 1.2 oz	2
Total Raisin Bran, 1 cup, 2 oz	3
Wheaties ¾ cup, 1 oz	3
Health Valley: Oat Bran O's, ¾ cup, 1 oz	3
Amaranth Flakes, ¾ cup, 1 oz	3
Bran Flakes w. Raisins, ¾ cup, 1.1 oz	5
Low-Fat Granola, ⅔ cup, 2 oz	5
Real Oat Bran Alm. Crunch, ½ cup, 1.7 oz	6
Golden Flax, ¾ cup, 1.9 oz	6
Kashi: Friends, 1 cup, 1.9 oz	5
GoLean Crunch!, 1 cup, 1.9 oz	9
7 Whole Grain Flakes, 1 c., 1.8 oz	6
Kellogg's: All-Bran: ½ cup, 1 oz	4
Complete Oat Flakes, ¾ c., 1.1 oz	3
Cocoa Krispies, ¾ cup, 1 oz	1
Corn Flakes, 1 cup, 1 oz	2
Low-fat Granola w. Raisins ⅔ c., 2.1 oz	4
Product 19, 1 cup, 1 oz	2
Raisin Bran, 1 cup, 2 oz	7
Rice Krispies, 1¼ cup, 1.2 oz	2
Smart-Start Healthy Heart, 1 c., 1.8 oz	6
Special K: Regular, 1 c., 1.1 oz	6
Protein Plus, ¾ cup, 1 oz	10
Post: Raisin Bran, ⅔ cup, 2 oz	4
Grape Nuts, ½ cup, 2 oz	6
Quaker: Crunchy Corn Bran, 1 cup, 1 oz	2
100% Natural Granola, ½ cup, 1.7 oz	5
Life, ¾ cup, 1.1 oz	3
Cap'n Crunch, ¾ cup, 1 oz	1
Oat Bran, ½ cup, 1.4 oz	7

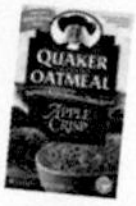

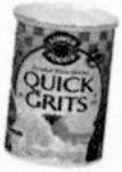

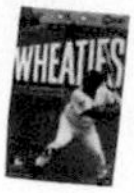

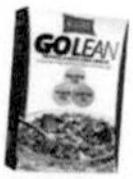

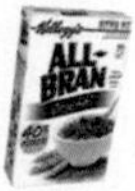

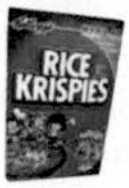

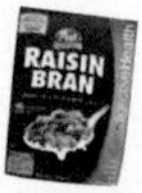

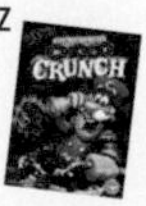

Brans & Wheatgerm — Pro

Oat Bran, raw, 1 Tbsp	2
Rice Bran, raw, 2 Tbsp	1
Wheat Bran, unprocessed, 2 T.	1
Wheat Germ, 2 Tbsp, ½ oz	4

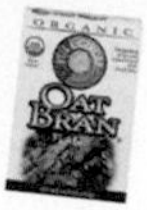

Grains & Flours, Yeast

Amaranth, ½ cup, 3.4 oz	14
Barley, ½ cup, 3.2 oz	12
Buckwheat Flour: Whole-groat, 1 cup	15
Carob Flour, 1 cup, 3.6 oz	5
Corn Flour, 1 cup, 4 oz	11
Corn Meal, 1 cup, 4½ oz	8
Flour: White, 1 cup, 5.6 oz	9
Wholegrain, 1 cup, 4¼ oz	16
Millet, wholegrain, 1 cup, 3½ oz	12
Rye Flour: Dark, 1 cup, 4½ oz	18
Light, 1 cup, 3½ oz	9
Soy Flour, full fat, 1 cup, 3 oz	29
Yeast: Brewers, 2 Tbsp, ½ oz	8
Nutritional Yeast Flakes *(Red Star)*, 1 heaping Tbsp, ½ oz	8

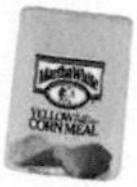

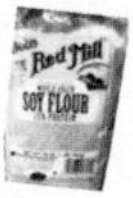

Rice, Spaghetti, Macaroni

Rice: Brown/White, average

1 cup cooked, 6½ oz	5

Spaghetti/Macaroni/Noodles (enriched):

Cooked, 1 cup, 4½ oz	7
Canned: in Tomato Sce, ½ cup	2
w. Meatballs, 1 cup, 8 oz	10
Macaroni & Cheese, 1 cup, 9 oz	8

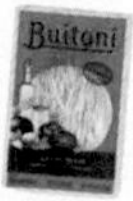

Soups

With Noodles/Vegetables, 1 cup	3
With Meat/Beans/Peas, 1 cup	8

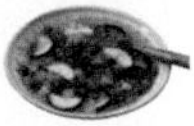

Fruit

Fresh/Canned:

Average, all types 1 medium/2 small fruit	1
Avocado, ½ medium	2
Dried Fruit: Apricots, 8 halves, 1 oz	1
Dates, 6 dates, 2 oz	1.5
Figs, 4 medium figs, 2 oz	2
Prunes, 5 medium, 1½ oz	1
Raisins, 1 oz	1
Fruit Juice: Average, 1 cup	0.5
Prune Juice, 6 fl.oz	1
Tomato Juice, 1 cup, 8 fl.oz	1.5

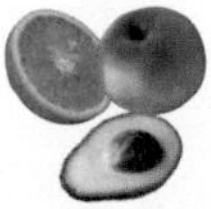

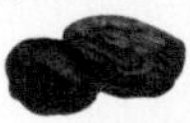

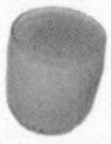

Vegetables | Pro
Beans: Snap/green, ½ cup, 2 oz	1
Dried: Average all types, cooked, ½ cup	7
Baked Beans, ½ cup 4½ oz	5
Bean Sprouts, mung, 1 c., 4 oz	3
Broccoli, 3raw, ½ cup, 1½ oz	1.5
Cabbage; Cauliflower, raw, 1 c. 3 oz	1.5
Corn, raw, ½ cup kernels, 3 oz	2.5
1 ear trimmed to 3½"	2
Lentils, cooked, ½ cup, 3½ oz	9
Mushrooms, raw, ½ c., sliced	1
Peas: Green, raw, ½ c., 2½ oz	4
Split Peas, cooked, 1 cup, 7 oz	16
Potatoes, cooked:	
1 medium, with skin, 5 oz	3.3
without skin, 4 oz	2.3
French Fries, small, 2.6 oz	2
Potato Salad, ½ cup, 4 oz	3.5
Pumpkin, ½ cup mashed, 4.3 oz	1
Seaweed, kelp, 1 oz	<1
Spinach, cooked, ½ cup, 3 oz	2.7
Squash, ckd, all types, ½ cup	1
Tomatoes, 1 medium, 4½ oz	1
Vegetables, mixed, ckd, 1 cup	2.5
Soybeans, cooked, ½ cup, 3 oz	14

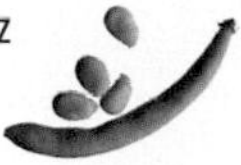

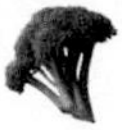

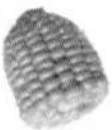

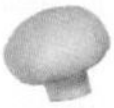

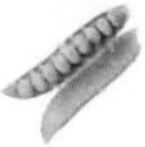

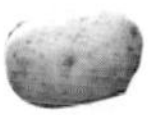

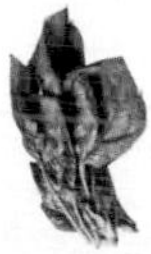

Tofu, Tempeh, Miso
Tofu, raw, firm, ½ cup, 4½ oz	10
Tempeh, ½ cup, 3 oz	16
Miso, ½ cup, 5 oz	16
Miso Soup, 1 cup	3
Soybean Protein (TVP), 1 oz	18

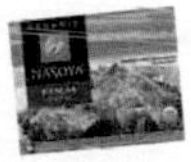

Cakes, Pastries, Pies
(Made with enriched flour)
Carrot w. cream cheese frosting, 4 oz	4
Cheesecake, 1 piece, 4 oz	6
Chocolate, 1 piece, 2 oz	2
Fruitcake, 1 piece, 3 oz	4
Plain, 1 piece, 3 oz	4
Croissant, plain, 2 oz	5
Danish Pastry, 1 pastry, 2¼ oz	4
Donuts, average, 2 oz	4
Muffins, average, 1 med., 1½ oz	3
Pancakes, 4" diam., two, 2 oz	4
Pies: Fruit, 1 piece, 5½ oz	4
Pecan, 1 piece, 5 oz	7
Puddings, average, ½ cup, 4½ oz	4
Waffles, 1 large, 2½ oz	7

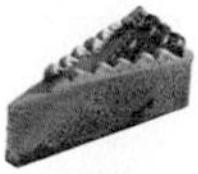

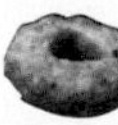

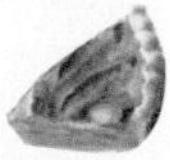

Peanut Butter | Pro
Regular: 2 Tbsp, 1.1 oz	8
Peter Pan Plus, 2 Tbsp, 1.1 oz	8

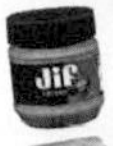

Sugar, Honey, Jam
Sugar: White	0
Brown, 1 Tbsp	0
Molasses: Light/Med., 1 Tbsp	0
Blackstrap, 1 Tbsp, ¾ oz	0
Corn Syrup, 1 Tbsp, ¾ oz	0
Honey, Jams, Jelly	0

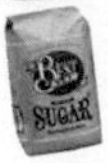

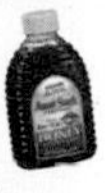

Candy, Chocolate, Carob
Candy, sugar-based	0
Chocolate: Plain, 2 oz bar	4
with nuts, 2 oz bar	6
Carob, plain, 2 oz	6

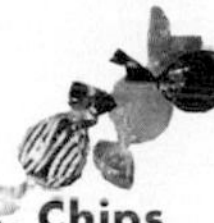

Cookies, Crackers, Chips
Cookies, average, 4 cookies	2
Crackers, Graham, 2½" sq., (2)	1
Rice Cakes, average, one	1
Corn/Potato Chips, 1 oz	2
Nuts: Almonds, shelled, 20-25 nuts	6
Brazil Nuts, 7-8 medium nuts, 1 oz	4
Cashews, 12-16 nuts, 1 oz	5
Macadamias, 1 oz	2
Peanuts, dry rsted, 40 nuts, 1 oz	6
Pecans, 24 halves, 1 oz	2
Walnuts, 15 halves, 1 oz	4
Seeds: Sesame Seeds, dry, 1 Tbsp	2
Pumpkin Kernels, dry, hulled, 1 oz	7
Sunflower Seeds, dried, hulled, 1 oz	6
Tahini, 1 Tbsp, ½ oz	2.5

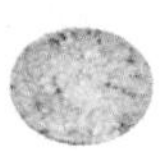

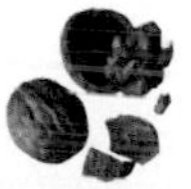

Granola & Food/Protein Bars
Granola Bars, avg., 1 bar, 2 oz	2
Anytime Health,	
Meal Bars, 80g	20
Snack Bars, 50g	12
Balance Bars, Orlg. 1.76 oz	14
Bariatrix Proti-Bars (1), 1.4 oz	15
Dr Soy Protein Bars, 1.76 oz	11
GeniSoy Protein Bar, 1.6 oz	15
Jenny Craig Bars, 1.8 oz	4
Met-Rx "Big 100", 3.5 oz	27
Myoplex Carb Sense Bar, 2.5 oz	26
Optifast Peanut Butter, 1.59 oz	8
PowerBar: Harvest	10
Performance Bar, 2.3 oz	10
ProteinPlus, 1 bar, avg., 2.75 oz	24
Slim-Fast: High Protein Meal, 1.7 oz	15
Optima Meal, 2 oz bar	8
Special K: Protein Meal, 1.6 oz	10
Protein Snack, 0.9 oz	4

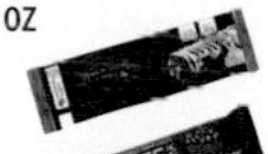

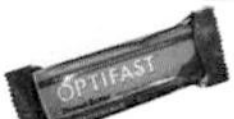

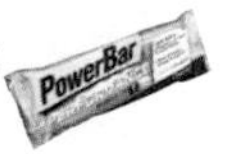

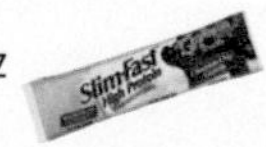

Protein Counter

High Protein Drinks   `Pro`

Anytime Health:	
Whey Protein Isolate,	
All flavors, 1 oz	25
Atkins Shakes, 11 fl.oz can	18
Boost High Protein, 8 oz	10
Carnation Instant Breakfast, 10 oz	13
Curves Protein Drink, 2 scoops, dry	15
dotFIT: FirstString, 4 scoops, 5.2 oz	42
Meal Replacement,	
Chocolate, 2 scoops, 2.2 oz	20
WheySmooth, Choc., 2 scoops, 2.2 oz	40
Ensure Plus, 8 oz can	13
Gatorade: Nutrition Shake, 11 oz	20
Protein Recovery Shake, 11 oz	20
GeniSoy Shake, 1 scoop, 1.2 oz	14
Kashi GoLean Shake, 2 sc., 2.1 oz	21
Met-Rx RTD 40	40
Myoplex, Original Nutrition Shake, 1 pkt	42
Optifast 800, made up, 8 fl oz	14
Resource (Novartis) Standard, 8 fl.oz	15
Slim-Fast Shakes: Meal, 11 oz can	10
High Protein, 11 oz can	15
Optima, 11 oz can	10
Special K₂O Protein Water, 16 fl.oz	5
Walgreens Slim For Less, 11 oz can	10
Weider Mass 1000, 4 scoops, 7 oz	34

Coffee, Tea, Soda

Coffee, Coffee Substitutes, 1 cup, 8 fl.oz	0
Coffee w. 2 oz milk, 1 cup, 8 fl.oz	2
Caffe latte, large, 16 fl.oz	12
Cappuccino, large, 16 fl.oz	8
Frappuccino, avg., 16 fl.oz	6
Hot Chocolate,	
with milk, 1 cup, 8 fl.oz	8
Soft Drinks/Soda	0
Tea (all types)	0

Beer, Wine, Spirits

Beer, 12 fl.oz	1
Wines, red/white, 1 glass	0
Spirits/Liquor	0

Fast-Foods/Burgers

Pancakes: Average all outlets, 3	8
Shakes, Chocolate, 16 fl.oz	12
Sundaes: Average all outlets	7
Arby's: Roast Beef Sandwich, regular	20
Chicken Club Salad	32
Roast Beef Sandwich, Super	21
Burger King: Whopper S/wich	29
Bacon Double Cheeseburger	32
BK Big Fish Sandwich	24

Fast Foods/Burgers (Cont)   `Pro`

Carl's Jr:	
Famous Star Hamburger w/ Cheese	27
Charbroiled Chicken Club Sandwich	39
Super Star Hamburger w/ Cheese	47
Domino's Pizza: Deep Dish (12")	
Beef, 2 slices	10
Cheese, 2 slices	12
Pepperoni, Sausage, 1 sl.	10
KFC: Original, Breast	42
Crispy Strips, 3 strips	33
Snacker, Regular	15
McDonald's: Big Mac	25
Cheeseburger	15
Chicken McNuggets (6)	14
Crispy Chicken Classic Burger	28
Filet-O-Fish	15
Hamburger	12
Quarter Pounder w. Cheese	29
French Fries: Small, 2.5 oz	3
Large, 5.4 oz	6
Salads w. Chicken, average	30
Triple Shake, average, 16 fl.oz	16
Breakfast: Egg McMuffin	18
Bacon, Egg & Cheese McGriddles	15
Sausage Burrito	12
Sausage McMuffin w. Egg	21
Pizza Hut: Per Medium, 1 slice, ⅛ Pizza	
Thin 'n Crispy, Supreme	10
Pan Pizzas, average	11
Hand Tossed, Pepperoni	10
Fit n' Delicious, Ham/Pineapple/Tomato	7
Subway (6" Subs): Roast Beef	26
Meatball Marinara	24
Roast Chicken Breast	23
Subway Club	26
Sweet Onion Chicken Teriyaki	26
Taco Bell: Bean Burrito	12
Chicken Quesadilla	28
Chicken/Steak Enchirito	21
Gordita Baja Beef	13
Steak Burrito Supreme	18
Taco Supreme	11
Wendy's: ¼ lb Single Burger	27
Chicken Club	37
Jr Hamburger	13

High Blood Pressure

High Blood Pressure

Many American adults have hypertension (high blood pressure), and are unaware of it. It is generally symptomless, so **have your blood pressure checked annually** – particularly if it runs in the family.

Untreated hypertension overworks the heart, damages arteries and promotes atherosclerosis. This in turn greatly increases the risk of heart disease, stroke, blindness, kidney disease and impotence. The earlier hypertension is detected, the sooner it can be brought under control.

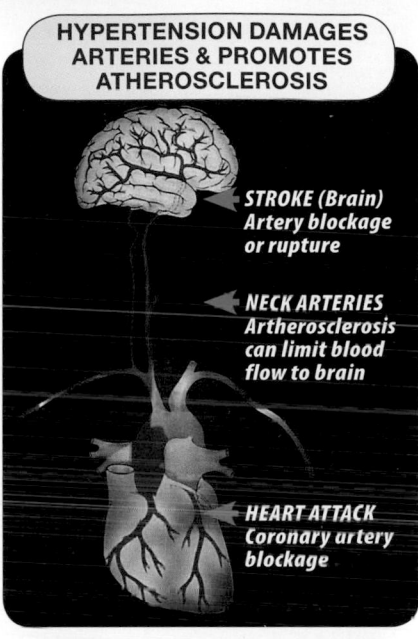

HYPERTENSION DAMAGES ARTERIES & PROMOTES ATHEROSCLEROSIS

STROKE (Brain) Artery blockage or rupture

NECK ARTERIES Artherosclerosis can limit blood flow to brain

HEART ATTACK Coronary artery blockage

BLOOD PRESSURE CLASSIFICATION

For Adults Age 18 & Older ~ Not Acutely Ill or on Medication (American Heart Association)

	DIASTOLIC		SYSTOLIC
Normal ➤	Below 80	and	Below 120
Prehypertension ➤	80-89	or	120-139
Hypertension:			
Stage 1 ➤	90-99	or	140-159
Stage 2 ➤	100 or more	or	160 or more

Treating Hypertension

Prehypertension (in the chart above) means you don't have high blood pressure now but are likely to develop it in the future.

You can take steps to lessen the risk by adopting healthy lifestyle habits such as:

- reducing sodium intake
- eating adequate fruit and vegetables
- losing weight if overweight
- limiting alcohol to 2 drinks or less daily
- quitting smoking
- exercising regularly, managing stress.

Stage 1 hypertension can often be treated with the above lifestyle changes.

Stage 2 hypertension usually requires drug therapy. However, salt restriction, abstaining from alcohol, and the above lifestyle changes will improve the success of drug therapy, and enable smaller drug doses to be prescribed.

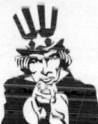

STROKE KNOW THE WARNING SIGNS

Stroke is a medical emergency! If you notice one or more of these signs, call 9-1-1 or your doctor immediately.

These signs may be signalling a possible stroke or transient ischemic attack:

- **Sudden weakness** or numbness in your face, arm, or leg on one side of your body
- **Sudden confusion,** trouble speaking or understanding
- **Sudden trouble seeing,** in one or both eyes
- **Sudden trouble walking,** dizziness, loss of balance or coordination
- **Sudden severe headache** - 'a bolt out of the blue' – with no apparent cause

Salt & Sodium Guide

Salt & Sodium

- **Sodium is a mineral element** most commonly found in salt (sodium chloride). It also occurs naturally in much smaller amounts in animal and plant foods, and water – normally sufficient for our needs without having to add salt to our diet.

- **Sodium is required** for nerve and muscle function, as well as to balance the amount of fluid in our tissues and blood.

  Sodium acts like a sponge to attract and hold fluids in body tissues.

- **Excess sodium** can cause water retention, and increase the risk of developing hypertension. Very high salt intake may also increase the risk of stomach cancer.

- **Too little sodium** may cause low blood pressure (hypotension), and decrease blood flow to the heart, brain and kidneys – especially during exercise. (A certain blood volume is required to sustain the blood pressure needed for adequate blood flow in the capillaries).

Salt-Sensitive Persons

- **Normally, our kidneys** excrete excess dietary sodium. The thirst we feel after a salty meal is the body calling for water to dilute the sodium, and enable the kidneys to flush out excess sodium.

- **However, 'salt - sensitive'** persons (up to 50% of adults) tend to retain excess sodium (above approximately 3000mg daily) instead of excreting it. Such persons are more likely to develop hypertension and would benefit most from sodium restriction. Assume you are susceptible if there is a family history of hypertension.

- **Although not everyone will benefit, all Americans are being asked to moderate their salt and sodium intake** as a public health measure – particularly because so many do not know whether or not they have hypertension, and also because we do not know just who is salt-sensitive.

SAFE SODIUM LEVELS

The American Heart Association recommends a **maximum sodium intake of 1500mg per day** for adults with normal blood pressure.

Persons with hypertension and kidney ailments are usually restricted to as little as **1000mg sodium per day**. Your doctor will discuss the correct sodium level for you.

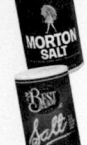

FINDING HIDDEN SODIUM

On average, **less than one third of our sodium intake comes from the salt shaker.**
The rest is hidden in processed foods that have salt added during manufacture.

Sodium compounds added to food or medicinals can also contribute significant sodium.

Sodium bicarbonate in particular is widely used in antacid tablets (such as *Alka Seltzer*) and powders. Sodium bicarbonate contains 27% sodium by weight. Each gram contributes 270mg sodium. Large amounts of sodium can be unwittingly consumed – up to 600mg per tablet. (See Antacids ~ Page 280)

Example: 2 *Alka-Seltzer* Tablets = 1000mg sodium

Other sodium compounds include monosodium glutamate (MSG), sodium ascorbate, sodium nitrite, and sodium citrate.

POTASSIUM BALANCES SODIUM

Potassium helps to balance sodium by helping the kidneys to excrete excess sodium. Fruit and vegetables are rich sources of potassium - another reason to ensure you have your 5-7 servings every day.

Nuts also provide potassium as well as magnesium and other heart-healthy nutrients and anti-oxidants. Eat them unsalted.

ALCOHOL DANGER

Excessive alcohol intake contributes to hypertension. Susceptible persons should limit alcohol intake to 1-2 drinks per day.

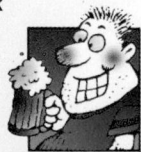

Salt Sodium Guide

Sodium accounts for only 40% of the weight of salt (sodium chloride). Examples:
1 gram (1000mg) Salt has 400mg Sodium
1 teaspoon (5g) Salt has 2000mg Sodium

HINTS TO REDUCE SODIUM

- **Cut down use of the salt shaker.** Start with an easy 50% cut in sodium by using Lite Salt (*Morton*) or *Cardia* Salt. Then gradually cut back until you can leave the salt shaker off the table. Sea salt is still high in sodium.

- **Use fresh herbs**, and salt-free seasonings to add flavor to food.

- **Choose low-sodium**, sodium-free, and reduced-sodium products in place of regular, salted products.

- **Check food labels for sodium levels.** FDA Guidelines for sodium descriptors are:
  - **Reduced Sodium:** At least 25% less sodium than the original product
  - **Low Sodium:** 140 mg or less/serving
  - **Very Low Sodium:** 35mg or less/serving
  - **Sodium Free:** Less than 5mg/serving
  - **No Salt Added:** Made without the salt normally added, but still contains the sodium that is a natural part of the food

- **Use reduced-sodium breads**, butter and margarine. Regular varieties are considered high in sodium in view of their significant contribution to our diet.

- **Go easy on salty condiments and sauces** such as ketchup, mustard, soy sauce, spaghetti sauces, and salad dressings. Use low-sodium varieties.

- **Limit pizzas and salty fast-foods.** Check **CalorieKing.com** food database.

- **Avoid salty snack foods** such as potato chips, corn chips, salted nuts, pretzels and cheesy-flavored snacks. **Choose unsalted** popcorn, nuts or seeds. Eat more fruit.

- **Don't salt children's food** to your taste.

- **Avoid antacids with** sodium bicarbonate (such as *Alka-Seltzer*). They are high in sodium. Look for low-sodium alternatives.

FOODS HIGH IN SODIUM

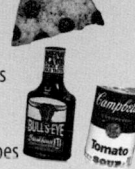
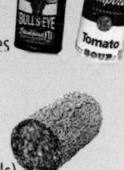

- Cheese, Butter, Margarine
- Pickles, Sauerkraut, Olives
- Condiments, Sauces
- Salad Dressings
- Canned vegetables/salads/beans
- Deli Salads (with dressing)
- Frozen/Packaged Meals/Entrees
- Soups: Canned/dry; bouillon cubes
- Meats: Ham, bacon, sausage, luncheon meats, smoked meats
- Canned Fish (in brine/salt)
- Sea Salt, Garlic/Celery Salt
- Snack Foods (potato chips, pretzels)
- Tomato Juice (Canned), V8 Vegetable Juice
- Fast Foods: Pizza, Burgers, Chicken
- *Alka-Seltzer* Antacid
- Bread (regular)

MODERATE SODIUM

- Meat, Fish, Poultry - Unprocessed
- Milk, Yogurt, Soy Drinks, Eggs
- Peanut Butter
- Breakfast Cereals (less than 200mg/serving)
- Chocolate Candy, Fruit/Nut Bars
- *Reduced Sodium & Low Sodium Products*

FOODS LOW IN SODIUM

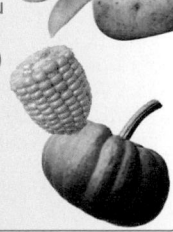

- Products labelled *Very Low Sodium*, or *Sodium Free*
- Bread (No Salt Added)
- Fresh fruits and vegetables
- Canned and Dried Fruits
- Potatoes, Rice, Pasta
- Dried Beans & Lentils, Tofu
- Nuts & Seeds (unsalted)
- Corn & Popcorn (unsalted)
- Pepper, Spices, Herbs
- Jam, Honey, Syrup
- Candy, Gum
- Hard & Jelly Candy
- Coffee, Tea, Alcohol
- Fresh Fruit Juices, Water

Sodium Counter

Milk & Dairy Products

	Sodium
Milk: Whole/lowfat/skim, average	
1 cup, 8 fl.oz	120
Whole, low sodium, 1 cup	5
Choc Milk, 1 cup	130
Soy Milk, 8 fl.oz	30
Buttermilk, cultured, 8 fl.oz	250
Dry/Powder, skim, ¼ cup, 1 oz	110
Yogurt, with fruit average, 8 oz	130
Cheese: Bleu, 1 oz	330
Parmesan, 1 oz	450
Kraft Cheddar, 2% milk, 1 oz	230
Philadelphia Cream Cheese, 1 oz	90
Process Cheese., average,1 oz	430
Swiss, 1 oz	40
Cottage Cheese, ½ cup, 4 oz	450
Ricotta Cheese, ½ cup, 4 oz	150

Ice Cream, Frozen Yogurt

Icecream, average, ½ cup	50
Frozen Yogurt, ½ cup	50

Fats/Oils

Butter/Margarine:	
Regular, 2 Tbsp, 1 oz	230
Unsalted, reg., 2 Tbsp, 1 oz	5
Mayonnaise, aver., 2 Tbsp, 1 oz	160
Oils/Lard/Drippings	0
Cream, average, 1 Tbsp	5
Coffee-Mate: Powdered, 1 tsp	2
Liquid, 1 Tbsp	5

Eggs

Whole, 1 large	70
Omelet, 2 egg, plain	220
w. cheese	400
Egg Beaters: Original, ¼ cup	115
Flavors, average, ¼ cup	230

Meats

Meat, average all types, cooked	
(Beef/Lamb/Veal/Pork), 4 oz	80
Corned Beef, cooked, 3 oz	800
Bacon, cooked, 2 sl., ½ oz	270
Ham, 3 oz	1100

Chicken & Turkey

Chicken/Turkey, cooked, unsalted, 4 oz	80
Stuffing Mixes, average., ½ cup	500
KFC ~ See Page 281 (Fast-Foods)	

Sodium ~ Sodium (mg)

Sausages & Meats

	Sodium
Bologna, 1 oz	280
Frankfurter, 2 oz	640
Ham, chopped, ¾ oz slice	290
Liverwurst (Braunschweiger), 1 oz	320
Pepperoni, 5 slices, 1 oz	570
Salami, cooked, 1 oz	350
dry/hard, 1 oz	600
Sausage, 1 oz link	220
Pork, 2 oz patty	260
Spam: Classic, 2 oz	790
25% Less Sodium, 2 oz	580
Turkey Roll, 1 oz	160

Fish:

Fresh Fish, average, plain	
Cooked, 4 oz (no bone)	60
Broiled w. butter, 4 oz	150
Breaded & fried, 4 oz	320
Fish fillets, batter-dipped 3 oz	350
Fish sticks, 1 oz stick	160
Gefilte Fish (w. broth), 1 pce, 1½ oz	220
Herring, pickled, 2 pces, 1 oz	260
Lobster, meat only, 4 oz	180
Oysters, fresh, 6 med., 3 oz	95
Salmon: Canned, 3 oz	460
No Salt Added, 3 oz	65
Smoked fish, average, 3 oz	650
Tuna: Canned, regular, 3 oz	330
No Added Salt, 3 oz	40
Spicy Flavored, 5 oz can	550

Entrees & Meals

Frozen Meals, average	600-900
Lean Cuisine, average	700
Stouffer's, average	580
Dinners, average	900-1200
Side Dishes, average	400-600
Pizza, frozen, ¼ large, 6 oz	800-1200
Microwave Cup Meals	900-1200
Cup O'Noodles, average	1500
Pizza ~ See Page 281 (Pizza Hut)	

More Sodium Counts:
www.CalorieKing.com

Soups

	Sodium
Condensed, 1 cup, 8 oz	800-1000
Low Sodium	70
Chicken Noodle, 1 cup	900
Bouillon Cube, average	950
Cup-A-Soup: Average	850
Lite, average	450
Soup Mixes, average, 1 cup	900

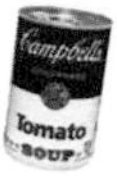

Condiments, Sauces, Dressings

A-1 Sauce, 1 Tbsp	280
Barbecue Sauce, 1 Tbsp	130
Bragg's Liquid Aminos, 1 tsp	220
Chili Sauce, 1 Tbsp	230
Ketchup: Tomato, 1 Tbsp	180
Low Sodium, 1 Tbsp	20
Mayonnaise, 1 Tbsp	80
Mustard, 1 tsp	70
Pizza Sauce, ½ cup	700
Salad Dressings, 2 Tbsp, 1 oz	160-400
Spaghetti Sauce, ½ cup	500
Soy Sauce: 1 Tbsp	900
Lite *(Kikkoman),* 1 Tbsp	600
Sweet & Sour, ½ cup	250
Tabasco, 1 tsp	25
Vinegar, Lemon Juice	0
Worcestershire, 1 Tbsp	200
Tomato: Sauce, 1 cup	1200
Paste/Puree (salted), ½ cup	1000
No Salt Added, ½ cup	25

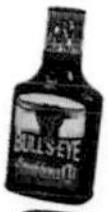

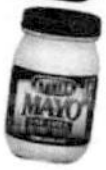

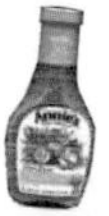

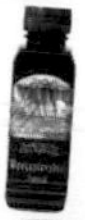

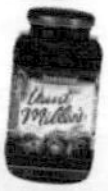

Salt & Salt Substitutes

Table Salt: 1 teaspoon, 6g	2400
Single Serve package, 1 g	400
Cardia Salt, 1 teaspoon	1080
Lite Salt *(Morton),* 1 teaspoon, 6g	1200
Morton/No Salt Substitute, 1 tsp	5
Garlic/Seasoned Salt 1 teaspoon, 4g	1300
Sea Salt, 1 teaspoon, 5g	2250

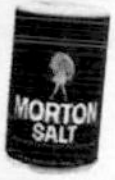

Seasonings, Herbs & Spices

Baking Powder, 1 tsp, 3g	340
Baking Soda (Sodium bicarb), 1 tsp, 3g	810
Accent (Flavor Enhancer), 1 tsp	600
Chili Powder, 1 tsp, 3g	25
Curry Powder	0
Lemon Pepper *(Lawry's),* 1 tsp	340
Meat Tenderizer, 1 tsp, 5g	1750
MSG (Monosodium glutamate), 5g	500
Mrs Dash Blends/Marinades	0
Old Bay, Seasoning (Less Sodium), 1 teaspoon, 2.4g	380
Pepper, Mustard (dry), 1 tsp	1
Yeast, Nutritional, 1 Tbsp	10

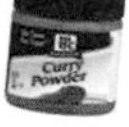

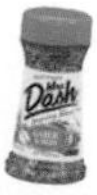

Breakfast Cereals

	Sodium
Kellogg's:	
All-Bran, ½ cup, 1 oz	80
Special K, 1 cup, 1.1 oz	220
Corn Flakes, 1 cup, 1 oz	200
Just Right, ¾ cup, 2 oz	240
Mini Wheats Frosted, 24 bisc., 1.8 oz	5
Health Valley Cereals, 1 serving	5
Quaker: Cap'n Crunch, ¾ cup, 1 oz	200
Crunchy Corn Bran, ¾ cup, 1 oz	230
100% Natural Granola, ½ cup, 1 oz	15
Puffed Rice/Wheat, 2 cups, 1 oz	1
General Mills: Total, ¾ cup, 1 oz	190
Oatmeal: Regular, ¾ cup	1
Instant *(Quaker),* ⅔ cup (1 pkt)	270

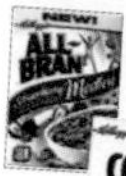

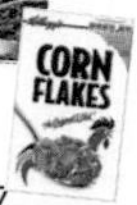

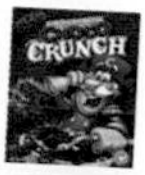

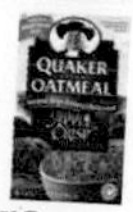

Breads, Bagels, Crackers

Bread: Thin Slice, average 1 oz	140
Thick Slice, 1½ oz	210
Low Sodium, 1 oz	10
Bagels: Plain, medium, 2 oz	200
Sara Lee, 3 oz	500
Biscuits, average, 1 oz	180
Bun/Roll: 1 medium, 1½ oz	200
Large, 4 oz	560
Crackers: Saltine, 2 crackers	70
Low Salt *(Premium),* 2	25
Graham, 2 regular	50
Croissant, Plain, average, 2 oz	280
Rice Cakes, average	25
Ritz **Crackers,** Low-Sodium, 1 oz	60
Ry-Krisp Crispbread, Sesame, 2	100

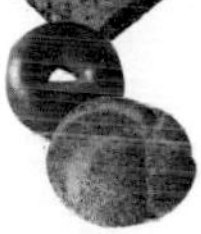

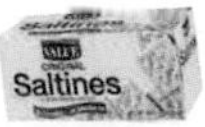

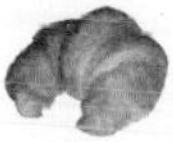

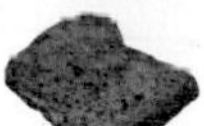

Cookies, Cakes, Desserts

Cookies: Average, 2-3 cookies, 1 oz	100
Average, 2½ oz	180
Baked Custard, ½ cup	100
Brownie, 1½ oz	130
Cake, average, 3 oz piece	250
Carrot Cake, 8 oz	650
Cheesecake, 7 oz	350
Cinnamon Sweet Roll, 2 oz	250
Danish, Apple/Fruit	250
Donut, average	150
Muffins: 1 medium, 2 oz	150
Pancakes, (4"), x 3	360
Fruit Pies, average, 7 oz	600
Pudding: Average, ½ cup	160
Jell-O (Mix), Instant, ½ cup	400
Waffles: Home-made, 7", 2½ oz	350
Frozen: Average, 1¼ oz	260
Aunt Jemima, avg, 2½ oz	565

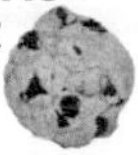

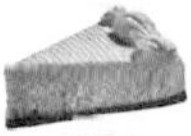

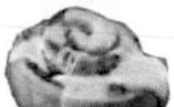

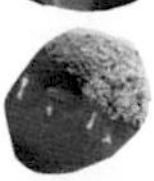

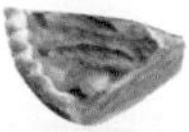

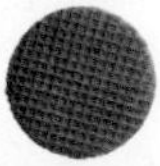

Sodium Counter

Fruit & Juices

	Sodium
Fresh Fruit, average all types, 1 serving	1
Dried/Canned Fruit, ½ cup	1
Fruit Juice: Fresh, sqz'd, 6 fl.oz	1
Commercial, aver., 6 fl.oz	20
Tomato Juice *(Campbell's)*, 6 fl.oz	570
Low Sodium (No Salt Added)	20
V8 Vegetable *(Campbell's)*: 5.5 fl.oz can	290
12 fl.oz bottle	630
Low Sodium, 5.5 fl.oz can	95

Vegetables

Fresh/Frozen (No Salt Added): *Per ½ Cup*

Asparagus, Bean Sprouts, Corn	3
Beets, Carrots, Celery, ½ cup	40
Broccoli, Cabbage, Cauliflower	10
Cucumber, Green Beans, Mushroom, Okra	3
Onions, Peas, Potato, Pumpkin, Squash	3
Peppers, Hot Chili, raw, each	3
Spinach, Turnips, ½ cup, ckd	40
Tomato, 1 medium, 5 oz	10
Canned: Asparagus, 4 spears	300
Beans, baked in tomato sauce	450
Beets, ½ cup, 3 oz	240
Corn Kernels, ½ cup, 3 oz	190
Creamed, ½ cup, 4½ oz	330
Mushrooms w. butter sce, 2oz	550
Peas, ½ cup, 3 oz	250
Sauerkraut, ½ cup, 4 oz	750

Pickles, Olives

Olives, pickled: Green, 1 large	90
Ripe/black, 1 large	40
Pickles: Bread & Butter, 4 sl., 1 oz	200
Dill, 1 pickle, 2½ oz	900
Sweet, 1 gherkin, ½ oz	130

Soybean Products

Miso (Soy Paste), ¼ c., 2½ oz	2500
Soybean Protein Isolate, 1 oz	280
Tempeh, Natural, ½ cup, 3 oz	5
Tofu, average, ½ cup, 4 oz	5

Jam, Honey, Syrups

Jam/Jelly, 1 Tbsp	2
Honey/Maple Syrup, 1 Tbsp	1
Log Cabin Syrup, 1 fl.oz	35
Lite, 1 fl.oz	90

Peanut Butter

Peanut Butter: Regular, 2 Tbsp, ½ oz	190
Low Sodium *(Jif)*, 2 Tbsp	65
Unsalted *(Trader Joe's)*, 2 Tbsp	5

Snacks, Nuts

	Sodium
Cheese Balls/Curls, 1 oz	280
Cheetos, 1 oz	290
Corn/Tortilla Chips, average, 1 oz	220
Fritos, Lightly Salted, 1 oz	80
Granola bars, average, 1 bar	80
Nuts: Plain, unsalted, 1 oz	1
Lightly salted, 1 oz	80
Salted or Honey Roasted, 1 oz	160
Popcorn: Plain (unsalted), 1 cup	1
Flavored, average, 1 cup	60
Salt added, 1 cup	180
Potato Chips: Plain, 1 oz	160
Lay's, Lightly Salted, 1 oz	90
Flavored, average, 1 oz	250
Pretzels: Regular, 3, 1 oz	450
Soft, salted, large	1000

Candy, Chocolate

Chocolate, milk, 1 oz	30
Fudge, chocolate, 1 oz	55
Candy Bars, average, 1½ oz	60
Hard Candy, Jelly Beans, 1 oz	10
Licorice, 1 oz	30

Beverages, Alcohol

Coffee, Tea, 1 cup	1
Cocoa, dry, plain, 1 Tbsp	0
Mix, average, 1 envelope	120
Quik *(Nestle)*, 2 tsp	35
Soft Drinks, average, 8 fl.oz	20
Mineral Water, Perrier, 8 fl.oz	5
Gatorade Thirst Quencher, 8 fl.oz	110
Red Bull, 8½ fl.oz can	200
Water, Average, 1 cup, 8 fl.oz	5
Alcohol: Beer, average, 12 fl.oz	15
Wines, average, 4 fl.oz	10
Spirits (distilled), 1½ fl.oz	1

Antacids ~ Alka-Seltzer

	Sodium
***Alka-Seltzer** (Per Tablet):*	
Original; Heartburn	570
Extra Strength	590
Lemon Lime	500
Gold	310
***Alka-Mints,** chewable*	0
***Bromo Seltzer,** ¾ capful*	760
***Rolaids,** All types*	0
***Tums,** Regular/Extra Strength*	0

Cold & Flu ~ Alka-Seltzer Plus

Effervescents, average, 1 tablet	480
Fast Crystal Packs; Liquid Gels	0

Fast-Foods & Restaurants | Sodium

Burger King:

Burgers: A1 Steakhouse XT	1930
Cheeseburger	740
Double Bacon Cheeseburger	1180
Hamburger	520
Whoppers: Original	1020
With Cheese	1450
Whopper Jr. with Cheese	750
Chicken, Original	1390
Sides: French Fries, medium, salted	670
Onion Rings, medium	630
Breakfast: Ham, Egg & Cheese Croissanwich	1110

Denny's:

Better Burgers: Classic Cheeseburger	1410
Western	1820
Sandwiches: Club	1530
Spicy Buffalo Chicken Melt	3820
Steak & Seafood: Lemon Pepper Tilapia	1520
T-Bone & Breaded Shrimp	1490
Soups, Salads & Sides: Chicken Noodle, 12 oz	1300
Clam Chowder, 12 oz	1820
Breakfast: Buttermilk Pancakes (3)	1770
Ham & Cheddar Omelette	1330
Southwestern Sizzlin Skillet	2140
Sides: Coleslaw, 3 oz	520
Everything H. Browns w/ Onions, Cheese & Gravy	3820
Garlic Bread, 2 pieces	350
Hash Browns, 5 oz	650
Vegetable Rice Pilaf, 5 oz	820
Desserts: Carrot Cake, 8 oz	660
Hershey's Chocolate Cake, 5 oz	400

Jack In The Box:

Burgers: Bacon Untimate Cheeseburger	1840
Hamburger	570
Jumbo Jack with Cheese	1250
Sandwiches: Homestyle Ranch Chicken Club	1940
Turkey, Bacon & Cheddar	2130

KFC:

Chicken Breast: Original	710
Extra Crunchy	1010
Grilled	460
Popcorn Chicken: Individual, 4 oz	1160
Value Box	1900
Strips, Crispy, 3 pieces	1280
Wings, Boneless Honey BBQ, 3 wings	1020
Sandwiches: Grilled Filet	850
Grilled Twister	1300
Snackers, average all varieties	700
Sides: Macaroni & Cheese	880
Mashed Potatoes with Gravy	530
Potato Wedges	740

Fast-Foods & Restaurants | Sodium

McDonalds:

Burgers: Angus Bacon & Cheese	2070
Big Mac	1040
Cheeseburger	750
Double	1150
Hamburger	520
McChicken	830
Quarter Pounder with Cheese	1190
McNuggets: 6 pieces	600
BBQ Sauce, 1 package, 1 oz	260
Sandwich: Prem. Grilled Chicken Ranch BLT	1440
French Fries: Small, 2.5 oz	160
Medium, 4.1 oz	270
Large, 5.4 oz	350
Ketchup, 1 package, 10g	110
Breakfast: Egg McMuffin	820
Big Breakfast, reg. size Biscuit	1560
Hash Browns, 2 oz	310
Hotcakes, with Syrup & Whipped Margarine	665
McSkillet Burrito, with Sausage	1390
Happy Meal: Cheeseburger/Fries/Choc. Milk	1060
Desserts/Shakes: Hot Fudge Sundae	180
Chocolate Triple Thick Shake, 16 fl.oz	250

Pizza Hut:

Pan Pizza, 12": Per ½ Pizza, 4 Slices	
Meat Lovers	3300
Cheese; Ham & Pineapple; Veggie, average	2100
Pepperoni; Hawaiian Luau; Dan's Original, av	2400
Supreme; Triple Meat; Spicy Sicilian, average	2800
Thin 'N Crispy -- *Add an extra 100mg to above figures*	

Subway:

6" Lowfat Sandwich: *W/o Condiments/Dressings/Cheese*	
Roast Beef/Chicken, average	800
Subway Club; Turkey; Ham	1150
Sweet Onion Chicken Teriyaki	1000
Veggie Delite	400
6" Sandwiches: *Without Condiments*	
BLT; Tuna, average	950
Philly Chsestk; Meatball Mar.; Subway Melt	1550
Italian B.M.T.; Spicy Italian, average	1800
12" Footlong ~ *Double above figures*	

Taco Bell: *Per Single Item*

Burritos: ½ lb Combo	1640
Supreme: Beef; Chicken; Steak, average	1400
Chapulas; Gorditas: Average	750
Nachos: Regular	520
BellGrande	1300
Specialties, Cheese Quesadillas	1120
Tacos: Chicken, Soft	660
Crunchy; Supreme, average	340

Other Restaurants ~ www.CalorieKing.com

Index A - C

FAST-FOODS INDEX
~ PAGE 175 ~

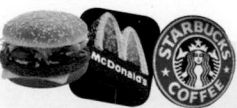

FAST-FOOD RESTAURANTS INDEX
~ SEE PAGE 175 ~

Index E - J

FAST-FOODS INDEX
~ PAGE 175 ~

FAST-FOODS INDEX
~ PAGE 175 ~

Index O - S

FAST-FOODS INDEX
~ **PAGE 175** ~

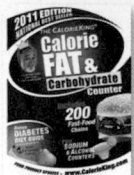
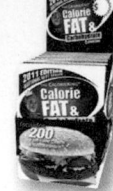
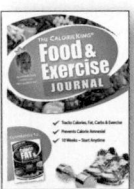
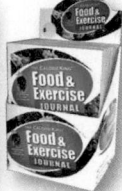
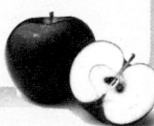
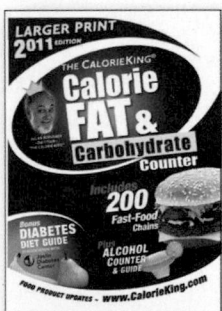
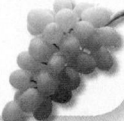

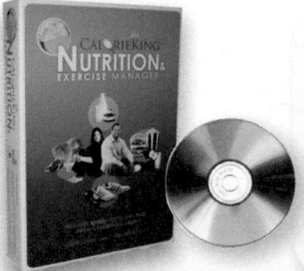